NASAL PLASTIC SURGERY

NASAL PLASTIC SURGERY

E. GAYLON McCOLLOUGH, M.D.
McCollough Plastic Surgery Clinic
The McCollough Aesthetic Medical Center
Birmingham, Alabama

Chapter 22 contributed by

DANIEL E. ROUSSO, M.D.
McCollough Plastic Surgery Clinic
The McCollough Aesthetic Medical Center
Birmingham, Alabama

FRED G. FEDOK, M.D.
Pennsylvania State University
Milton S. Hershey Medical Center
Hershey, Pennsylvania

W.B. SAUNDERS COMPANY
A Division of Harcourt Brace & Company
PHILADELPHIA, LONDON, TORONTO, MONTREAL, SYDNEY, TOKYO

W. B. SAUNDERS COMPANY
A Division of Harcourt Brace & Company
The Curtis Center
Independence Square West
Philadelphia, PA 19106

Library of Congress Cataloging-in-Publication Data

McCollough, E. Gaylon.
Nasal plastic surgery / E. Gaylon McCollough.
p. cm.
ISBN 0-7216-4067-2
1. Rhinoplasty. I. Title.
[DNLM: 1. Rhinoplasty—methods. WV 312 M477n 1994]
RD119.5.N67M33 1994
617.5'230592—dc20
DNLM/DLC 93-26436

Cover illustrations from Alinari/Art Resource, NY. Michelangelo, Three female heads. Gabinetto Disegni e Stampe, Florence, Italy.

NASAL PLASTIC SURGERY ISBN 0–7216–4067–2

Printed in the United States of America.

Last digit is the print number: 9 8 7 6 5 4 3 2 1

PREFACE

Admittedly, rhinoplasty is a difficult art to master. Like most young surgeons in training, I struggled to reduce to the lowest common denominator the volume of material and personal bias about nasal plastic surgery. Only after this has been done, I concluded, can a novice develop confidence in his or her ability to perform a complex surgical procedure.

In the 1990s, learning how to practice and perform nasal plastic surgery is becoming easier because experienced surgeons from several disciplines share new ideas and information with one another. The willingness of colleagues to teach one another coupled with audiovisual technology make it possible for surgeons to expand their knowledge base by drawing on the experience of the masters.

Nasal Plastic Surgery addresses practical issues and deals not only with the hows but also the whys of advocated technical options that are available to the nasal plastic surgeon. It also provides the essentials and establishes a foundation on which one can build a plastic surgical practice composed of a high volume of nasal surgery.

I have attempted to demonstrate time-tested methods on how a rhinoplastic surgeon searching for answers might accomplish the following:

1. Select and inform patients appropriately.
2. Acquire a better appreciation of both the surgical anatomy and the physiology of the nose.
3. Prepare the patient so as to allay anxiety and instill confidence in the surgeon.
4. Systematically anesthetize the nose to alleviate pain.
5. Surround himself or herself with a competent and caring staff.
6. Acquire and/or develop an appropriate physical plant for building a successful plastic surgical practice.
7. Approach the operation with a systematic plan based on analysis and diagnosis of the specific problems to be corrected.
8. Develop the surgical skills required to adapt the initial plan in the event that correction of unforeseen intraoperative problems becomes necessary.

9. Acquire permission to obtain and use grafts and/or implants if they should become necessary during surgery.
10. Treat the tissues in and around the nose with finesse and respect.
11. Develop a postoperative treatment plan (coupled with printed instructions and medications) designed to minimize discomfort, edema, and ecchymosis.
12. Provide convenient, comfortable accommodations for the patient throughout the surgical experience.
13. Give each patient the care and consideration expected.

Today's surgeons may see more situations than did our forefathers and many understand them more clearly only because our generation sits atop a huge mass of knowledge produced by pioneers who have passed before. Two thousand years ago, Lucan recognized, in *The Civil War* (A.D. 39–65), that "dwarfs seated on the shoulders of giants can see farther than the giants."

This book is based on a philosophy of prudence and pragmatism. It is dedicated to our teachers, past and present . . . the "giants" whose experience has provided contemporary rhinoplastic surgeons with both the opportunity and the responsibility to become the best that they can be.

I express my gratitude to my mentors, Jack R. Anderson, M.D., Walter E. Berman, M.D., Richard C. Webster, M.D., and James J. Hicks, M.D., for their encouragement and guidance. A special acknowledgment is owed to Dr. Anderson, who was one of the first to develop patient information materials. Because I have found them beneficial in my own practice, these materials have been incorporated into the philosophies and recommendations shared in this publication.

E. GAYLON MCCOLLOUGH, M.D.

CONTENTS

SECTION 3
SURGERY

PREOPERATIVE CONSIDERATIONS

CHAPTER 1

General Concepts

Healthy people request cosmetic surgery to improve their *quality* of life, even though they are aware of the potential for serious complications. According to a national survey conducted by *Psychology Today,* 40 per cent of Americans are dissatisfied with the shape of their noses and 25 per cent are dissatisfied with their chins and necks. The survey also revealed that 25 per cent of all cosmetic surgery is performed on men, with that percentage increasing.

In 1992 almost 3 million people in the United States alone underwent elective surgery to improve their appearance (Figs. 1–1 and 1–2). Many more elected to undergo reconstructive procedures after an accident or tumor surgery or procedures to correct a congenital defect (Fig. 1–3).

Those seeking surgery include not only people in the upper socioeconomic bracket but also people who live on a budget. Many people save for plastic surgery just as they would for a vacation, a new piece of jewelry, or an automobile. They view it as an investment in themselves. When their appearance is improved, their self-esteem increases and they perform better.

Madison Avenue advertising firms understand how important personal appearance is to Americans. People in the United States spend billions of dollars each year on cosmetics, accessories, fashionable wardrobes, vitamins, health food, and weight control products. These are the same people who have plastic surgery.

Text continued on page 7

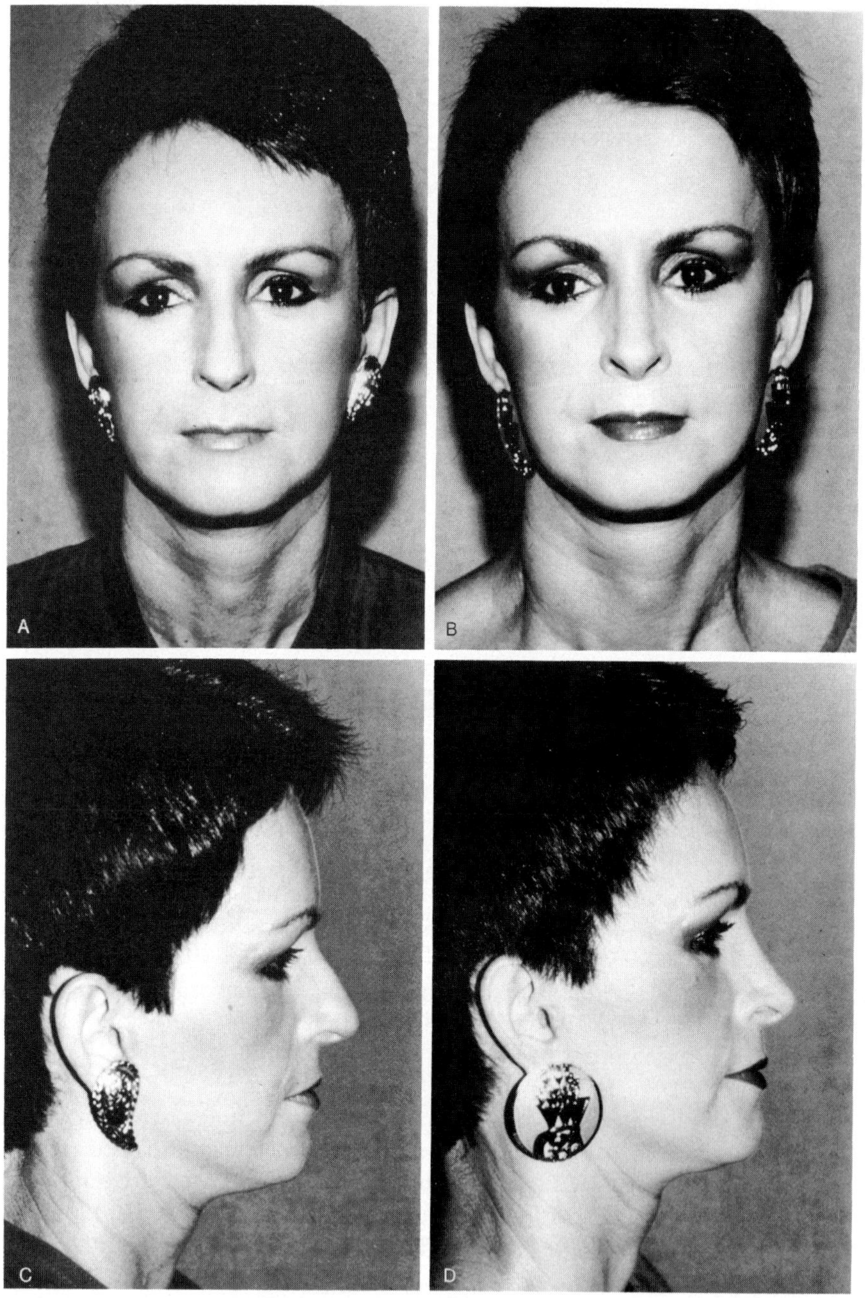

FIGURE 1–1. (*A* and *B*) Some patients' self-esteem is enhanced when minimal improvements are made in the shape of their noses. (*C* and *D*) Small dorsal humps may pose large concerns for patients who have a perfectionist focus on their faces.

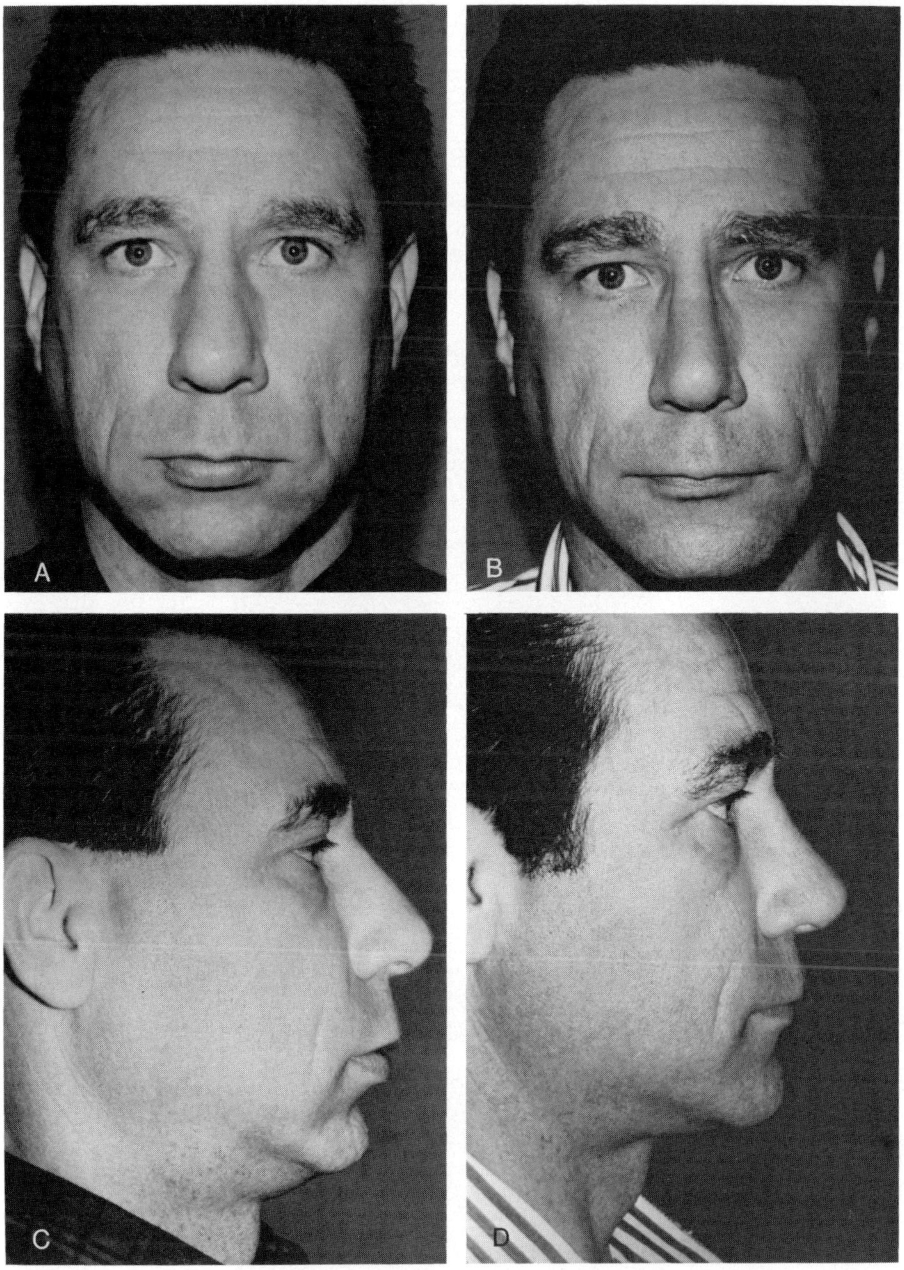

FIGURE 1–2. (*A* and *B*) Many patients desire surgery to establish facial balance. (*C* and *D*) A small or receding chin can be improved with an alloplastic implant, but reduction in the size of the nose provides even better harmony.

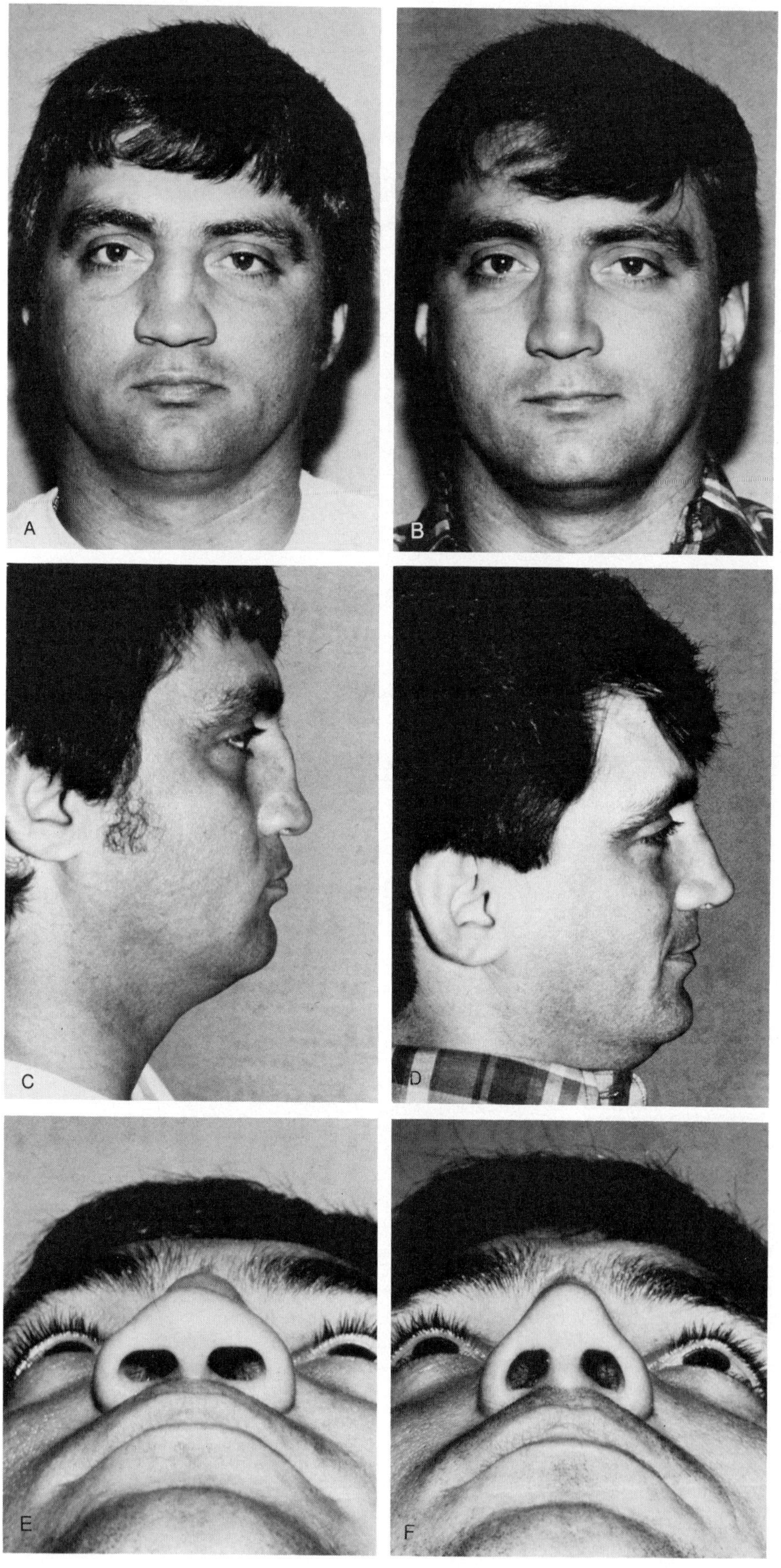

FIGURE 1–3. (*A* and *B*) Reconstructive plastic surgery helps to restore the nose and face to a state similar to the one that existed before injury. (*C* and *D*) Noses with multiple deformities may require more aggressive measures. Augmentation with multiple cartilage grafts and alloplastic implants may be required. (*E* and *F*) Extreme loss of tip projection may necessitate a subtotal reconstruction of the tip through an external approach.

ART AND SCIENCE

The purpose of *plastic surgery* is to restore and repair external defects, malformations, injured bones, body organs, and tissues. *Cosmetic* (or aesthetic) plastic surgery can improve one's appearance by correcting deformed or unsightly facial or body features and by eliminating some of the conspicuous manifestations of the aging process. *Reconstructive* plastic surgery attempts to restore portions of the body to the state that might have existed before an injury, infection, tumor removal, or previously unsuccessful surgery. The correction of many congenital defects also falls under this category.

Of all the procedures performed in plastic surgery, rhinoplasty may be the most challenging. The operation is more than a surgical exercise: It may be the ultimate merger between art and science. Dr. Gustav Aufrict had this to say about this sometimes deceptive adventure: "Rhinoplasty appears to be an easy operation, but it's hard to produce consistently good results." Yet consistently good results are the very key to a successful practice.

MASTER SURGEON

The nasal plastic surgeon occupies a unique position among his peers. He is first a physician and bound to consider both the medical and the psychological factors involved in subjecting a healthy patient to surgery. He is also a sculptor. Like Michelangelo, who could visualize his masterpieces surrounded by stone and needed only to chip away the bonds to release his creations, the master rhinoplasty surgeon develops the vision and technical skills to "release" his creation on each patient's face. It has been said about Dr. Jacques Joseph, the father of modern rhinoplasty, that "there was hardly any part of the human face he could not reconstruct and enhance."[1]

Experience Begets Humility

As the surgeon's career progresses, he gains even greater respect for nasal plastic surgery. He becomes humbled by the vagaries of healing and the sometimes unpredictable events that occur after the final suture has been placed into the nasal tissues.

The natural course of a medical practice that consists of a high volume of nasal plastic surgery eventually brings even the most arrogant surgeon to the reality that no one specialty possesses a monopoly on competence, or incompetence. The surgeon also comes to recognize that there is more than one way to address a problem nose, and that even when the operation *appears* to be successful, unforeseen complications might arise and/or the patient might be dissatisfied with the results.

A prudent surgeon learns to become more critical of his own results as well as those of his colleagues because without intellectual honesty there can be no progress. Sooner or later the credible investigator realizes that surgeons who claim to have all the answers (1) do not follow their patients long enough postoperatively, (2) have yet to develop eyes keen enough to recognize imperfections, (3) adhere to lower aesthetic and functional standards, or (4) choose to turn away from the facts.

Cause and Effect

For almost 15 years I have taught rhinoplasty to younger surgeons serving fellowships through the American Academy of Facial Plastic and Reconstructive Surgery as well as to colleagues attending postgraduate seminars. I often am impressed with the lack of understanding and/or the misconceptions relative to the dynamics and long-term effects of the operative maneuvers that constitute the so-called "classic" rhinoplasty. The principles of cause and effect that physicians learn in basic sciences are not always correctly applied during rhinoplasty, yet nowhere are they more applicable. This book deals with the cause and effect of maneuvers that should be incorporated into the armamentarium of all surgeons who perform nasal plastic and reconstructive surgery.

Systematic Approach

Nasal plastic surgery is a graduated and prudent progression composed of building blocks that, when selected appropriately and performed predictably, improve form and function. Each step in the rhinoplasty operation either moves one closer to his intended goal or creates a condition that must be overcome to obtain the optimal result possible in any given case. This "building block" approach to the complex subject of primary and revisional rhinoplasty is designed to assist both the novice and the advanced surgeon to achieve more predictably good postoperative results while making the patient's surgical experience as convenient and comfortable as possible. By following a sequential treatment plan, the surgeon should also become more efficient in the operating theater.

Case Studies

Cases that demonstrate both common and unusual circumstances are presented for the purpose of sharing my experiences with the reader. Some cases with less than optimal results were selected to demonstrate the imponderables and limitations associated with a practice composed of a high volume of nasal plastic surgery. Case studies include an evaluation of the problem and a description of the techniques used for correction (Figs. 1–4 through 1–6).

BEAUTY AND HANDSOMENESS: PUBLIC SCRUTINY AND SELF-IMPROVEMENT

The international society of the 1990s is both appearance- and youth-oriented. Although the definition of beauty has changed through the ages, favors have always been granted to those considered beautiful or handsome. According to Aristotle, "beauty is a greater recommendation than any letter of introduction." One's appearance can affect school grades, the chances of getting a good job, who will become one's friends, the probability of prosperity, and (believe it or not) how long one may be detained in a mental hospital. From baby face to mature physiognomy, beauty has its benefits.

Although beauty may be in the eye of the beholder, psychologists have identified the criteria people use to judge good looks. Simply, beauty is a creative blend of physical appearance, facial expressions, self-esteem, and status cues.

Text continued on page 12

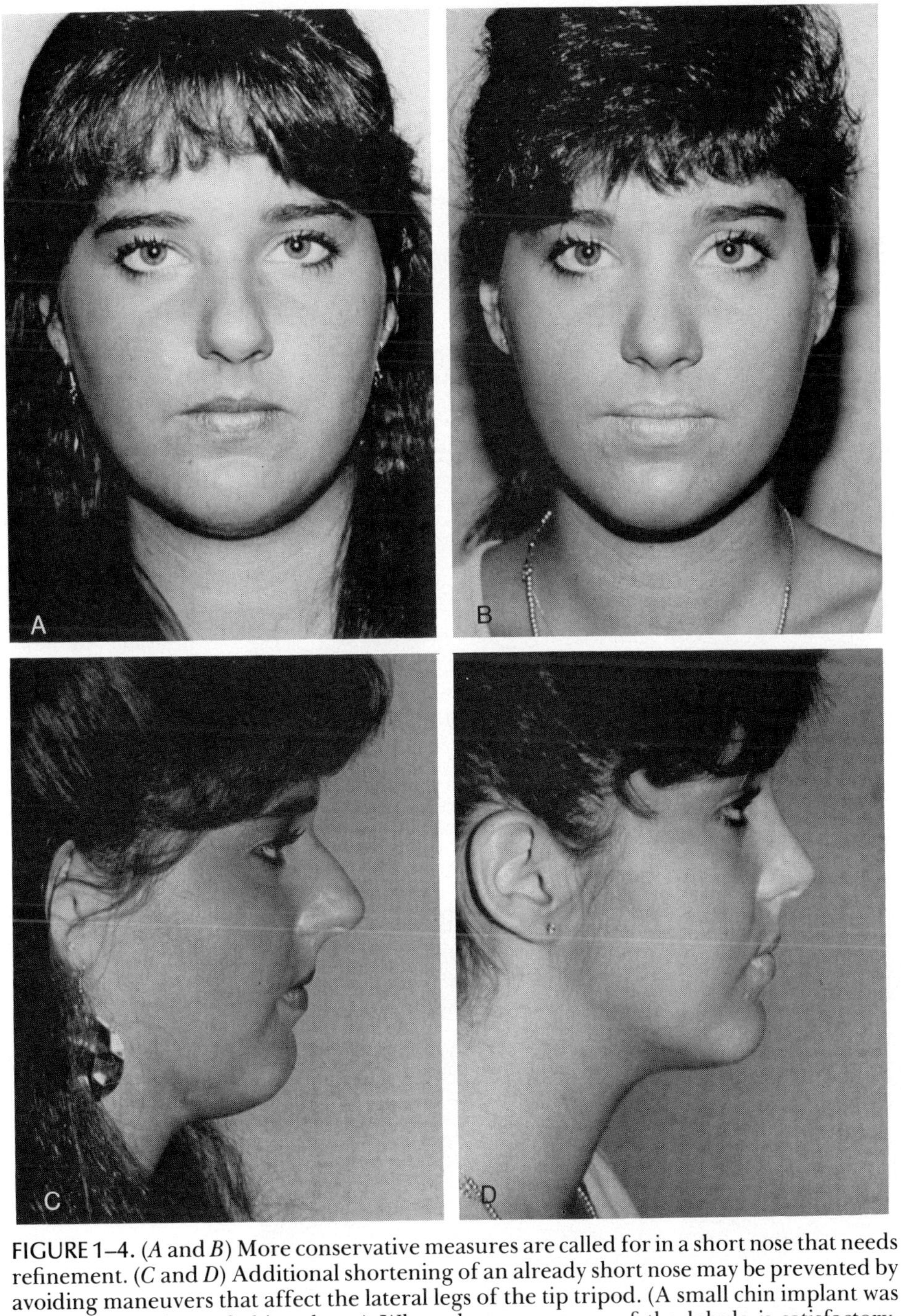

FIGURE 1–4. (*A* and *B*) More conservative measures are called for in a short nose that needs refinement. (*C* and *D*) Additional shortening of an already short nose may be prevented by avoiding maneuvers that affect the lateral legs of the tip tripod. (A small chin implant was placed at the time of rhinoplasty.) When the appearance of the lobule is satisfactory, preservation of the integrity of tip anatomy is desirable.

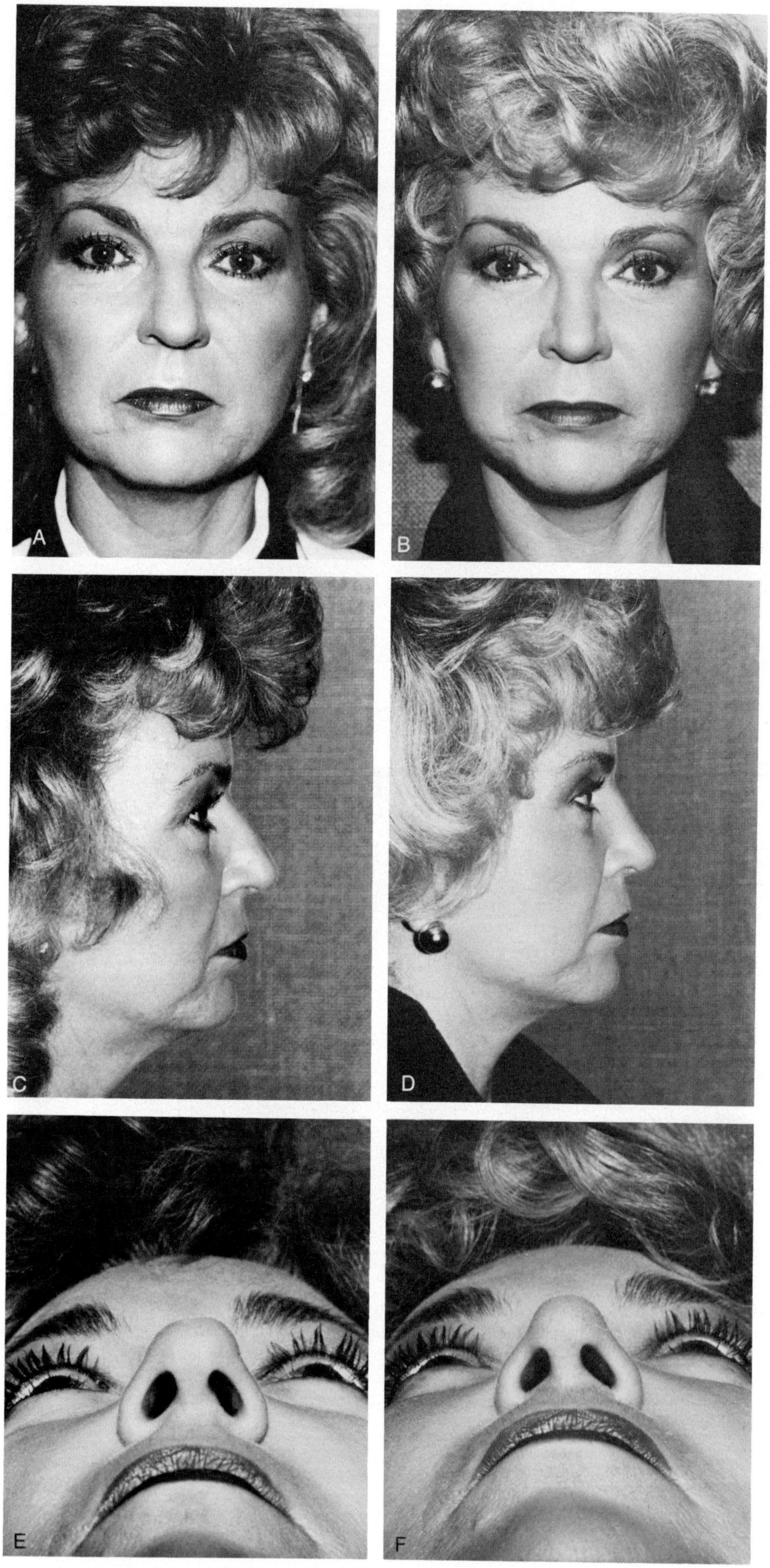

FIGURE 1–5. (*A* and *B*) Many patients who present for facial rejuvenation also desire improvement in the appearance of their noses. (*C* and *D*) A straighter nasal dorsum is desirable in more chronologically mature patients. Correction of tip ptosis usually is indicated. (*E* and *F*) As the nose ages, the feet of the medial crura settle to the base of the columella. Central support with a strut or plumping graft may avoid this phenomenon.

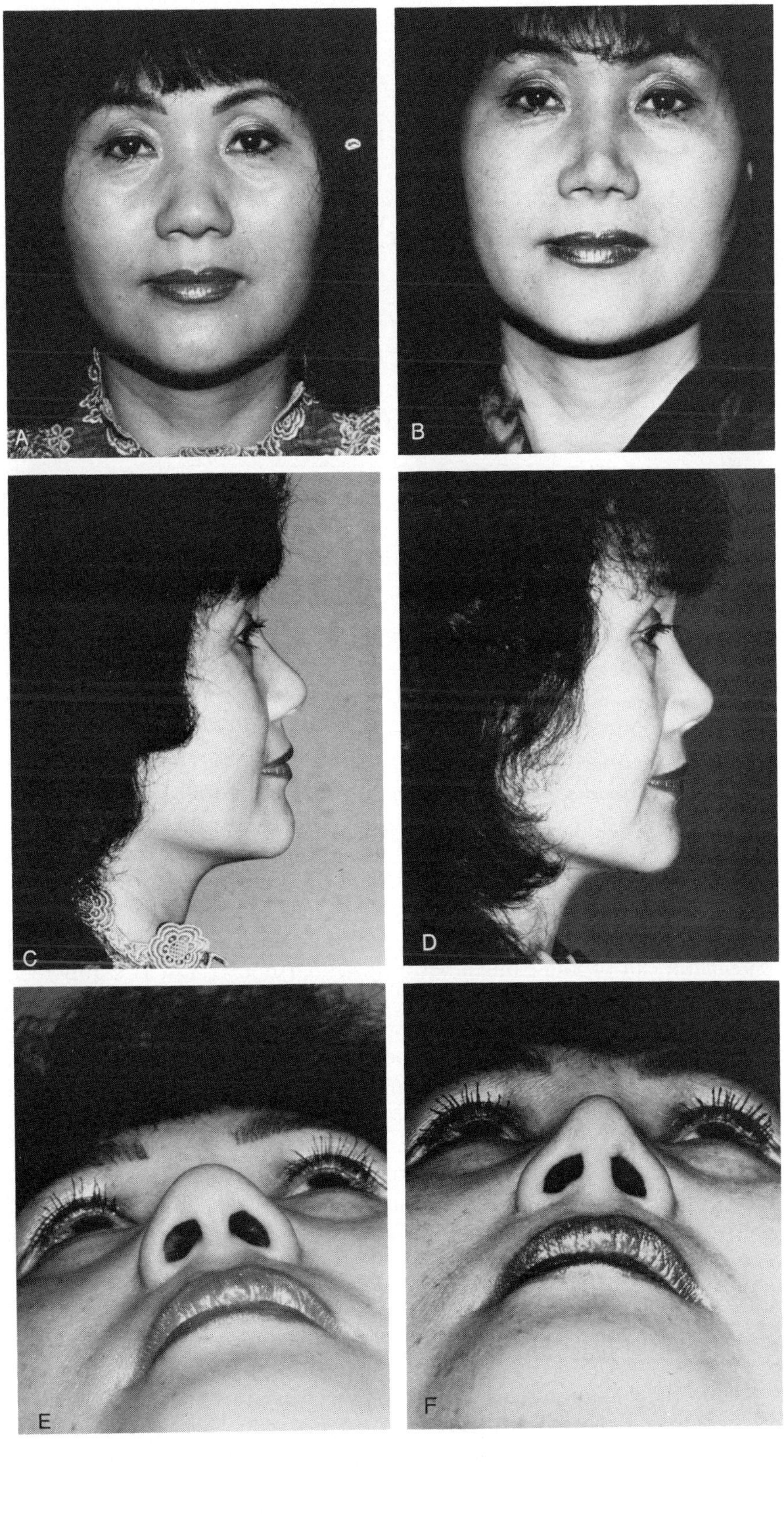

FIGURE 1–6. (*A* and *B*) The platyrrhine, or "non-Caucasian," nose lacks much of the structural and skeletal integrity of the leptorrhine nose. The wide nose lacks dorsal height. (*C* and *D*) Augmentation of the dorsum and premaxilla usually is required. (*E* and *F*) Tip cartilages typically are small and soft. Projection may be obtained with aggressive tip maneuvers that require columellar graft.

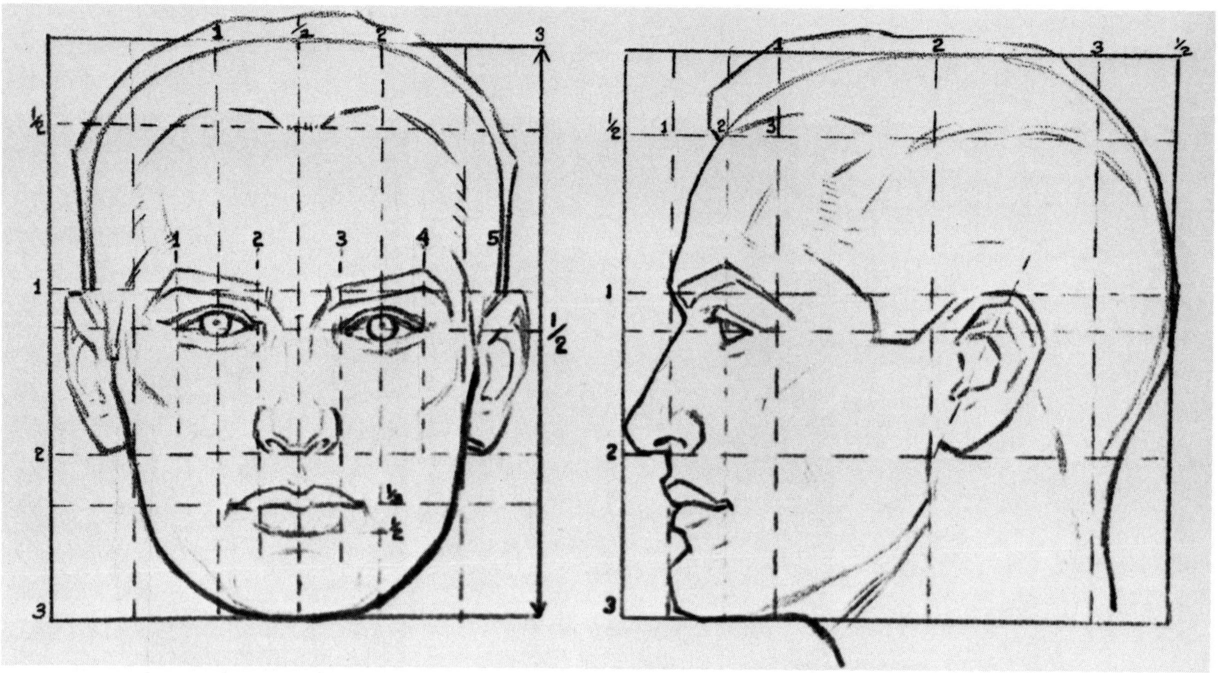

FIGURE 1–7. Leonardo da Vinci's criteria for ideal facial proportions provide the surgeon with guidelines from which to plan to reestablish facial harmony through sophisticated surgical techniques.

Perhaps Leonardo da Vinci was one of the first to record that the "ideal" face can be divided into proportional sections. Horizontal lines drawn through the forehead hairline, the brows, the base of the nose, and at the lower margin of the chin determine how these sections are related. Additionally, the face should be five eyes wide (i.e., five times the width of one eye; (Fig. 1–7).

If the nose or chin is "out of proportion" to the other facial features, correction can produce much better facial harmony (Figs. 1–8 and 1–9). In profile view the projection of the chin should be in line with the lower lip. A deficiency can be improved with chin augmentation or genioplasty.

Some criteria may be gender-specific. The nasal dorsum in a male should be higher and straighter than in a female and the naso-labial angle ought to be about 95 degrees; the same angle in the female ought to be about 105 degrees.

A receding or protruding chin frequently needs to be corrected at the time of nose surgery to provide harmony of the facial features. A "strong" or projecting chin is a masculine characteristic; conversely, a smaller or receding chin feminizes.

Psychological Factors

Dr. Michael Cunningham, associate professor of psychology at the University of Louisville in Kentucky, has mathematically quantified beauty. He asked 150 college students to rate the attractiveness of 50 women (27 of whom were finalists in an internationally recognized beauty pageant.) After the ratings were completed, he mathematically calculated physical

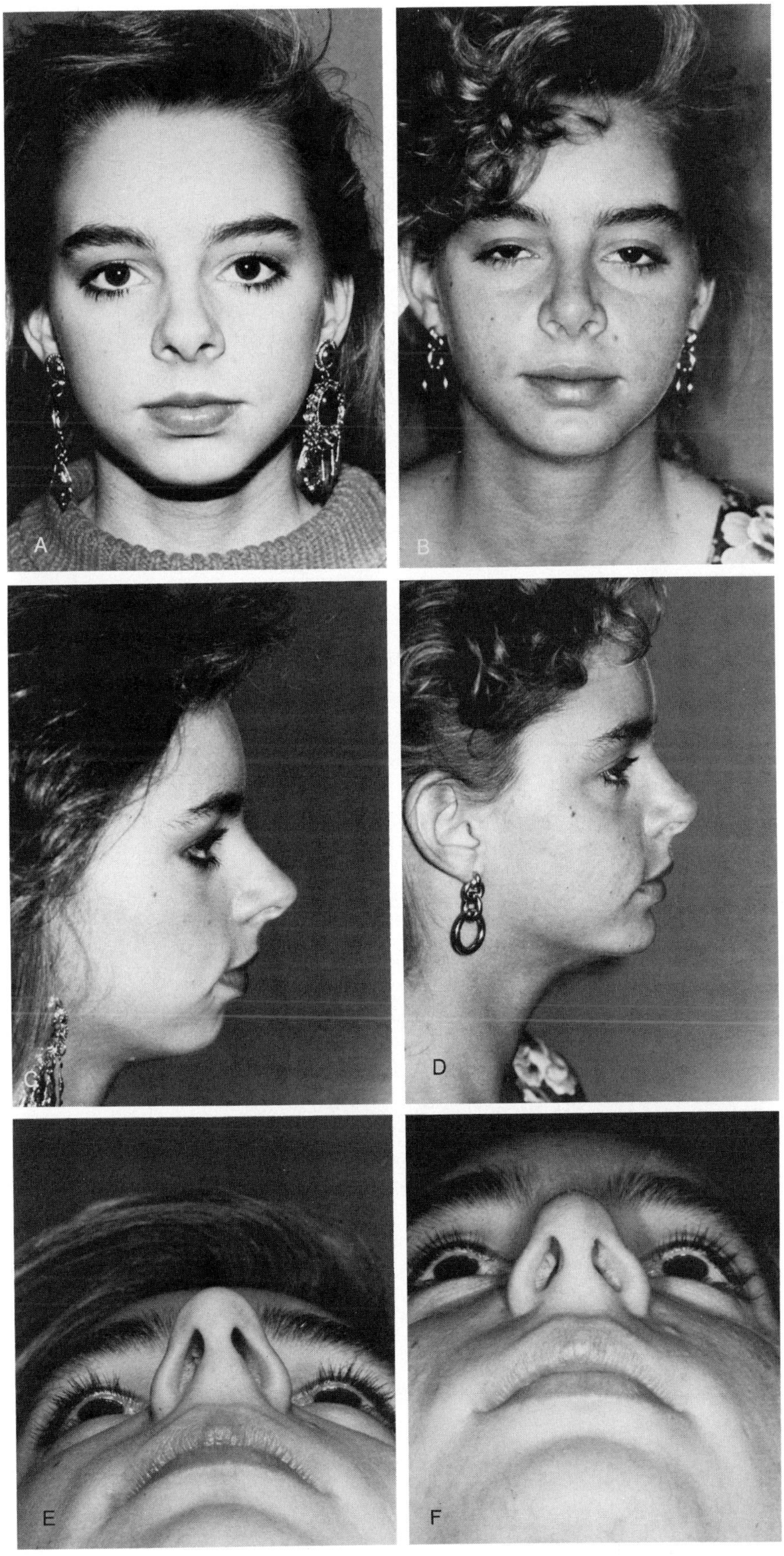

FIGURE 1–8. (*A* and *B*) Severe facial imbalance may not be evident from some angles. (*C* and *D*) Although some experts might recommend repositioning of the facial skeleton with orthognathic surgery, a rhinoplasty and alloplastic chin implant can restore harmony. (*E* and *F*) Retrodisplacement of the tip can be accomplished by techniques that alter the tip tripod.

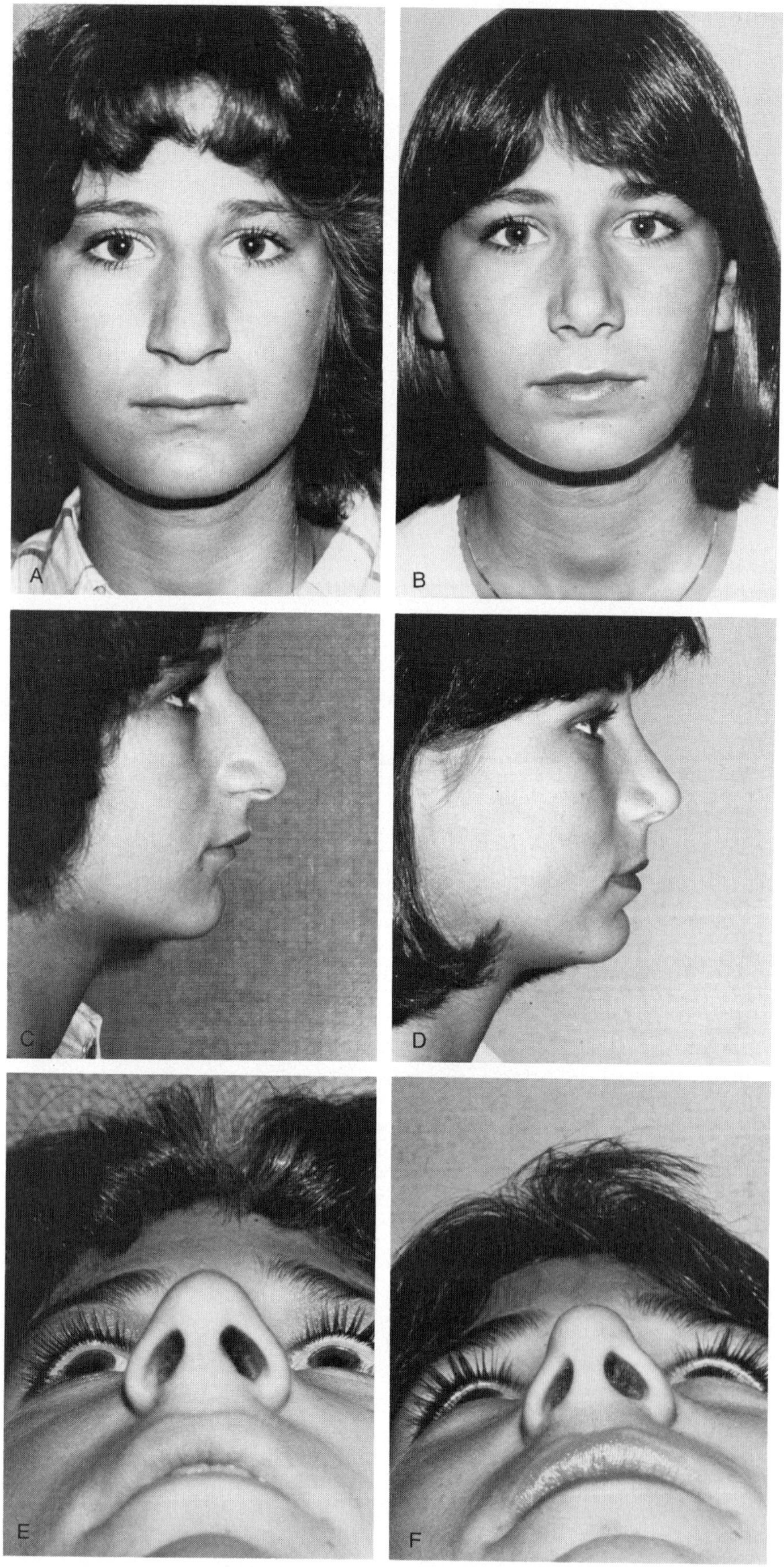

FIGURE 1–9. (*A* and *B*) Vertical disharmony may be secondary to a long middle one-third of the face. Shortening the nose can produce balance. (*C* and *D*) In some cases, the nose overpowers other facial features. When its size is diminished, other procedures often are unnecessary. (*E* and *F*) When a projecting tip is retrodisplaced, the alae may flare, necessitating an alar base resection. The scars usually are imperceptible.

beauty. His findings suggest that large eyes, a small nose and chin, bigger cheekbones, and large smiles are the physical attributes of a beautiful female face. Concerning male facial attractiveness, Cunningham says that the handsome male face "includes large eyes, a relatively small nose, bushy eyebrows, high cheekbones, and a large chin. A large smile is a requirement for both (genders)." Cunningham's theory is based on the premise that the ideal face is a blend of child-like and mature elements. The idea is that child-like beauty, which he calls neonate features (large eyes and small nose and chin) also holds true in adulthood.

This theory has been confirmed by Dr. Leslie Zebrowitz, Manual Yellen professor of social relations and chair in the department of psychology at Brandeis University. Dr. Zebrowitz has studied attractiveness—specifically baby-faced looks—and beauty since the late 1970s.

Research has demonstrated that people are sensitive to small changes in the ability to recognize the age of a face. Structural changes can also influence perception of other traits—not just age but also psychological traits. People whose faces have child-like qualities are perceived as having more child-like traits than those who have mature faces (i.e., small eyes, a broad chin, and angular shape).

Concerning social consequences of the baby face, Zebrowitz documented a number of factors. When applying for a job, having a baby face or a mature face has certain advantages, depending on the nature of the job the applicant is seeking. A baby face is advantageous for positions that require warmth and submissiveness; a mature face is advantageous when shrewdness and leadership skills are required.

Cunningham found that certain maturity features are also indicators of good looks. The most attractive face always contains maturity features, specifically high cheekbones and narrow cheeks for women and some men. In addition, men are seen as being more attractive if they have large chins and bushy eyebrows. Maturity features are more desirable for men than for women. For women, beauty is associated with highly arched eyebrows, which play a bit of a psychological trick, suggesting that people look more interested than they might really be.

Self-Esteem and Desirability

Another facet of expressiveness relates to self-esteem. The expression of self-worth has been linked with a person's perception of another's beauty.

Dr. Jay Hewitt, associate professor at the University of Missouri, has been studying beauty and self-esteem for more than 20 years. He explains:

> In our study, we were interested in finding out if men with high self-esteem would be seen as more attractive than women with high self-esteem. What we found was that the people tend to show an equal preference for a man with higher self-esteem and a man with equal self-esteem. They split their preferences. When it comes to a woman, everyone preferred females with equal rather than higher self-esteem.[2]

Hewitt's research is consistent with other social psychological studies that suggest that superiority and popularity are more attractive traits for men than for women. Cunningham has concluded that men do not want women with lower self-esteem than they have, but they are not as attracted to women with greater self-esteem.

In addition to physical attractiveness, facial expressions, and self-esteem, both Cunningham and Hewitt note research trends indicating that, besides self-esteem, expressiveness has another component: "status cues."

Because public awareness of the advantages of attractiveness, good grooming, and enhanced self-esteem is heightening, many more patients are having cosmetic plastic surgery for economic reasons. This is true not only for the fashion model, television or movie personality, corporate executive, and professional person but for anyone whose work or life-style requires that they interact with the public. In a service-oriented economy, few are exempted from public scrutiny.

References

1. Natvig, P. Jacques Joseph, Surgical Sculptor. Philadelphia: W.B. Saunders Co., 1982.
2. Hewitt, J. Perfection, stress and vulnerability. In Buffington, P.W. (ed). Your Behavior Is Showing. Nashville: Hillbrook House, 1988, p. 170.

Suggested Readings

Anderson, J.R. Cosmetic Facial Surgery. New Orleans: published privately, 1974.
McCollough, E.G. Plastic Surgery. Birmingham: Ebsco Publishing, 1991.

CHAPTER 2

Effective Communication with the Patient

PATIENT INFORMATION BOOK

Misconceptions about plastic surgery abound. They have been fostered by media portrayals and by plastic surgeons themselves, who have failed to make the facts about plastic surgery readily available to the public.

A book containing pertinent information about the surgery being considered should be given to the patient before consultation with the surgeon (Fig. 2–1). This enables the patient to become familiar at leisure with the facts about the procedure and to be better able to understand the surgeon's explanation of the procedure. When consulting with an informed patient, the surgeon can spend more time discussing the specifics of the operation and establishing a common goal that is both realistic and obtainable (Figs. 2–2 and 2–3).

In addition to preparing the patient for the consultation visit, the patient information book serves as a reference after the surgery has been performed.

The following material is contained in the patient information book distributed to patients of the McCollough Plastic Surgery Clinic in Birmingham, Alabama, and has been adapted for this book. The author has

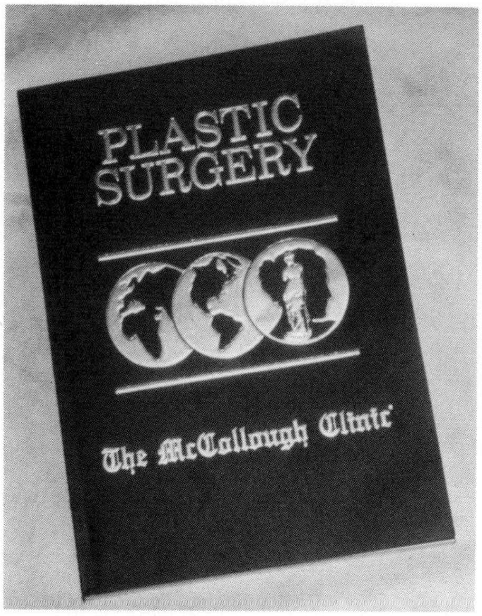

FIGURE 2–1. Printed materials and instruction books allow the surgeon to inform and instruct patients before and after surgery.

attempted to answer many questions that should be asked by patients contemplating nasal surgery.

EXPECTATIONS: RISKS AND IMPONDERABLES

Misunderstandings and misconceptions often can be avoided when the involved parties enter into a venture with mutual trust and realistic expectations. When patients are given the facts before surgery, they, as consumers, can make more informed decisions regarding the services they are about to purchase.

It is important that patients understand that plastic surgery is an art. In both planning and performing a procedure, the surgeon-artist has myriad options from which to choose. It is not always possible to predictably alter human tissues to achieve the outcome desired by patients seeking self-improvement. The surgeon's goal is to enhance the patient's appearance through carefully planned operations. How successful he is in satisfying this goal is determined largely by training, experience, knowledge, and dexterity—all highly variable factors. Most nasal plastic surgeons develop insight based on past experience.

The imponderables of healing and an individual patient's response play a major role in the eventual outcome of any surgical experience. Ethical surgeons cannot guarantee the outcome of surgery; they can only pledge to put forth their best efforts. A high level of communication and cooperation between medical personnel and the patient is required. By following instructions and using good judgment, the patient can promote healing and contribute to the successful outcome of his operation.

If a problem arises, the surgeon and his staff should be notified so that the situation can be evaluated and action taken, if necessary. Most dilemmas can be resolved satisfactorily when the involved parties are committed to maintaining good relationships and working toward a common goal.

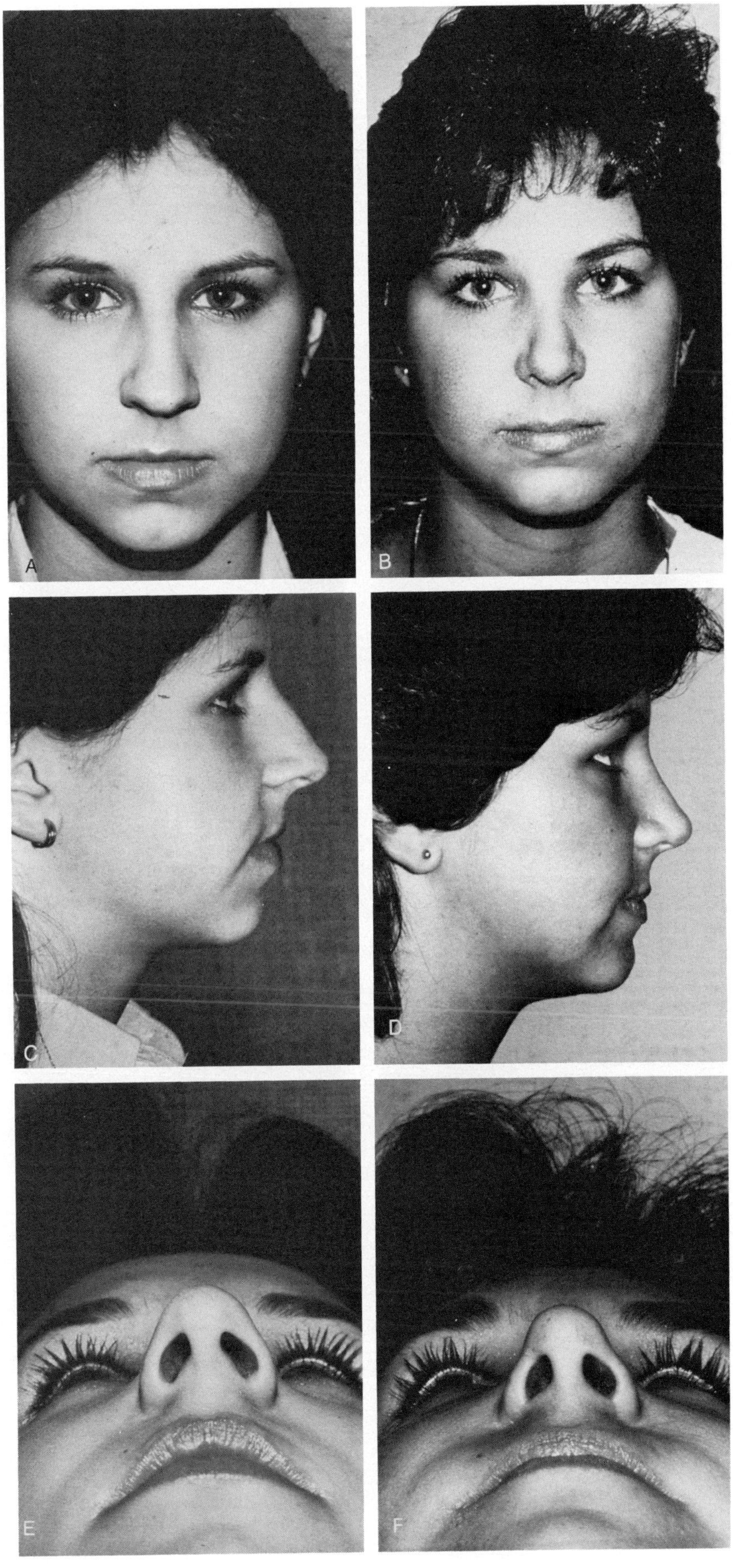

FIGURE 2–2. (*A* and *B*) The surgeon's goal should be to correct the undesirable features of the nose and face but leave the patient with a natural or "unoperated" nose. (*C* and *D*) Predictable, conservative rhinoplasty allows the surgeon to maintain control of the operation and make the necessary corrections in a prudent and pragmatic manner. (Chin augmentation was also necessary in this patient.) (*E* and *F*) When minimal tipplasty is indicated, minimal surgery should be performed.

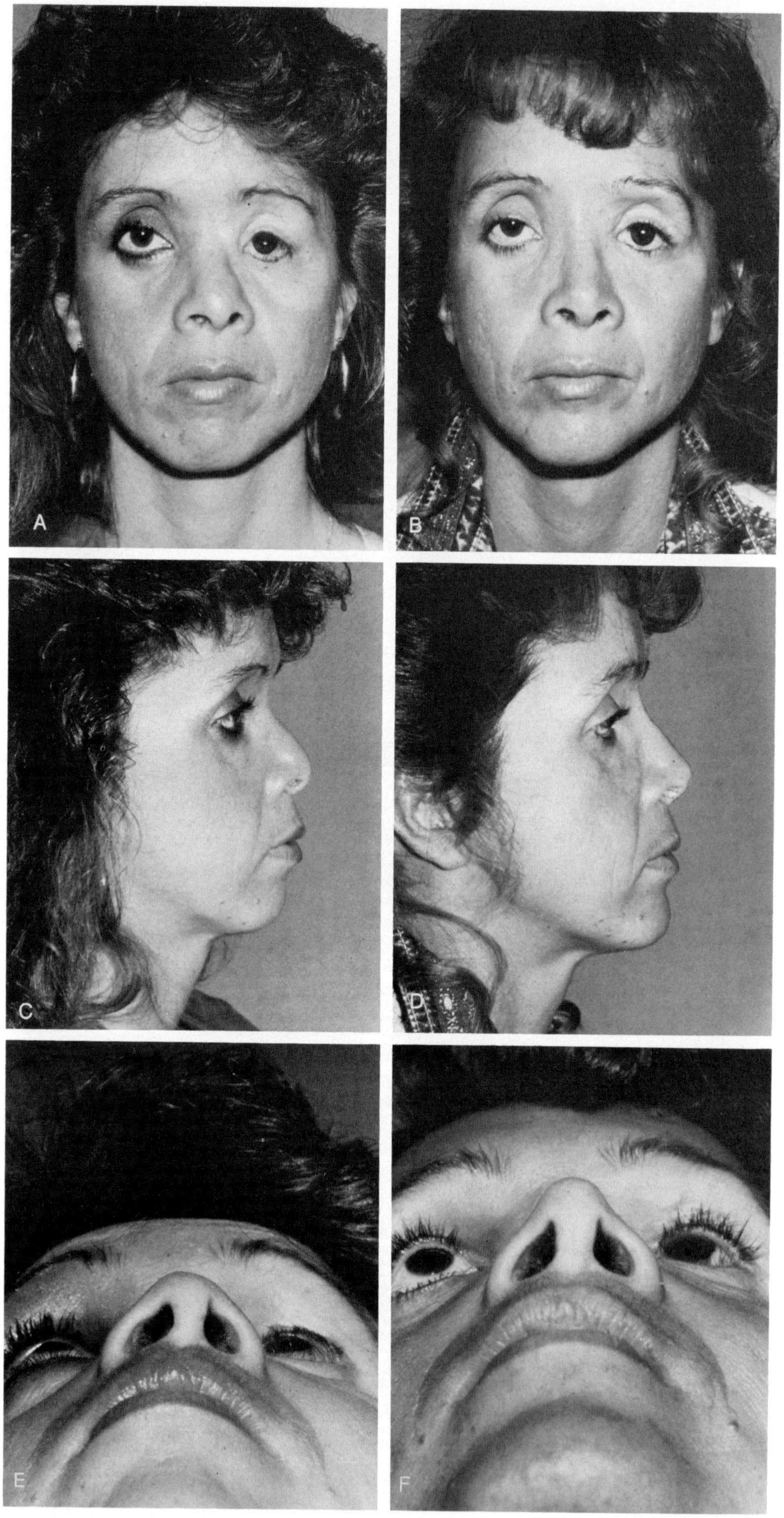

FIGURE 2–3. (*A* and *B*) Patients with familial and iatrogenic deformities present a special challenge. Some conditions are correctable; others are not. More than one operation may be necessary to achieve improvement. (*C* and *D*) The surgeon's goal is to help provide *improvement* by restoring the nasal architecture with grafts and implants. (*E* and *F*) Scar contracture and tissue loss provide special challenges and can limit the degree of improvement that is achievable. Perfection is unobtainable.

Risks

A prerequisite for undergoing any surgery is a sense of realism born of emotional maturity. The following facts should be accepted by any patient in advance of surgery.

1. Every patient is not a good candidate for surgery for one reason or another, nor is surgery recommended for every patient who requests it.

2. The goal of any operation should be improvement, not perfection. If the patient expects perfection, he or she should not have surgery (Fig. 2–4).

3. The degree of success in any surgeon's hands depends not only on his skill but also on the age, health status, skin texture, bone structure, and specific problems and expectations of the patient—all widely variable factors. In other words, the surgeon is limited by the materials given to him with which to work.

4. There is a limit to the corrective procedures possible or recommended. Some of the limiting factors in rhinoplasty are as follows:

- The existing size and shape of the nose (Fig. 2–4)
- The contour and shape of the face (see Fig. 2–8)
- The texture and thickness of the skin (Fig. 2–5)
- The inclination of the chin, lip, and forehead (Fig. 2–6)
- The depth of the angle between the forehead and the nose (Fig. 2–4)
- The height and age of the individual (Fig. 2–7)
- The healing powers of patient's tissues (scar formation, poor blood supply, immunity against infection, and other factors) (Fig. 2–3)
- Facial asymmetry (i.e., differences in the right and left halves of the face) (Fig. 2–8)

5. A nose that has been severely injured (e.g., from an athletic injury or an accident), that is markedly crooked, or that has previously been operated and has left the patient with an unsatisfactory result is technically more difficult to correct. Some surgeons approach these complex problems by scheduling two operations about six months apart. However, most contemporary surgeons try to make the necessary corrections in one operation and succeed in the vast majority of cases. Sometimes additional procedures are required six months to one year later.

6. Most faces are asymmetrical. The surgeon must recognize asymmetries and explain that some are not correctable with surgery: others are (Fig. 2–8). Both the surgeon and the patient must realize the limitations of potential improvement in each case.

7. The following progression of words is referred to as the "one-step theory for plastic and reconstructive surgery":

GREAT
GOOD
AVERAGE
DEFORMITY
MONSTROSITY

Assuming that the surgeon is skilled in myriad techniques used in nasal plastic surgery and that all variables surrounding the operative experience fall on the positive side of the equation, there is a reasonable chance that the end result might be one or two steps higher than the condition that existed before surgery. But the reverse is also possible (Fig. 2–9).

Text continued on page 28

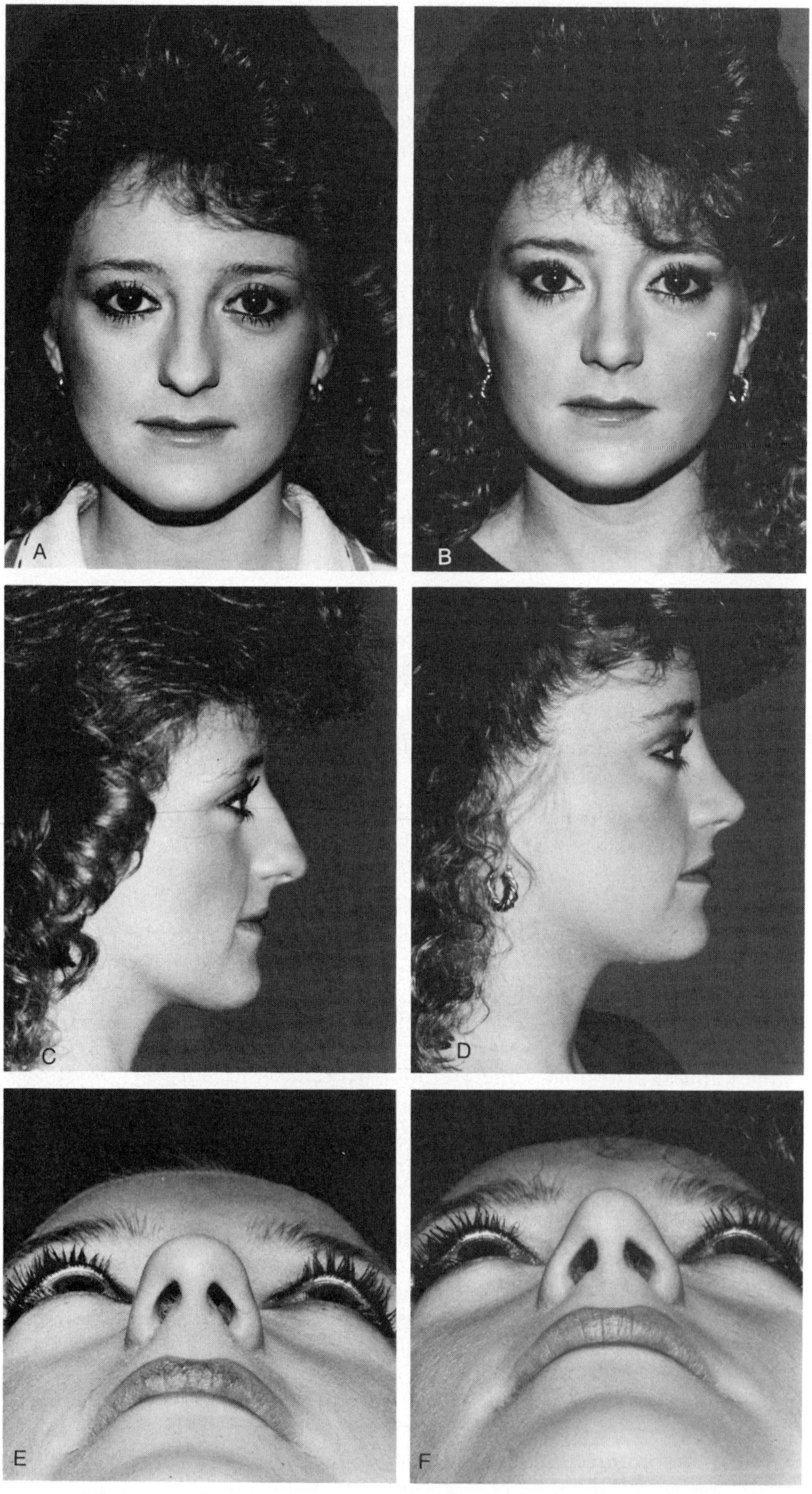

FIGURE 2–4. A petite young woman with a short, projection nose may be able to have a greater inclination to the nasolabial angle and a more retroussé dorsum.

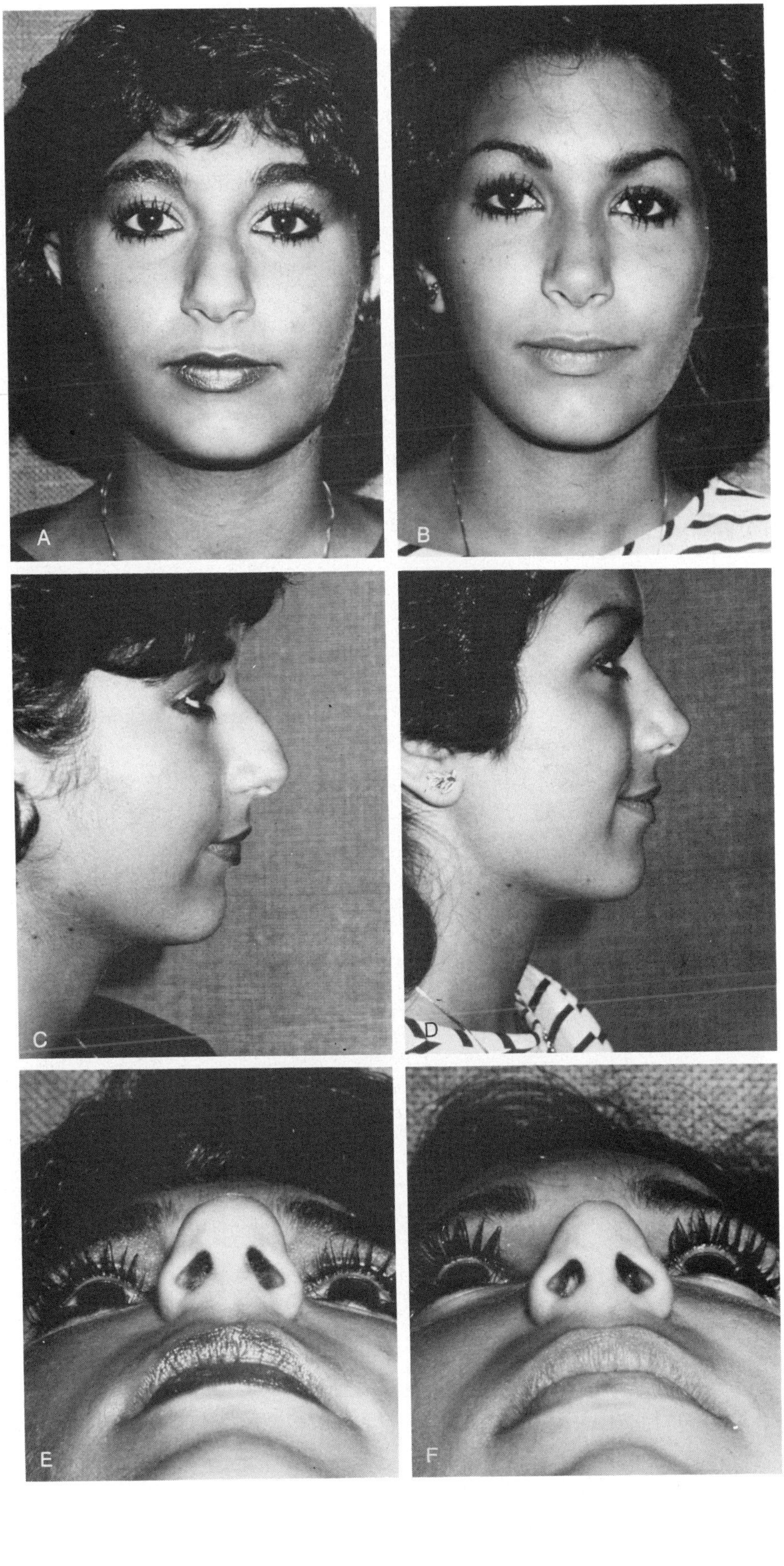

FIGURE 2–5. (*A* and *B*) Patients with thick skin may require more aggressive tip-plasty techniques to provide noticeable refinement. (*C* and *D*) In thick-skinned patients, it is imperative to maintain (or restore) dorsal height. (*E* and *F*) The thickness of the alae is an indication of skin thickness.

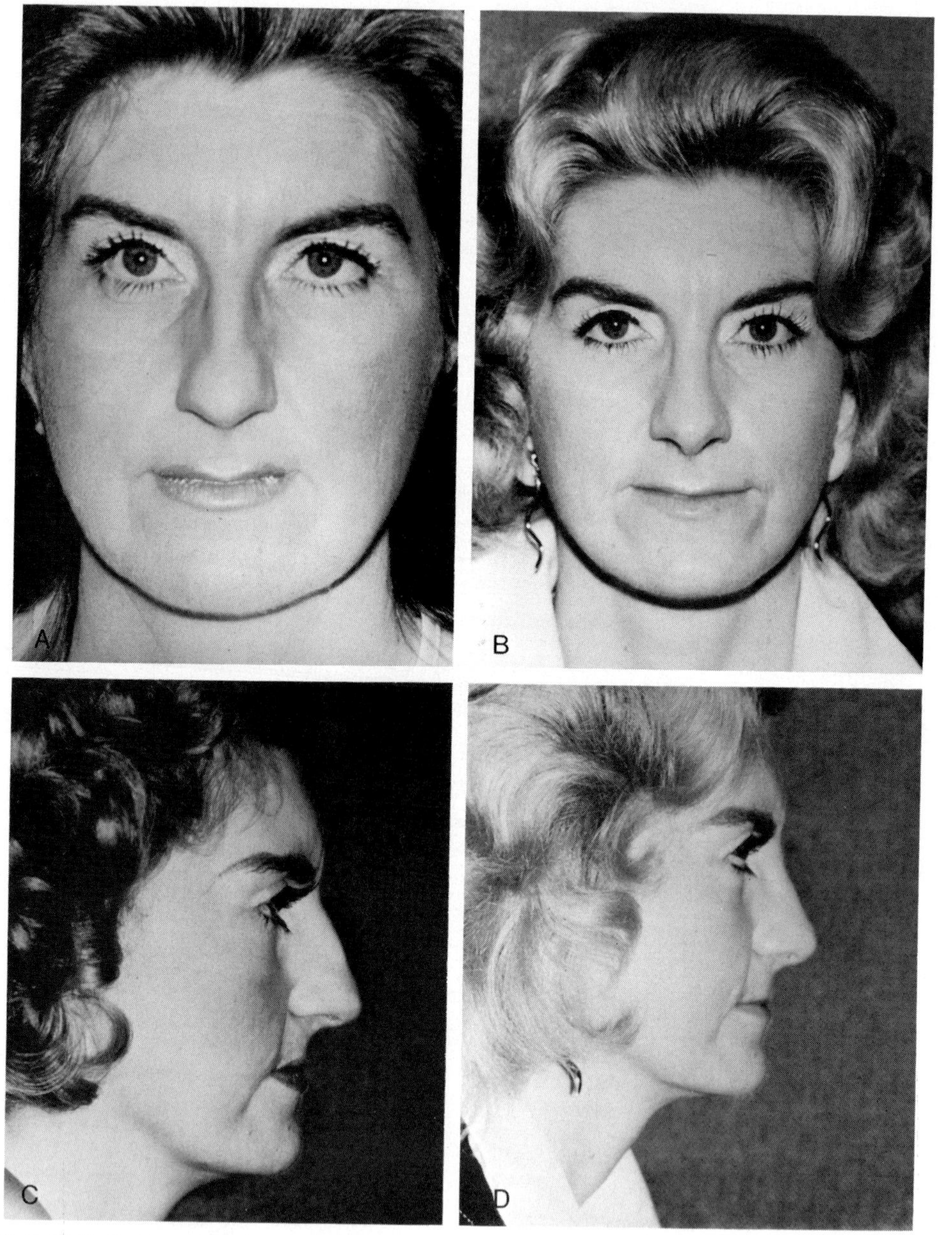

FIGURE 2–6. (*A* and *B*) A prominent chin, particularly in a female, presents a dilemma to the surgeon during the analysis phase. (*C* and *D*) Shortening the nose and increasing the nasolabial angle help to offset a pointed chin.

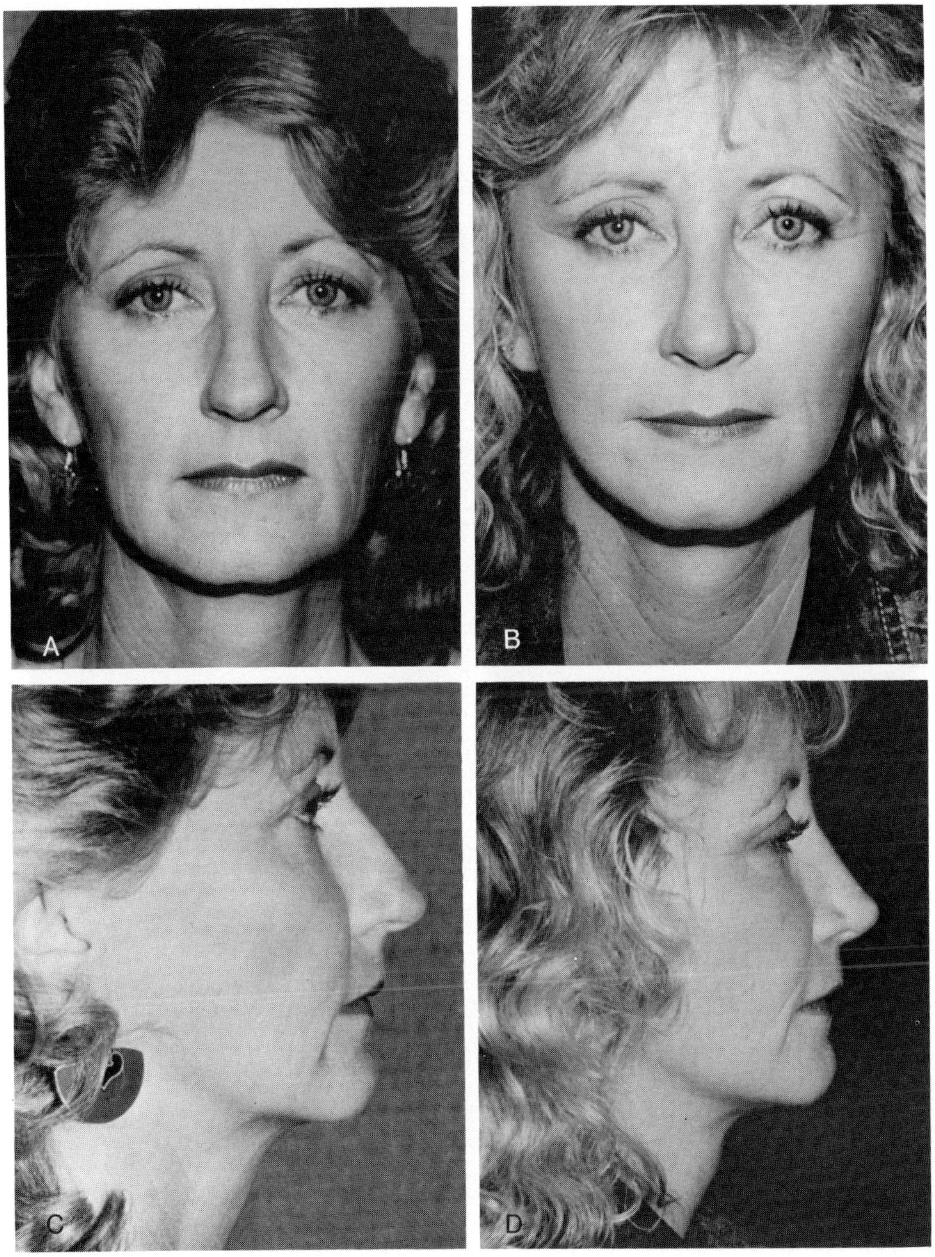

FIGURE 2–7. (*A* and *B*) Many patients over age 40 seek to improve their appearance with nasal plastic surgery. (*C* and *D*) A more youthful look can be achieved when tip projection and rotation are accomplished along with reduction of a dorsal hump.

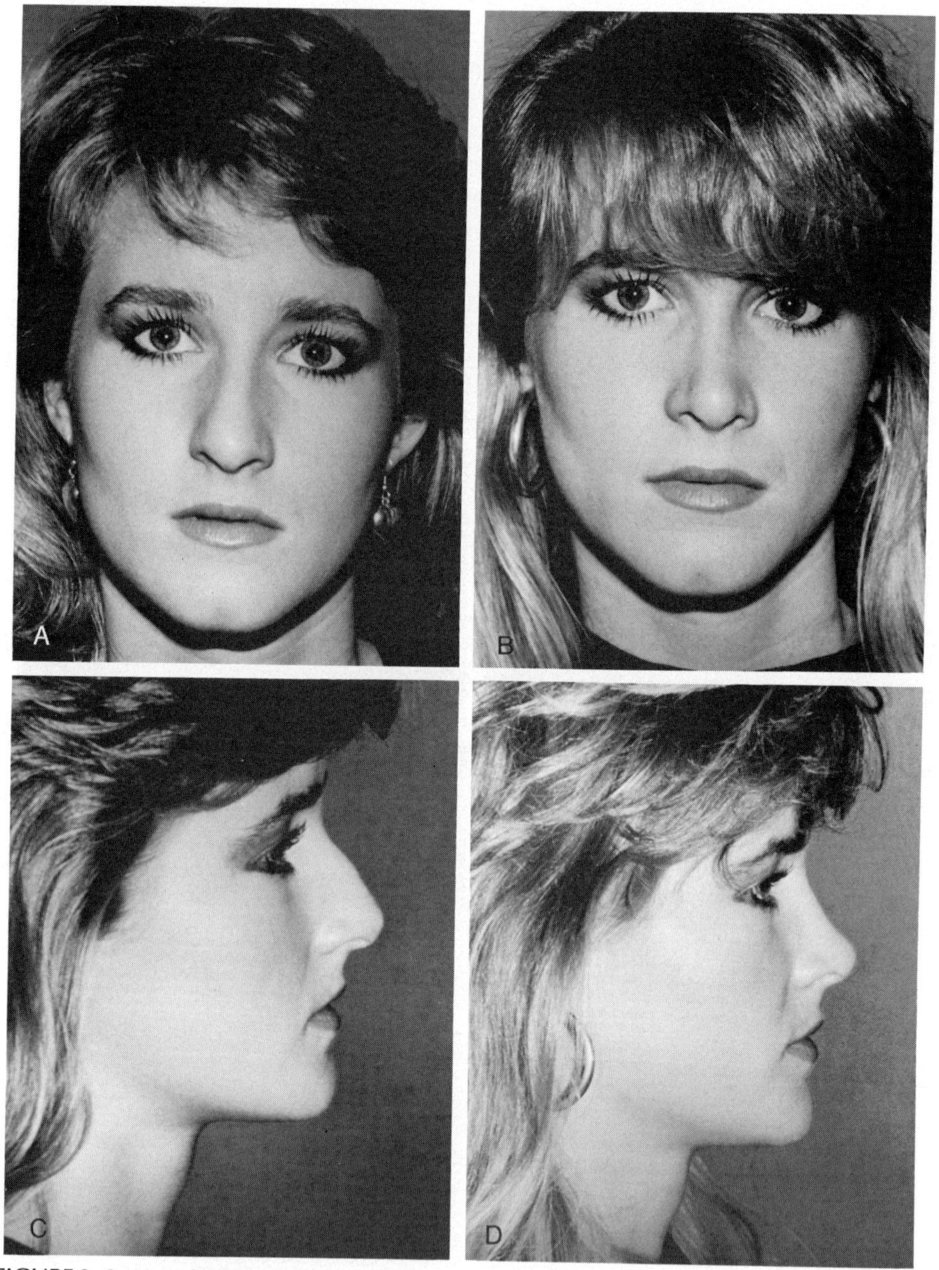

FIGURE 2–8. (*A* and *B*) Every person has some degree of facial asymmetry. The right and left halves of the face seldom are mirror images. The surgeon must demonstrate the *preoperative* relation of facial structures to the patient and explain which can be corrected with surgery. The postoperative photographs demonstrate *improvement* in each of the conditions—an upward progression of one or two steps. The patient shown has multiple challenges. Her nose is crooked, too long, and asymmetric, and she has airway obstruction. (*C*) Preoperative lateral view. (*D*) Postoperative photograph shows reduction in hump and tension in the nasolabial angle.

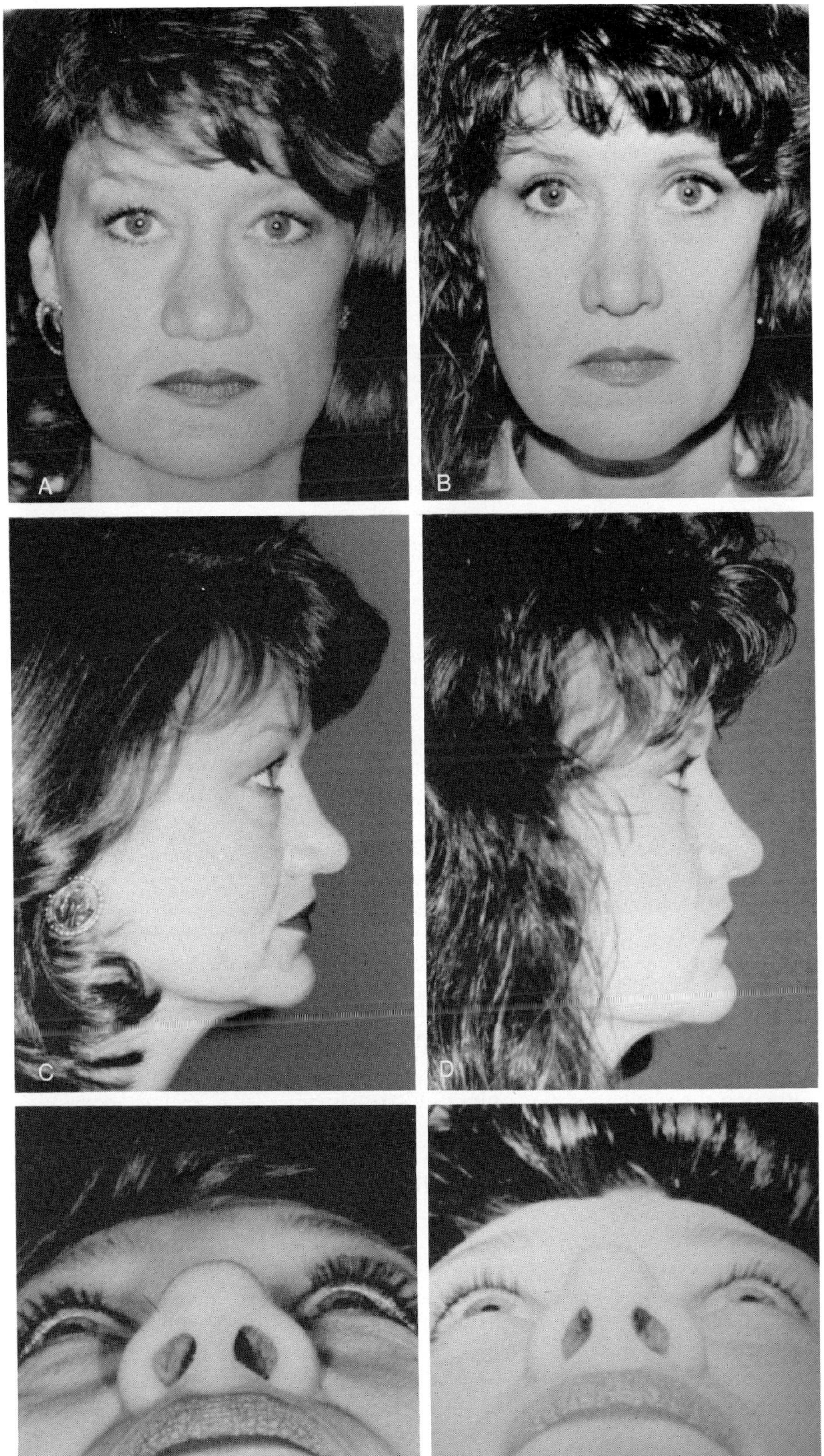

FIGURE 2–9. (*A* and *B*) Multiple conditions (a long, crooked nose with a deviated septum, thick skin, bulbous tip projection, and wide alae) were improved in this patient. (*C* and *D*) Facial harmony was established by narrowing the bony and cartilagenous vault, augmenting the nasal dorsum and nasolabial angle, and performing tip-plasty rhinoplasty. (*E* and *F*) Asymmetric, deformed alar cartilages were corrected and tip projection was increased. Those measures, coupled with alar base narrowing, corrected the wide lower one third of the nose.

8. The motive that impels a patient to seek surgical aid should be realistic. Plastic surgery is not a panacea or a cure-all for every problem one might have. Any resulting improvement in appearance may be psychologically beneficial because it increases self-esteem and self-confidence. Surgery will not solve all a patient's problems, particularly if the appearance is blamed for lack of success or happiness in life. Nor will the patient receive universal approval from family members, friends, and acquaintances after the surgery has been performed. A surgeon often cannot match what the patient has in mind in connection with the operation requested; it may be that the outcome the patient envisions is surgically unattainable or inadvisable. If the surgeon suspects that a deep-seated emotional problem exists, he must not hesitate to recommend that the patient consult with a therapist such as a psychiatrist or psychologist.

9. Plastic surgery usually is accompanied by a minimal amount of pain, incapacity, and discomfort. The patient should be prepared to accept what little there is.

10. Every surgical procedure—even such a simple one as the removal of a mole—entails some degree of risk, both in terms of serious complications and in the sense that the results may not match the patient's expectations.

To put things into perspective about risks, a patient should approach surgery as if it were a journey. There are risks and imponderables associated with automobile or airplane travel, but the possibility of a catastrophe or mishap occurring on a particular trip is statistically unlikely. A prudent and pragmatic driver or pilot can reduce the odds even further.

Some of the risks of surgery the patient must accept are untoward reactions to anesthesia or other medical preparations used for treatment, infection, injury to muscles or nerves, numbness, swelling, discoloration, excessive scarring, dissatisfaction and others. One must also accept risks that are statistically unlikely, such as blindness, paralysis, or even death. Patients are encouraged to inquire further about the risks of the surgery they are contemplating.

11. It would be unethical for a physician or surgeon to guarantee the results of any treatment he performs. He should strive to do the best he can to help each patient achieve a satisfactory result.

12. Some degree of swelling follows any surgical procedure. Every attempt should be made to keep it to a minimum. The increased blood supply to the region is responsible for the pink color of the skin and some of the discoloration associated with surgery. Bruises, too, are due to the residual red blood cells that have been deposited in the surgical regions as a result of trauma and postoperative dissection into the perisurgical areas. Although the swelling and discoloration are visually disconcerting, most people view them as negligible inconveniences for the physical and psychological improvement they obtain.

13. When an incision is made through the full thickness of the skin, the wound heals by way of a scar forming that joins the two edges together. Surgeons attempt to keep scars narrow and camouflaged in natural facial folds and creases or hidden in inconspicuous places.

During the initial healing period, scar lines are pink and somewhat swollen and lumpy. They usually become less conspicuous with time as they "mature." In most cases, facial scars eventually become barely visible to the casual observer, but it may take 6 to 12 months for them to mature.

The much-feared scar, or *keloid,* is rare on the face. Some people are more prone to scarring than are others, as are some anatomic areas. Anticipated incisions usually are drawn on the consent form so that the patient may know the extent and location of postoperative scars.

14. The patient's overall attitude and health play an important role in

the results of any surgery. Patients should see their personal physicians for a preoperative medical workup (see Chapter 4).

An integral part of the art of practicing nasal plastic surgery is establishing a solid physician-patient relationship. Dealing with the ever-changing socioeconomic and medicolegal issues has become an undesirable but necessary part of practicing medicine and surgery. Today, more than ever, documentation is an essential element of medical practice. Physicians who are able to practice "defensive medicine" and at the same time establish a long-term physician-patient relationship reduce their exposure to malpractice claims and enhance their odds of winning in the courtroom if a suit should be filed against them.

A special acknowledgement is owed to Dr. Jack R. Anderson, New Orleans, who pioneered the concept of a patient information book, for introducing me to much of the material contained in this chapter.

Personal Communication

1. Wright, W. K. Personal communication.

Suggested Readings

American Academy of Facial Plastic and Reconstructive Surgery. The Face Book: The Pros and Cons of Facial Plastic Surgery. Washington, D.C.: Acropolis Books, 1988.

Goldstein, R. E. Change Your Smile. Chicago: Quintessence Publishing Co., 1988.

McCollough, E. G. Rhinolasty: A humbling experience. Oral Maxillofacial Surgery 47:1132–1141, 1989.

McCollough, E. G. Plastic Surgery. Birmingham: Ebsco Media, 1991.

CHAPTER 3

Consultation

PRELIMINARY EXAMINATION

First impressions are important when attempting to establish long-term relationships. At consultation, both the patient and the surgeon are contemplating entering into a contract for delivery of medical services.

The patient is considering putting his or her life into the hands of the surgeon (and his staff) while asking for a change in appearance and/or function. Altering a person's appearance is serious business, especially the nose, which is the most prominent feature of the face. Therefore, it is crucial that the surgeon's demeanor convey quiet confidence and professionalism.

Of equal importance, the surgeon should feel untroubled about accepting a patient for surgery. In a litigious society, every patient represents a potential lawsuit. The surgeon must also consider that an unhappy patient can be detrimental to the art of practice building. If, for any reason, the surgeon receives "bad vibes," the surgeon ought to refuse to perform surgery on that patient.

The consultation period provides an opportunity to build a physician-patient relationship based on mutual trust and realistic expectations. At the time of consultation, the surgeon's staff reviews the medical history and questionnaire and makes sure all questions have been answered (see Fig. 4–4). The surgeon also reviews the information provided by the patient and notes whether or not the patient information book was read and understood. He then proceeds to address any concerns he or the patient might have.

When the surgeon is satisfied that the patient's goals and expectations are realistic, he takes the patient to a three-way mirror and *together* they discuss the changes desired or anticipated. An internal nasal examination is carried out, and the proposed alterations are demonstrated in the mirror to the patient (and family) (Fig. 3–1). Facial proportions and asymmetries are reviewed.

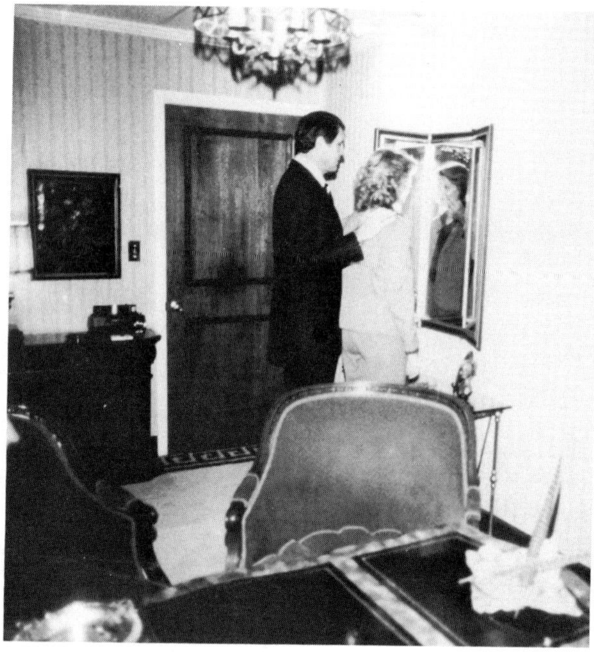

FIGURE 3–1. A three-way mirror allows the patient and surgeon to discuss the patient's desires and the surgeon's limitations before surgery.

For nasal plastic surgery, consideration must be given to correcting any septal thickening and/or deviation found on examination because after hump removal and osteotomies the nasal vault becomes smaller and more narrow. A preoperative, nonsymptomatic deviation or excessive width, particularly at the bony-cartilagenous junction, could become a problem postoperatively. Any proposed "functional" surgery is addressed at this time.

Patients are urged to study their faces in a mirror or old photographs before the consultation. The surgeon must assure his patient that some facial asymmetry is normal. One eyebrow, nostril, or corner of the mouth might be higher than the other; one ear, cheek, or side of the chin might project more than its counterpart. The surgeon might remind the patient that in the embryonic stage, the face initially develops as a bilateral structure and later merges at the midline. It is easy to understand, then, how the two "halves" of the face can be different (Fig. 3–2). Most patients are aware that one foot or hand usually is different from the other one and have no difficulty correlating that the failure of a midline merger leaves some children with a cleft lip or cleft palate deformity.

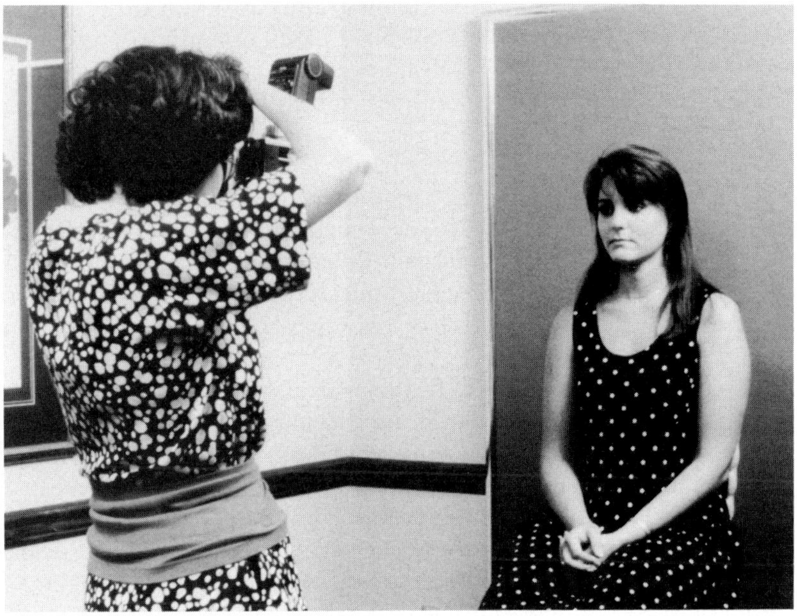

FIGURE 3–8. Photographs are a crucial part of the medical record. They provide accurate patient identification and precisely record the conditions present in the patient seeking appearance enhancement.

Storage cabinets in plastic surgeons' offices commonly are filled with cameras, flashes, and devices that were recommended to "solve" photographic problems. Despite the abundance of equipment, consistently good photographs are frequently not obtained. Like the instruments used to perform surgery, the camera is but another device until it is placed into the hands of a skilled artist and he exercises his acquired skills. Equipment failure and the imponderables associated with development and transfer of film products may be beyond the artist's control.

Photographic areas in a plastic surgery office may range from an elaborate system of cameras mounted on tripods with overhead and rear-mounted "slave" flashes coupled with umbrella reflectors to an Instamatic flash bulb, tourist-type camera. The equipment shown in Figure 3–9 is used in my office.

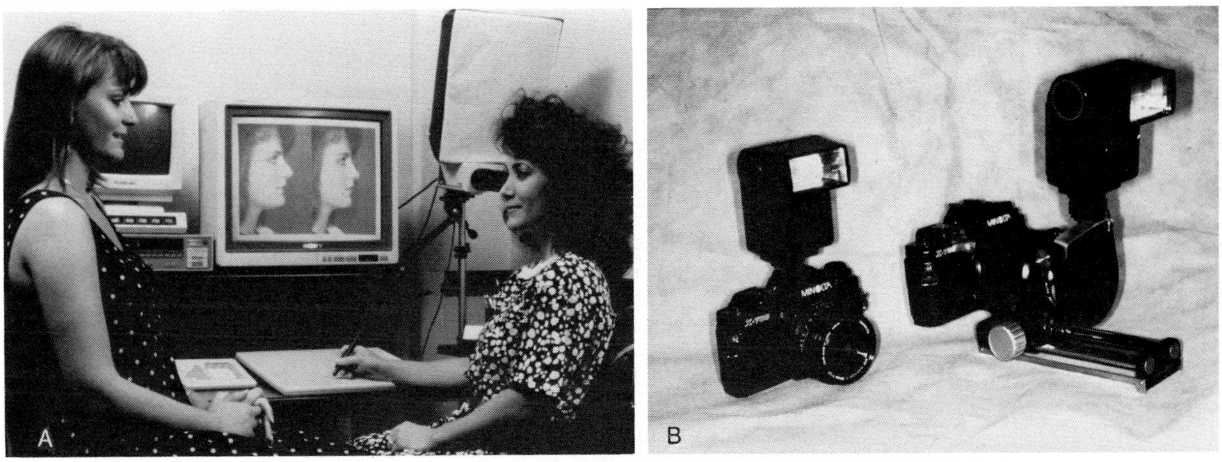

FIGURE 3–9. (*A*) Computer imaging allows the patient to visualize anticipated changes before consenting to surgery. (*B*) Standard 35-mm cameras with zoom lens capability and single side-mounted flash attachments can produce adequate photographs for plastic surgery.

The vast subject of medical photography is beyond the scope of this book. The recommendations given are based not only on my own experiences but also those of my colleagues, who have invested countless hours and untold dollars in pursuing predictable photography.

The standard equipment for plastic surgery photography should include (at a minimum) a quality 35-mm camera with a 100-mm lens and a single, side-mounted flash. Lenses with less than 100-mm focal length are not acceptable for plastic surgery purposes. Parallax, or distortion of facial features, commonly occurs with lenses of shorter focal length.

Although convenient and less cumbersome, most "ring" flashes produce red pupils when the subject is photographed while looking into the camera.

A hand-held system offers flexibility and cost savings when one's practice dictates that he take photographs in several areas of the office, in the operating room, and at more than one surgical facility. If the cost of equipment is not a concern, multiple systems can be developed.

Not unlike most of the maneuvers in rhinoplasty, medical photography is encumbered by compromises. The surgeon often must choose between convenience and cost, time-saving measures and quality. A backup system based on some of these alternatives is essential because equipment failure is a reality of life.

FILM

Kodachrome film provides the truest colors and affords an element of comfort relative to fading over many years. A major disadvantage, however, for many surgeons is that the *undeveloped* roll of film may have to be mailed to another city for developing. The imponderables of such a transfer must be considered. Ektachrome film is an acceptable substitute and offers the convenience of "local" development in most areas of the United States. When turn-around time is crucial, local developing capabilities must be factored into the system.

BACKDROP

Most experts agree that a light blue background is the most complimentary to skin tones.

SHADOWS

Rotating the camera or camera-mounted light source can hide the shadow behind the head. Moving the patient 3 to 4 ft away from the backdrop also helps to reduce shadows.

WHY ARE PHOTOGRAPHS NECESSARY?

It is risky business to perform an operation designed to alter a person's appearance without having preoperative photographs in hand before commencing the operation. Photographs not only enhance the medical record, accurately record the preoperative state of the patient's conditions to be altered, and build one's teaching library; they also allow the surgeon to study his patient's features before surgery and help him plan the operation. It is beneficial to bring the photographs to the operating room so that they may be referred to during the operation as the patient's appearance changes.

Most ear surgeons would refuse to operate on the tympanic membrane or ossicular chain without a reliable audiogram. Contemporary orthopedic surgeons would refuse to manipulate a fractured limb without quality radiographic documentation. It stands to reason that a surgeon about to alter a patient's appearance by changing the size and shape of her nose ought to make every effort to document, photographically, the preoperative state of the nose.

Most rhinoplasties are elective, and the surgeon has ample time to obtain a set of preoperative photographs. In emergency situations or as a backup of last resort, Polaroid prints may provide documentation of the preoperative state. Nasal injuries should be photographed before any treatment is undertaken—even before debris and dried blood are washed from the nose and face.

GRADING THE SURGEON'S WORK

A frequently overlooked benefit of photography is that postoperative photographs taken under identical technical conditions as preoperative photographs (e.g., film, positioning, lighting, distance) allow the surgeon to *critically* evaluate the results of his surgery. Unless a rhinoplastic surgeon periodically reviews his preoperative and postoperative photographs, he may acquire misconceptions about the quality of his work.

EVERY CASE A TEACHING CASE

A surgeon should consistently produce better results if he addresses every case as a teaching case. Imagining that the preoperative and postoperative photographs of each case might be projected on a giant screen before hundreds of his peers at a specialty convention helps to establish standards of excellence and prudence not practiced by many of his colleagues.

A PHOTOGRAPHIC PORTFOLIO

It may be desirable for the surgeon to take *both* prints and slides of patients before surgery. A number of options exist. Slides alone may be sufficient because prints can be made (at a cost) from slides. The reverse is also true. A slide can be made by photographing a color print. I give each patient a set of preoperative black and white prints the day his nasal dressings are removed. After trial and error, the most time-efficient and cost-effective method of obtaining *both* 35-mm slides and 3 × 5 black and white prints seems to be to have two cameras: one loaded with slide film (Ektachrome 100 or Agfachrome 100RS) and one loaded with print film (Kodak Plus-X Pan 125).

A Polaroid system for immediate documentation is advisable. Additionally, Polaroid black and white prints can be made from slides with a Vivitar Slide Printer system (Figs. 3–10 through 3–13).

STANDARD PREOPERATIVE VIEWS

The following views are desirable to document the interrelations of the nasal and facial features. Standardization with respect to positioning the patient to center his face in the frame, light source, and camera is essential in obtaining consistency.

Anteroposterior View. An anteroposterior photograph taken with the patient holding his chart showing the chart number and name can help to avoid incorrect labeling and filing of photographs. This identification

Text continued on page 44

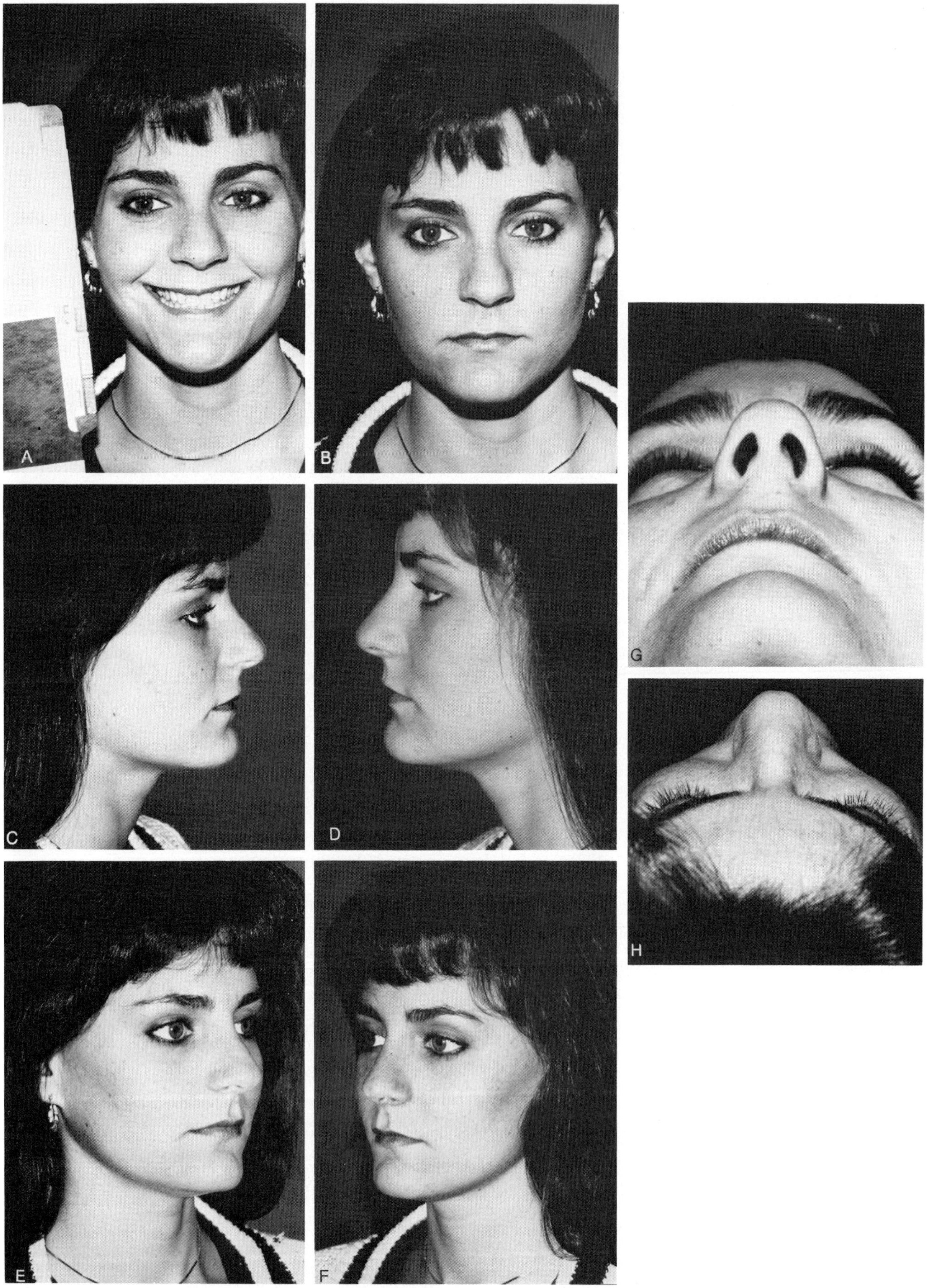

FIGURE 3–10. For nasal plastic operations, the standard views shown are taken. Slides are labeled with the patient's name, surgeon's name, and date. In *A*, the patient's chart showing her name and number is incorporated into the photographic field for accurate identification. (*B*) Anteroposterior view. (*C* and *D*) Lateral views. (*E* and *F*) Oblique views. (*G* and *H*) Base views.

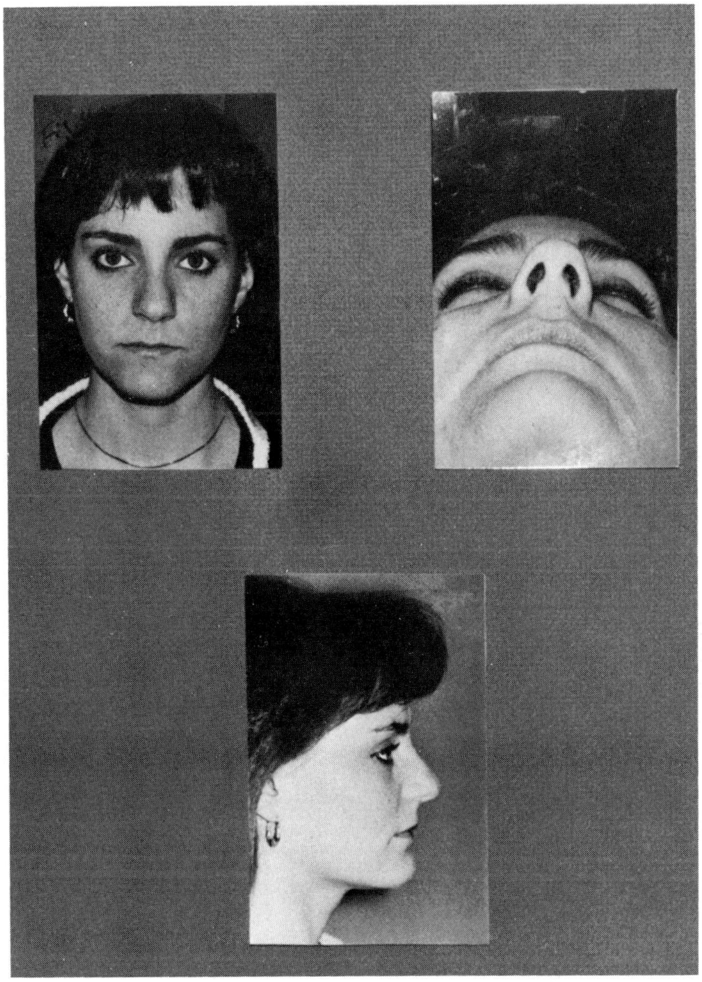

FIGURE 3–11. Black and white prints are displayed in the operating room during surgery for the surgeon to refer to preoperative conditions.

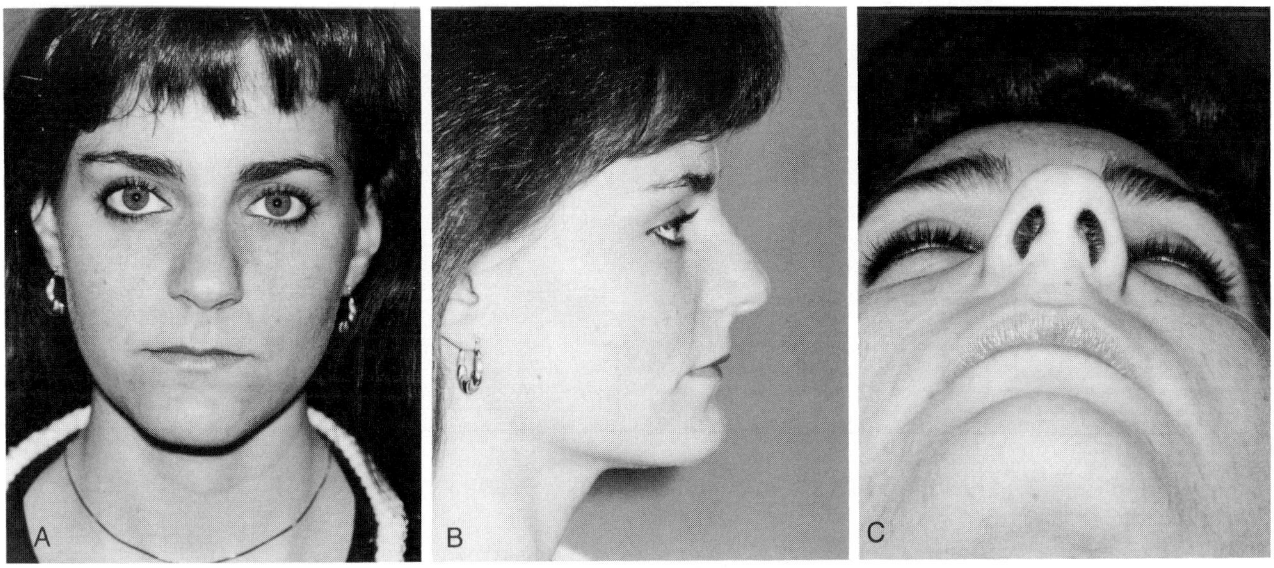

FIGURE 3–12. Black and white prints (5 × 7) are also taken. A set of these prints is given to the patient when the nasal dressings are removed on the 7th postoperative day.

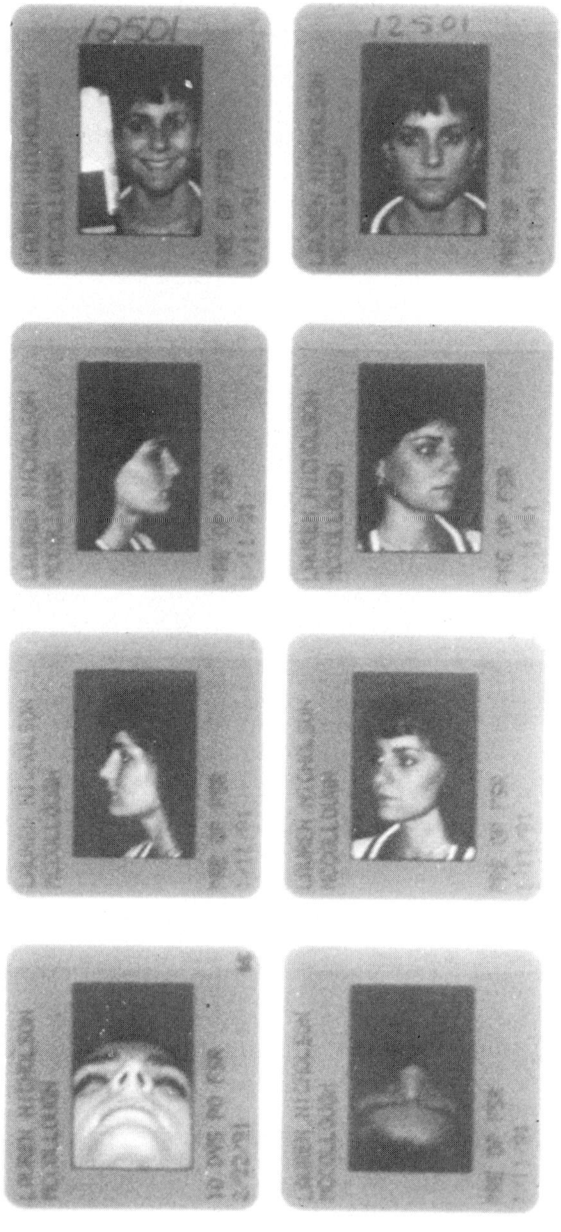

FIGURE 3–13. Polaroid prints can be made from 35-mm slides with special film and equipment.

view allows the surgeon-artist to evaluate symmetry. It is desirable to include the entire face, along with the hair and part of the neck in the frame.

Lateral Views. The patient's face is turned toward (or away) from the camera until the brow uncovers the glabellar skin. An imaginary line extended through the chin and forehead should be parallel to the lateral margin of the frame. The lateral view of the face and head should occupy about three-fourths of the frame. Right and left lateral views are recomended.

Oblique Views. With interest in cheek augmentation increasing, the oblique view is becoming a more important part of the rhinoplasty photographic portfolio.

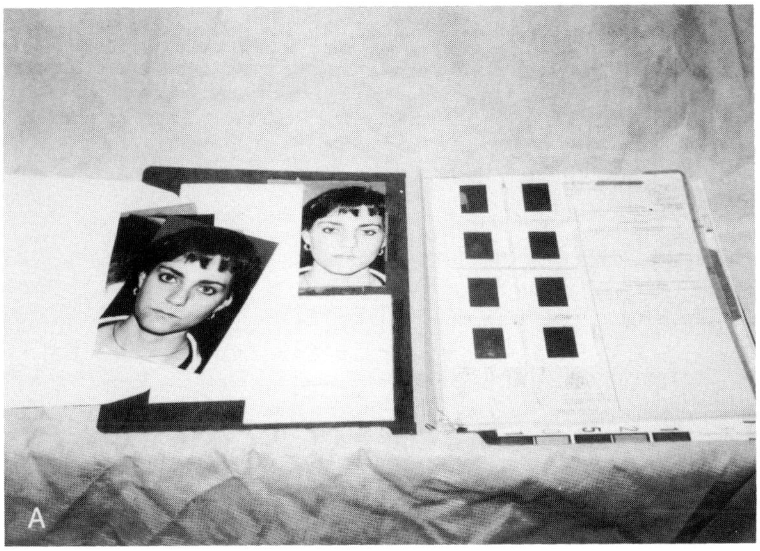

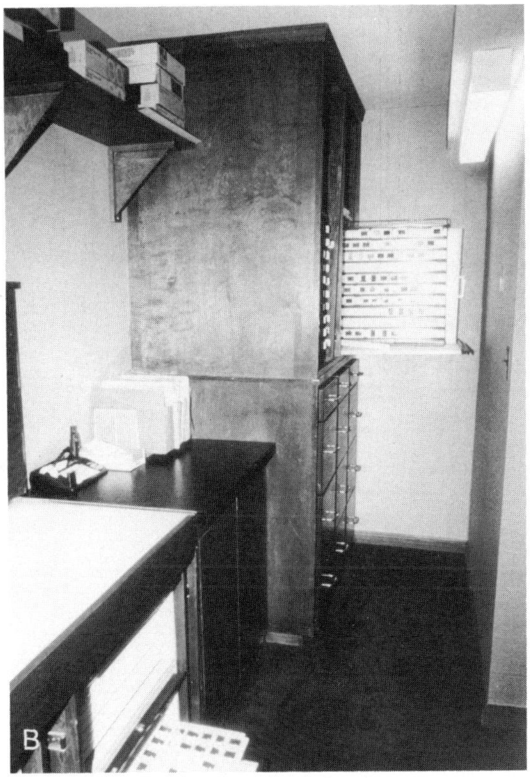

FIGURE 3–14. A special filing system should be established for surgeons who teach. Duplicates of original slides are used for lectures. Originals should remain in the patient's chart. Large, lighted viewing surfaces provide convenient work stations.

Base View. Valuable information is gained from studying the base of the nose. Skin thickness, columellar and nostril symmetry, and septal dislocations are easily recorded. Ideally, the tip of the nose should be centered in the frame and placed in line with the brows.

Overhead View. This view helps the surgeon to evaluate the symmetry of the lateral nasal walls and lower lateral cartilages.

FILING PHOTOGRAPHS

Although myriad systems for filing photographs exist, only that used by the McCollough Plastic Surgery Clinic is discussed.

The most efficient method of filing slides is to keep them in the patient's chart in 8 × 10-inch transparent jackets. Prints are filed in an envelope fastened to the inside flap of the chart. A print of the identification photograph is attached to the inside of the patient's chart (Fig. 3–14*A*).

TEACHING FILE

When a case represents subject matter that qualifies for teaching purposes, the 35-mm slides are duplicated and the duplicates are filed in a special cabinet (Fig. 3–14*B*).

SUMMARY

Attention to detail and commitment to quality photography are essential to the practice of nasal plastic surgery. High-quality equipment should be used, but the humanistic characteristics of the photographer ultimately determine whether or not the photographs are suitable to be shared with one's peers.

Personal Communications

1. Anderson, J. R., 1974.
2. Berman, W. R., 1974.
3. Webster, R. C., 1974.

Suggested Readings

American Academy of Facial Plastic and Reconstructive Surgery. The Face Book: The Pros and Cons of Facial Plastic Surgery. Washington, D.C.: Acropolis Books, 1988.

Stevens, A. The Persuation Explosion. Washington, D.C.: Acropolis Books, 1985.

Wright, M. R. How to recognize and control the problem patient. Dermatol Surg Oncol 10:389–395, 1984.

Wright, M. R. Surgical addiction: A complication of modern surgery. Arch Otolaryngol Head Neck Surg 112:870–872, 1986.

CHAPTER 4

Consummating the Contract

After the consultation, the surgeon obtains an informed consent form for surgery and, if applicable, sketches anticipated incisions on the form.

Fees and expenses are discussed, and the contract for surgery is finalized. There should be no unanswered questions or misconceptions about the financial arrangements. Throughout the world, payment in advance is customary for cosmetic plastic surgery. In some circumstances, expenses incurred for functional, medically necessary, or reconstructive surgery are guaranteed by third-party providers.

Blue Cross and Blue Shield of Alabama has formulated the following definitions of these sometimes misunderstood terms.

> "Cosmetic surgery" (sometimes referred to as "aesthetic surgery") and related services are performed to reshape structures of the body in order to alter the individual's appearance or to alter the manifestations of the aging process. Cosmetic surgery means any surgical procedure that primarily improves or changes appearance and does not primarily improve physical bodily functions or correct deformities resulting from disease, trauma, and congenital anomalies. Improvement of physical bodily function does not include improvement of psychological effects caused by physical defects or conditions.
>
> "Reconstructive" procedures and related services are performed on structures of the body to improve/restore bodily function or correct deformity resulting from disease, trauma, congenital or developmental anomalies, or previous therapeutic processes. Certain procedures can be either cosmetic or reconstructive, based on the condition of the patient and on the purpose and intent of the procedure.

"Medically necessary" means the use of a hospital or the furnishing of other services or supplies which are necessary to treat illness or injury. To be medically necessary, the services and supplies furnished must, as determined by the company (BC/BS of Alabama):

1. Be appropriate and necessary for the symptoms, diagnosis or treatment of member's condition, disease, ailment, or injury;
2. Be provided for diagnosis or direct care of the member's medical condition;
3. Be in accordance with the standards of good medical practice accepted by the organized medical community;
4. Not be solely for the convenience of the member, his family, his physician, or another provider of services;
5. Not be experimental or investigative; and,
6. Be performed in the least costly setting the member's medical condition requires.

CONSENT FORM

The consent form shown in Figure 4–1 is offered as a guideline for colleagues who want to develop their own form.

ABOUT MEDICATIONS

Prescribing medications is part of the art and science of practicing nasal plastic surgery. Some drugs have a specific scientific purpose (e.g., analgesics, antiemetics, and antibiotics), whereas others, although they may not have a proven scientific basis, are perceived by patients as an attempt on the part of the surgeon to do everything he can to help them through their surgical experience with minimum problems.

Informing the patient about which medications should be avoided may be as important as enumerating which to take (Table 4–1). Salicylate-like drugs affect clotting and should be avoided. Because they increase the tendency for bleeding, aspirin and aspirin-related products should *not* be taken for at least 14 days before or after surgery (Fig. 4–2; Table 4–2). For this reason, the contents of any over-the-counter preparations should be carefully checked before they are used. Many headache preparations, cold remedies, and hangover cures contain aspirin (acetylsalicylic acid).

LABORATORY TESTS

Examples of two forms used in laboratory testing before plastic surgery are shown in Figure 4–3.

Laboratory test results are reviewed before surgery. Consultation with the patient's personal physician, especially for patients with known medical problems, is advisable so that medical clearance can be obtained.

When the consultation appointment is scheduled, a medical history form (Fig. 4–4) is mailed to the patient. This form should be completed, signed, and returned to the office as soon as possible.

Suggested Readings

Belli, M. M., Belli: For Your Medical Defense. Oradell, N.J.: Medical Economics, 1986.
Stevens, A. The Persuasion Explosion. Washington, D.C.: Acropolis Books, 1985.
Wright, M. R. The elective surgeon's personality and role confusion. Otolaryngology Head and Neck Surgery 89:776–779, 1981.

Name: John Doe Date: 7-19-93 Time: 8:10 A.M./P.M.

1. I hereby request and authorize Dr. ______________, aided by any assistants he may designate, to perform in the presence of qualified medical personnel, the following procedure(s):
Nasal and septal reconstruction

2. I also authorize Dr. ______________ to perform any other procedures he may deem necessary or desirable in attempting to improve the condition(s) stated in paragraph 1 or any unhealthy or unforeseen condition that he may encounter during the time I am under his care.
3. I consent to the administration of medications and anesthetics to be applied by or under the direction of Dr. ______________ and/or an anesthetist and to the use of such anesthetics and medications as may be deemed advisable in my case.
4. I have been advised that part of this surgery (is or may be) performed through external incisions in the skin and that any penetrating wound to the skin will leave permanent scars, which have been described and demonstrated to me. I have been advised that scars could take one year or more to mature. The changes in their appearance that ordinarily occur have been described to me.
5. I have been told that medical-grade implants may be used in the above-mentioned operation and have been advised of the possible risks as well as alternative methods of treatment.
6. I have been informed that the operation above may require transplantation of *cartilage/bone/skin* from other areas of my body or from other people.
7. I understand that if Dr. ______________ judges at any time that my surgery should be postponed or cancelled for any reason, he may do so.
8. I hereby state that the information furnished to Dr. ______________ and his staff during my comprehensive preoperative evaluation is correct and that I have disclosed all known medical conditions, allergies, or adverse reactions to medical preparations.
9. I agree to follow the instructions given to me by Dr. ______________ and his staff to the best of my ability before, during, and after the above-named surgical procedures, and that I will, as soon as possible, notify him of any questionable conditions that may arise.
10. I have read the parts of the booklet titled *Plastic Surgery* pertinent to the proposed surgery, and I understand them. Furthermore, Dr. ______________ and his staff have fully explained in terms clear to me the effect and nature of the operation(s) to be performed, forseeable risks involved, and alternative methods of treatment.
11. I know that the practice of medicine and surgery is not an exact science and that, therefore, reputable physicians cannot guarantee results. I acknowledge that no guarantee or assurance has been made by anyone regarding the operation I have herein requested and authorized. In this connection, I have been advised that the goal of the operation I have requested is improvement in appearance and/or function, that there is a possibility that imperfections might ensue, and that the results might not live up to my expectations or the goals that have been established.
12. I hereby give permission to Dr. ______________ or any assistant he might designate to take photographs for diagnostic purposes and to enhance the medical record; I agree that these photographs will remain his property. I further authorize him to use such photographs for teaching purposes or to illustrate scientific papers, books, or lectures if, in his judgment, medical research, public interest, education, or science will be benefited by their use.
13. I understand that the operating surgeon and his staff must obtain information about the status of my health. In that regard, I hereby authorize him or his staff to contact my personal physician(s) and to obtain medical records that might assist him in his comprehensive preoperative evaluation. I also authorize the staff of the ______________ Clinic to obtain the necessary laboratory studies before my surgery, including studies to evaluate the clotting and immunological defense systems, such as HIV and/or Western Blot for acquired immunodeficiency syndrome.
14. I attest that I am proceeding with surgery of my own free will and that I have requested and authorized treatment consistent with the goals of the surgery to be performed.
15. I have been given an opportunity to ask any questions I desired regarding the treatment I am requesting as well as the matters covered in the preceding paragraphs, and these questions have been answered to my satisfaction.

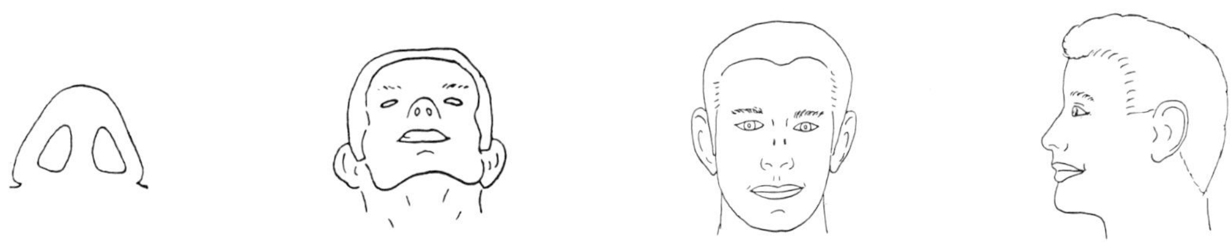

Witness: ______________ Signed: ______________ Date: ______________
(Not a family member) (Patient or person authorized to give consent for the patient)

_____ This informed consent for surgery was signed in my presence.
_____ The patient acknowledged to me that the signature is his/her signature.

FIGURE 4–1. Request and informed consent form for surgery.

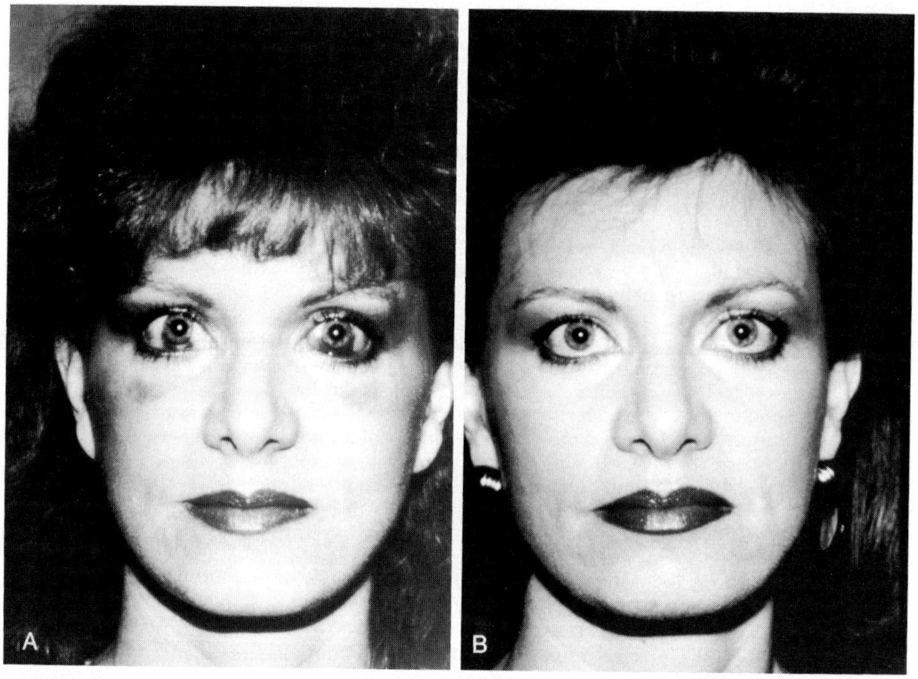

FIGURE 4–2. (*A*) Postoperative edema and ecchymosis are unpredictable. Even though measures may be taken to eliminate or reduce these effects, some patients bruise more easily. (*B*) Although disconcerting, bruising eventually subsides.

TABLE 4–1. PRESCRIPTIONS

The following instructions concerning prescriptions are given to the patient before surgery:

Take your prescription to the pharmacist about two weeks before surgery. Bring all your medications with you the day of the surgery. If you have trouble having the prescriptions filled, call our office for help.

Multivitamins: A multivitamin should be taken twice daily beginning the day before surgery and every day afterward for 2 weeks. This vitamin may be taken, however, for as long as desirable. No prescription is needed.

Vitamin C: Take 500 milligrams twice daily beginning the day before surgery and before 7:00 A.M. the day of surgery. Continue this for 2 weeks after surgery. No prescription is needed.

Diazepam: Take one or two tablets 1 hour before bedtime and the night before surgery and one or two tablets as needed for sleep after surgery.

Hydrocodone bitartrate: Take one tablet every 4 hours as needed for pain after surgery.

Promethazine hydrochloride: This suppository is prescribed for relief of nausea and vomiting. One suppository can be used every 6 hours as needed after surgery.

Cefadroxil monohydrate: Take this antibiotic twice daily beginning the evening after surgery and every day after surgery until the prescription is gone. It is important to take all the medication, if prescribed. [A Duricef capsule is also administered by the nurse before surgery.]

Tetracycline: This antibiotic is substituted for Duricef if an allergy is suspected. There is some evidence that patients with true penicillin allergy might demonstrate cross-sensitivity to cephalosporins. Take a capsule ________ times a day beginning the day before surgery and every day after surgery until all have been taken. Don't take this medication with dairy products. It is important to take all the medication, if prescribed.

Contac: This over-the-counter-medication can be taken every 12 hours as needed for nasal congestion or mucus drainage before or after surgery. No prescription is needed.

TABLE 4–2. DRUGS TO AVOID BEFORE SURGERY

The following drugs contain salicylates:

Acetidine	Bufferin	Liquiprin
Alka-Seltzer	Coricidin	Midol
Anacin	Darvon Compound	Pepto-Bismol
Anahist	Dristan	Persistin
APC	Ecotrin	Sal-Sayne
Aspirin	Empirin Compound	Stanback
BC	Excedrin	Theracin
Bromo-Quinine	4-Way Cold Tablets	Trigesic
Bromo-Seltzer	Inhiston	

Examples of aspirin-related products (ibuprofen, indomethacin, naproxen, tolmetin) are as follows:

Advil	Indocin	Nuprin
Anaprox	Motrin	Tolectin
Feldene	Naprosyn	

These products should *not* be taken for 14 days before or after surgery. Acetaminophen can be substituted for these drugs.

Encourage patients to check with their pharmacists if they are not sure the medicine they are taking contains aspirin or ibuprofen.

Beta Blockers

Patients taking propranolol (Inderal or Inderide) for mitral valve prolapse, high blood pressure, or headaches should receive special attention. Interactions with epinephrine have been shown to cause serious cardiovascular complications in some patients. The patient's physician should consider substituting another medication for Inderal or Inderide at least 1 week before surgery that might require the use of epinephrine.

Please complete the following tests *as marked* on the attached form.
CBC (complete blood count)
Chemistry profile—routine chemistries
Total protein/albumin/calcium/phosphorous/bilirubin/alkaline phosphatase
Albumin/globulin ratio—calculation
Globulin
Liver enzymes
LDH/GOT/GPT/GGT
Electrolytes
Sodium/potassium/chloride/CO_2
Anion gap—calculation with lytes
BUN/creatinine—calculated ratio
Chloride/triglyceride/ionized calcium—calculation
Urinalysis (clean-catch)
PT (prothrombin time)
PTT (partial thromboplastin time)
HIV antibody (acquired immunodeficiency syndrome)
VDRL
Pregnancy test (only if marked on the attached form)
The tests above should be done at a time when the patient has *not* eaten in 6 hours.
Lab work should be done 1 month before surgery. This is important to confirm the scheduled surgery date.
Have lab tests done on this date: ____________
The results of these tests are due in our office no later than 2 weeks before surgery.

HIV Antibody Testing

Date: ____________________
Physician: ____
Patient: ____
(Last name) (First name)
Address: ____
(Street)
____
(City) (State) (Zip)
Date of Birth: ____________________
Billable party (please circle):
Patient Client Medicaid Medicare PMD
\# _______ # _______ # _______
Responsible party: ____
I give my consent for HIV antibody testing.

____
Signature of patient

I verify that the above-named patient has given informed consent to the performance of HIV antibody testing.

____
Signature of attending physician

FIGURE 4–3. Laboratory tests administered before plastic surgery.

CONSULTATION AND MEDICAL HISTORY DATA

Name ________________ Date of Birth ________ Today's Date ________

Address: Home ________________
street city state zip telephone

Business ________________
street city state zip telephone

Marital Status: S, M, D, Sep., Widowed Spouse's name ________ Ages of Children ________

Your Occupation/Employer ________ Spouse's Occupation/Employer ________

How were you referred to us? ________ Names of family members who are our patients ________

In which surgical procedure(s) are you interested? (please circle)

Rhinoplasty (nose) ______ Chin ______ Face or Neck Lift ______ Eyelids ______
Chemical Peel ______ Dermabrasion ______ Scar Revision ______ Protruding Ears ______
Removal of Cysts, Warts, Moles, Etc. ______ Hair Transplantation ______ Breast Surgery ______
Body Contour Surgery (tummy tuck) ______ Suction Lipectomy ______ Other ______

What **specifically** do you wish to have corrected: (i.e. what don't you like about the above condition(s)?) ________

Do you desire improvement in both appearance and function? Yes ______ No ______

When did you begin to consider surgical correction? ________

Why have you decided to have it done at this point in time? ________

Have you consulted any other doctor about this? (when?) ________

Have you discussed this surgery with your family? **Yes** **No** Are they agreeable? **Yes** **No**

Have you had **any** previous cosmetic, plastic or reconstructive surgery? **Yes** **No** When, and what, if anything was done? ________

Who performed the surgery? ________ Where was it performed? ________

Were you satisfied with the results? ________ If not why? ________

Have you had any other surgery, or an injury, to the face. nose, neck or eyes? ________

When? ________ Describe. as best you can ________

Has anyone in your family or a close friend had cosmetic, plastic or reconstructive surgery? ________

What was done? ________ By whom? ________

Have you had **any other** prior surgery? (What was done & when was it performed?) In the head & neck area? ________

On your skin? ______ On your teeth or gums? ______ In your chest? ______ In your abdomen? ______

On the reproductive system? ______ On your back, arms, or legs? ______ Other: ______

Were there any complications? **Yes** **No** Did you have a normal recovery? **Yes** **No**

Did the results meet your expectations? ________ Please explain ________

MEDICAL HISTORY (circle appropriate response)

No Yes Are you now taking any drugs or medications? (How Often?)
List them if you can ________

No Yes Are you allergic to any medication, creams, tape, make-up, etc.?
List them if you can ________

When was your last physical examination? ________

Who is your family doctor? ________ Address ________

No Yes Would you object to our contacting him for additional information pertaining to your health?

(continued on back)

FIGURE 4–4. Medical history form. *Illustration continued on following page*

MEDICAL HISTORY (continued)

No Yes Have you ever received local anesthesia ("Novacaine, Xylocaine" etc.) by a dentist or doctor? (circle appropriate response)
No Yes Did you have a "reaction" to any anesthetic? Explain ____
No Yes Are you considered a healthy person?
No Yes Do you take vitamins regularly? Explain ____

Do you or any family members have: (indicate who)

Heart trouble ____ Excessive bleeding tendencies ____ Psychiatric or "nerve" problems ____
High blood pressure ____ Diabetes ____ Thyroid problems ____
Excessive bruisability ____ Excessive scarring ____ Delayed or poor healing ____

Do you have any history of bleeding: (indicate which)

From the nose ____ In the urine ____ Vomiting blood ____
From the rectum ____ Coughing up blood ____ Other? ____

No Yes Do you have hay fever, nasal allergies or asthma? Explain ____
No Yes Do you have or have you had any problems with your eyes or vision? Explain ____
No Yes Do you have frequent pains in the chest?
No Yes Has a doctor ever said you had "heart trouble"? Explain ____
No Yes Do you have "stomach trouble" or ulcers? Explain ____
No Yes Do you have or have you had chest or lung problems? Explain ____
No Yes Have you ever had liver, gall bladder trouble or "yellow jaundice"? (circle which one)
No Yes Have you been bothered by kidney or bladder problems? Explain ____
No Yes Do you or any family members suffer from "arthritis"?
No Yes Do you experience poor circulation in your fingers or toes?
No Yes Do you have frequent skin infections, irritations or rashes (circle which one)
No Yes Have you ever had fever blisters or "cold sores" or Canker sores on your face, lips or in your mouth or Genital Herpes? (circle which one)
No Yes Do you often have severe headaches or dizzy spells? (circle which one)
No Yes Has any part of your body ever been paralyzed or numb? Explain ____
No Yes Did you ever have a convulsion or seizure? Explain ____
No Yes Have you ever received treatment for your genital area? Explain ____
No Yes Were you ever told you had any venereal disease or AIDS? Explain ____
No Yes Are you frequently sick or ill?
No Yes Do you worry about your health?
No Yes Were you ever treated for anemia or any problems with your blood? Explain ____
No Yes Have you ever taken hormones or thyroid medication? Explain ____
No Yes Do you smoke more than 10 cigarettes a day?
No Yes Do you drink more than 6 cups of coffee a day?
No Yes Do you usually take two or more alcoholic drinks a day?
No Yes Have you ever received treatment for abuse of alcohol or drugs? Explain ____
No Yes Do you often get depressed?
No Yes Do you usually feel unhappy or depressed?
No Yes Are you considered a nervous person?
No Yes Did you ever have a "nervous breakdown"? Explain ____
No Yes Have you ever received medical treatment for a "nervous breakdown"? Explain ____
No Yes Are you easily upset or irritated?
No Yes Do you tend to hold a "grudge" when someone angers you?
No Yes Have you ever considered consulting a psychiatrist or psychologist? Explain ____
No Yes Have you ever been under the care of a psychiatrist or psychologist? Explain ____

Women Only: When was your last menstrual period? ____

No Yes Are your periods often irregular?
No Yes Have you had "female" or GYN problems? Explain ____
No Yes **Men Only:** Have you ever had prostate problems?

No Yes Do you have any other medical problems that have not been covered? Explain ____

No Yes Do you accept the fact that every medical and surgical treatment is associated with risks and other imponderables?
No Yes Have you read our patient reference book, **"Plastic Surgery"** including the patient's Bill of Rights/Responsibilities?
No Yes Do you give consent and authorize the recommended diagnostic, medical, surgical, anesthetic and other diagnostic services that the clinic deems beneficial while you are under their care?

Signed ____ Date ____

Thank you,

The information you have provided is essential in our comprehensive evaluation in your case. Please re-read the book **"Plastic Surgery"** and write down any questions you may have so that we may discuss them in detail during your Consultation period. If you do not have the book please ask for one; it is an important part of informing you about your surgery.

FIGURE 4–4. *Continued*

CHAPTER 5

Rhinoplasty: An Overview

In nasal plastic surgery, undesirable "excess" bone and/or cartilage is carefully removed and the remainder is rearranged or reshaped. Sometimes it is necessary to use reconstructive techniques such as grafts and implants, especially after severe accidents or unsuccessful primary operations.

Most rhinoplasties are performed because the patient desires an improvement in appearance or nasal function. The patient may simply want a nose that is in harmony with the rest of the face rather than one that is out of proportion with respect to the other facial features (Fig. 5–1). Or, as the patient ages, the nose may become progressively more disfigured until breathing difficulty occurs (Fig. 5–2). Some patients have deformities of the inside of the nose that impair breathing, cause headaches, or contribute to sinus infection. These problems cannot be satisfactorily treated without simultaneously straightening the external nose (Fig. 5–3).

Like faces, every nose is different; some noses are too long, some are too wide, some have large humps, some project away from the face, and so on (Figs. 5–4 through 5–6). Because rhinoplasty surgery is as much an art as it is a science, seldom should any two patients' noses be identical after surgery. It is not possible, nor is it desirable, to duplicate the nose of a model in a magazine photograph. The surgeon must strive to make each patient's nose fit his or her face, blending harmoniously with the other features.

Text continued on page 62

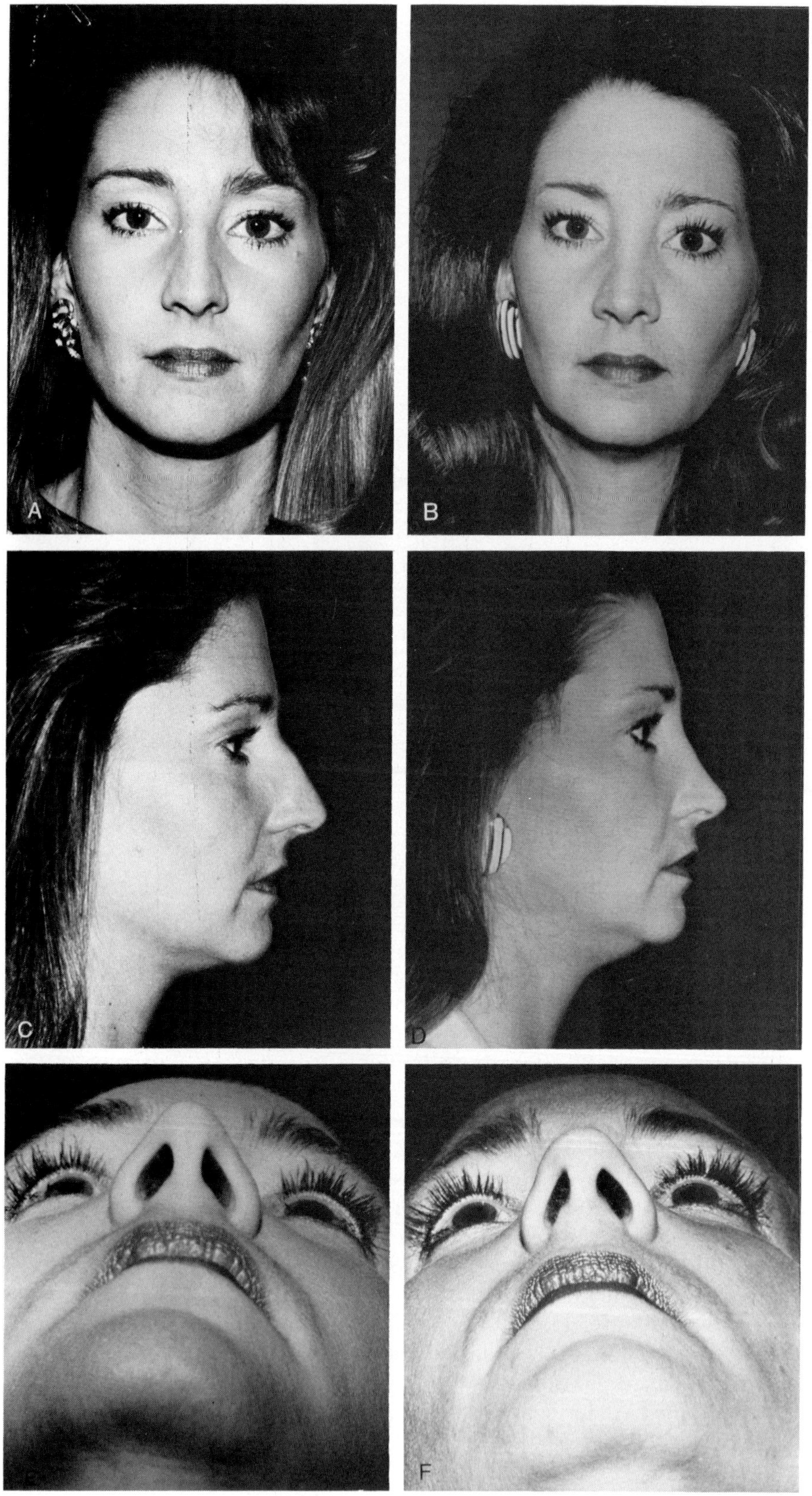

FIGURE 5–1. (*A* and *B*). An ideal candidate for septorhinoplasty, this patient has good facial harmony and relatively thin skin. (*C* and *D*) She requested reduction of a dorsal hump but wanted a straight dorsum. (*E* and *F*) Nostril and columellar asymmetry may be secondary to a caudal dislocation of the nasal septum, asymmetrical alar cartilages, or both.

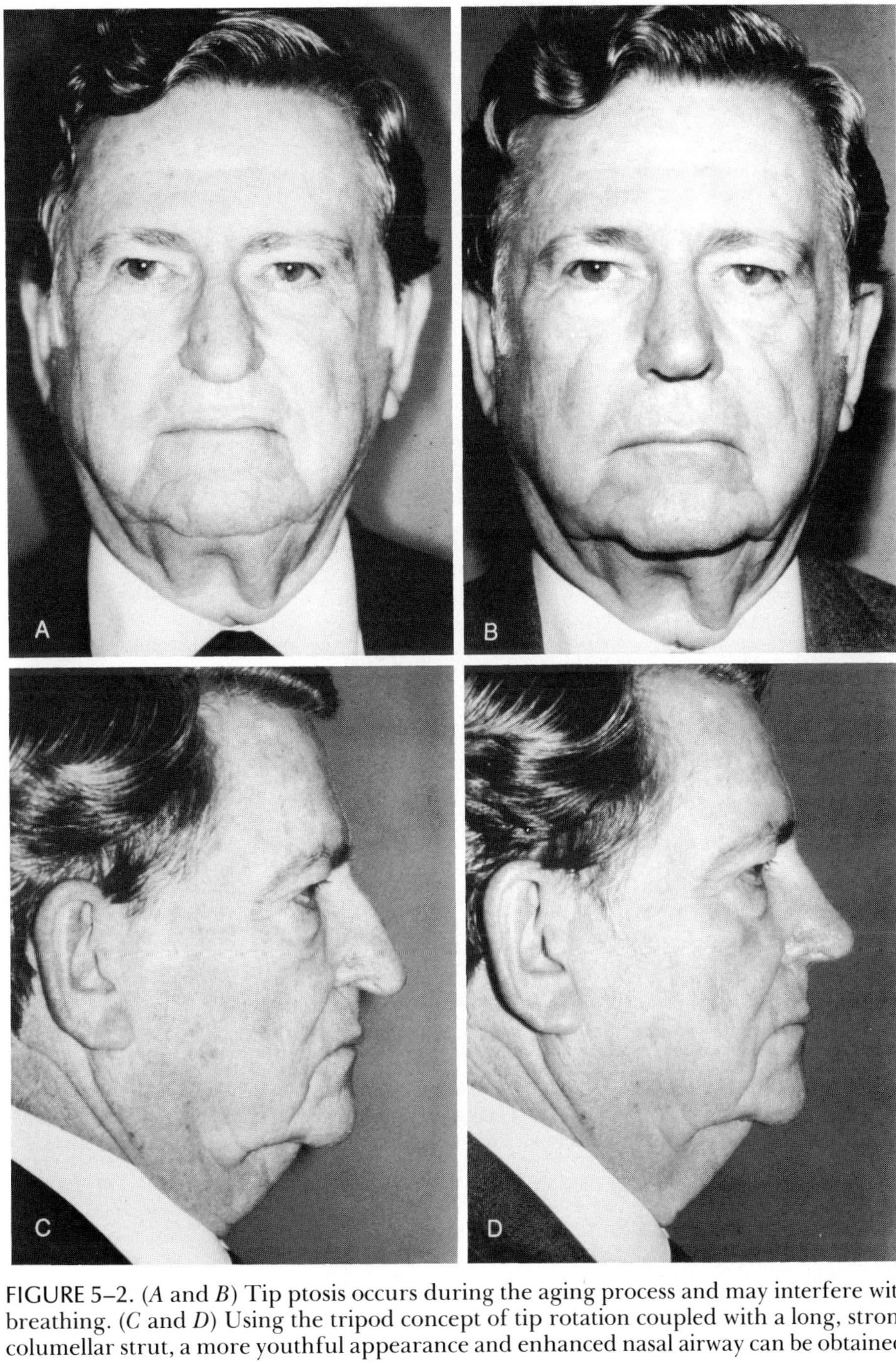

FIGURE 5–2. (*A* and *B*) Tip ptosis occurs during the aging process and may interfere with breathing. (*C* and *D*) Using the tripod concept of tip rotation coupled with a long, strong columellar strut, a more youthful appearance and enhanced nasal airway can be obtained.

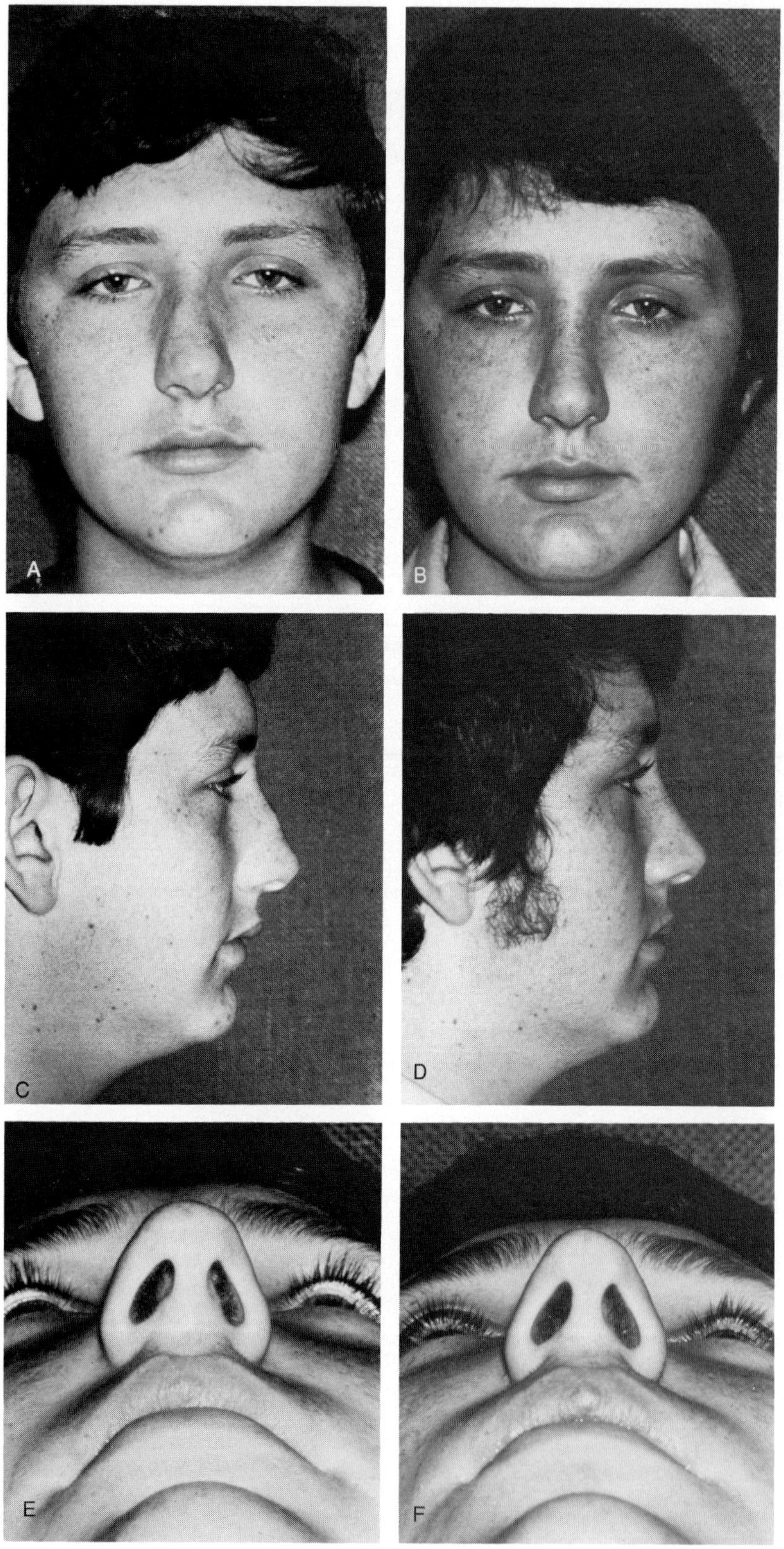

FIGURE 5–3. (*A* and *B*) Nasal injuries may produce deformities of both internal and external nasal structures, requiring reconstructive rhinoplasty. (*C* and *D*) A small hump can be removed when functional surgery is performed. (*E* and *F*) No tip surgery was performed on this patient.

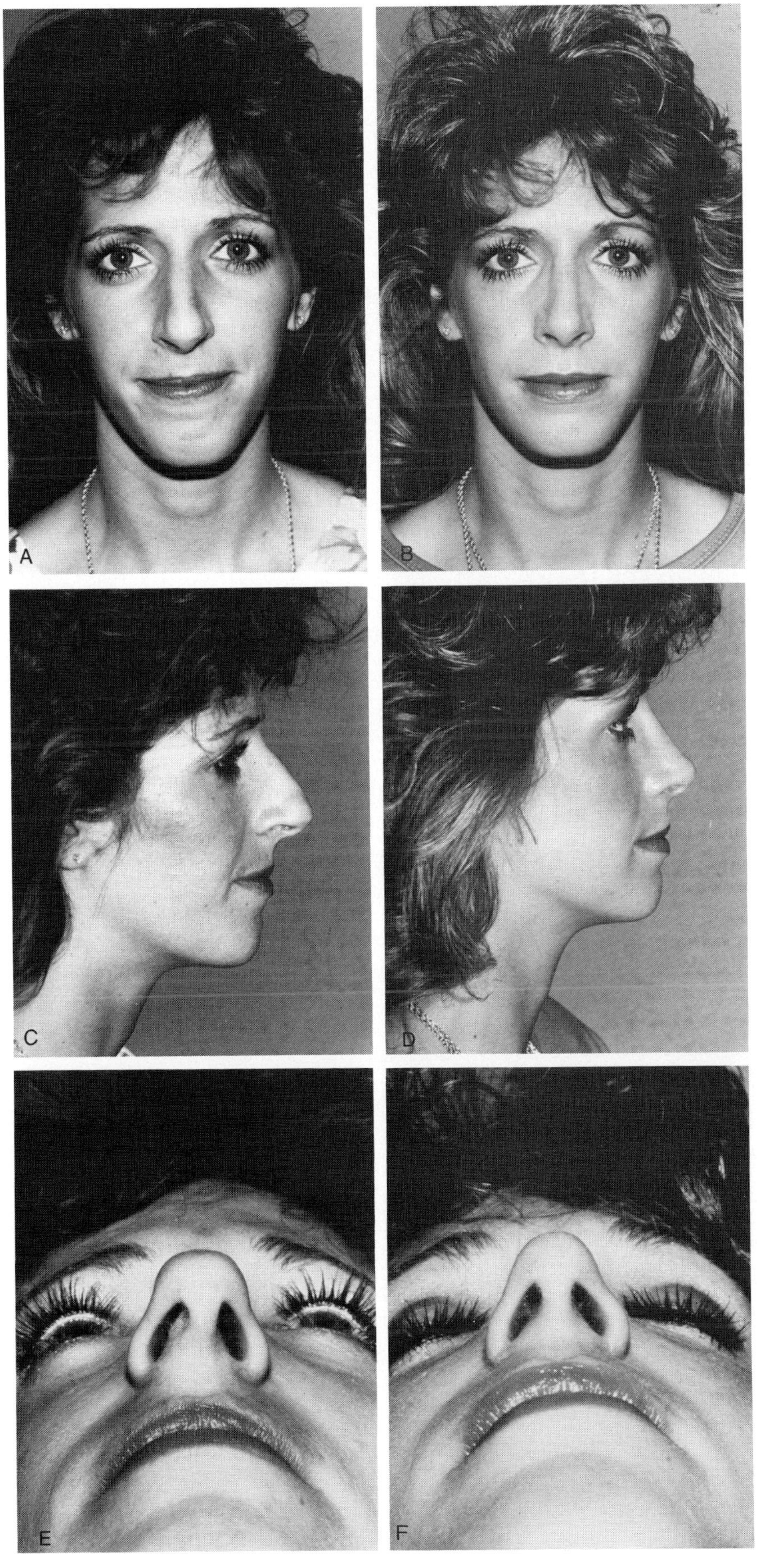

FIGURE 5–4. (*A* and *B*) A large nose in a patient with small features and a thin face can produce disharmony. (*C* and *D*) No surgery was performed on the chin, but a smaller, less projecting nose restores the balance. (*E* and *F*) Tipplasty was accomplished with a double-dome technique.

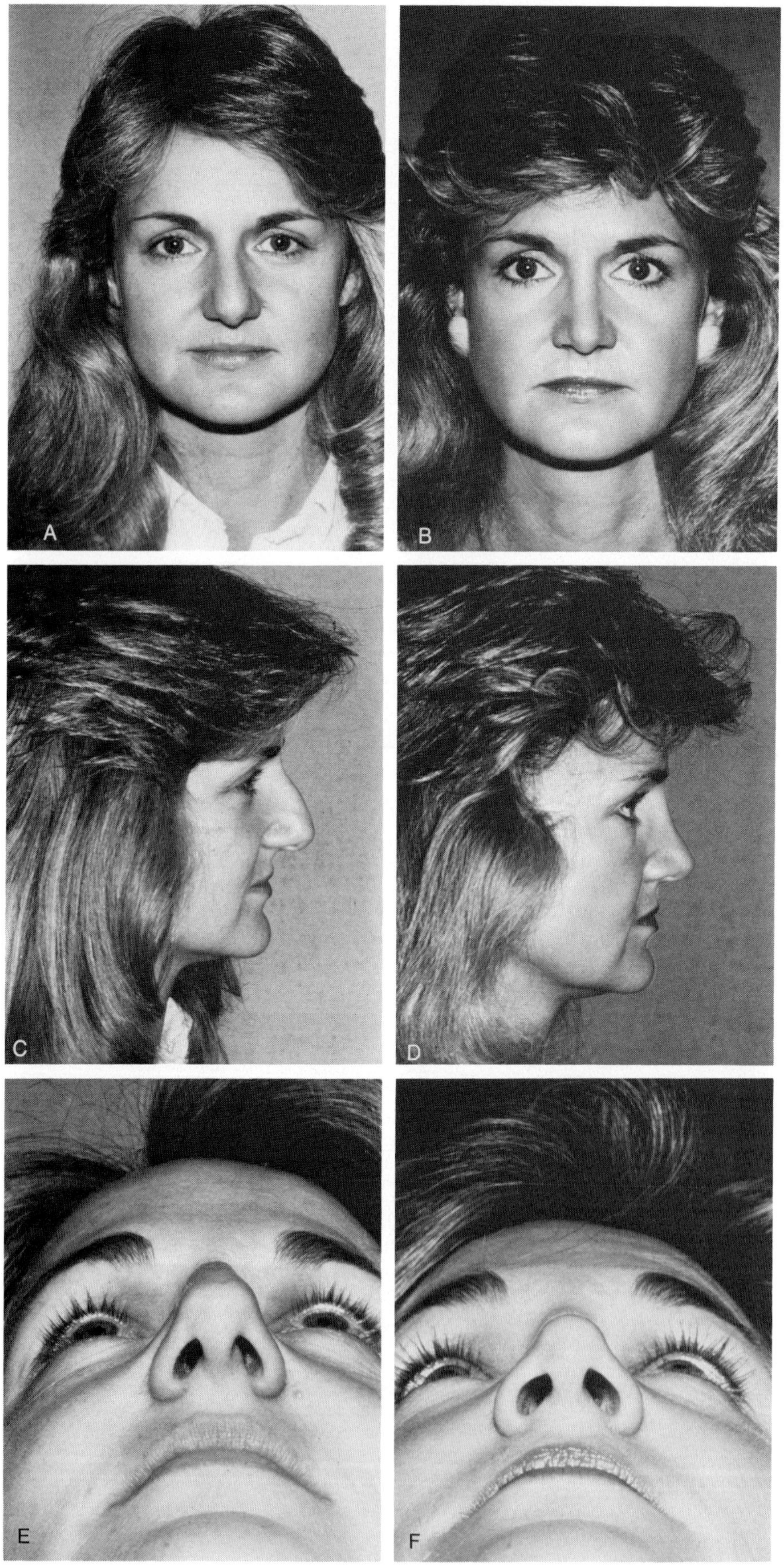

FIGURE 5–5. (*A* and *B*) Patients with a short middle one-third of the face pose a unique challenge. (*C* and *D*) Removing the hump and correcting an acute nasolabial angle without producing tip rotation and the illusion of further shortening are the surgeon's challenge. (*E* and *F*) Double-dome maneuvers can produce tip refinement while preventing rotation.

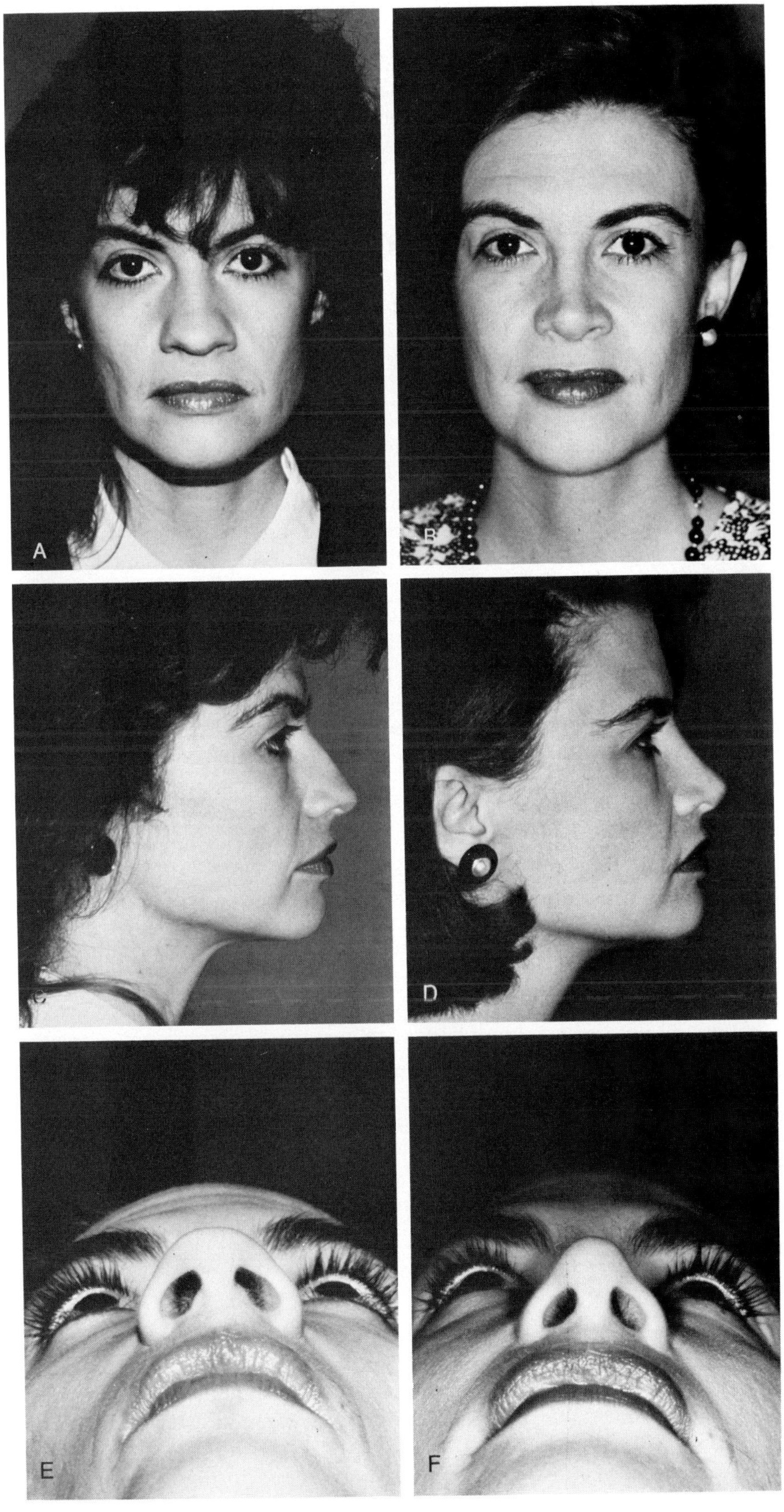

FIGURE 5–6. (*A* and *B*) A wide nose requires medialization of the lateral nasal walls with osteotomies and tip techniques, which provide projection and narrowing. (*C* and *D*) Maintaining or producing tip projection allows the surgeon to leave the nasal dorsum higher—the key to noses that appear narrow from the front. (*E* and *F*) Dome division with central I beam grafts and alar base resections was performed.

The alterations recommended are determined by many factors, including height, age, skin thickness, ethnic background, and configuration of other features, such as the forehead, eyes, and chin. All in all, the nasal plastic surgeon strives to achieve a natural-looking nose rather than one that appears to have been operated on. No patient wants an assembly-line "nose job"; he wants a nose individually tailored to his own features, personality, and station in life.

AT WHAT AGE CAN SURGERY BE DONE?

An often-asked question is: At what age can nasal plastic and reconstructive surgery be performed? If a severe breathing problem exists, even in a child, the airway obstruction should be corrected. With children, additional surgery at maturity may be required to obtain the best result. Certain limitations exist in children that preclude performing the definitive correction before puberty. Most girls are mature enough by age 15 (boys at age 18) to have surgical correction. However, it is necessary to individualize this factor because some boys and girls mature at earlier ages.

So that growth and maturation can be monitored, young men and women should consult a surgeon when they decide they want to have rhinoplasty, even though surgical correction may be deferred (Fig. 5–7). When an adolescent's height, weight, and shoe size have remained unchanged for 6 to 12 months, one can assume that maturation is complete. Palpating the tip cartilages can help to determine if the patient has achieved the bulk and rigidity associated with maturation. When young women have been menstruating regularly and young men shaving regularly for about 12 months, I will perform a septorhinoplasty, provided that the young person is emotionally prepared to undergo surgery. The criteria may be met at different ages because each person has his or her own biological clock. Some young women are mature at 13 and some young men at 15.

Early correction of nasal deformities can give young people more self-confidence and improve their self-esteem at a crucial time in their lives when they are discovering not only who they are but also who they may want to become.

A parent should come with a minor to the consultation visit.

About 30 per cent of rhinoplasties are performed on patients over age 40. Many remark that they have disliked their noses for much of their lives and finally are in a position to have corrective surgery. Provided that the patient is in good health, it is never too late to have a rhinoplasty (Fig. 5–8). It often is done as part of a facial rejuvenation program to minimize the undesirable signs of aging (Fig. 5–9). Repositioning or lifting the tip of a nose that is drooping can result in a more youthful appearance.

ANXIETY AND PAIN

Nasal surgery does not have to be an unpleasant experience, but in many unfortunate incidences it has been. Because most patients are apprehensive about surgery, an anesthetic program must be designed to make patients as comfortable as possible before, during, and after their operation.

In my practice most septorhinoplasties are performed under local anesthesia with sedation. The patient must be given appropriate medication to help ensure amnesia to much of the operating room experience.

Text continued on page 66

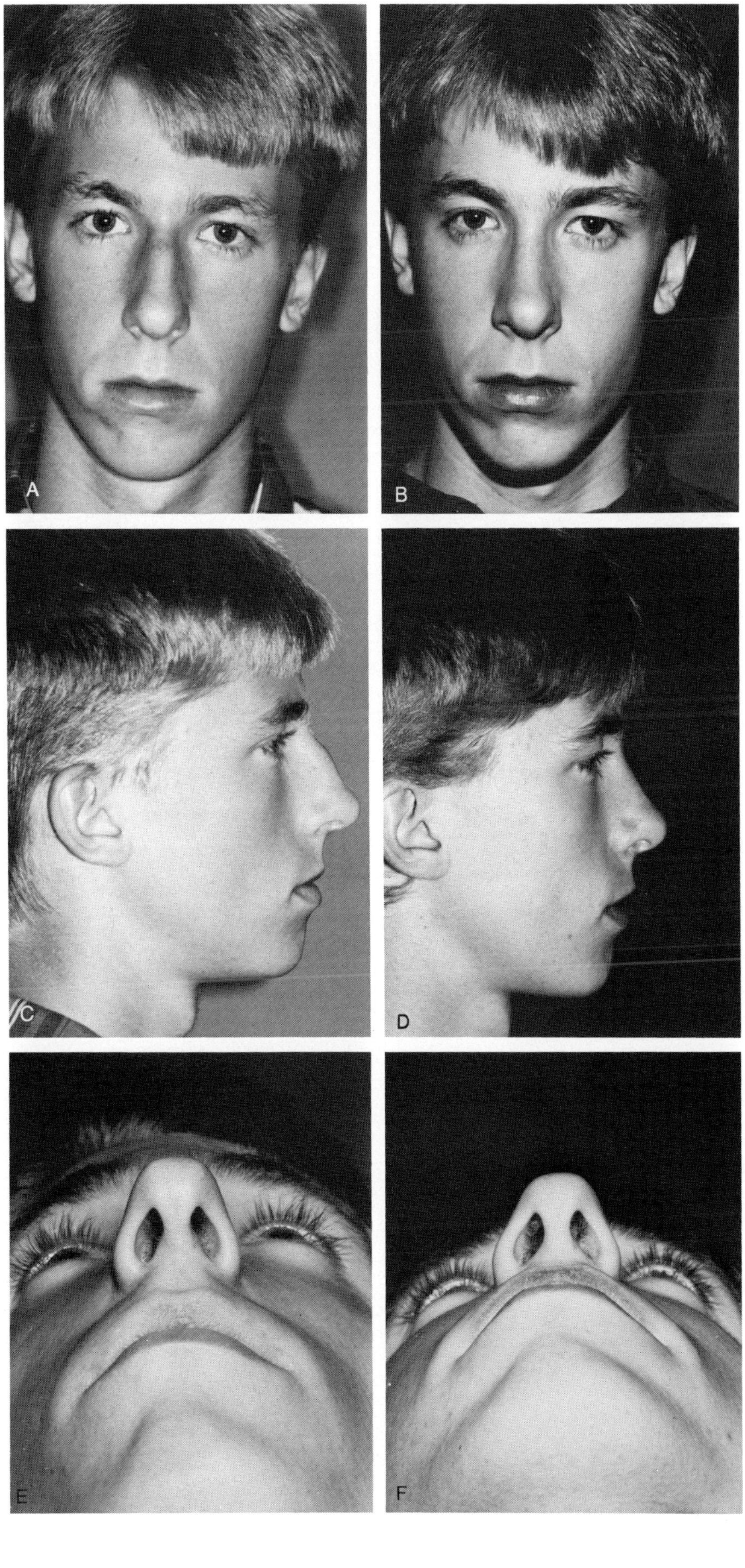

FIGURE 5–7. (*A* and *B*) At 16, many young men are mature enough to undergo aesthetic nasal surgery when reconstructive surgery is performed to correct a nasal fracture. (*C* and *D*) Small humps can be removed by gentle rasping, especially if surgery is delayed for 2 to 3 months. (*E* and *F*) A complete strip technique was used for tip-plasty.

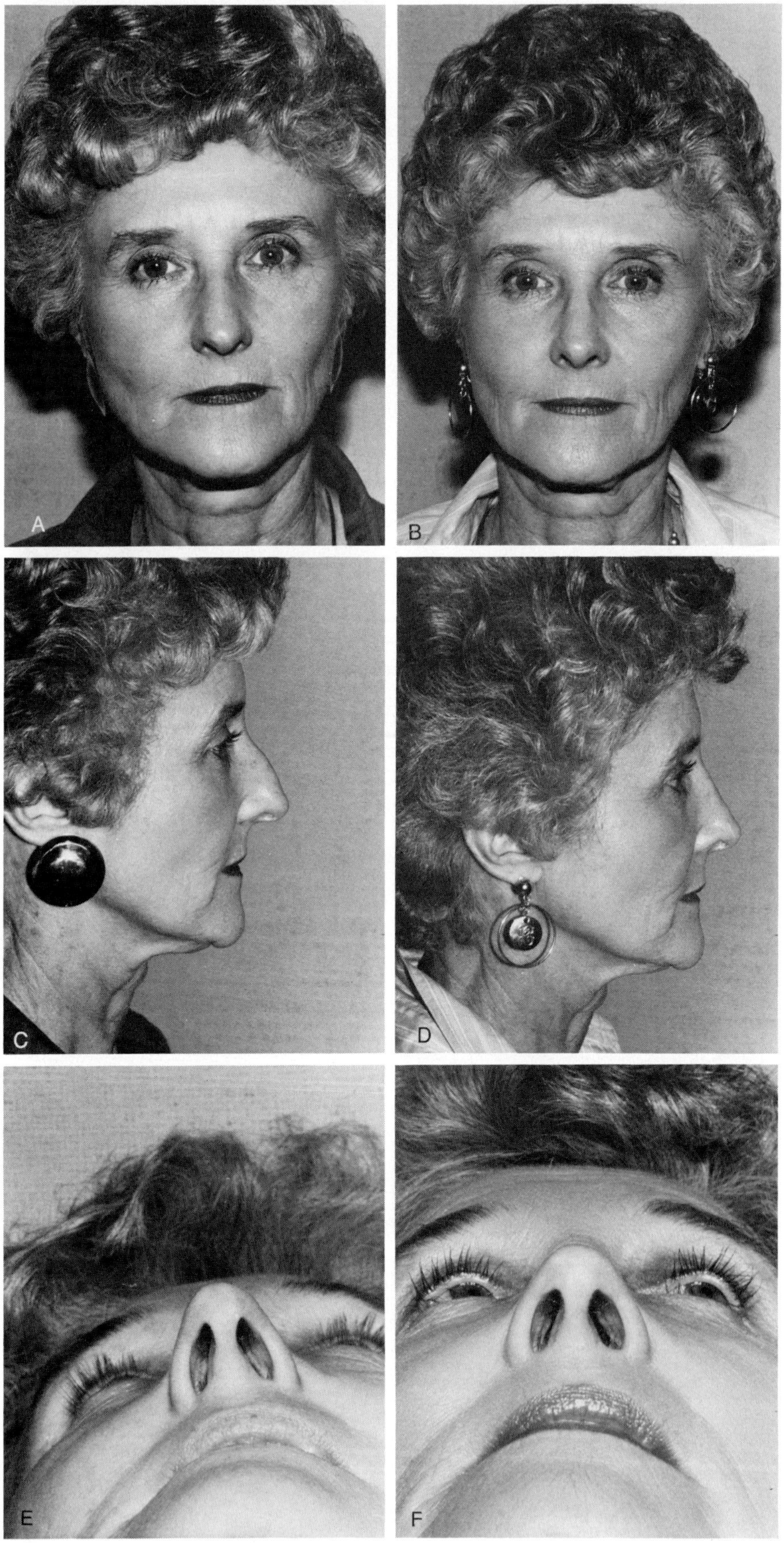

FIGURE 5–8. (*A* and *B*) Conservative rhinoplasty is recommended for the aging patient who desires refinement. (*C* and *D*) Tip support and correction of an acute nasolabial angle is accomplished with cartilagenous plumping grafts. (*E* and *F*) Tip-plasty was carried out with a complete strip technique.

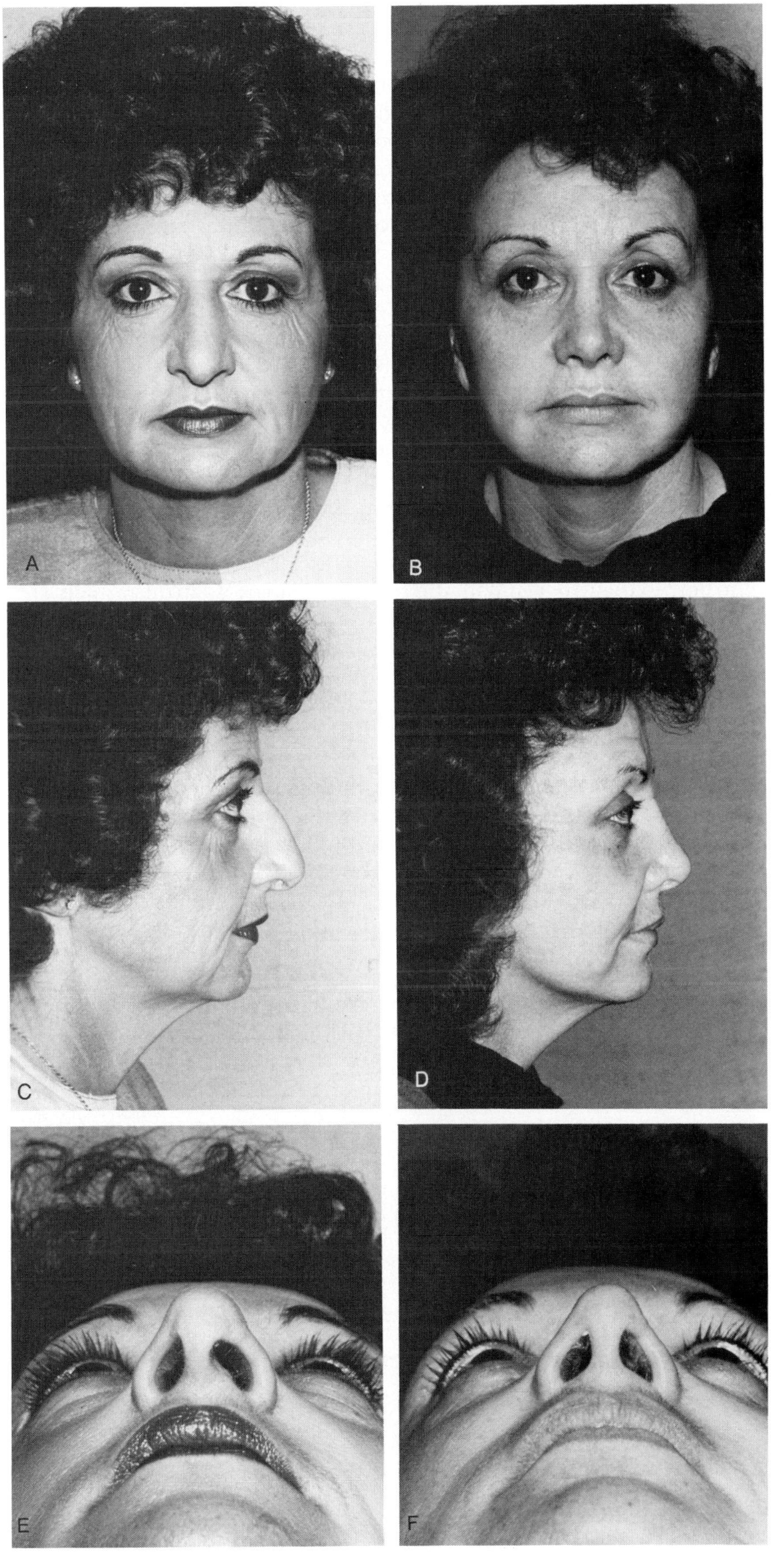

FIGURE 5–9. (*A* and *B*) Rhinoplasty is an integral part of facial rejuvenation. It can be done at the same time rhytidectomy and blepharoplasty are performed. (*C* and *D*) Minimal hump removal is recommended; however, increased tip projection and rotation are necessary. (*E* and *F*) Tip-plasty was accomplished with a double-dome unit with dome division.

This technique is known as "twilight sleep." It is helpful to tell patients that twilight sleep is similar to the state that exists during the night when the patient is in the deepest stages of natural sleep. If someone nudges him and asks him to roll over, he complies and appears to wake up. The next morning he can barely recall the incident.

Anesthetics, sedatives, and hypnotics are given in a graduated, programmed manner. When patients are apprehensive, sedatives and hypnotics are prescribed the night before surgery and oftentimes on arising the morning of surgery. By the time the patient arrives at the surgical facility, much of the anxiety is greatly reduced. Shortly after arrival, additional medication is given so that before going to the operating room, the patient is very relaxed.

When in the operating room, intravenous medication is given to finalize the twilight sleep. After the patient has reached this state of sedation, topical and local anesthetics (usually lidocaine) are given to produce anesthesia in the areas to be operated. Local anesthetics sting as they spread through the tissues. After the local anesthetic has taken effect, the patient should experience *no discomfort* during surgery. With twilight sleep, most patients do not remember receiving the local anesthetic. Supplementary medication may be given if necessary.

Although most people have amnesia to the operation, they are alert on returning to their rooms. With this type of anesthesia, patients usually are ambulatory sooner and the likelihood of potential complications is reduced. In children and some patients who insist on it, a general anesthetic may be used.

Uncomplicated septorhinoplasty should take about 1 hour. Dissection should proceed in a systematic, unhurried manner. Quality must not be sacrificed for speed, nor should recognized internal deformities be left untreated. The master nasal plastic surgeon is as concerned about function as he is form. As the surgeon gains experience, fewer unnecessary surgical moves naturally result in shortened operative time.

Local anesthetics are effective for about 1 hour. If the surgeon anticipates that the operation might take 2 hours or more, general anesthesia should be considered.

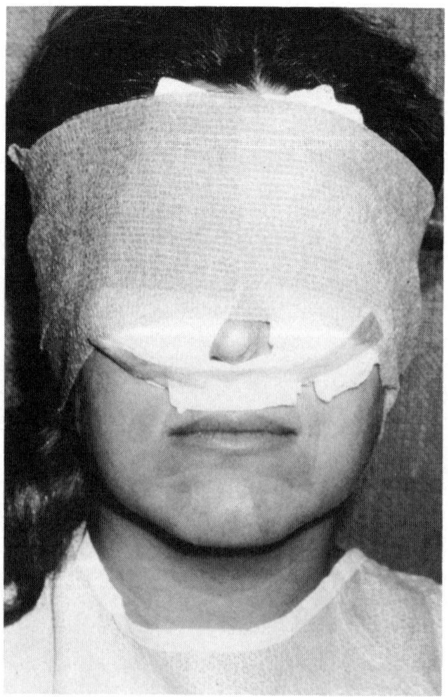

FIGURE 5–10. Pressure dressings, when correctly applied and left in place for 4 hours, help to reduce postoperative ecchymosis.

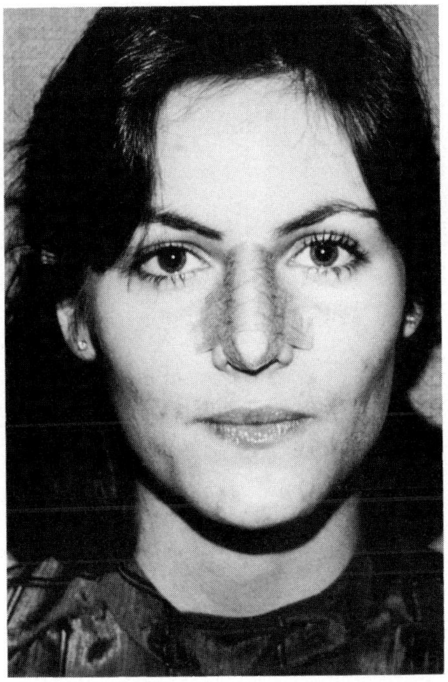

FIGURE 5–11. An external nasal splint and tapes should be undisturbed for about 7 days.

At the completion of surgery, a small protective adhesive dressing and splint is applied to the nose; then a bulky dressing is placed over the eyes and nose (Figs. 5–10 and 5–11). The bulky dressing (along with the premedication taken before surgery) plays an important role in reducing postoperative swelling and discoloration. The bulky dressing is removed after 4 hours; the external protective splint and tape remain in place for about 1 week.

Although a tiny Surgicel drip dressing is applied at the nasal introitus and obstructs the nostrils, *the nose is not packed after surgery*—even extensive septal surgery. Patients, therefore, are more comfortable and less swelling occurs. With the elimination of nasal packing, postoperative pain, swelling, bleeding, discoloration, and so forth are dramatically reduced, making the recovery period much more tolerable for the patient. A special technique of suturing the internal nasal tissues (mucoperichondrial flaps) and intercartilagenous incisions with absorbable sutures eliminates the necessity of internal packing. This technique has been a landmark advancement in nasal surgery and reduces much of the postoperative discomfort experienced by patients whose noses are packed (see Chapter 10).

Many patients contemplating rhinoplasty ask, "Do you have to break my nose?" The answer is no. When the bones need to be repositioned, an internal osteotomy incision is made into the nasal bones along the desired mobilization tract, thereby eliminating the more traumatic and less predictable technique of breaking the bones. This method allows for better control of the operation and reduces the anxiety of many patients about to undergo nasal surgery.

AFTER NASAL SURGERY

After discharge, the patient is urged to remain out of bed because being in an upright position decreases swelling and accelerates healing.

The protective splint and dressings on the nose are removed 7 days after surgery. At the end of 1 week, most of the swelling and discoloration have

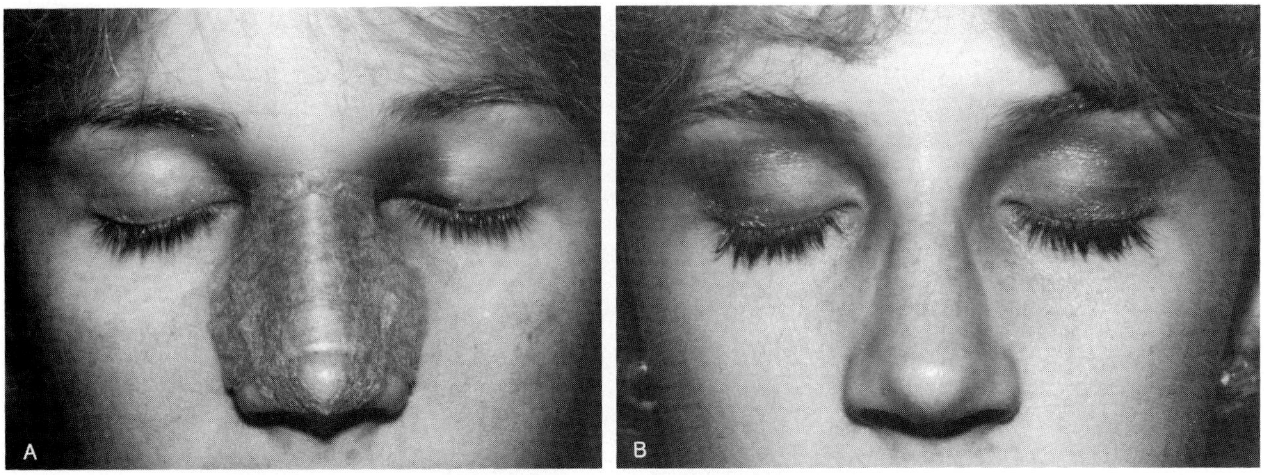

FIGURE 5–12. (*A*) This patient underwent septorhinoplasty 7 days earlier. For 4 hours after surgery, light pressure dressings were applied over the eyes and operative areas. (*B*) The patient's appearance 7 days after the dressings were removed.

disappeared. Patients can use makeup, if applicable, and in most cases they can return to work or school at this time.

Some swelling of the nose (which patients feel more than they or anyone else see) is present but progressively diminishes over the next several weeks. When the dressings are first removed, the nose appears turned up because the effects of the bandage and the swelling of the tissues (Fig. 5–12). Because of this, the patient who expects to see a perfectly shaped nose as soon as the dressings are removed will suffer disappointment. The surgeon and his staff must reinforce this point to patients *before* the dressings are removed.

Additional swelling disappears within 3 to 4 days after the bandage is removed, and the nose begins to take on its eventual appearance. It usually takes at least 1 year for the last 1 to 2 per cent of the swelling to disappear; this does not bother most patients or distract from the appearance of the nose; rather, the nose seems to acquire improved definition as the last bit of swelling subsides. This is especially true for the tip of the nose and along the lateral nasal walls (Figs. 5–13 and 5–14).

The tissues inside the nose also remain swollen after surgery; therefore, progressively decreasing amounts of nasal blockage should be expected for a time after the average uncomplicated nasal operation. About 80 per cent of the swelling disappears by 2 weeks; 90 per cent is gone by 2 months. The remainder disappears at the rate of about 1 per cent per month. The final result is not seen for about a year. In patients with thicker skin, it takes longer for the nose to assume its final shape. Thicker skin, like a sponge, holds on to the swelling. (Each case is different, and in my preoperative evaluation, I attempt to explain the limitations associated with a particular person's skin.)

When patients have associated breathing problems that require work to be done on the nasal septum and turbinates, there may be varying amounts of nasal blockage for several weeks after surgery. If allergy, vasomotor rhinitis, and excess mucus production are contributing factors, sometimes antihistaminic decongestants can provide symptomatic relief. Because these medications make some patients drowsy, they should not be taken unless mucus production and drainage are excessive.

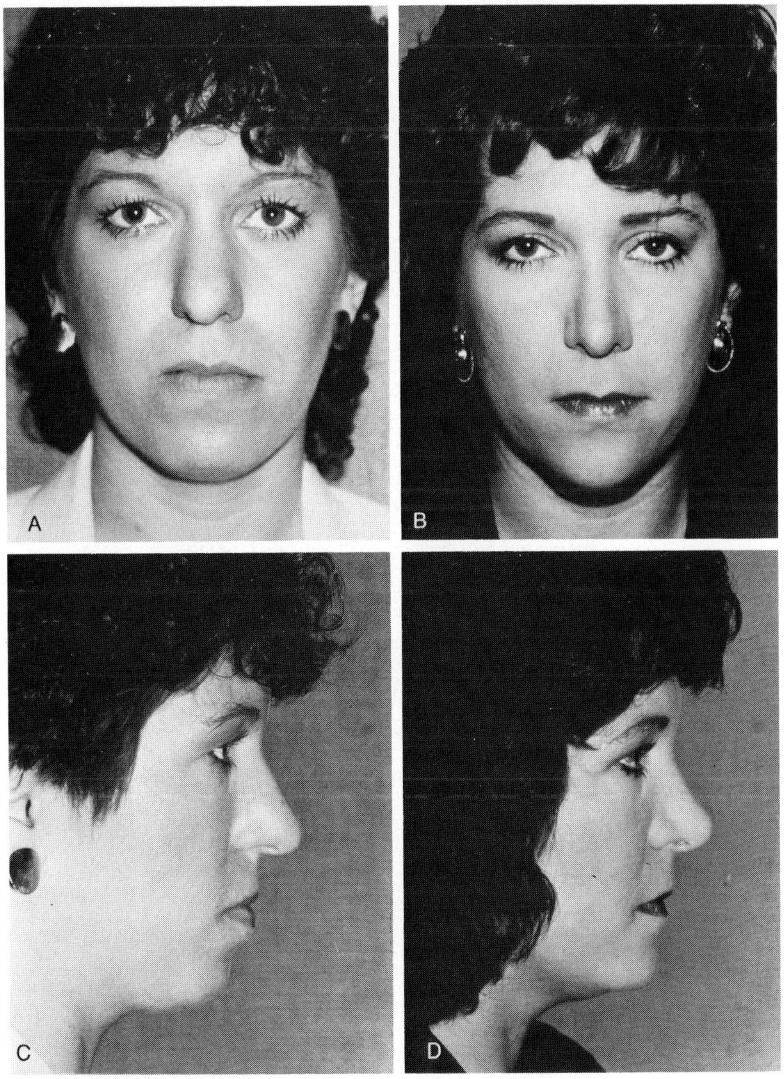

FIGURE 5–13. (*A* and *B*) In this thick-skinned nose, refinement continued to occur for 5 years, especially in the tip. (*C* and *D*) Supratip definition may be the last change to occur, provided tip support is adequate. Tip-plasty was accomplished by a complete strip and cartilagenous plumping grafts placed beneath the feet of the medial crura.

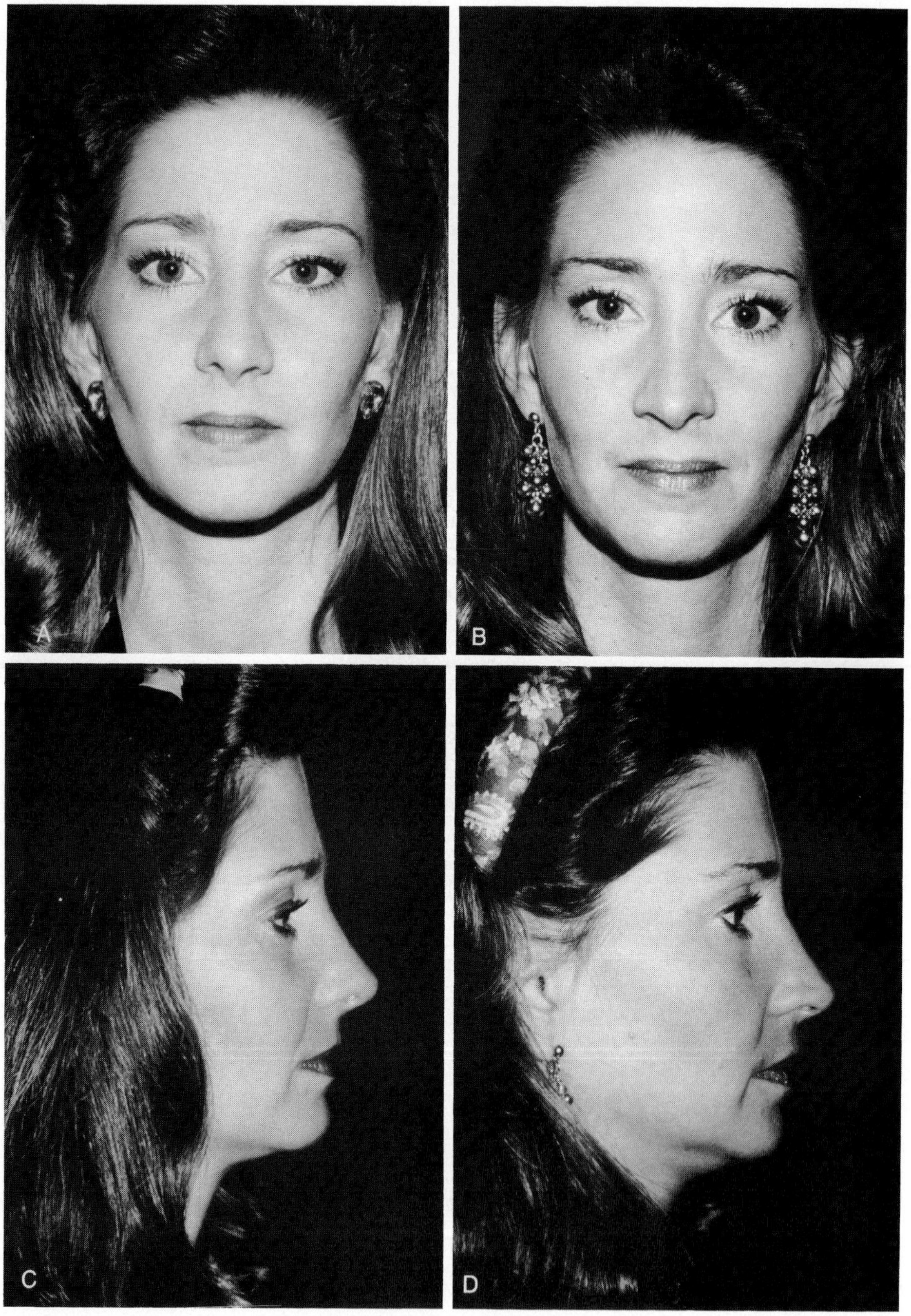

FIGURE 5–14. (*A* and *B*) Patient shown in Figure 5–1A 6 weeks after surgery. (*C* and *D*) Same patient 6 months after surgery. Note the definition of the tip and lateral nasal walls with the passage of time. (See Figure 5–1 for long-term result.)

CAUSE OF NASAL BREATHING PROBLEMS

One of the common causes of breathing difficulties is a deviated, or crooked, nasal septum. A nasal septum that is excessively thickened, dislocated, or bowed to one side can interfere with the flow of air through one or both sides of the nose (Fig. 5–15).

Many patients whose septums are not deviated have a dominant nostril (airway passage). Most people have a dominant eye, hand, or foot; it is not unusual for one nasal airway to be more patent. The prudent nasal surgeon attempts to improve the airway at the time of rhinoplasty if he thinks that it might be helped with corrective surgery.

Although surgery often can straighten or remove the offending portions of the crooked bones and cartilages and improve breathing, the membrane lining inside the nose can become swollen from one or more of the following conditions:

- Allergies (hay fever)
- Changes in temperature (vasomotor rhinitis)
- Viral infections
- Bacterial infections
- Emotional disturbances
- Addiction to nasal sprays (rhinitis medicamentosa)
- Exposure to irritants in the air (hair spray, smoke, etc.)
- Pregnancy

Patients must understand beforehand that none of these membrane conditions are corrected by conventional surgery. If, however, the patient has a deviated septum *plus* one of these problems, correction of the septum may make it easier for the patient to tolerate membrane swelling.

Enlarged turbinates can also be reduced in size to help enlarge the air passages. The surgeon often can reduce the size of the turbinate and place it in a more desirable location, but the membranes may continue to swell in response to the conditions previously mentioned.

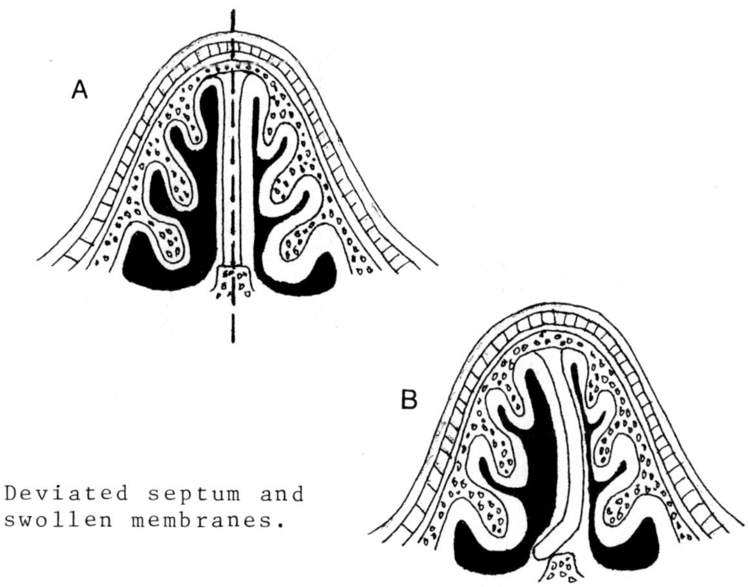

FIGURE 5–15. (*A*) Normal thickness of internal nasal passages. (*B*) Thickened membranes obstruct the airway.

If the patient has one of the medical conditions listed above, the surgeon might recommend that the patient see a colleague who specializes in allergy or medical rhinology. It is also helpful to inform patients that because of positional shift of body fluids, almost everyone's nose is stuffier at night or when they are lying down.

TRAUMATIC NASAL INJURY

The nasal bones or cartilages may be fractured or dislocated when the nose is injured. As long as considerable swelling is present, it is difficult to diagnose these conditions. Radiographs are of limited value because cartilaginous deformities are not visible with conventional x-ray studies. About one-half of nasal fractures involve the cartilaginous portions of the nose.

As the swelling subsides, the nose may appear to be growing crooked or look deformed, and airway obstruction may persist. These conditions commonly are a result of underlying fractured or dislocated bones and cartilages (Fig. 5–16).

Septal hematomas and compound fractures require immediate attention; uncomplicated nasal fractures do not require emergency surgery but probably should be repaired, within 6 weeks. The nasal surgeon must consider each case individually and make specific recommendations, depending on existing circumstances.

Sometimes desired changes in the size or shape of the nose can be made while the fractures are being corrected. In other cases, the surgeon may not feel comfortable attempting aesthetic surgery at the time of nasal fracture repair. Patients should be asked if they want to have such alterations when the appointment is made for evaluation, so that the doctor may refer the patient to a colleague, if appropriate.

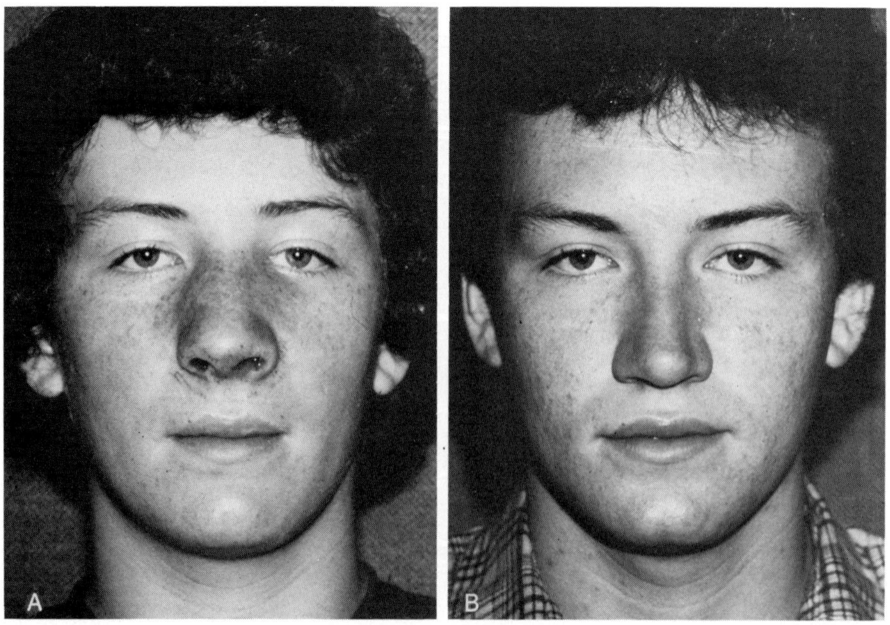

FIGURE 5–16. Acute nasal injuries are best corrected with a planned open reduction, including bilateral osteotomies of the lateral nasal walls and septal reconstruction. The photographs show an acute injury in a 13-year-old male (*A*) and postoperative results 2 years later (*B*).

SCARS FROM NASAL SURGERY

Most surgical maneuvers are performed inside the nose (through the nostrils). There are two exceptions: If it is necessary to make flaring or wide nostrils smaller, an incision can be made in the crease where the side of the nostril joins the upper lip and cheek (Fig. 5–17). Because this is located in a natural body fold, the scar is practically invisible within a few weeks (see B in Fig. 5–17).

In severely deformed noses or in reconstructive or revisional (secondary) rhinoplasty, a small incision may be made below the tip of the nose in the central portion, *between* the nostrils. With time, these incisions associated with external, or open, rhinoplasty become inconspicuous (see A in Fig. 5–17).

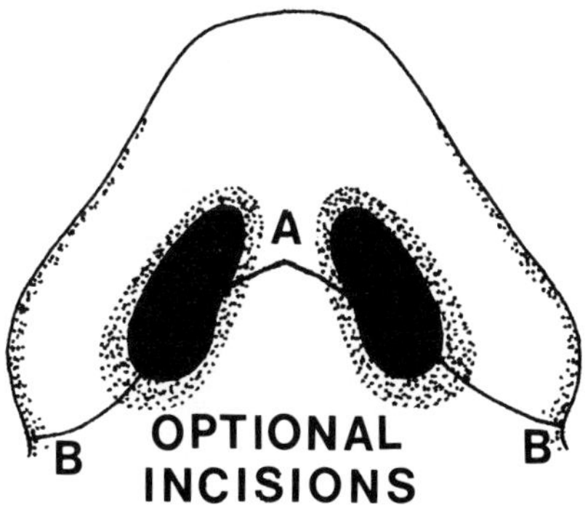

FIGURE 5–17. A columellar incision (*A*) is made in certain difficult noses. An alar incision (*B*) is made when nostril width is reduced.

Suggested Readings

Anderson, J. R. Cosmetic Facial Surgery. New Orleans, 1974.

McCollough, E. G. Plastic Surgery. Birmingham: Ebsco Media, 1991.

Stucker, F. J. Gender identity in rhinoplasty. Plastic Surgery of the Head and Neck. Proceedings of 5th International Symposium. Toronto, Canada, 1988. Philadelphia: B. C. Decker, 1991.

Wright, M. R., and Wright, K. A psychological study of patients undergoing cosmetic surgery. Arch Otolaryngol 101:134–151, 1975.

CHAPTER 6

Postoperative Instructions

Practically every question that may arise regarding the do's and don'ts after surgery is covered in this chapter. The instructions are based on experience with thousands of nasal operations, and both the patient and his family should read them several times and become thoroughly familiar with them.

The postoperative treatment program outlined here also favors healing and, statistically, leads to more predictable results.

GENERAL GUIDELINES FOR PATIENT

1. Remain upright (sitting, standing, walking around) as much as possible.
2. Avoid bending over or lifting heavy objects for one week. Besides aggravating the swelling, this may raise the blood pressure and cause bleeding.
3. Avoid hitting or bumping the nose. It is wise not to pick up young children and advisable to sleep alone for 2 weeks after the operation.

4. Sleep with the head of the bed elevated until all dressings have been removed. To accomplish this, place two or three pillows under the head of the mattress and one or two on top of it. Try not to roll over on the nose.
5. Ice compresses consisting of moistened, cold wash towels (not an ice bag) should be applied in an inverted V across the top of the nose and covering the inner corners of each eye as much as possible during the first 3 days after surgery (Fig. 6–1).
6. Avoid sunning the face for prolonged periods for 1 month; ordinary exposure is not harmful.
7. Do not tweeze the eyebrows for 1 week.
8. Do not sit under the type of hair dryer used in beauty salons; use a hand-held blow dryer.
9. When bathing, avoid getting the nasal dressing wet; if the dressing becomes loose, contact the surgeon.
10. Avoid sniffing. Forcibly attempting to pull air through the nose will not relieve the sensation of blockage—it will only aggravate it by causing more swelling. It also may produce bleeding.
11. Avoid constantly rubbing the nostrils and the base of the nose with tissues or a handkerchief. Not only will this aggravate the swelling but it could cause infection or bleeding or prematurely disrupt the dissolvable sutures placed inside the nose at surgery. If the discharge is excessive, continue using a moustache dressing.
12. Report excessive bleeding that persists after applying pressure to the face along the sides of the nose, using a nasal spray, and lying down for 15 minutes.

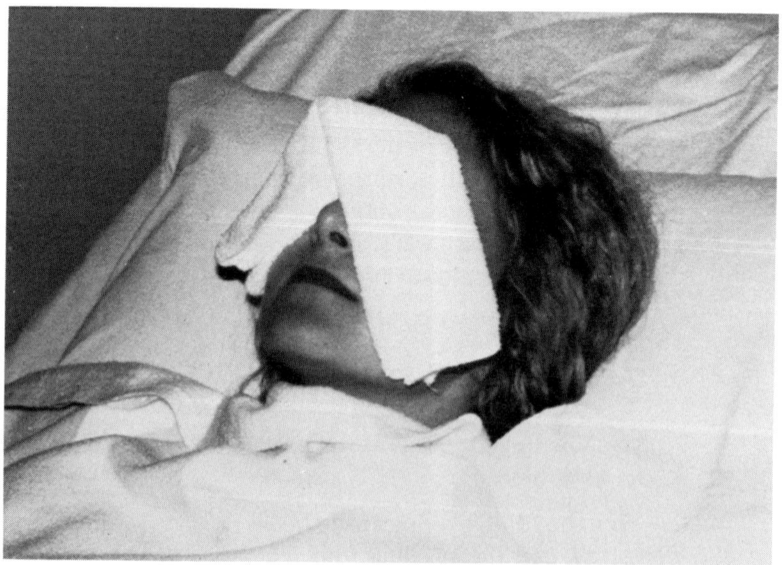

FIGURE 6–1. Cold compresses placed over the eyes and nose after surgery may minimize postoperative edema and ecchymosis.

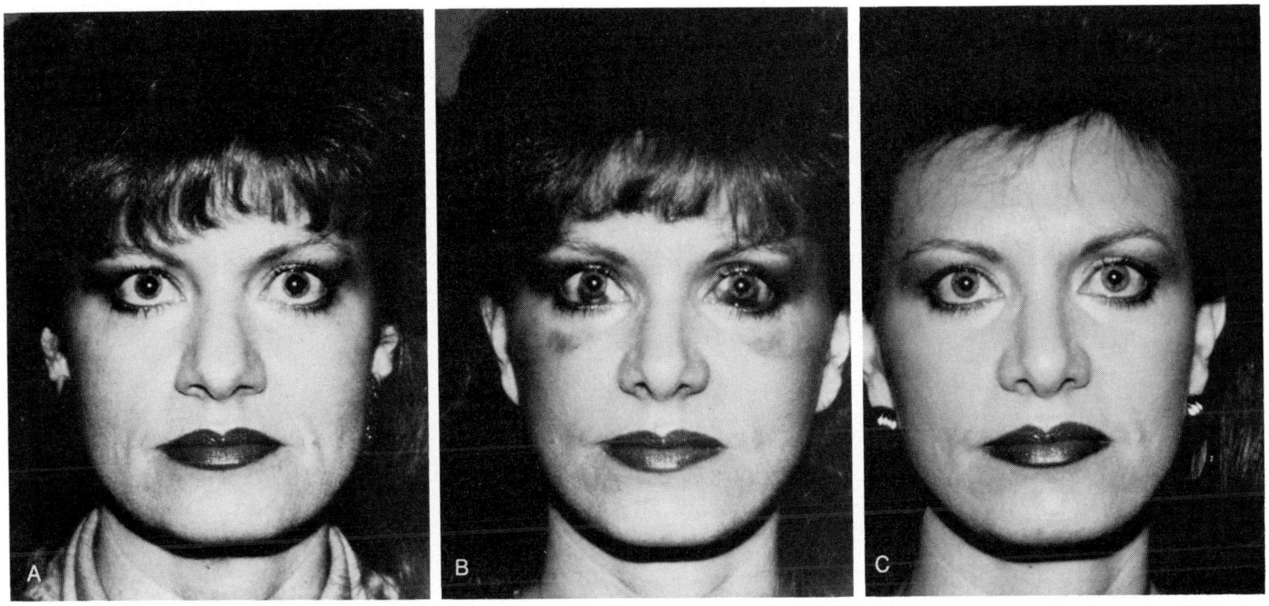

FIGURE 6–2. (*A*) Preoperative appearance. (*B*) Extreme ecchymosis and scleral chemosis are still evident 2 weeks after nasal and septal surgery. (*C*) Effects are completely resolved several weeks later.

SWELLING AND DISCOLORATION

Every operation—no matter how minor—is accompanied by swelling of the surrounding tissues. The amount of swelling that occurs varies from person to person. It is more noticeable in the face because the looseness of the tissues makes the features appear distorted. Swelling usually is greater when both the inside (septum) and the outside of the nose have been operated on than when surgery is done on the inside only. Patients may be given medications (e.g., steroids, vitamin C) before the operation to keep swelling at a minimum. Steroids tend to reduce the initial inflammatory reaction while vitamin C may help reverse capillary fragility.

Swelling is caused by an increase in the volume of fluids that are brought into the injured area to promote healing. The increased blood supply to the region is responsible for some of the discoloration associated with surgery. When the healing fluids are no longer required, the tissues release them and they are absorbed through the bloodstream. Dark bruises are caused by residual red blood cells that dissected into the tissues around the nose. The body eventually should absorb them.

Patients must be willing to accept the temporary swelling and discoloration that occurs postoperatively. Although such effects usually are visually disconcerting, most people think that they are a negligible inconvenience to endure for the physical and psychological improvement they receive.

Sometimes the swelling increases the first and second days after surgery, reaching its peak on the third day. It may also become more pronounced along the jaw line and usually is worse when the patient first arises in the morning (proof that it is better to stay up as much as possible during the day!). This type of swelling is not serious and does not indicate that there is a complication (Fig. 6–2).

As with the swelling, discoloration may become more pronounced for 1 to 2 days after the patient has been discharged; it usually does not last for more than a week, all the while decreasing in intensity (Fig. 6–3).

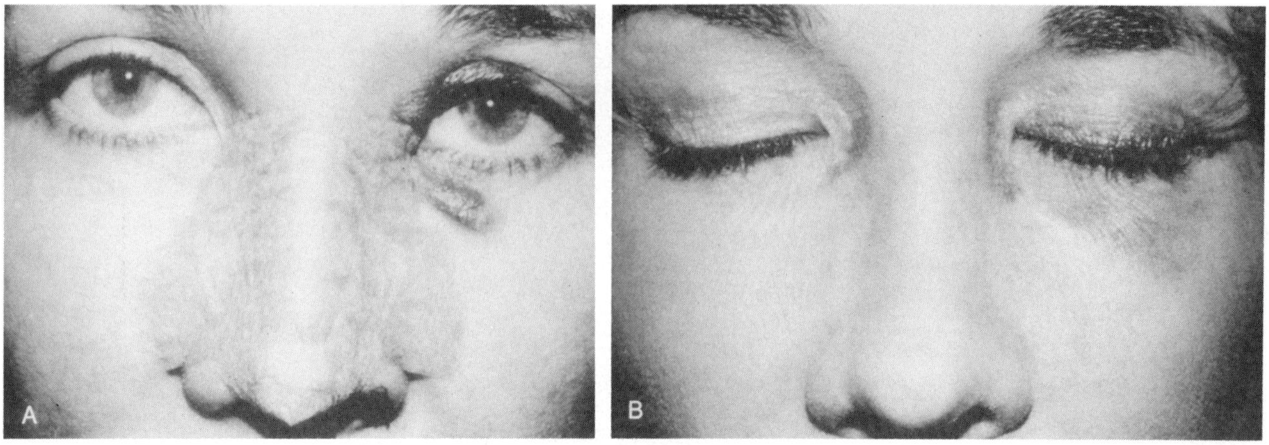

FIGURE 6–3. (*A*) Postoperative day 1. (*B*) Seven days postoperative.

Patients can camouflage the discoloration by using makeup. The makeup can be applied anywhere on the face except where sutures have been placed.

HEMORRHAGE

Whenever the nasal passages are blocked, the nasal glands produce more mucus. Nasal blockage is to be expected after rhinoplasty, and one can expect more mucus drainage for several days. The drainage typically is blood-tinged and should cause no concern unless it becomes frankly bloody and flows profusely.

If hemorrhage does occur, the patient should lie down, use a nasal spray, elevate the head, apply ice compresses about the nose, neck, and face, and notify the surgeon. If the bleeding persists, the surgeon usually can control it by placing Surgicel over the site of the bleeding. Sometimes light chemical cautery with a silver nitrate–tipped applicator is all that is required. Only rarely are more invasive measures necessary.

Nasal Spray

Nose drops and sprays should not be used unless bleeding occurs. Long-term abuse leads to rhinitis medicomentosum and may damage the membranes and delay healing. "Rebound vasodilatation" might also invite postoperative bleeding.

PAIN

When internal nasal packing is omitted, there usually is little pain after rhinoplasty. The patient may, however, experience a deep bruised sensation as a result of postoperative swelling. The pain may seem worse at night and when the patient becomes nervous.

Most pain medication causes light-headedness, especially in the immediate postoperative period. Therefore, it is better to apply cold compresses to relieve pain before resorting to drugs. If the compresses are not effective, a nonaspirin pain reliever may be ordered.

INSOMNIA

If the patient is having difficulty sleeping in the period before the dressings are removed, the surgeon may prescribe a sedative. Such medications also cause light-headedness and weakness and delay recovery.

DEPRESSION

Patients commonly are depressed for a few days after surgery. Anesthetics, analgesics, and sedatives produce a hangover effect when they wear off and contribute to depression and fatigue on the second or third postoperative day. In addition, no matter how much they wanted the operation and how much they were told about what to expect postoperatively, patients are disturbed when they see their swollen and/or discolored faces.

Patients must be reminded that this is a temporary condition that will shortly subside. The best "treatment" consists of busying one's self with the details of postoperative care and trying to divert one's attention to other activities.

LIP MOVEMENT AND DRYNESS

Patients are urged not to move the upper lip excessively after nasal surgery to avoid tension on the surgical incisions during the early stages of healing. Some do's and don't's for the patient to observe are as follows:

1. *Don't* grin or smile excessively.
2. *Don't* pull the upper lip downward (as when applying lipstick). Lipstick should be applied with a brush.
3. *Don't* chew gum or eat foods that are hard to chew. Soups, mashed potatoes, stewed chicken, hamburger steak, or any easily chewed food is permissible.
4. *Do* clean the upper teeth with toothpaste on a face cloth; the lower teeth may be brushed as usual.
5. *Do* wear the moustache dressing if drainage continues. If the dressing is hard to remove, it may be loosened with a few drops of hydrogen peroxide. Micropore paper adhesive tape should be used because it is less irritating to the skin.

If the lips become dry from breathing through the mouth, coat them with a petroleum-based lip balm (e.g., Chapstick).

CLEANING THE NOSE

The nose should not be blown for 10 days; then blowing through both sides at once is allowed but the patient must not compress one side.

The nostrils and the upper lip may be cleaned with a cotton-tipped applicator moistened with hydrogen peroxide. Vigorous rubbing is not recommended. After 1 week the inside of the nostrils may be cleaned with white petroleum jelly applied with a cotton-tipped applicator. This lubricant helps to soften crusts and usually makes the inside of the nose feel better. The nose may be cleaned this way for several weeks.

After the bandage has been removed, the outside of the nose may be cleaned in the usual manner twice daily to remove the oily material produced by the sebaceous glands. The nose can withstand gentle cleaning at this time. A mild soap (e.g., Neutrogena or Ivory) and cotton balls are recommended. Pimples can develop in the nasal skin if it is not thoroughly cleaned. If pimples do develop, they should first be scrubbed vigorously with a cotton-tipped applicator and soap and water and then bathed with hydrogen peroxide.

RESUMING ACTIVITIES

The patient may sleep without the head of the bed elevated after 2 weeks.

Until the bandages are removed, she should wear clothing that fastens either in the front or in the back, rather than the type that must be pulled over the head.

Swimming, gym, or strenuous athletic activity is not permitted for 2 weeks; diving or skiing is not allowed for 2 months. *No contact sports are permitted for 4 months.* Joggers may walk after 2 weeks and jog after 3 weeks. They should start slowly and work their way back to their presurgery routine. Tennis players may hit ground strokes in 2 weeks and resume competition after 3 weeks. They should not play doubles for 6 weeks.

Sneezing should be avoided until the bandage is removed. If the patient must sneeze, he should let it come out like a cough—through the mouth. If sneezing becomes a problem, medication can be ordered to alleviate the condition.

Eyeglasses can be worn as long as the protective dressings remain on the nose, usually the first postoperative week. After that, the glasses must be suspended from the forehead for about 6 weeks because the pressure of the glasses may change the new contour of the nose. The staff can show the patient how to do this if glasses must be worn. Contact lenses may be inserted the day after surgery.

Tub bathing or showering can be resumed as soon as the patient feels strong enough to do so. It is best to have assistance standing by for the first few baths.

The patient may wash his or her hair with help after 3 or 4 days. Hot water should not be used. Care should be taken not to wet the nasal bandage. The head can be laid back in a lavatory or sink as long as the dressings are in place. A cap-type dryer or hand-held blow dryer may be used for drying.

Returning to Work or School

The average patient can return to school the day the bandages are removed, that is, 7 days after surgery. Some hearty souls have done so earlier.

When the patient should return to work depends on the amount of physical activity and public contact his job involves, in addition to the amount of swelling and discoloration that is present. The average patient may return to work by the 8th to 10th postoperative day.

TEMPERATURE

The body temperature does not rise much above 100°F after rhinoplasty. This rise is caused by patients' becoming mildly dehydrated because they do not generally want to drink enough fluid.

Some patients think that they have a fever because they feel warm. To be sure, they should measure their temperature either rectally or in the armpit; the rectal temperature is 1°F above and the armpit temperature is 1°F below the oral temperature. Persistent temperature readings above 100° should be reported.

MEDICATIONS

The patient may resume taking the medication ordered by the surgeon preoperatively until the supply is exhausted; these prescriptions need not be refilled.

Several other medications may also be ordered, including a sedative, pain medication, an antihistamine-decongestant, and an antibiotic. The patient should not take the antihistamine unless sneezing or having excessive mucus drainage because it may cause drowsiness and add to depression.

Patients routinely taking medications prescribed by their medical doctor should continue them. Because of cross-reactions between some beta-blockers and epinephrine, it may be wise to check with the patient's family doctor for a suitable substitute.

After receiving an anesthetic or undergoing surgery, it is not unusual for a patient to experience weakness, have a rapid pulse rate, break out in "cold sweats," or feel dizzy. These effects gradually subside in a few days without medication.

THE FIRST POSTOPERATIVE CLINIC VISIT

Before the patient is discharged he or she should make an appointment to see the surgeon about a week after the surgery. The patient should be informed about what will be done at this first visit to avoid anxiety. The tape and splint will be removed; a special tape-removing solution is used to ensure that these come off easily. Likewise, any material inside the nose will be softened to facilitate removal. No stitches will be removed from inside the nose because the sutures will dissolve. If the nostrils were narrowed, those stitches also will dissolve.

INJURY TO THE NOSE

Many people sustain accidental hits on the nose during the early postoperative period. One need not be too concerned unless the blow is hard or hemorrhage or considerable swelling ensues. The patient should report the incident at the next clinic visit or by telephone if sufficiently concerned.

PATIENT REMINDERS

Review with the patient the information given preoperatively.

1. When the bandage is first removed, the nose will appear swollen and turned up too much; this is due to operative swelling over the nose and in the upper lip. The swelling will begin to subside within

1 week; it will take at least 1 year for all the swelling to dissipate and for the nose to assume its final shape. With thicker and oilier skin it takes longer for the swelling to subside.

2. In most cases, the discoloration will gradually disappear in 7 to 10 days. We have yet to encounter a case in which it persisted permanently.
3. The upper lip may feel stiff for awhile and may interfere with smiling. This will disappear within a few weeks.
4. Sometimes the tip of the nose feels numb after rhinoplasty, but this numbness eventually disappears.
5. Patients who have oily skin may use rubbing alcohol and cotton balls to remove excess oils from the nasal skin for 2 to 3 days after the dressings have been removed.
6. A nose that is crooked, has sustained injuries, or has had previous surgery is more difficult to correct. Additional improvement may be obtained with a relatively minor procedure later.

Suggested Readings

Anderson, J. R. Rhinoplasty Emphasizing the External Approach. New York: Thieme, 1988.
McCollough, E. G. Surgical anatomy of the skin and wound healing. In Otolaryngology, English, G. M. Volume 4, Chapter 3. Philadelphia: Harper & Row, 1979.
McCollough, E. G. Outpatient surgery: A proven method of cost containment. Ala Med 52:53–54, 1983.
McCollough, E. G., Chatham, D. R. The art and science of wound healing: The physician can influence the process. Ala Med 54:26–38, 1985.
McCollough, E. G. Plastic Surgery. Birmingham, 1991.

ANESTHESIA

CHAPTER 7

Techniques of Effective Anesthesia

Intraoperative comfort and convenience are essential elements in a successful rhinoplasty practice. Surgeons who acquire a reputation for making the surgical experience more tolerable for their patients build their practices more rapidly. Rhinoplastic surgeons are challenged to dispell the horror stories that have become associated with nasal surgery.

The groundwork for successful local anesthesia is laid long before the patient enters the operating room—at the initial consultation. Once the patient develops complete confidence in his surgeon, preoperative anxiety is diminished. The patient who *anticipates* pain naturally is more anxious about the surgical experience and requires more medication at the time of surgery.

With the assistance of a staff psychologist, I have developed an audiocassette that is given to the patient at the consultation. The patient is instructed to listen to the tape several times a day for 1 week before surgery. Relaxation tapes provided by the surgeon maintain contact with the patient up to the time the anesthetic is administered—another aspect of the art of practicing nasal plastic surgery.

The following protocol is my approach to anesthesia for nasal surgery.

GENERAL COMMENTS

Most patients are apprehensive about surgery. For this reason I have developed an approach to anesthesia based on my own and others' experience that is designed to make patients as comfortable as possible before, during, and after their operations. This type of anesthesia, called twilight anesthesia or twilight sleep, is similar to the deepest stages of natural sleep. The patient is heavily sedated and has amnesia to much of the operating room experience but usually is alert on returning to the room. This approach to anesthesia allows patients to be up and around sooner and reduces the likelihood of complications.

The regimen is administered in a graduated, programmed manner. If the patient is apprehensive, a sedative (flurazepam) or an antianxiety agent (diazepam) is ordered the night before surgery and on arising the morning of surgery.

Shortly after the patient arrives at the surgical facility on the day of surgery, additional medication (diazepam and dimenhydrinate) is given. Then patients listen once more to the "relaxation" surgery preparation tapes in the preoperative areas while awaiting surgery.

In the operating room, intravenous medication is given to finalize the twilight sleep. After the patient has reached this state of sedation, topical and injectable anesthetics are administered to the areas to be operated. Patients should be forewarned that local anesthetics cause a stinging sensation as they are injected into the tissues and while they are anesthetizing nerve endings. After the local anesthetic has taken effect, the patient should experience no discomfort. If the surgeon tells his patient "This won't hurt" and then proceeds to induce pain, the patient will lose confidence and believe little else the surgeon tells him.

Although twilight anesthesia is used in the vast majority of cases, general anesthesia is recommended for patients younger than 15.

PREOPERATIVE MEDICATIONS

A successful outcome with local anesthesia begins with the first physician-patient encounter and is reinforced on the morning of surgery when preoperative medications are given and before anxiety builds. The following medications are administered for specific reasons. Each has been chosen because of its unique pharmacologic properties.

Sedatives. Diazepam (10 to 20 mg) given 1 to 2 hours preoperatively usually produces adequate sedation before the patient enters the operating room. Narcotics are best avoided in the preoperative period because they may cause nausea and vomiting when the ambulatory patient is moved from one area to another.

Antiemetics. Preloading with antiemetics reduces nausea and potentiates the effect of most sedatives. Dimenhydrinate (100 to 200 mg orally) seems to be sufficient for most cases. Theoretically, the antihistaminic effect of dimenhydrinate may counter some of the edema and discomfort produced as histamine release occurs at the cellular level in the injected areas.

Steroids. To minimize intraoperative and postoperative edema in the perioperative regions, prednisone (20 mg) can be given orally 1 to 2 hours before surgery.

Antibiotics. The debate over the efficacy of prophylactic antibiotic therapy for nasal surgery continues. If the decision to use antibiotics is made, the medication should be circulating in the patient's bloodstream at the time the first incision is made. Broad-spectrum coverage may be obtained with cephalosporins. If a medication allergy is suspected, erythromycin or tetracycline may be substituted. When prescribed for prophylaxis, antibiotic therapy should continue for 7 days.

INTRAOPERATIVE PERIOD

Intravenous Steroids

Steroids may help to reduce postoperative edema. Dexamethasone (Decadron; 12 mg) may be injected *slowly* intravenously in the operating room just before surgery. The patient may experience an intense burning sensation in the perineum *if* dexamethasone is injected rapidly. The discomfort lasts for only a few seconds, but it is wise to warn every patient that this phenomenon might occur.

Intravenous Sedation

After a cardiac monitor and a pulse oximeter are connected to the patient and an intravenous line is established, diazepam is injected in 1- to 2-mg increments at 1- to 2-minute intervals until adequate sedation is obtained. Physostigmine (0.25 to 0.5 mL) may help to reverse the effects of diazepam if oversedation should occur.

If after a total of 20 mg of diazepam has been injected and more sedation is desired, hydromorphone is added to the regimen in 0.20-mg increments every 5 to 10 minutes. To reduce the incidence of nausea, dimenhydrinate (25 mg) is given intravenously each time a narcotic supplement is added. To reduce intravenous discomfort, dimenhydrinate is diluted with 5 mL of sterile saline solution. Only in rare instances is more than a total dose of 2 mg of hydromorphone recommended or required. The maximum effect of hydromorphone is not realized immediately. It often does not peak for 5 to 10 minutes, so caution is advised. Naloxone (Narcan) may be used for overdose, but the effect of hydromorphone may continue after that of naloxone has subsided, so close observation by qualified personnel is recommended.

If a trained anesthesiologist or anesthetist is present, fentanyl (Sublimaze) may be substituted for hydromorphone.

When the patient responds inappropriately to questioning, the desired level of sedation has been achieved.

Topical Anesthetics

In preparation for intranasal injections and topical cocainization, the nose is sprayed with a mixture of 12.5 mg of ephedrine and 100 mL of 0.5 per cent dyclonine hydrochloride.

After 5 minutes have elapsed, 5 per cent topical cocaine solution is placed in key positions. The intranasal membranes are first bathed with a 5 per cent cocaine solution. Cotton-tipped applicators are recommended. Then, four cocaine-saturated applicators are strategically placed for 5 minutes: Two are placed high in the nasal vault under the nasal bones in the region of the anterior ethmoid nerves and the other two are placed in

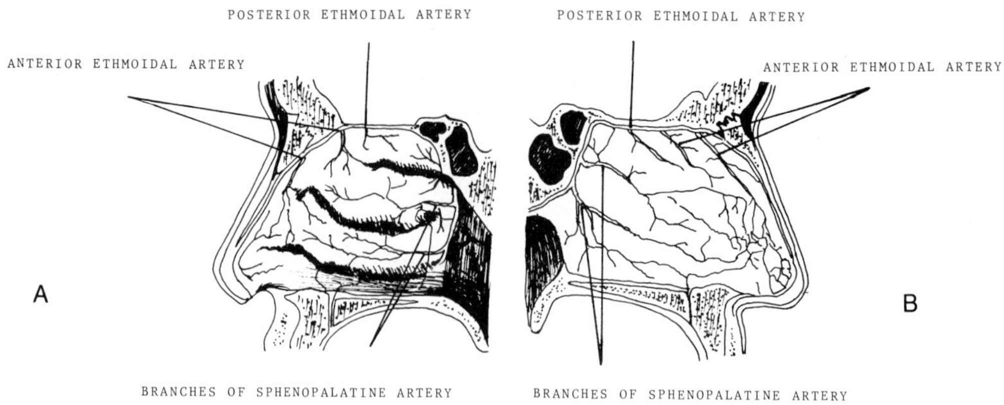

FIGURE 7–1. (*A*) Sensory nerve supply to the lateral walls. (*B*) Innervation of the nasal septum.

the region of the sphenopalatine ganglion. Both vasoconstriction and anesthesia are potentiated when this routine is appropriately followed (Fig. 7–1).

Injectable Anesthetics

The surgeon should have two objectives in mind when he administers local anesthetics. First and foremost is to eliminate pain. Effective injection also reduces intraoperative bleeding.

Lidocaine (2 per cent) mixed with 1:75,000 or 1:100,000 epinephrine is the preferred anesthetic for nasal surgery. The combination is formulated by adding 0.15 cc of epinephrine (1:1,000) to 30 cc of 2 per cent lidocaine with 1:100,000 epinephrine. In hypertensive patients or those with cardiac arrhythmias, the concentration of epinephrine can be reduced. Every attempt is made to keep the total volumn of anesthetic to a minimum. The entire nose usually can be anesthetized with 10 to 12 mL of anesthetic, including intranasal injections.

Once the anesthetic has been injected, the surgeon may have from 60 to 90 minutes before rebound vasodilatation occurs and the anesthetic loses its effect. If additional time is required, the *entire* nose should be reinjected. The surgery can then be completed under much more desirable circumstances for both patient and surgeon.

Technique

To obtain the maximum degree of anesthesia with the minimum volume, the proper technique of injection is essential (Figure 7–2). A 1 1/2 inch disposable 27-gauge needle is recommended for nasal injections; 10-mL syringes are more than adequate.

The anesthetic is deposited in each strategic site as the needle is slowly withdrawn from the track.

When topical anesthetics are used properly, the discomfort of the intranasal injections may be lessened. Injection should progress from previously anesthetized regions to nonanesthetized areas (i.e. from mucous membranes affected by cocainization to vestibular skin and then to the external skin).

The first injection is placed in the mucous membrane at the anterior end of the inferior turbinate, so that the anesthetic can begin to diffuse toward the floor of the vestibule and, laterally, the nasofacial angle.

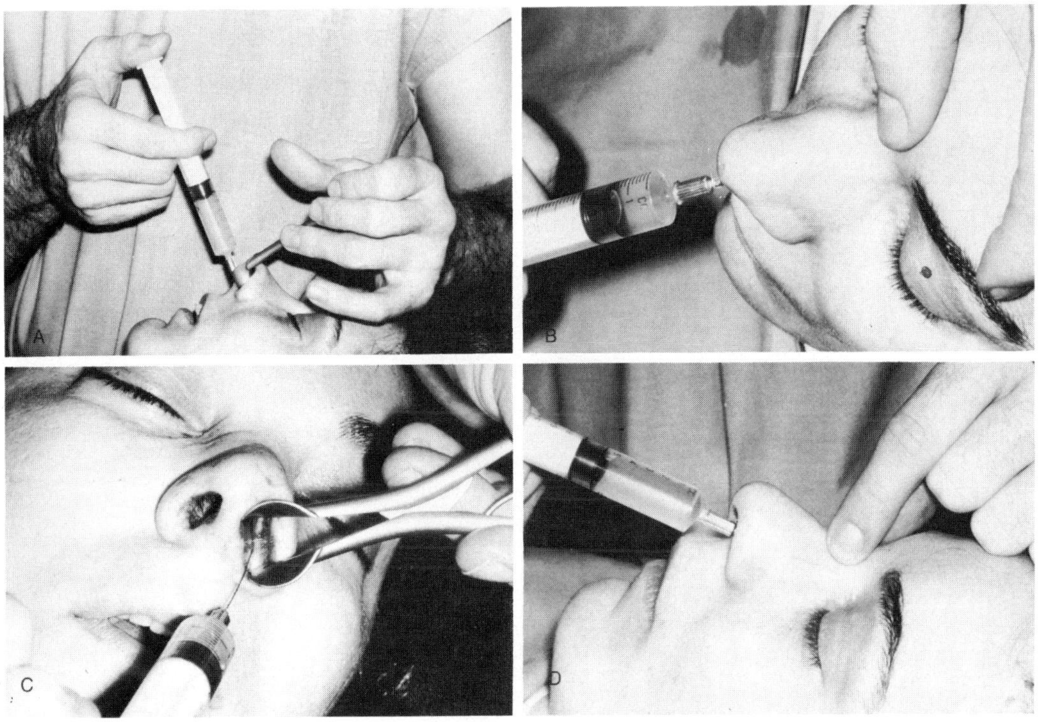

FIGURE 7–2. (*A*) Lidocaine (1 per cent) and epinephrine (1:75,000) are injected using a 10-mL syringe and a 27-gauge needle. (*B*) The needle tract should be placed between the perichondrium (ostium) and the nasal musculature. (*C*) To avoid injury to the angular vessels, the lateral walls can be adequately anesthetized by depositing anesthetic halfway between the nasal dorsum and the nasofacial angle. (*D*) Anesthetization of the tip begins with an injection at the mucovestibular junction at the anterior end of each inferior turbinate.

Illustration continued on following page.

Next, a bolus of anesthetic is placed *submucosally* high under the nasal bones in the region of the anterior ethmoid nerve branches. These nerves provide sensory innervation to the lateral nasal walls, middle and interior turbinates, and, with a more midline branch, the skin over the nasal dorsum. A bolus placed posteriorly and superiorly in the septum anesthetizes the distal branches of long septal nerves.

Within 1 to 2 minutes these field blocks should help to diminish discomfort that might result from additional injections in the regions supplied by the preceding nerves and, equally importantly, produce vasoconstriction to the large vessels that course through the region.

The next series of injections are made into the skin along the floor of the vestibule and in the mucous membrane at the caudal end of the septum. This sets the stage for tip and columellar injections that should follow momentarily.

After the initial, strategically placed septal injections have taken effect, the remainder of the septum is infiltrated with 2 to 3 mL of anesthetic. Anesthesia to the lateral walls of the external nose is completed when, after a small bolus of anesthetic is deposited in the limen vestibuli regions, the needle is passed along a line that dissects the dorsal midline and the nasofacial groove.

To avoid injury to the nasal vessels, the needle should course in the immediate perichondrial and periosteal planes. It is *not* necessary to violate the nasofacial groove or perform an infraorbital nerve block to obtain complete anesthesia for the osteotomy tracks and other maneuvers performed to the lateral aspect of the nose.

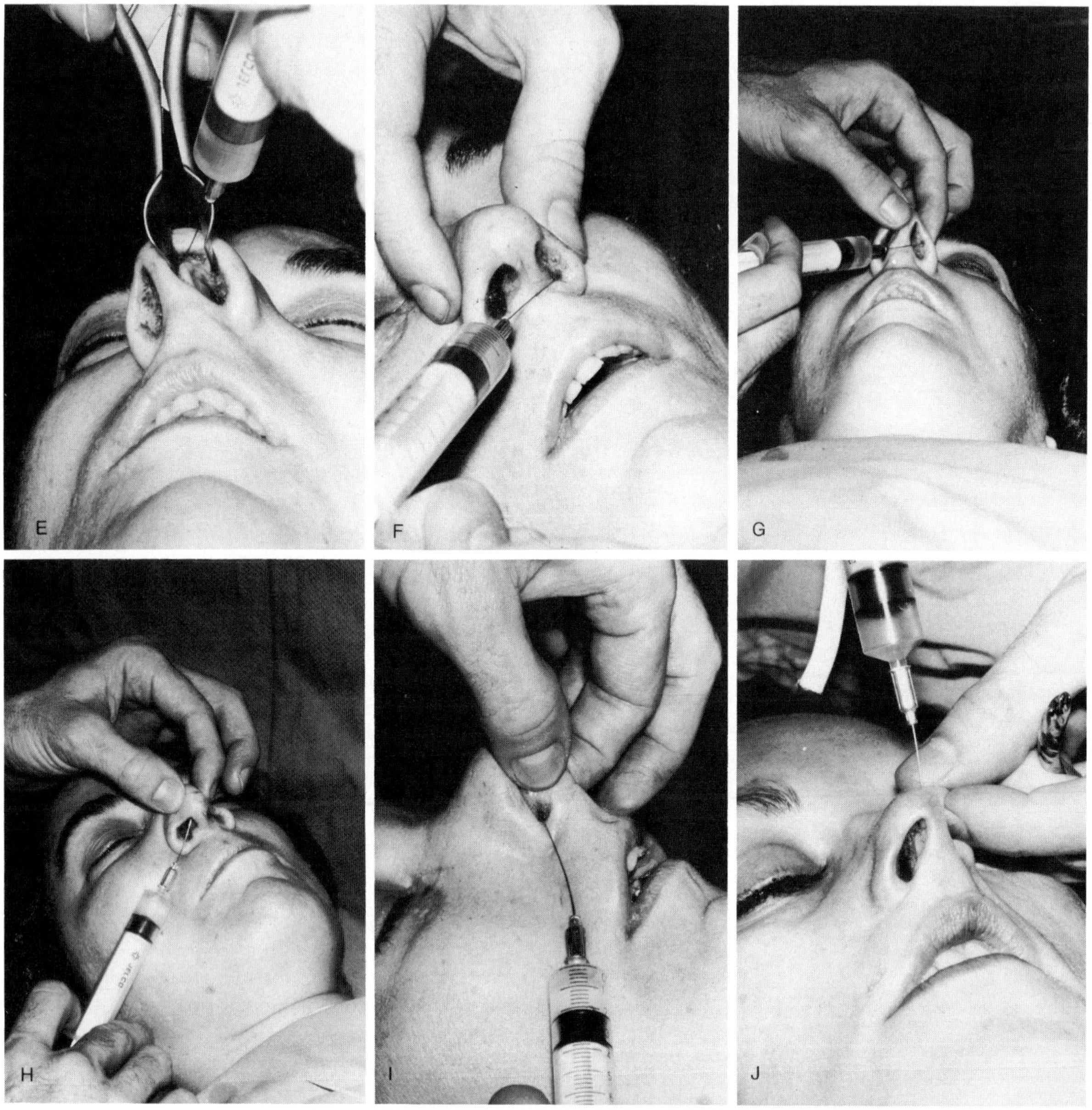

FIGURE 7–2 *continued* (*E*) The region of the superior septal angle is injected. (*F*) The nasolabial region is infiltrated. (*G*) The alar margin is injected. (*H*) Anesthetic is injected between the domes of the alar cartilages. (*I*) The membraneous septum on both sides is injected. (*J*) Anesthetic is injected between the medial crura to complete anesthesia of the external nose.

Anesthesia to the dorsal two-thirds of the nose is completed when the needle is passed in the midline over the superior septal angle to the rhinion and, finally, to the nasion to deposit a small amount of anesthetic along the nasal dorsum. Every attempt should be made to keep the plane of injection deep to the procerus muscle to avoid injury to the small penetrating vessels in the region.

Anesthesia of the tip proceeds from inferiorly to superiorly and from laterally to medially (see Fig. 7–2). Injection sites are spaced at 1-cm intervals along the alar rim until the tip is outlined. Waiting a few seconds between injections and alternating sides seem to produce tiny field blocks and help to minimize discomfort.

The columella is anesthetized by passing the needle externally through the previously anesthetized skin of the lobule and between the medial crura to the base of the columella.

Care must be taken to minimize the volume of anesthetic placed in the nasolabial region; otherwise, the tip of the nose will be artificially projected during surgery.

Even though lidocaine is one of the most diffusable local anesthetics available, gentle massage in each region seems to help potentiate diffusion. Hyaluronidase (Wydase) is not necessary for nasal anesthesia when lidocaine is used. The extreme diffusibility of lidocaine enables the number of injection sites to be kept to a minimum and the discomfort associated with the injection to be lessened.

Some observers contend that warming the solution to body temperature before injection or adding sodium bicarbonate to lidocaine changes the pH of the solution and reduces the pain of injection. There is some question, however, concerning the longevity of buffered lidocaine.

One of the most important aspects of effective local anesthesia is to *wait* until both amnesia and vasoconstriction have occurred before commencing the operation. When lidocaine is used, anesthesia is obtained within seconds; maximum vasoconstriction produced by epinephrine usually is not obtained for 10 to 12 minutes.

Suggested Readings

McCollough, E. G. Local anesthetic reactions and treatment. Emerg Med, August, 1974, p. 121.

McCollough, E. G., Beeson, W. H. Aesthetic Surgery of the Aging Face. St. Louis: C. V. Mosby, 1986, pp. 13–21.

McCollough, E. G., Langsdon, P. R. Dermabrasion and Chemical Peeling. New York: Thieme Publishing, 1988, p. 60.

SURGERY

CHAPTER 8

Anatomy

No discussion of nasal plastic surgery would be complete without clarification of terminology and anatomic relationships.

Directional indicators can be confusing to the novice. These anatomic borders originally were described in lower animal forms that walked on all fours. For surgical purposes, Figure 8–1 describes the directional borders that are discussed throughout this book, as well as the landmarks dividing the nose into its three component parts.

Figures 8–2 and 8–3 show the basic anatomy needed for an understanding of the surgical procedures described in subsequent chapters.

The nose can be divided into thirds. The upper one-third comprises the bony vault; the middle one-third, the cartilagenous vault; and the lower one-third, the tip cartilages.

The external nose contains several critical anatomic landmarks: the nasion, rhinion, supra-alar, supratip, and infratip regions and the alae, lobule, and columella (Fig. 8–2).

Internally, the nasal septum is composed of bony and cartilagenous structures, namely the vomer and perpendicular plate of the ethmoids, maxillary crest, and quadrangular cartilage. Externally, the middle one-third is composed of the paired upper lateral cartilages and the dorsum (or anterior) surface of the cartilagenous septum. The lower one-third contains the paired lower lateral (or alar cartilages), which, for surgical purposes, are subdivided into the medial and lateral crura. The crura meet at a dome (or apex), which is defined as the cartilage that lies between the external and internal soft triangles (or facets).

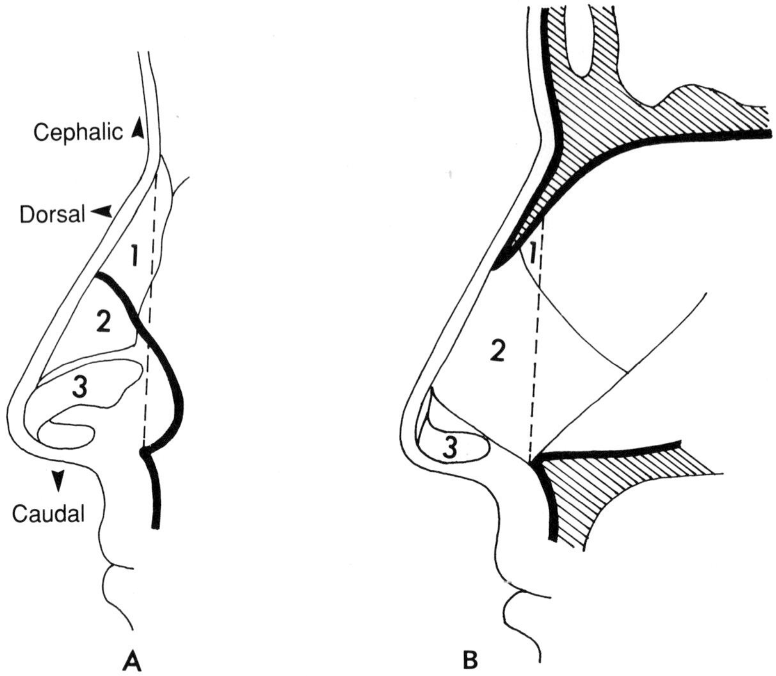

FIGURE 8–1. (*A, B*) The nose can be divided into thirds: the bony vault (1), the cartilagenous vault (2), and the tip (3).

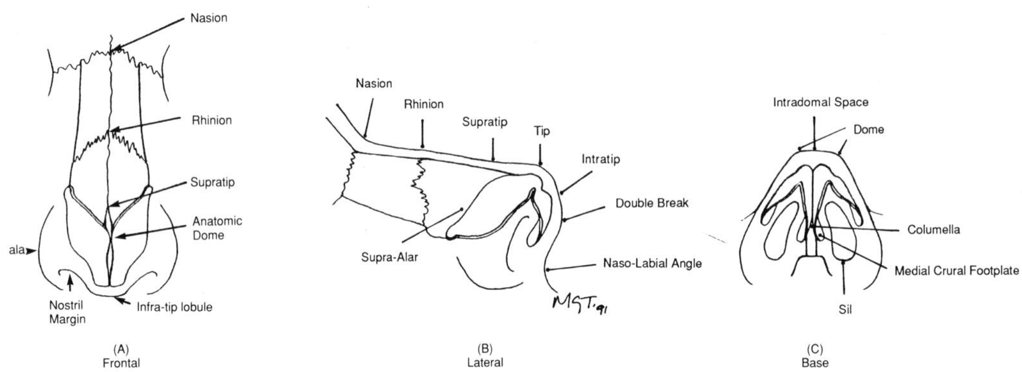

FIGURE 8–2.

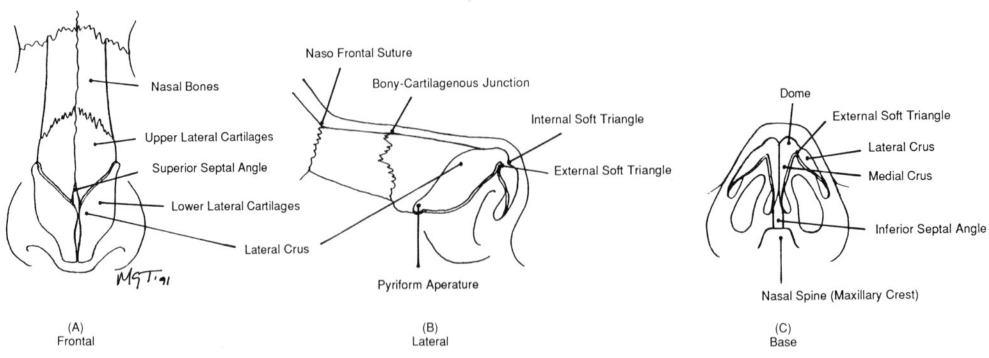

FIGURE 8–3.

Along the internal surface of the lateral walls, the bony middle and inferior turbinates (conchae) may come into play as the surgeon strives to improve the patient's airway.

In the vestibule, the internal nasal lining is composed of stratified squamous epithelium that gives way to pseudo-stratified columnar epithelium (mucosa) at the limen vestibuli.

Suggested Readings

Denecke, H. J., Meyer, R. Plastic Surgery of the Head and Neck. Vol. 1. New York: Springer-Verlag, 1967, pp. 3–9.

McCollough, E. G., Beeson, W. H. Aesthetic Surgery of the Aging Face. St. Louis: C. V. Mosby, 1986, p. 300.

CHAPTER 9

Nasal Incisions

An incision should neither restrict nor limit which technique a surgeon chooses to use. An experienced surgeon recognizes that each time an incision is made, the structure of the nose may be altered. Interrupting the soft tissue connections between the cartilagenous components of the nose destroys the structural framework. In some cases it may be desirable to retrodisplace the tip or change the relationship between the upper lateral cartilages and the septum. If that is the surgeon's objective, multiple or extended incisions can help predictably to accomplish it. In most cases the objective is to *preserve* tip support; therefore, the prudent rhinoplastic surgeon makes only those incisions that are necessary to expose the structures he wants to modify.

TECHNIQUES

Perhaps there are no clearly defined types of rhinoplasty (i.e., open, closed, external) but various approaches or building blocks that constitute the whole.

Some variation of a transfixion incision is made at the caudal margin of the septum. When it is desirable to *maintain* the preoperative projections of the tip, as much soft tissue attachment of the medial crura to the septum as possible should be preserved.

Modified Transfixion Incision

In those rare cases in which no surgical correction of the nasal septum is required, the transfixion incision need only extend 2 to 3 mm inferiorly to the superior septal angle (Fig. 9–1).

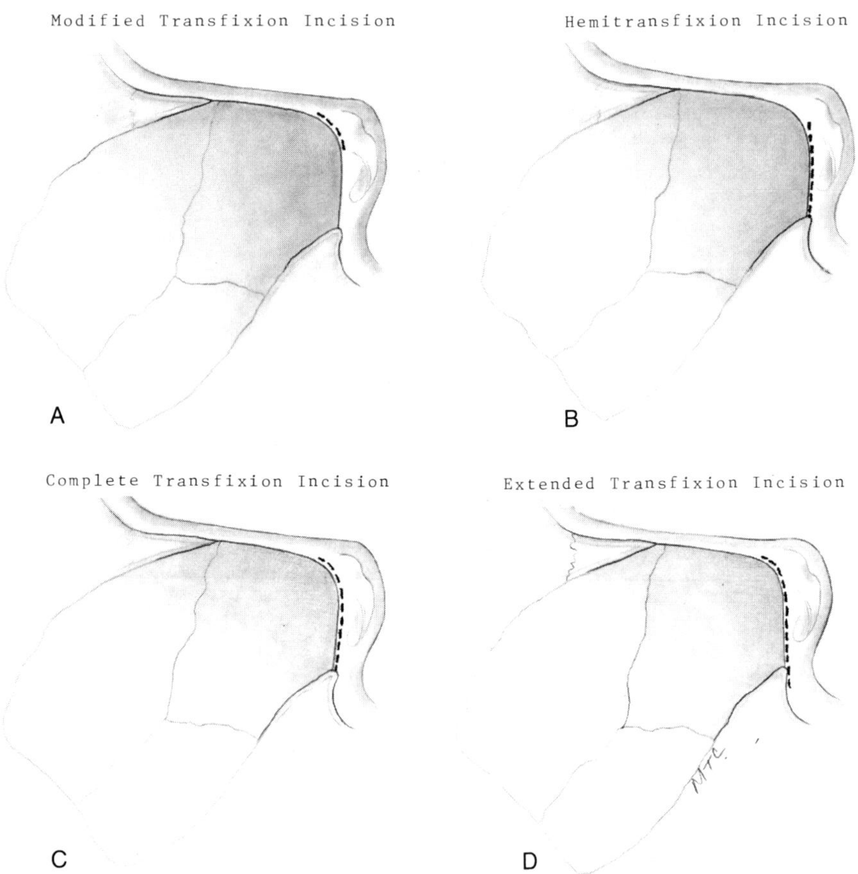

FIGURE 9–1. (*A*) Modified transfixion incision. Unilateral or bilateral incision that does not extend beyond the medial crural–septal attachment. (*B*) Hemitransfixion incision. Unilateral incision that may extend beyond the medial crural–septal attachment but leaves the opposite attachment intact. (*C*) Complete transfixion incision. Bilateral (through and through) incision that extends beyond the medial crural–septal attachment but stops short of the nasal spine. (*D*) Extended transfixion incision. Bilateral (through and through) incision that extends beyond the medial crural–septal attachment and the nasal spine and may interrupt the depressor and nasi muscles.

Hemitransfixion Incision

When the caudal end for the septum is in the midline but a deviation exists posteriorly, the incision is extended inferiorly on *one side only* to allow for exposure of the caudal margin of the septal cartilage. A hemitransfixion incision interrupts only one medial crural–septal attachment and helps to preserve some support for the tip.

Complete Transfixion Incision

Most long-standing caudal septal deviations necessitate a bilateral transfixion incision so that cicatricial contractures can be released and midline fixation can be established by some variation of a "swinging-door" procedure.

Complete transfixion interrupts *both* medial crural–septal attachments and results in a loss of tip projection (Fig. 9–2).

Extended Bilateral Transfixion Incision

An overly projecting tip can be permanently retrodisplaced by extending the transfixion incision not only beyond the medial crural–septal attachment but beyond the *inferior* septal angle and posteriorly into the floor of the vestibule (Fig. 9–3).

Killian Incisions

When an isolated septal deformity is recognized deep in the nose, especially if a radical submucous resection has been performed previously, vertical (Killian) incisions can be made immediately anterior to the deformity and the appropriate amount of bone and/or cartilage removed. Because the Killian incisions do not disturb the medial crural–septal attachment, changes associated with altering the attachment are not expected (Fig. 9–4).

Marginal Incision

The marginal incision follows the inferior margin of the lower lateral cartilages from about mid-columella to mid-ala on each side. Care should be taken in the external soft triangle area (facet) to stay close to the cartilage edge to prevent undue postoperative scarring. This incision is made in preparation for either a "delivery" approach or an external rhinoplasty conversion (Fig. 9–5).

Intercartilagenous Incision

The intercartilagenous incision is made at the mucosal-vestibular skin junction *between* the upper and lower lateral cartilages and connected to the incision made at the superior septal angle. This incision usually is coupled with a marginal incision for delivery; the cephalic border of the alar cartilage can be excised using a retrograde approach through a limen vestibuli incision (Fig. 9–6).

In rare instances a tip-plasty incision is made through both the vestibular skin and the alar cartilage (cartilage-splitting incision). The location of the incision depends on how much lateral crus the surgeon intends to remove. Although in the past I have used this approach to tip-plasty extensively, for the most part it has been replaced by delivery and "open" approaches (Fig. 9–7).

Text continued on page 105

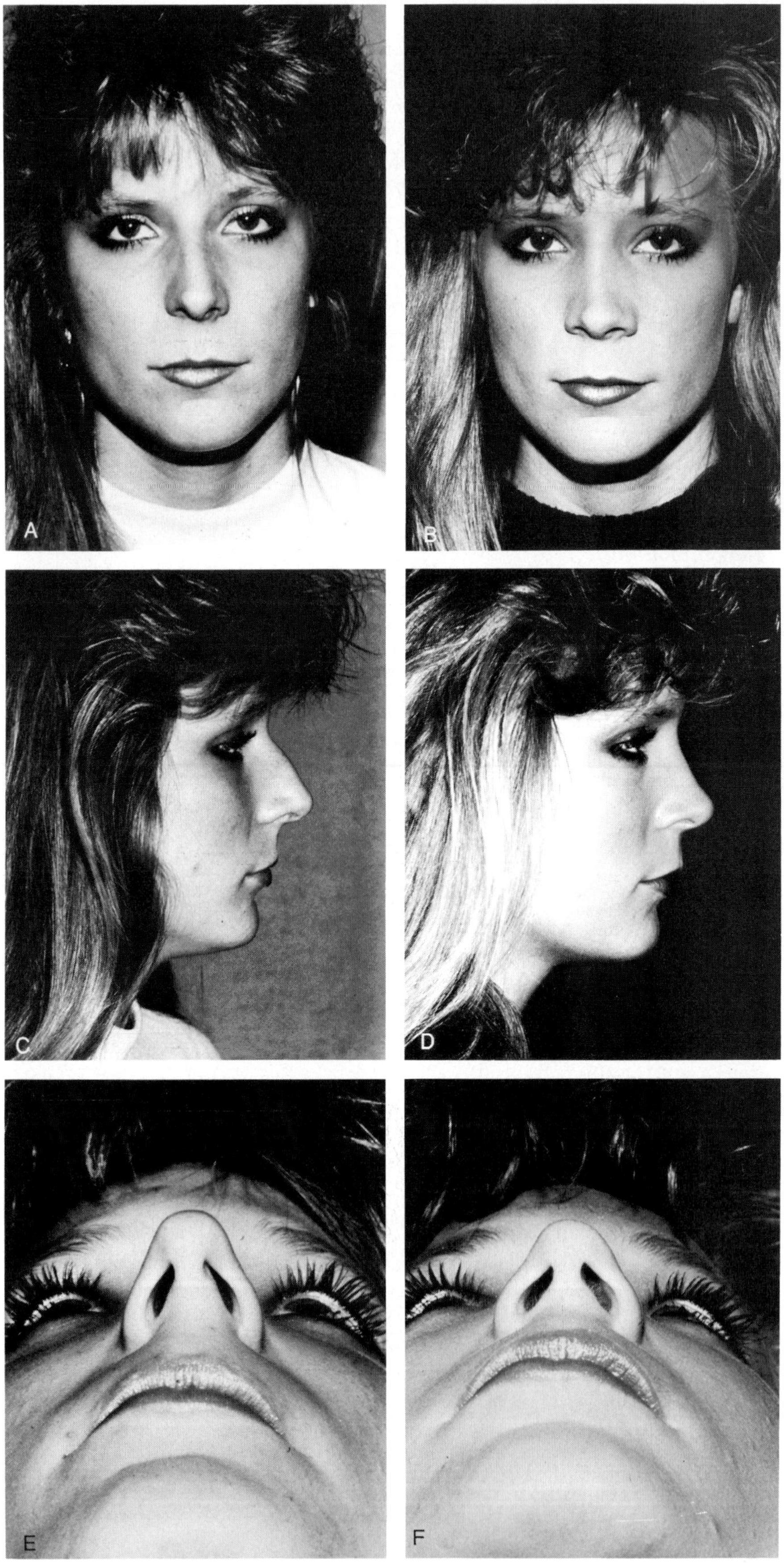

FIGURE 9–2. (*A–F*) When tip retrodisplacement is desirable, a bilateral complete transfixion incision allows the feet of the medial crura to settle until they come to rest at the base of the columella.

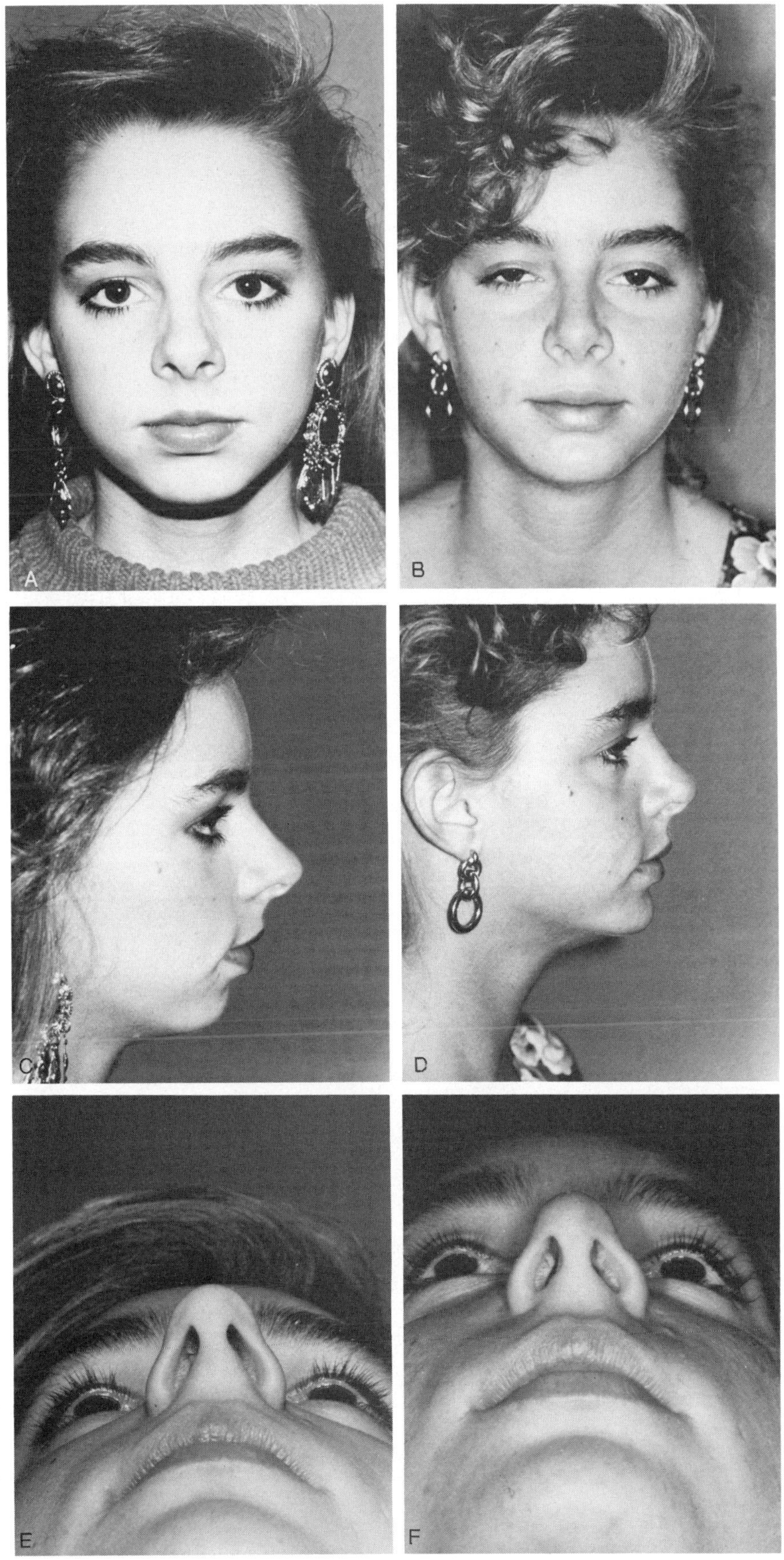

FIGURE 9–3. Extended bilateral complete transfixion incision produces significant tip retrodisplacement in the overly projected nose.

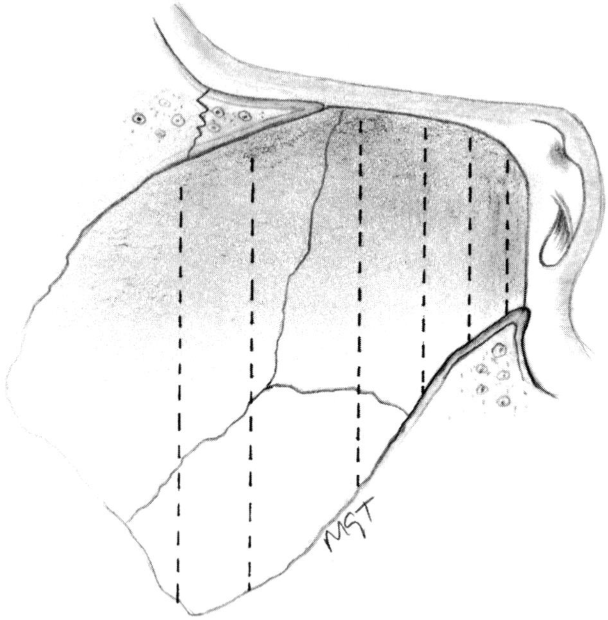

FIGURE 9–4. Killian described incisions that allow access to the cartilagenous and/or bony septum. This incision may be made wherever necessary cephalically to the caudal end of the septum.

FIGURE 9–5. Marginal incision is made as close to the caudal edge of the alar cartilage as possible. It may extend from the medial crural footplate to the pyriform aperature, if indicated.

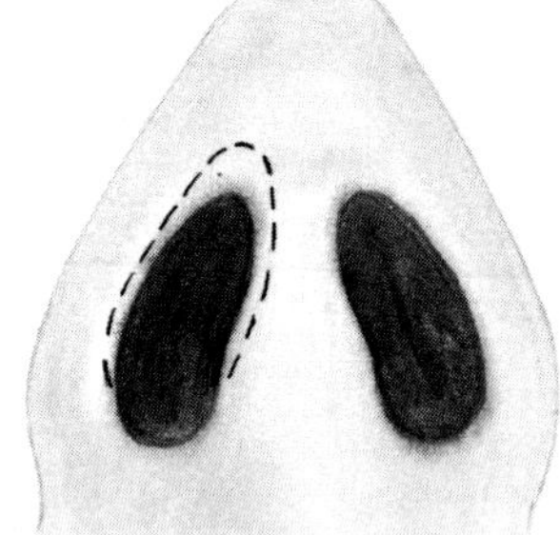

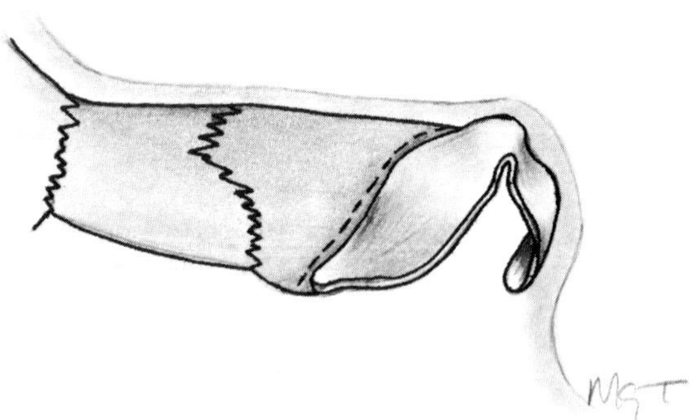

FIGURE 9–6. Limen vestibuli intercartilagenous incision is made between the upper and lower lateral cartilages.

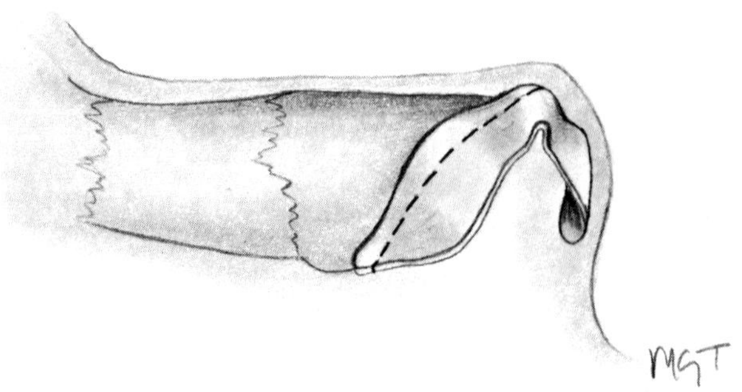

FIGURE 9–7. Cartilage-splitting intercartilagenous incision is made horizontally into the lateral crus, thereby producing horizontal division of the cartilage at same time the incision is made into the internal nasal lining.

Transcolumellar (External Rhinoplasty) Incisions

If at any point in the operation the surgeon desires additional exposure of the tip cartilages or nasal architecture, the two columellar portions of the marginal incisions can be connected with an inverted V made in the thinner skin of the columella. It is best made at about one-half the distance from the apex of the nostril to the base into the thinner skin overlying the medial crural extension of the lower lateral cartilages (Fig. 9–8).

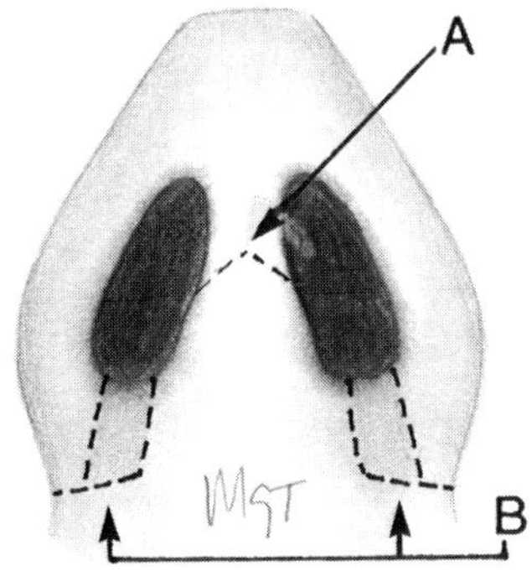

FIGURE 9–8. (*A*) Transcolumellar incision connects the two marginal incisions whenever external rhinoplasty conversion is indicated. The inverted V design follows the aesthetic lines of the base of the nose. (*B*) Alar sil incisions are designed to excise the desired portion of the nostril floor when narrowing of the base of the nose is desired.

Alar Sil Incisions

When it is desirable to narrow or alter the alar base, sections of the alae and/or floor of the vestibule can be removed so that the alae can be advanced and rotated medially. I seldom use the classic weir incisions in which crescent-shaped sections of tissue are removed in the nasofacial crease (Figs. 9–9 through 9–11). For more detail in alar base narrowing, see Figures 9–12 and 9–13 and Chapter 11.

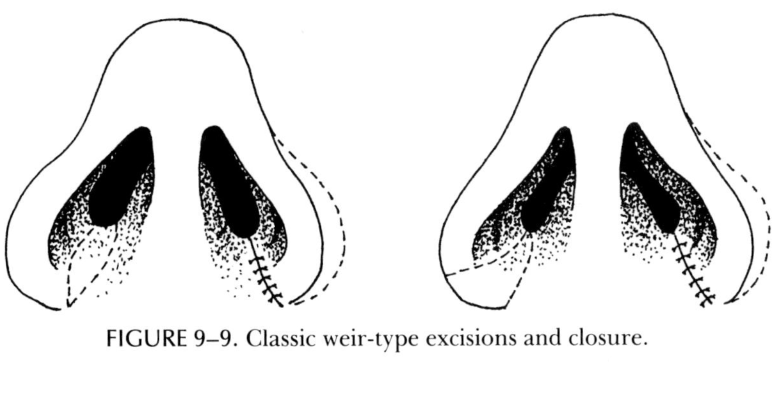

FIGURE 9–9. Classic weir-type excisions and closure.

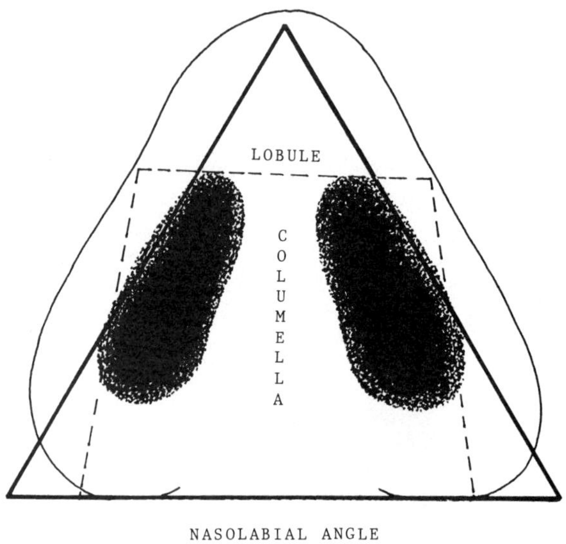

FIGURE 9–10. Ideal relation between component parts of the base of the nose.

FIGURE 9–11. In the classic Weir procedure the excision extends laterally into the nasolabial groove.

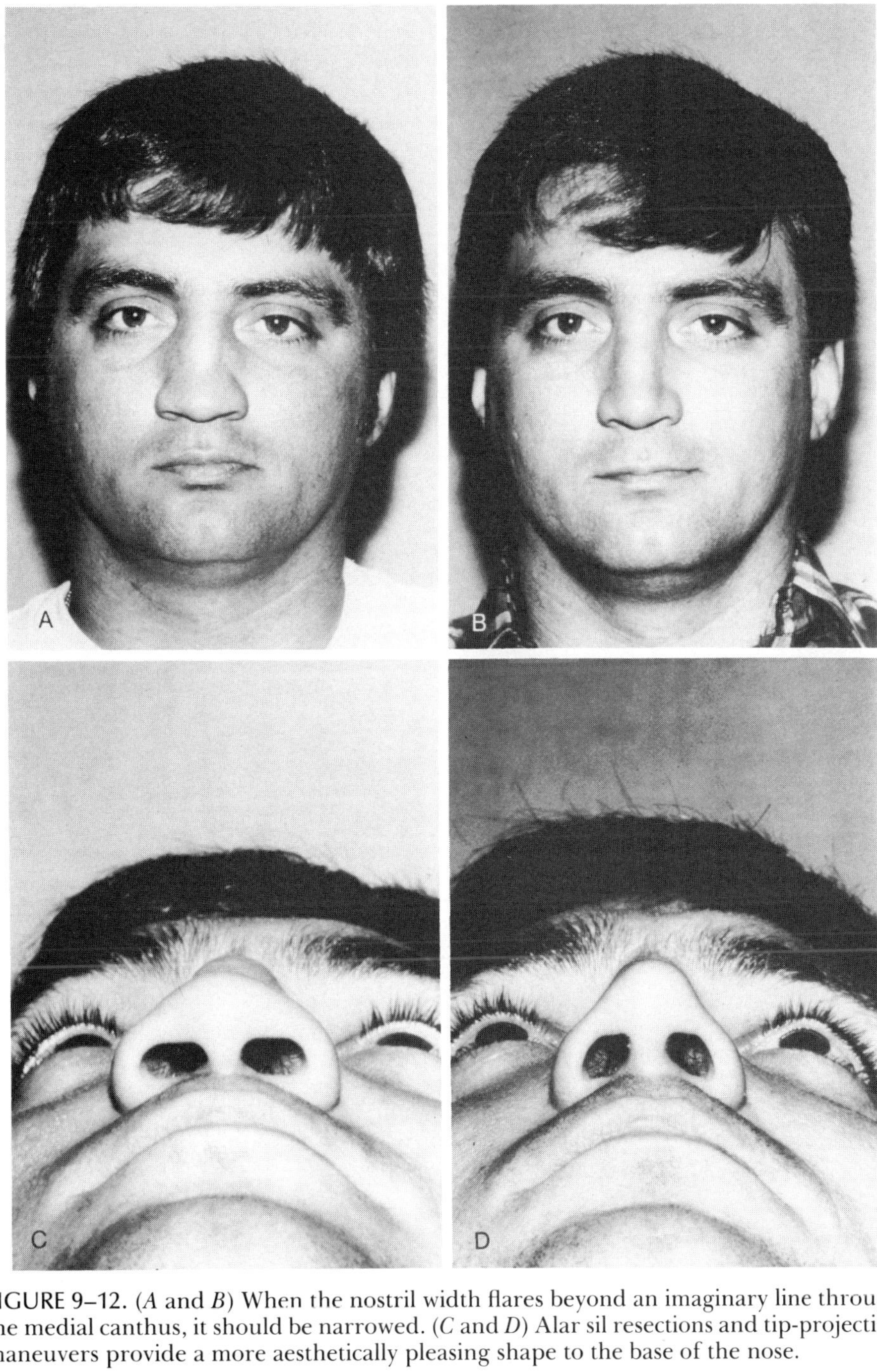

FIGURE 9–12. (*A* and *B*) When the nostril width flares beyond an imaginary line through the medial canthus, it should be narrowed. (*C* and *D*) Alar sil resections and tip-projecting maneuvers provide a more aesthetically pleasing shape to the base of the nose.

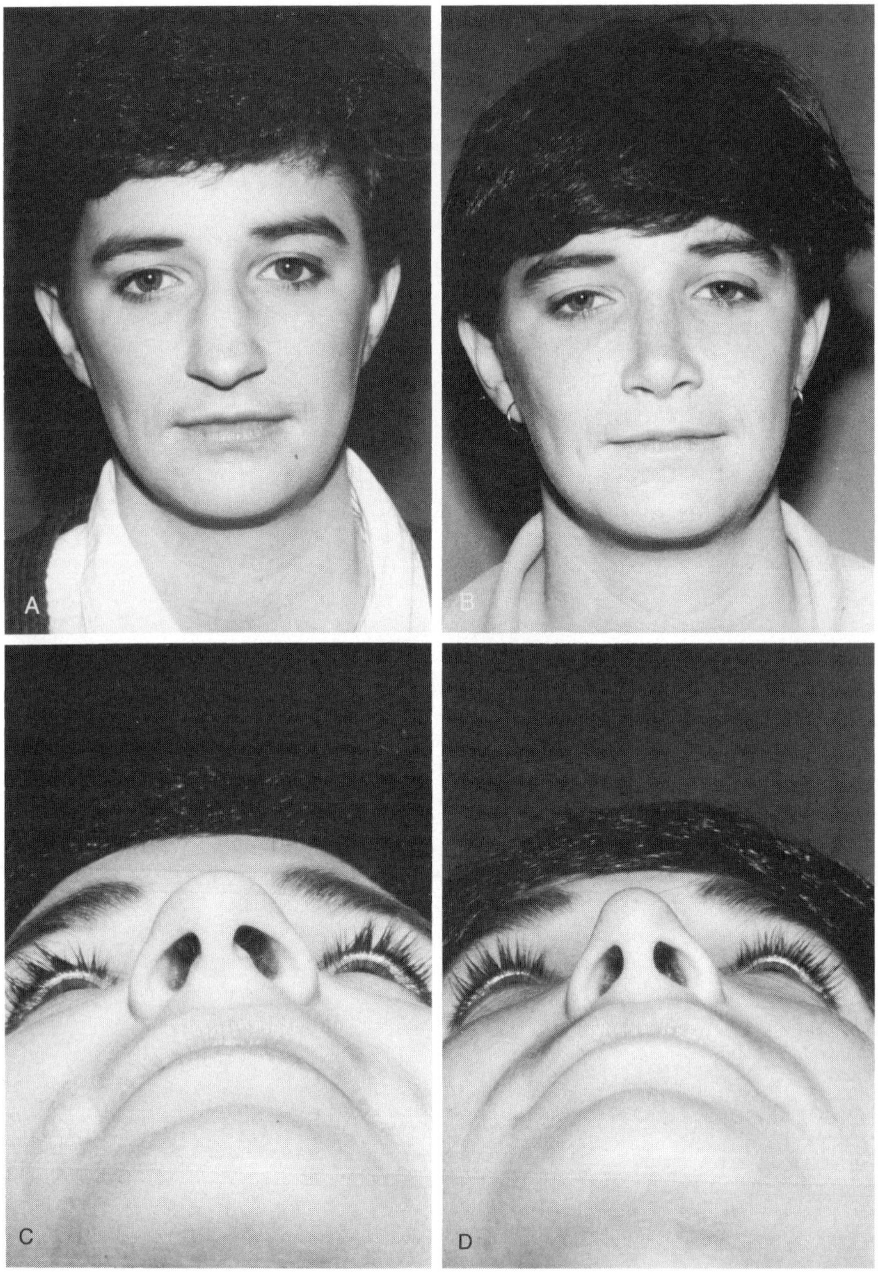

FIGURE 9–13. (*A* and *B*) A wide nose may require the narrowing of all components: bones, cartilages, and soft tissues. (*C* and *D*) Tip-plasty was performed with vertical dome division and I-beam columella graft. Alar sil resections corrected the flare of the nostrils.

Personal Communications

1. Anderson, J.R. 1974.
2. Berman, W.E. 1974.
3. Webster, R.E. 1974.

Suggested Readings

Denecke, H.J., Meyer, R. Rhinoplasty. New York: Springer-Verlag, 1976, pp. 40–43.

Joseph, J. Rhinoplasty and Facial Plastic Surgery. Reprint of 1931 ed. Phoenix: Columella Press, 1987.

Simons, R.L. Aesthetic Surgery of the Aging Face. St. Louis: C.V. Mosby, 1986, pp. 311–315.

CHAPTER 10

Surgery of the Nasal Septum

The objective of the nasal plastic surgeon should be two-fold: to produce a nose that is not only aesthetically pleasing but also functionally competent (Fig. 10–1). When airway compromise is due to a septal deformity (and the surgeon is trained in techniques designed to correct the internal pathology), appropriate septoplasty procedures should be performed at the time of rhinoplasty. Even minor deviations (or deformities) of the nasal septum deserve attention. As the lateral walls are mobilized and displaced medially toward the septum to close the open roof created by hump removal or to narrow a wide pyramid, the internal nasal vault becomes smaller. With this maneuver a preoperative asymptomatic deviation or superior thickening might become symptomatic, requiring the patient to undergo another operation at a later date.

MUCOPERICHONDRIAL FLAP ELEVATION

The mucosa, with its attached perichondrium and periosteum, can be freed with the following technique. Once the appropriate transfixion incision has been made, sharp scissors are used to dissect the mucosa from the initial 2 to 3 mm of the caudal septum.

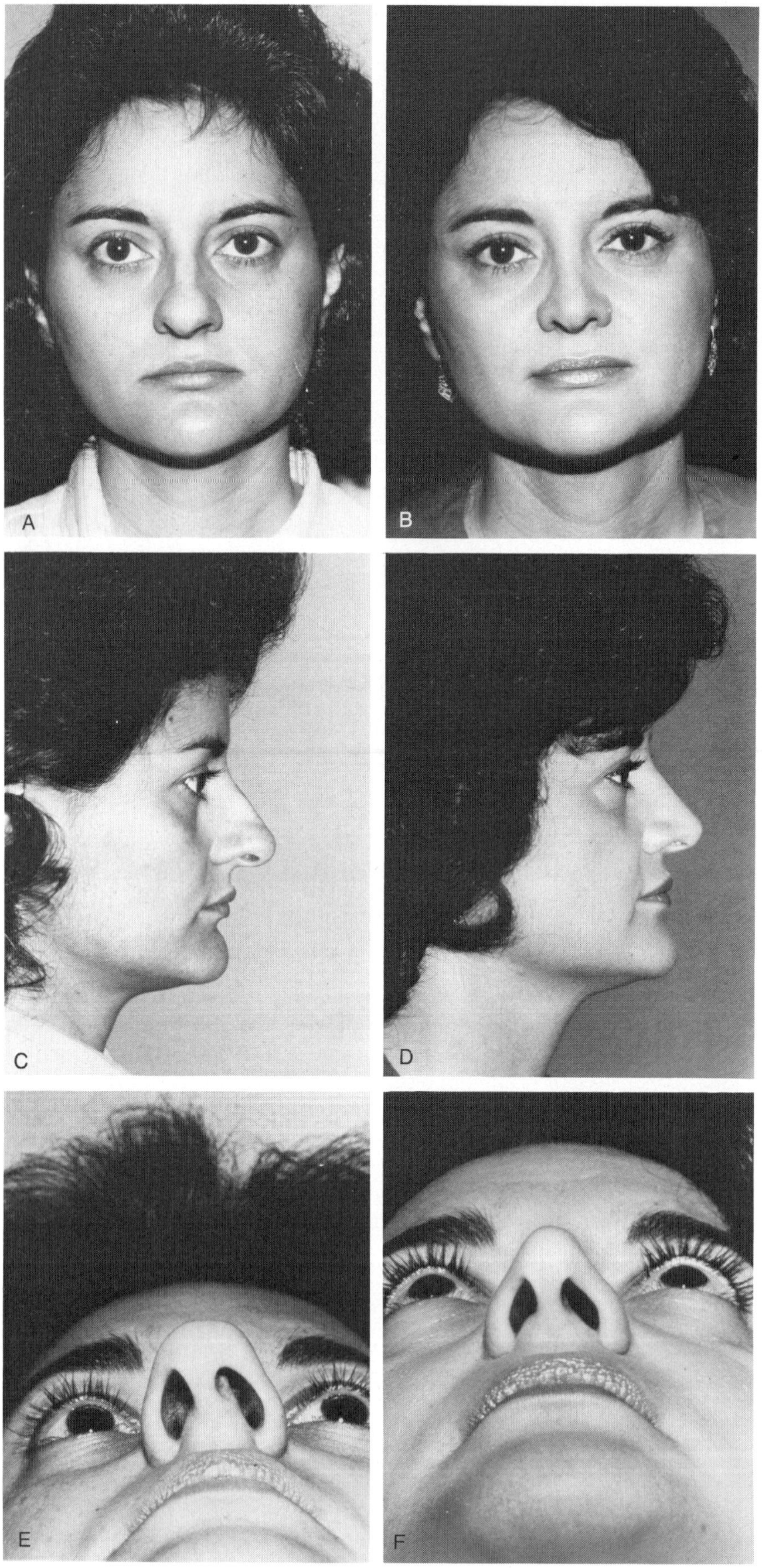

FIGURE 10–1. (*A* and *B*) Many patients who desire aesthetic improvement have an associated internal deformity. (*C* and *D*) Cosmetic enhancement can be accomplished at the time of septal reconstruction. (*E* and *F*) A deviated, dislocated septum may produce asymmetry as well as distortions of the columella and nostrils.

A no. 15 blade is used to make several crisscrossing incisions *into* the perichondrium (but not the cartilage). A dental amalgam packer (no. 0/1) is used to scratch a small section of the frayed perichondrium from the septal cartilage (Fig. 10–2).

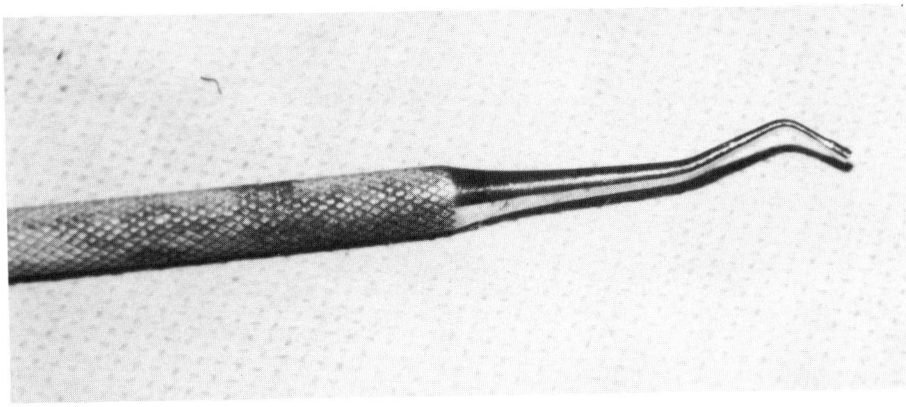

FIGURE 10–2. An amalgam packer is helpful in the initial steps of developing the septal mucoperichondrial flap.

When the correct plane has been established with the previous maneuvers, a McCollough-Anderson nasal elevator is used to dissect the remainder of the mucoperichondrial (-osteal) flap (Figs. 10–3 and 10–4*A* and *B*). Establishing the correct plane of dissection minimizes intraoperative and postoperative bleeding and lowers the risk of tearing the mucosal flaps, which could lead to unwanted sequelae (bleeding, synechiae, and septal perforations).

Flap elevation may be carried out unilaterally or, in the case of complicated septal reconstructions, bilaterally.

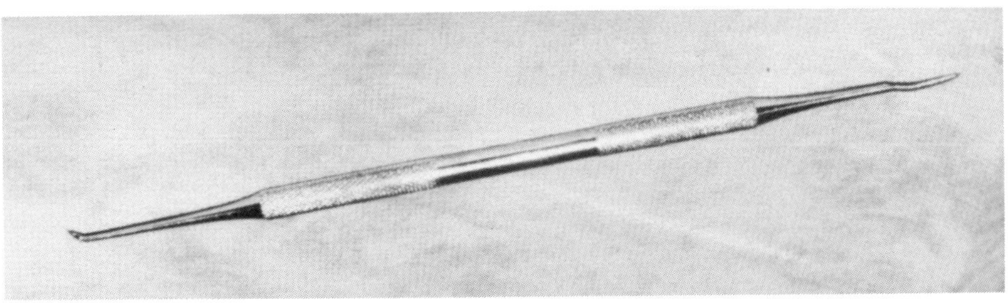

FIGURE 10–3. The McCollough-Anderson nasal elevator was specially designed for nasal surgery. At one end (*left*) there is a perichondrial (osteal) elevator that may also be used to make incisions into cartilage. At the other end (*right*) there is an angulated Rosen flap knife (an otologic instrument), which is helpful for cutting through periosteum and cartilage in tight spaces.

TECHNICAL CONSIDERATIONS

Like rhinoplasty, septoplasty should be approached in a progressive manner from the simplest submucous resection to total septal reconstruction. The following discussion is arranged in that progression.

MODIFIED SUBMUCOUS RESECTION

When the pathology is limited to a portion of the cartilagenous or bony septum, only the offending portion is removed through a hemitransfixion or Killian-type incision, followed by *unilateral* elevation of the mucoperi-

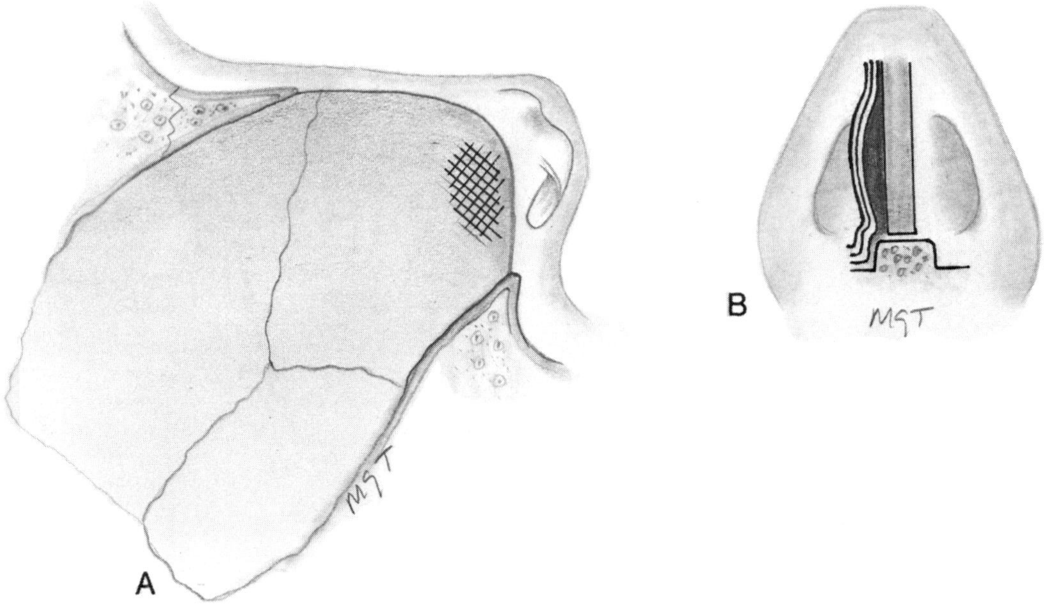

FIGURE 10–4. (*A* and *B*) After initial mucosal elevation, crisscrossed incisions into the *superficial* surface of the septum allows complete perichondrial elevation in continuity with nasal mucosa.

chondrium (-ostium). Under direct vision (Fig. 10–5) the least amount of bone and/or cartilage possible should be removed to relieve the obstruction.

SUBTOTAL SUBMUCOUS RESECTION

Many posterosuperior deviations comprising bony and cartilagenous components, especially those secondary to trauma, require removal of large amounts of both. It is desirable to leave at least 1.5- to 2.0-cm dorsal and caudal cantilever of bone and/or cartilage to avoid dorsal saddling or, caudally, retraction of the columella.

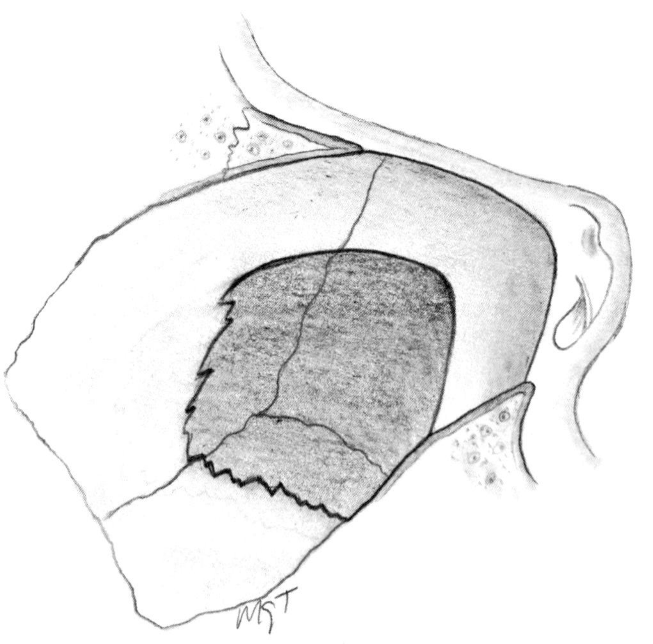

FIGURE 10–5. Only the offending portions of cartilage and/or bone are removed, leaving behind at least a 2-cm caudal and dorsal cantilever for support.

CAUDAL REALIGNMENT

When the caudal septum is dislocated to either side of the maxillary crest and the deformity is long-standing, bilateral mucoperichondrial elevation usually is necessary to free the cartilage from cicatricial forces. It usually is necessary to free the quadrilateral cartilage from the vomer and ethmoid bones (except for a dorsal segment of 1.5 to 2.0 cm) and from the maxillary crest by excising a strip of cartilage along the floor of the nose (Fig. 10–6). This maneuver creates a "swinging door" so that the caudal septum can be realigned and secured in a midline position.

A 3-0 chromic suture is placed in the manner described by Wright[1] to secure the cartilage into the correct position, as shown in Figure 10–7.

It is desirable to place internal bilateral sandwich septal splints, which help to hold the cartilage in a midline position during the initial healing period. The splints can be made from *exposed* x-ray material or Silastic. One or two mattress sutures are used to hold the splints in place for 7 to 10 days (Fig. 10–8.)

SEPTAL DISARTICULATION WITH FIXATION

In severely twisted noses the septal deviation may extend to and through the nasal dorsum. The pathology may be a result of overriding positions of cartilage and/or bone (Fig. 10–9).

Separation of the cartilagenous septum from *all* its attachments, including the ethmoid, vomer, maxilla, and upper lateral cartilages, may be necessary. When all the components mentioned above are involved, I usually approach the deformities through an external rhinoplasty conversion. This approach helps the surgeon to identify the multiple pathologic conditions and allows him to make the necessary corrections and suture the structures into a more normal anatomic position. The caudal deflection is treated in the manner described in the section on caudal realignment.

If cartilagenous-ethmoid disarticulation becomes necessary, its integrity can be reestablished by submucosal suture fixation using 4-0 polyglactin 910 (Vicryl) sutures. A small hole can be drilled in the ethmoid bone with an 18-gauge needle. Manually rolling the Luer-Lok end of the needle between the thumb and index finger creates a defect through which the needle can be passed (see Fig. 10–8).

Dorsal integrity can be reinforced by suturing both upper lateral cartilages back to the dorsal ridge of the septal cartilage. One or two 4-0 or 5-0 Vicryl sutures usually suffice (see Fig. 10–8). When the dorsal cantilever of cartilage is curved, *gentle* morselization (softening of the cartilage) coupled with upper lateral cartilage suture fixation may be adequate.

More severe deformities may require both morselization and/or vertical interruption of the cartilagenous dorsum and placement of a cartilagenous graft, which, when sutured in place with 5-0 Vicryl, provides additional support (Figs. 10–10 and 10–11). Upper lateral cartilage attachment is carried out as described in the preceding section.

CARTILAGENOUS DEVIATIONS

Numerous maneuvers for straightening cartilage have been described, including extensive morselization, vertical and horizontal cartilagenous strip excision, and crosshatching. In my experience these measures have produced varying and unpredictable results. The conversion of a single block of curved cartilage to independent segments, as shown in Figure 10–10 (*A* and *B*), followed by suture fixation, support grafting, and

Text continued on page 117

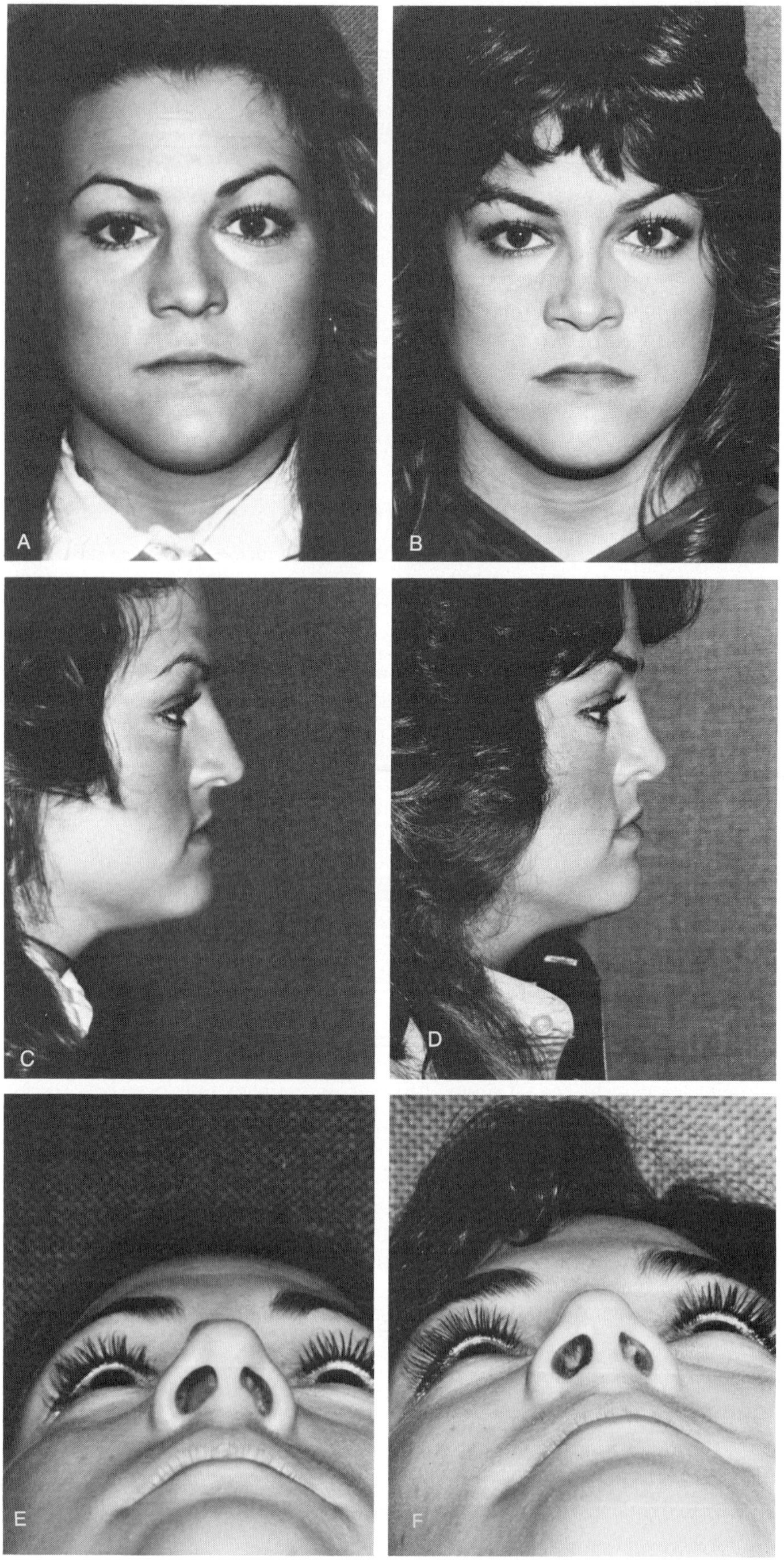

FIGURE 10–6. (*A* and *B*) Severely twisted noses commonly are associated with dislocation-deviation septal deformities. (*C* and *D*) Dorsal height can be maintained when the cantilever is treated as described in Figure 10–5. (*E* and *F*) Reconstructive septoplasty, as described in Figure 10–8, was necessary to realign the septum.

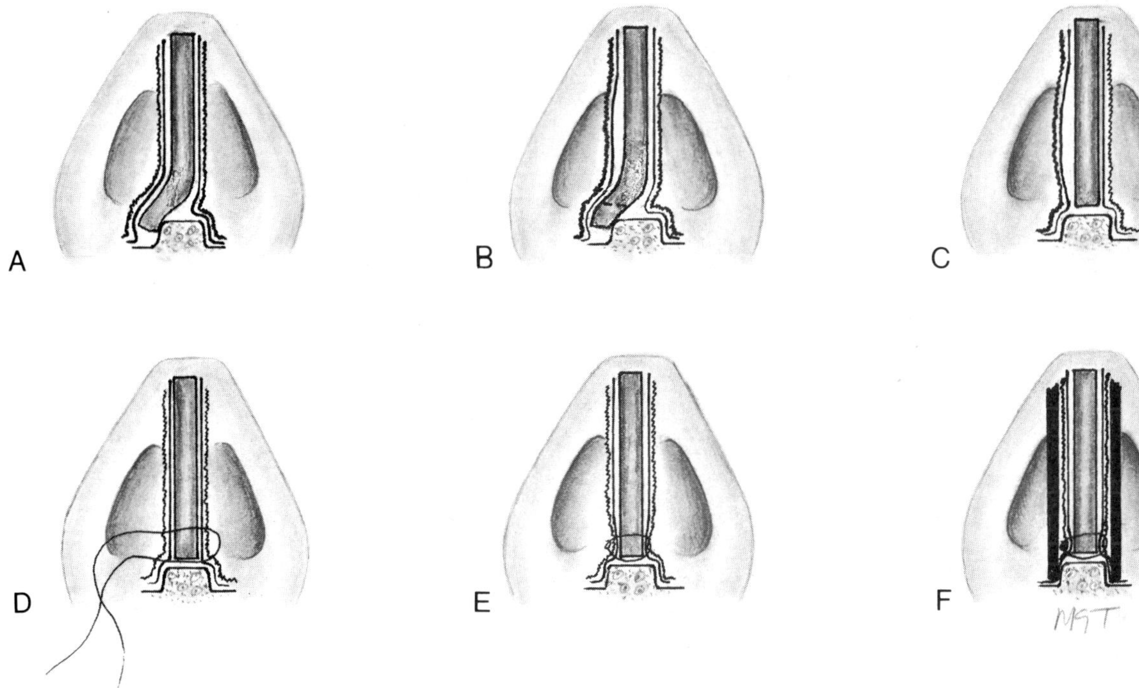

FIGURE 10–7. (*A*) Dislocated caudal septum. (*B*) After submucous resection, the dislocated inferior portion of the remaining cantilever is excised. (*C*) When the caudal septum is free, it can "swing" back into a more midline position. (*D*) A 3-0 chromic suture is passed. (*E*) When the suture is tied, it helps to cinch the septal cartilage perichondrium and mucosa to the maxillary crest. (*F*) Bilateral internal splints provide additional support until healing is established.

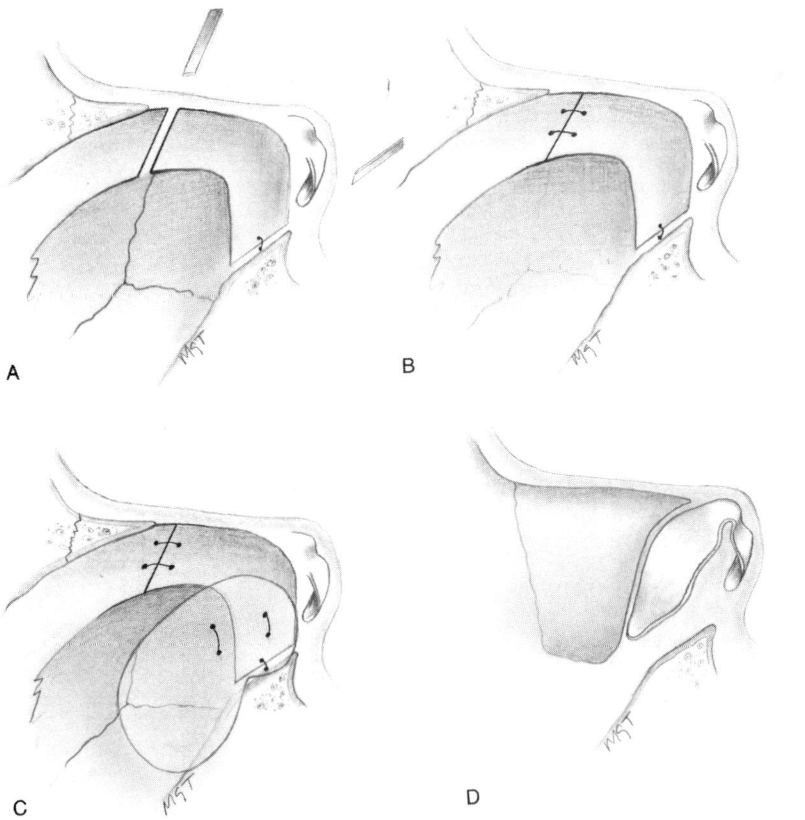

FIGURE 10–8. (*A*) In severely crooked noses it might be necessary to disarticulate the cartilagenous cantilever. (*B*) The integrity of the cantilever can be reestablished with sutures. (*C*) Internal splints provide additional support. (*D*) The upper lateral cartilages, when resutured to the dorsal cantilever with horizontal mattress sutures, help to straighten and support the nasal dorsum.

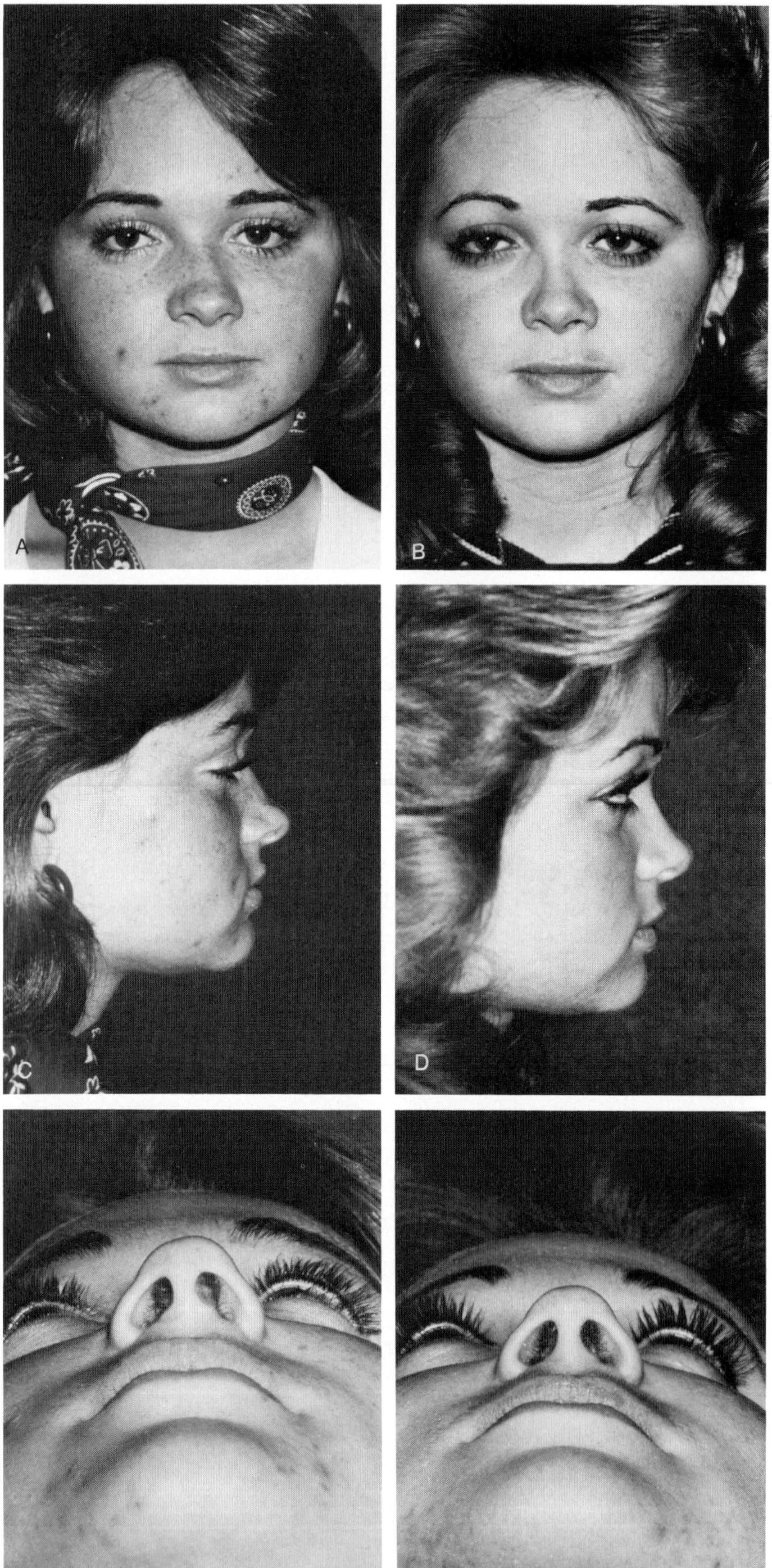

FIGURE 10–9. (*A* and *B*) When the septal deformity extends through the nasal dorsum to the bony-cartilagenous junction, disarticulation may be necessary (see Fig. 10–8). (*C* and *D*) Preoperative and/or intraoperative saddling should be corrected with morselization septal cartilage onlay grafts. (*E* and *F*) Caudal realignment was carried out with a swing-door maneuver. No tip-plasty was performed.

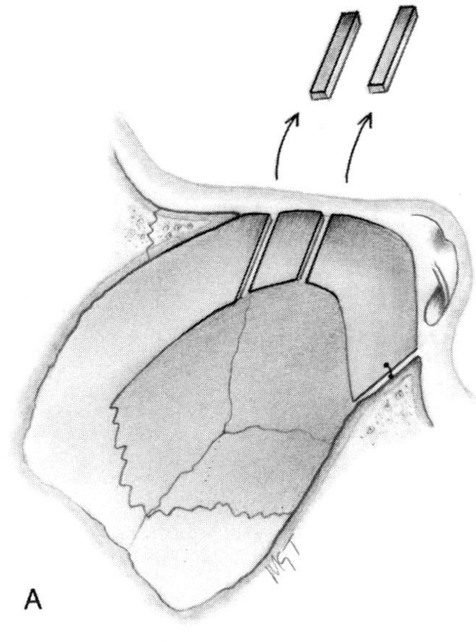

FIGURE 10–10. (*A*) The dorsum can be reconstructed by suturing a septal cartilage graft adjacent to the interrupted cantilever. Internal splinting is also indicated. (*B*) When the dorsal cantilever contains multiple fracture sites or is severely crooked, it might be necessary to interrupt its integrity at more than one site.

internal splinting, is the most effective method of permanently correcting deformities that result from curved cartilage.

BONY DEVIATIONS

The most effective and safest method of correcting a bony deviation is to remove the deviant portions of bone. Fracturing or displacing the ethmoid bones toward the midline could produce an iatrogenic defect in the cribriform plate and lead to cerebrospinal fluid rhinorrhea and its associated sequelae.

TURBINATE REDUCTION

Sometimes the nasal airway can be improved by reducing the size of the inferior and/or middle turbinates. The spongy bone of the turbinates can be compressed with a blunt instrument (Bard-Parker handle) and displaced laterally (see Fig. 10–11). Thickened, boggy membranes can be

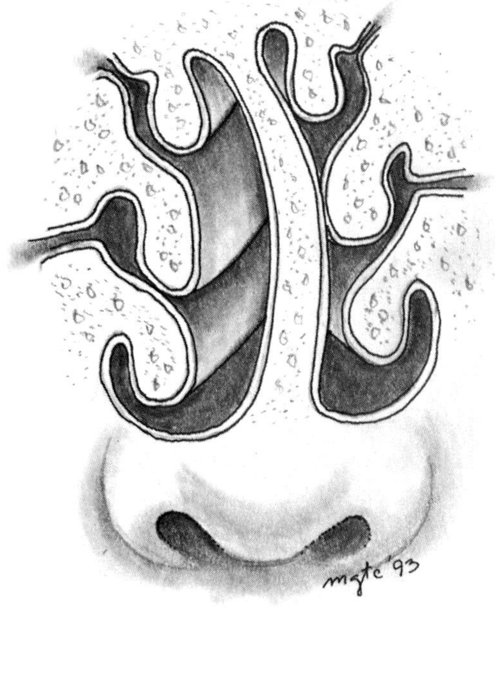

FIGURE 10–11. A deviated septum, when combined with large turbinates compounds airway and sinus troubles. Both are a frequent but overlooked cause of headaches.

cauterized with electrical cauterization. Caution is encouraged because overzealous cauterization could lead to ozena. In rare cases resection of a portion of either the middle or the inferior turbinate may be indicated.

NASAL POLYPS

Distinct allergy-related polyps can be surgically avulsed under direct vision. Pathologic investigation is recommended for any polypoid lesion removed from the nose. The application of a large piece of Surgicel to avulsed surfaces usually prevents bleeding and eliminates the need for extensive intranasal packing.

Suspicious intranasal lesions should be addressed with caution. Consultation may be indicated.

NASAL PACKING

After septal correction the mucoperichondrial (-osteal) flaps can be reapproximated with mattress sutures, thereby eliminating traditional internal nasal packing. A 4-0 plain catgut suture on a straight needle (Ethicon 1824 cutting SC-1 needle) is placed in a continuous elliptic manner (Fig. 10–12).

INTERNAL SPLINTS

Silastic or previously exposed x-ray splints are used for midline fixation purposes only—not to reapproximate mucoperichondrial flaps.

Splints should be just large enough to pass through the nostril openings with ease. If they go in with difficulty, they will be difficult to remove and cause the patient discomfort (Figs. 10–13 and 10–14 [*A* and *B*]). If internal nasal splints are used, they must extend to the floor of the nose and overlap the maxillary crest, which helps to secure them in the midline (see Fig. 10–8*C*). A notch should be created at the point where the splints rest over the pyriform aperture (see Fig. 10–13).

Splints are secured with one or two mattress sutures of 2-0 silk or 3-0 chromic. The sutures should not be tied too tightly; strangulation of the mucoperichondrial flaps could result in septal perforation.

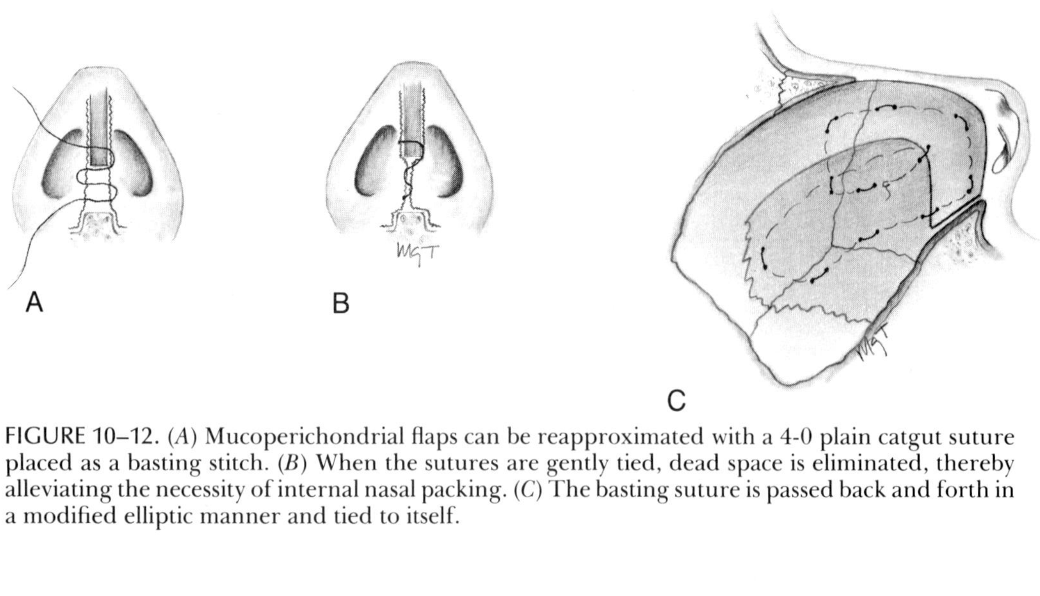

FIGURE 10–12. (*A*) Mucoperichondrial flaps can be reapproximated with a 4-0 plain catgut suture placed as a basting stitch. (*B*) When the sutures are gently tied, dead space is eliminated, thereby alleviating the necessity of internal nasal packing. (*C*) The basting suture is passed back and forth in a modified elliptic manner and tied to itself.

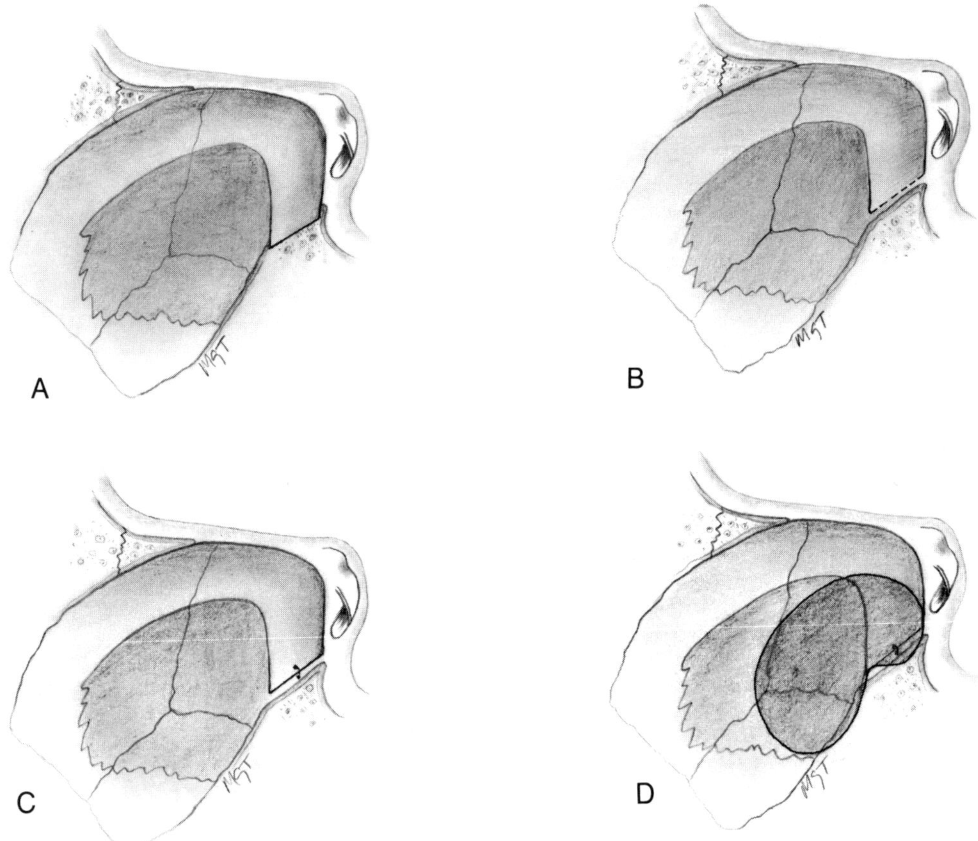

FIGURE 10–13. (*A*) Large boggy turbinates produce airway obstruction. (*B*) Turbinates can be displaced laterally and the spongy bone component compressed. (*C*) Unipolar cauterization can produce fibrosis, which helps to eliminate membrane bogginess. (*D*) When healed, the nasal airway is improved. Bilateral intranasal splints can help to stabilize and support a reconstructed septum.

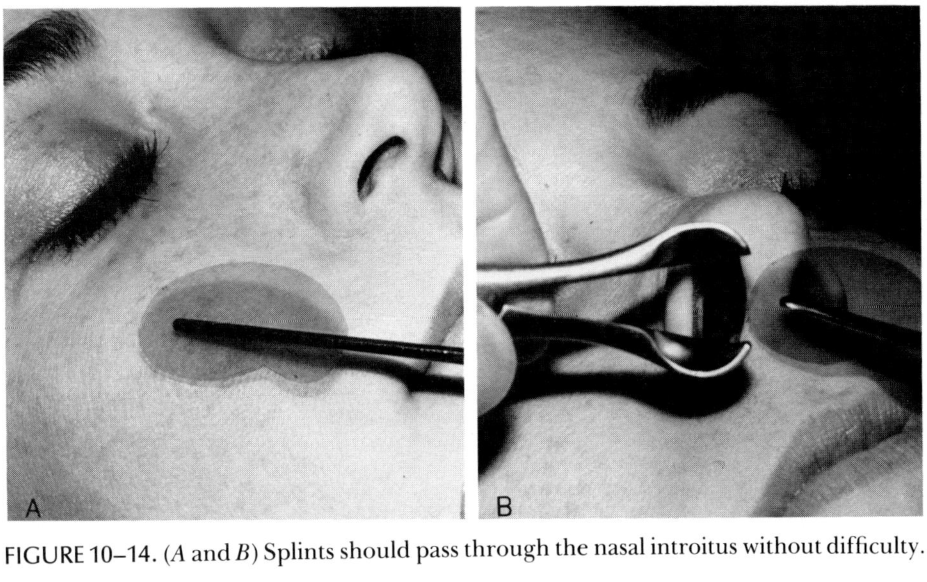

FIGURE 10–14. (*A* and *B*) Splints should pass through the nasal introitus without difficulty.

SYNECHIAE

When intranasal synechiae are lysed, internal splints placed in the traditional manner against the septum and between the raw mucosal edges may help to prevent reattachment of the medial and lateral components. After 7 days the splints usually can be removed.

AFTERCARE

On the morning after surgery the Surgicel is removed from the nasal vestibule and the nose is gently cleaned. Careful suction may remove debris, but overzealous manipulation might promote epistaxis.

Patients should be given written and specific instructions relative to activities and wound care (see Ch. 6). Most patients return at 1 week for a postoperative checkup. Any remaining debris, splints, and/or Surgicel can be gently removed at this time. Spraying the nose with a decongestant–topical anesthetic before manipulation may reduce discomfort.

When internal packing has been avoided, the postoperative course is more pleasant and postoperative visits less eventful. Many patients who have been packed after a previous nasal procedure comment that removal of the packing was the most uncomfortable part of their surgical experience.

Some internal edema remains for several weeks, but the airway usually continues to improve for up to 8 weeks. Follow-up visits at 6 and 12 months are advised to check the status of the septum and airway.

Personal Communications

1. Wright, W. K. 1975.
2. Beelkuis, J. 1975.
3. Anderson, J. R. 1974.

Suggested Reading

Bull, T. Septoplasty vs. submucous resection. J Laryngol Otol [Suppl] 8:108, 1983.

Colton, J., Beekhuis, G. Correction of the crooked nose. Otolaryngol Clin North Am 20:200 1987.

Courtias, E. Diagnosis and treatment of nasal airway obstruction due to interior turbinate hypertrophy. Clin Plast Surg 15:11–13, 1988.

Denecke, H.J., Meyer, R. Rhinoplasty. New York: Springer-Verlag, 1976.

CHAPTER 11

Preparing for Hump Removal: Dorsal Dissection

Exposure of the nasal dorsum is accomplished in three stages. First, the superior septal angle is identified and the supratip soft tissue is freed from the cartilagenous dorsum for a distance of 1 to 2 cm with a curved sharp scissors.

Then bilateral intracartilagenous (limen vestibuli) incisions are made between the upper and lower lateral cartilages with a no. 15 blade. The plane of dissection is created as close as possible to the perichondrium of the upper lateral cartilages and deep to the vessels of the dorsal nasal skin and muscle (Fig. 11–1). Lateral dissection is carried toward the nasal dorsum to join the pocket previously created with scissor dissection.

Sharp dissection is continued cephalically over the left upper lateral cartilage superiorly toward the nasal bones with a no. 15 blade or scissors, always staying close to the cartilage to reduce bleeding.

The dissection is continued to a point just superior to the caudal margin of the left nasal bone. Then an incision is made through the periosteum of the dorsal aspect of the nasal bone, and a periosteal elevator is used to lift the periosteum from the nasal bones (Fig. 11–2). Periosteal elevation should extend superiorly and laterally only far enough to allow for removal of the necessary portions of bones. The process is repeated on the opposite side and connected in the midline.

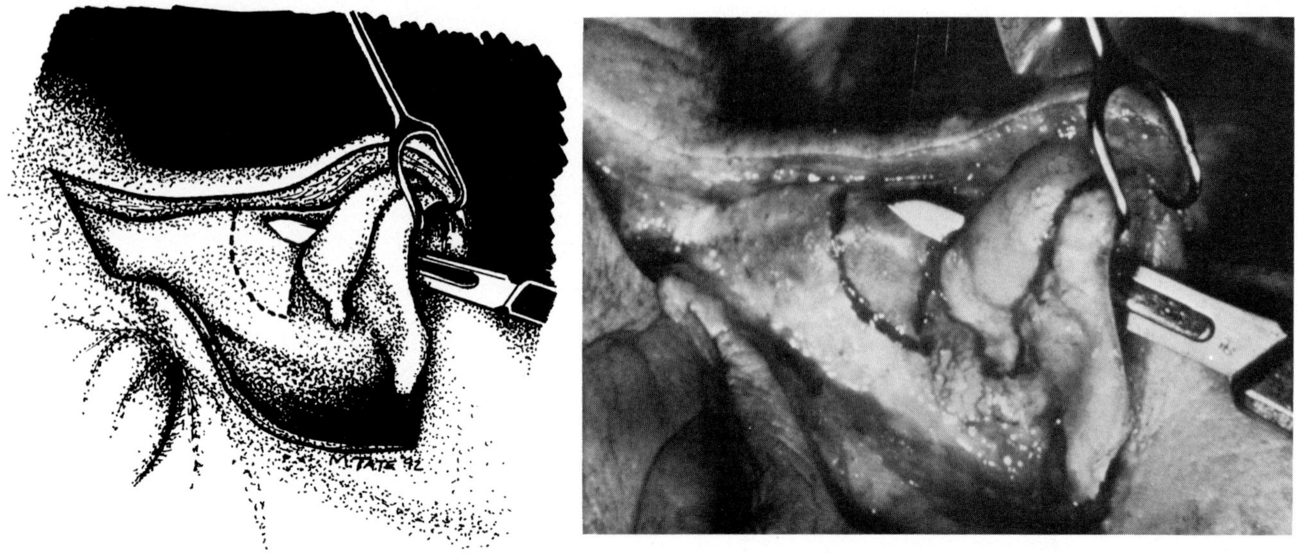

FIGURE 11–1. (*A* and *B*) Intercartilagenous incisions are performed with a no. 15 blade. The soft tissue is dissected from the upper lateral cartilages in the immediate supraperichondrial plane.

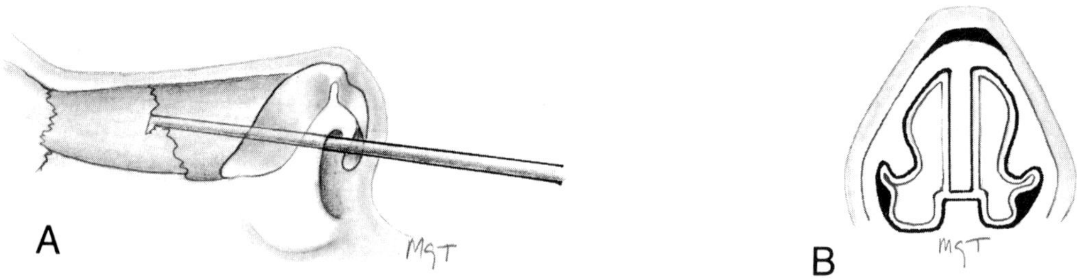

FIGURE 11–2. (*A*) An incision is made through the periosteum so that a precise plane of dissection can be developed. (*B*) The periosteum is lifted in continuity with the skin and/or mucosa only far enough to allow for hump removal (or osteotomies).

It is desirable to keep the dissection as close as possible to the nasal skeleton not only to reduce bleeding but also to leave behind a more uniform and thicker "blanket" of soft tissue, which can help to camouflage small irregularities.

In older patients who have large humps and less elastic skin, undermining may be carried more laterally over the upper lateral cartilages to allow for better draping of redundant skin. Dorsal periosteal elevation should still be limited.

Dorsal periosteal elevation should *not* communicate with any anticipated periosteal elevation for lateral osteotomies; otherwise, the lateral bony walls might prolapse into the nasal vestibule when mobilization is accomplished after osteotomies.

Suggested Reading

Denecke, H.J., Meyer, R., Rhinoplasty. New York: Springer-Verlag, 1976.

CHAPTER 12

Hump Removal

The goal in rhinoplasty is to create a natural-looking nose and avoid the "operated" look. The ideal height of the nasal dorsum may vary with the patient's age, gender, and height. Taller people should have straighter dorsums; conversely, shorter people may need a slightly retroussé dorsum (Figs. 12–1 through 12–3). In a male the dorsum should be slightly convex; in a woman the tip can be slightly higher than the rhinion. Patients over age 50 should also have straighter noses to avoid the operated look (Fig. 12–4).

Hump removal can be the most dramatic step in rhinoplasty, but it should be approached with prudence and pragmatism. An overly aggressive excision of bone and/or cartilage might convert an aesthetic rhinoplasty to one that requires most of the surgeon's *reconstructive* skills. The end result then depends on the imponderables of healing.

In three-dimensional art, height and width are inseparable. Noses that appear narrow and are aesthetically pleasing from the frontal view typically consist of strong, straight dorsums (Fig. 12–5). Wide noses often are associated with a paucity of dorsal height (Fig. 12–6).

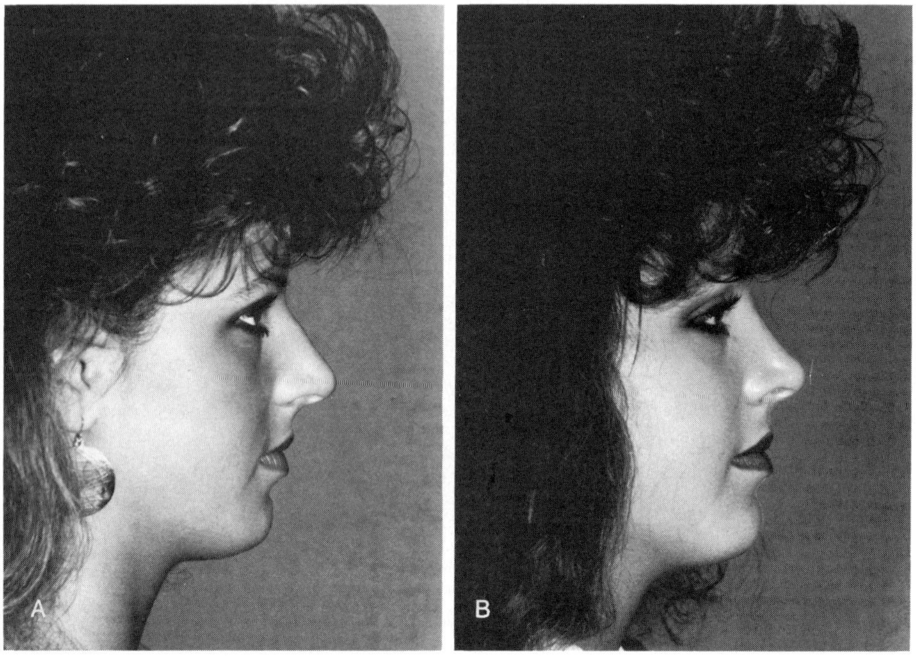

FIGURE 12–1. (*A* and *B*) In younger, shorter females the tip should sit 1 to 2 mm higher than the nasal dorsum.

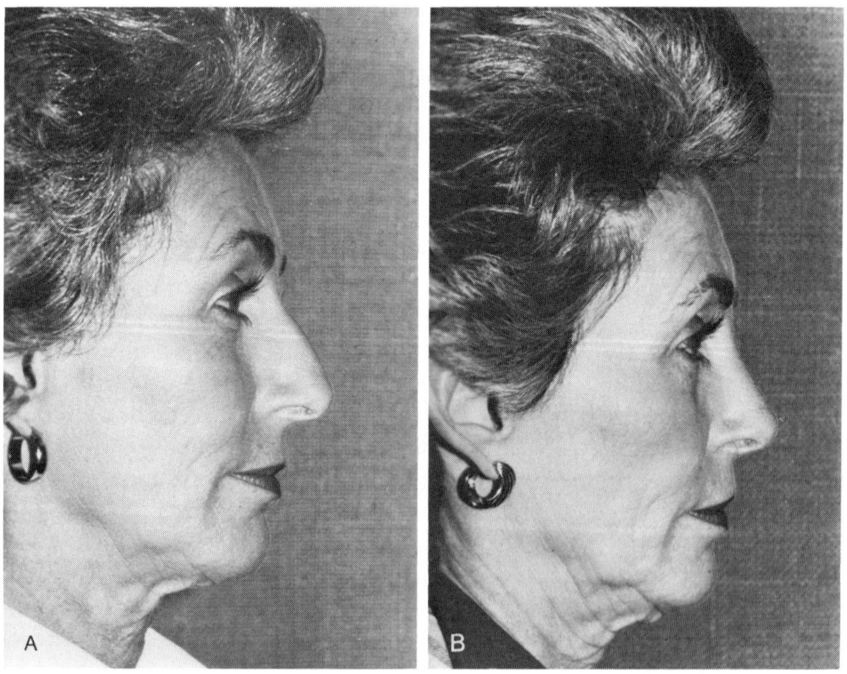

FIGURE 12–2. (*A* and *B*) In patients over age 50 a straighter nasal dorsum is preferred.

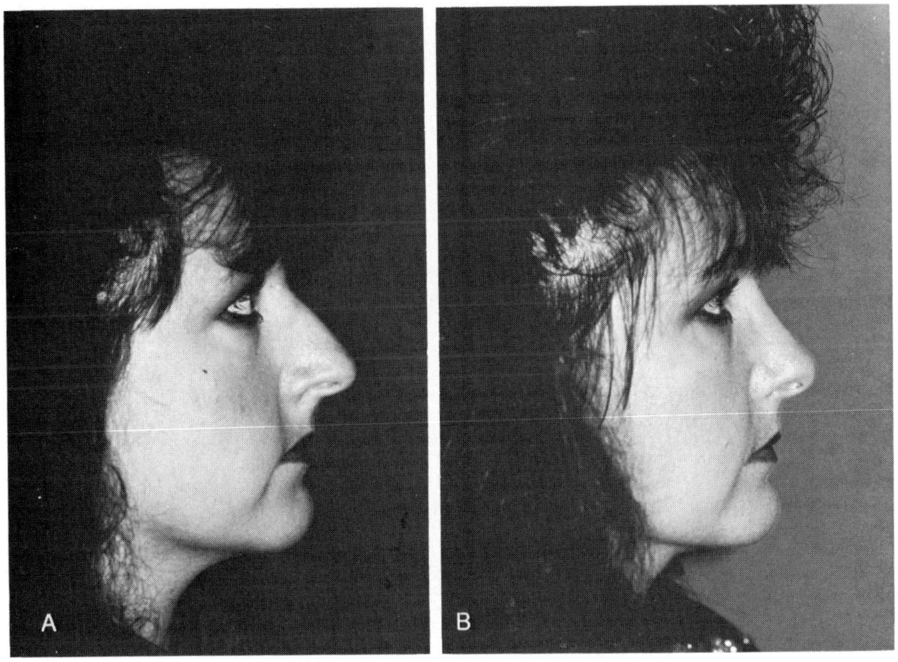

FIGURE 12–3. (*A* and *B*) Straight nasal dorsums are preferable in taller patients.

TECHNIQUE

Removal of the dorsal hump is accomplished in two stages.

CARTILAGENOUS HUMP REMOVAL

The cartilagenous hump usually is incised as a single unit (i.e., both upper lateral cartilages and the attached septum) under direct vision with a no. 11 blade. Once the anticipated amount of cartilagenous hump to be removed has been determined, the bony-cartilagenous junction is visualized. Mucosa is not ordinarily elevated from the undersurface of the upper lateral cartilage–septal junction; nor are the upper lateral cartilages routinely separated from the septum before hump removal.

The tip of the no. 11 blade is passed through all three components of the cartilagenous hump: the left and right upper lateral cartilages and the septum. Dissection is continued inferiorly toward the superior septal angle. The underlying mucosa moves aside as the blade passes over.

With the first pass of the blade it is best to remove about 1 mm less than one eventually intends to remove. Depending on the surgeon's experience and the size of the hump, the cartilagenous hump can be removed at this point with angulated scissors, or it may be removed in conjunction with the bony component with an osteotome.

Text continued on page 129

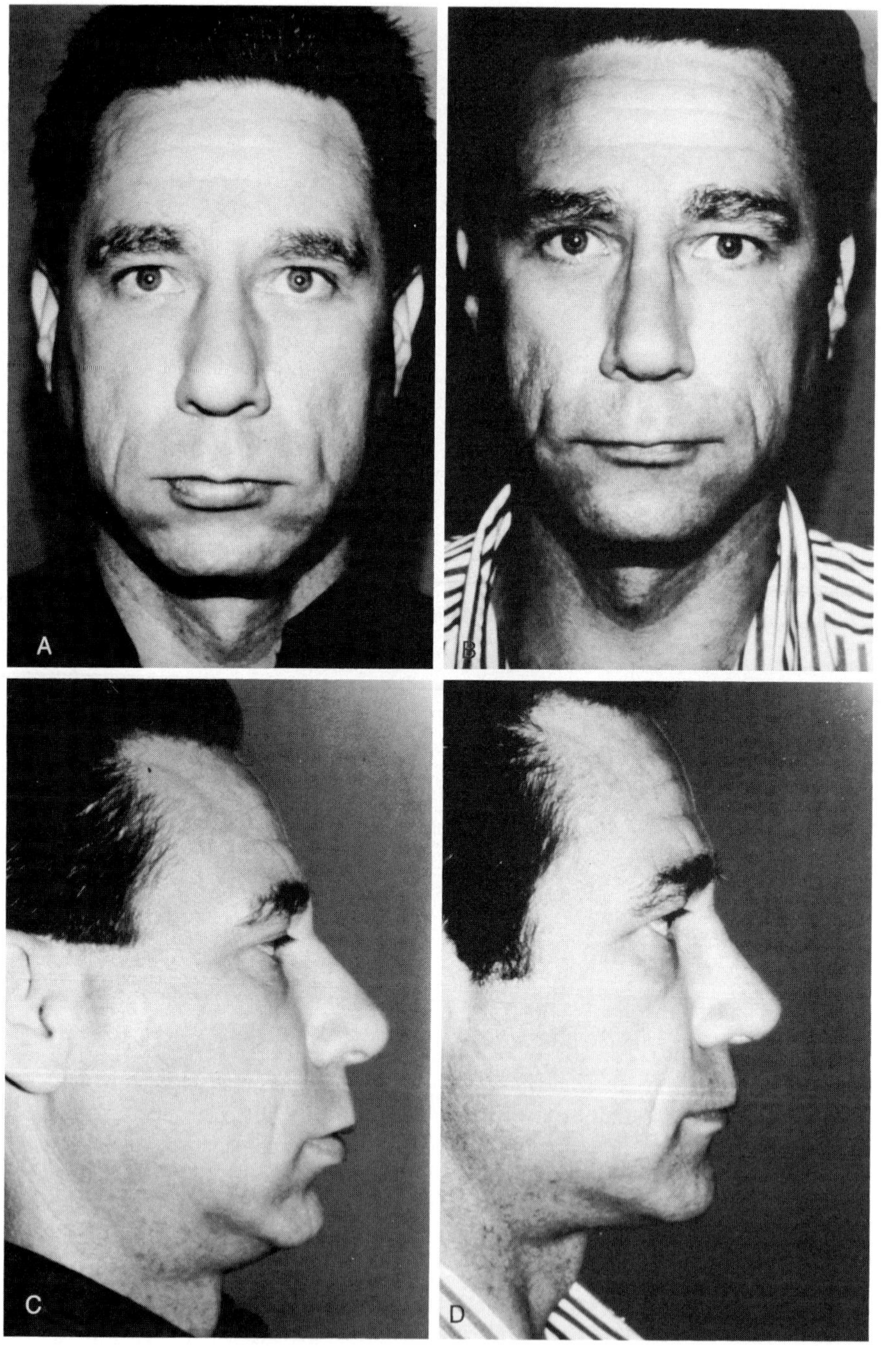

FIGURE 12–4. (*A–D*) A masculine appearance can be maintained by leaving a strong dorsum that is in line with the tip. Chin augmentation may help to provide a more masculine appearance in some cases.

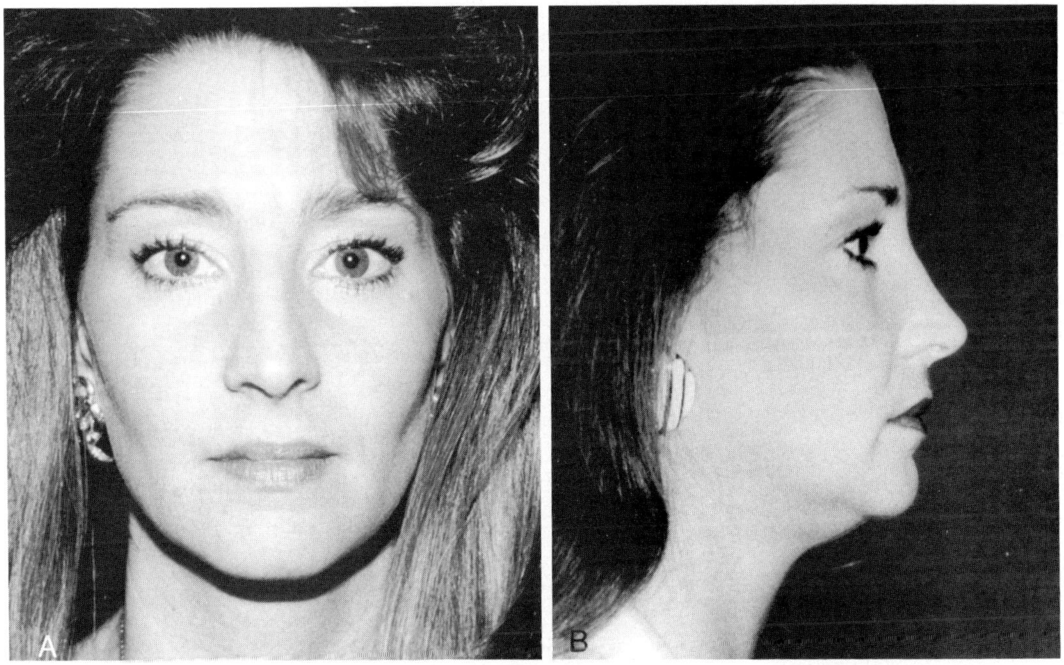

FIGURE 12–5. (*A*) Leaving a higher nasal dorsum in a patient who already has a narrow nose is necessary to avoid a widened postoperative appearance. (*B*) A strong, straight bridge on the profile view can be left, provided tip support is assured.

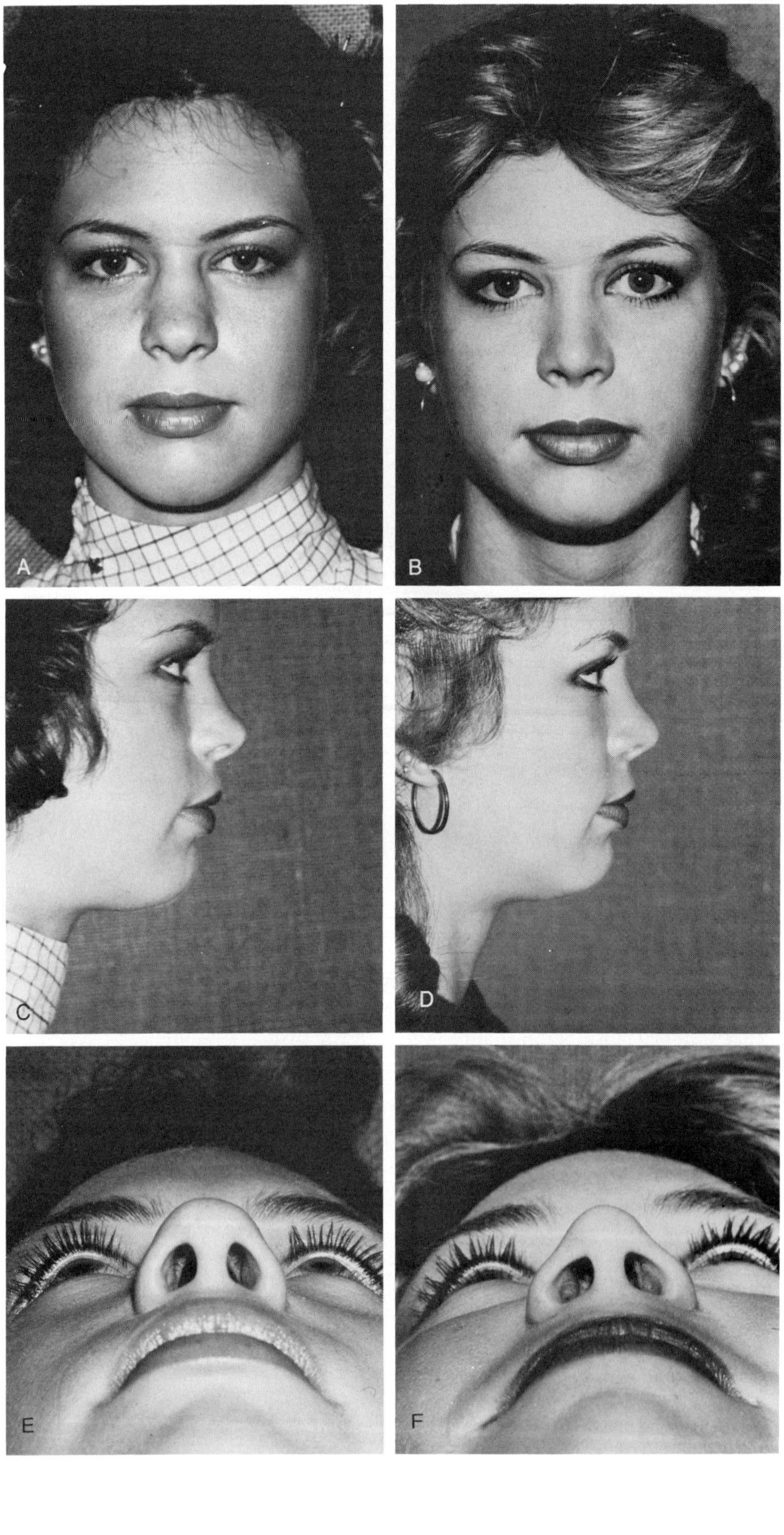

FIGURE 12–6. (*A* and *B*) Wide noses are associated with a paucity of dorsal height. Narrowing the bony and cartilagenous pyramid alone may help in some cases. (*C* and *D*) Hump removal was not performed in this patient. (*E* and *F*) Tip-plasty was performed with vertical division followed by suturing the transected medial crura to themselves in the midline.

DORSAL SHAPING

The skin and subcutaneous covering are thickest at the nasion and in the supratip region and thinnest at the rhinion. Therefore, when hump removal is complete, the dorsal skeleton should *not* be straight (Fig. 12–7). Because the thickness of the soft tissue covering of the nasal dorsum varies at different anatomic sites, the underlying skeleton must be adjusted accordingly.

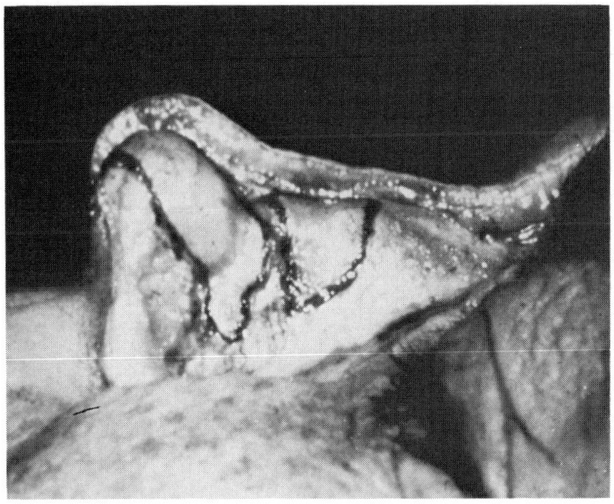

FIGURE 12–7. Anatomic configuration of the nasal skeleton of the nose with a straight dorsum.

FINGER TEST

At the conclusion of cartilagenous hump removal, the superior septal angle must not be visible when the tip of the nose is depressed (Fig. 12–8). If it is, a cartilagenous "polly-beak" could appear a few months postoperatively (Figs. 12–9 and 12–10).

UPPER LATERAL CARTILAGES

Projection portions of the upper lateral cartilages are trimmed with angulated (Fomon) scissors until they lie at the same height as the altered septal dorsum.

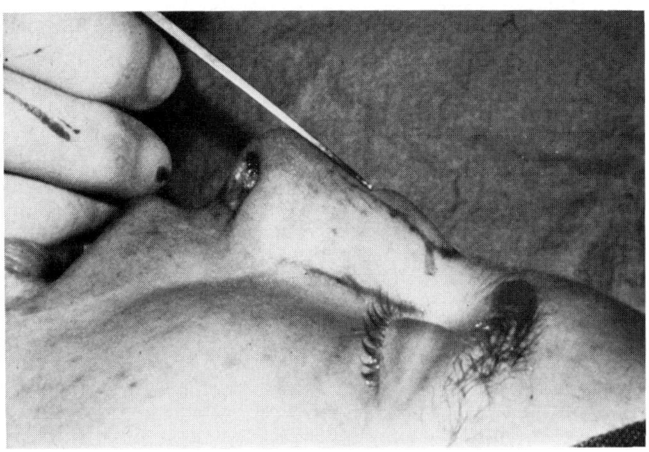

FIGURE 12–8. The superior septal angle is visible when the tip is depressed.

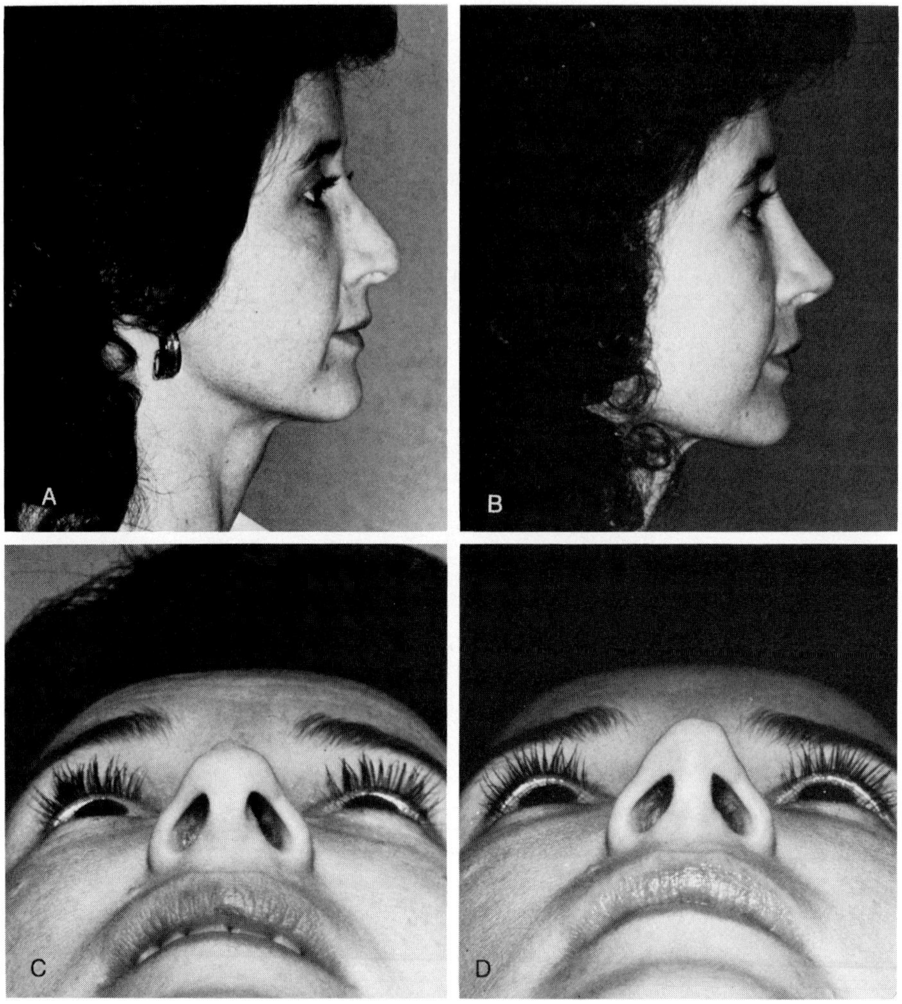

FIGURE 12–9. (*A* and *B*) Prevention and correction of "polly-beak" requires proper tip support and adequate excision of the superior septal angle. (*C* and *D*) Tip-plasty required vertical dome division with I-beam cartilage graft.

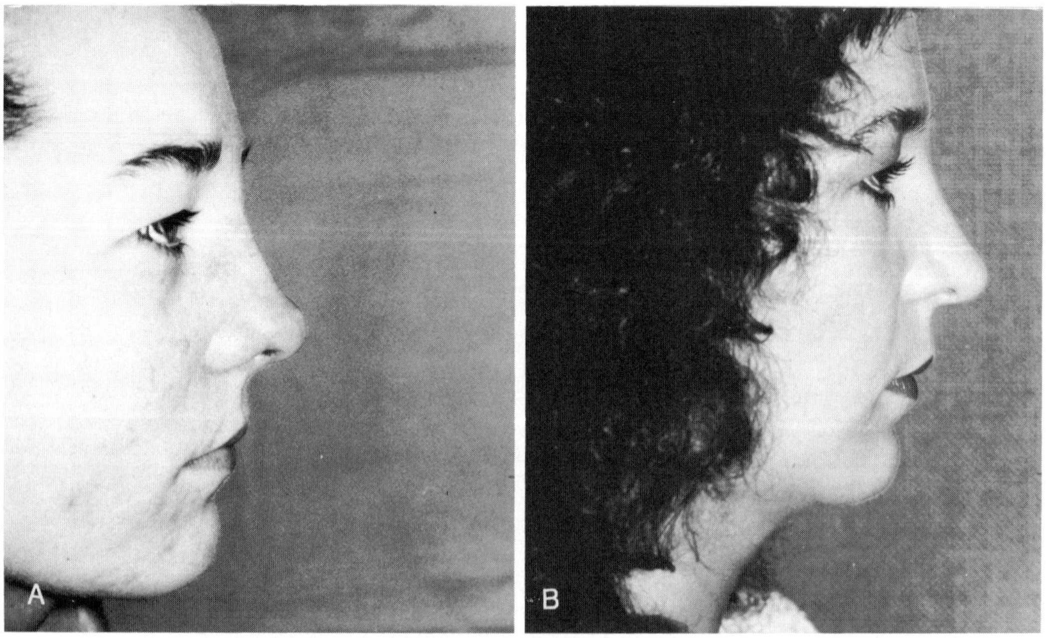

FIGURE 12–10. (*A*) Preoperative lateral. (*B*) Postoperative lateral. At the conclusion of the operation the tip should sit 2 to 3 mm higher than the nasal dorsum to allow for intraoperative edema. As healing takes place over the next 12 months, some loss of projection occurs, leaving the patient and surgeon with the desired result.

BONY HUMP REMOVAL

If the cartilage component is excised independently, the bony hump can be removed by a variety of techniques. Two are described below.

RASP TECHNIQUE

Until the surgeon has gained a great deal of experience, or in previously traumatized noses, it is safer to incrementally remove bony humps with sharp rasps. The rasp technique is also preferred for smaller humps.

Before rasping and after the periosteum is elevated, the cortical bone can be "prepared" by creating several superficial incisions into it with a straight nasal saw (Fig. 12–11). Even large humps can be removed in this manner.

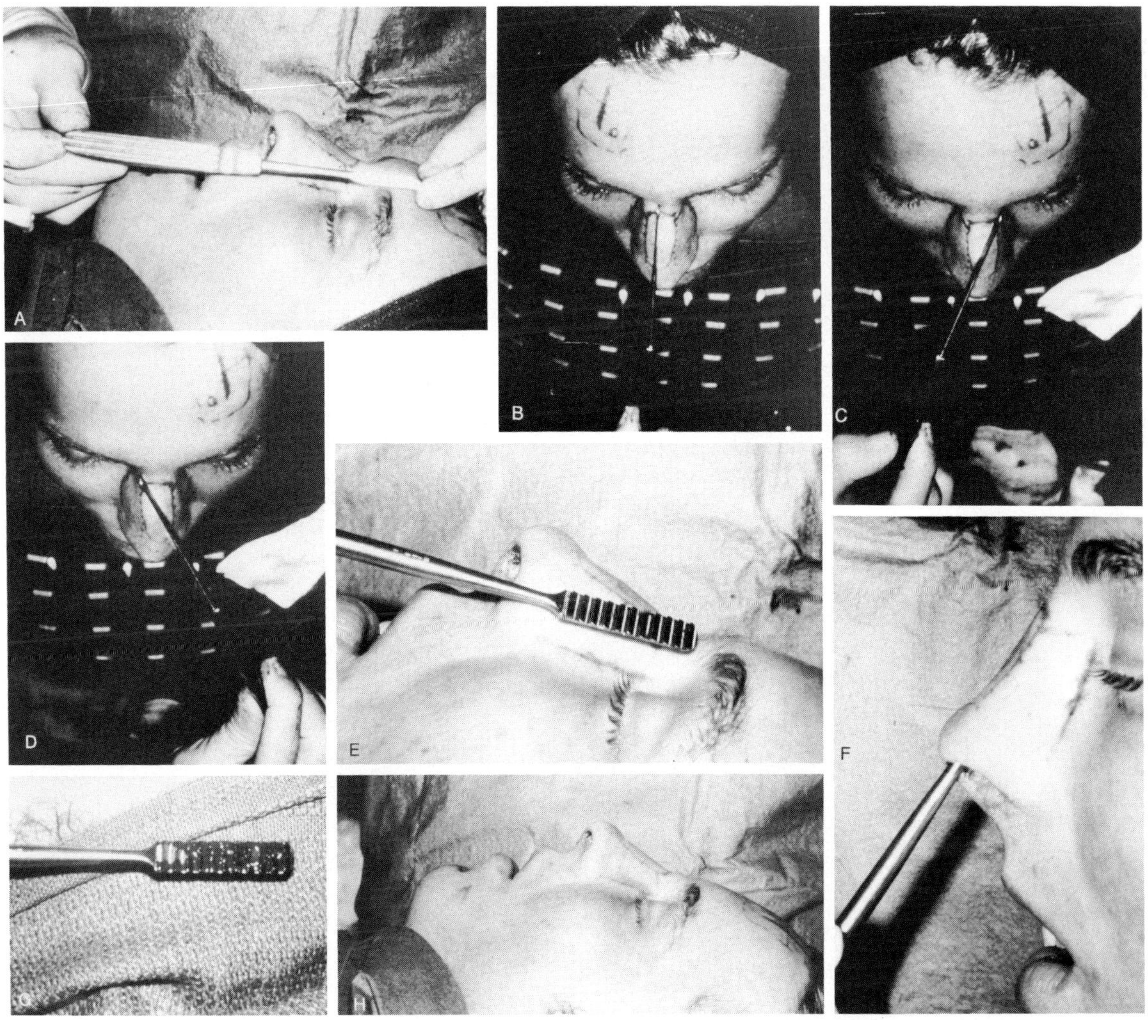

FIGURE 12–11. (*A*) A straight Joseph saw can be used to assist hump removal with a rasp. (*B*) A saw cut is made vertically into the cortical bone. (*C*) The saw is turned to make another angulated cut. (*D*) A third cut helps to produce a roughened surface for the rasp. (*E* and *F*) A large-toothed rasp is used first to remove most of the large hump. (*G*) Bone dust is inspected throughout hump removal. (*H*) Large humps can be removed predictably and quickly using this technique. *Illustration continued on following page*

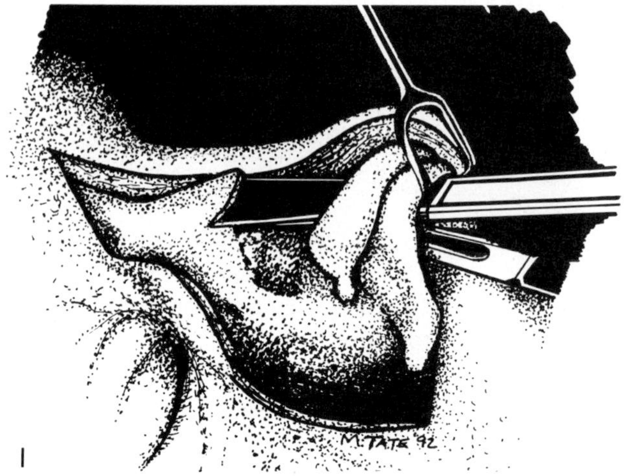

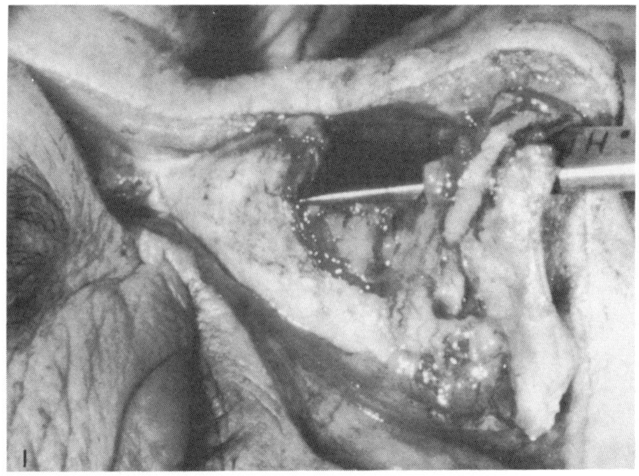

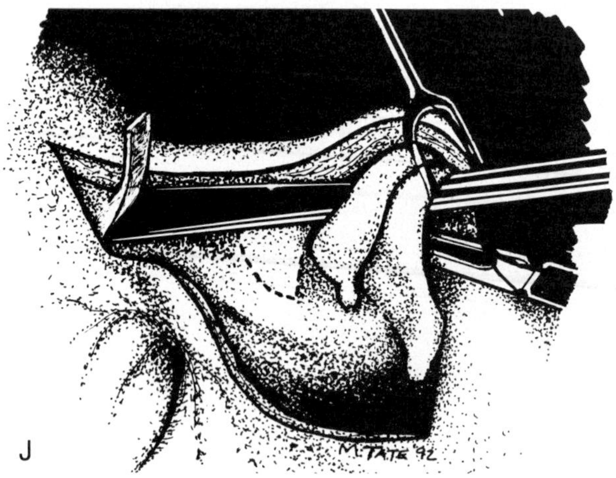

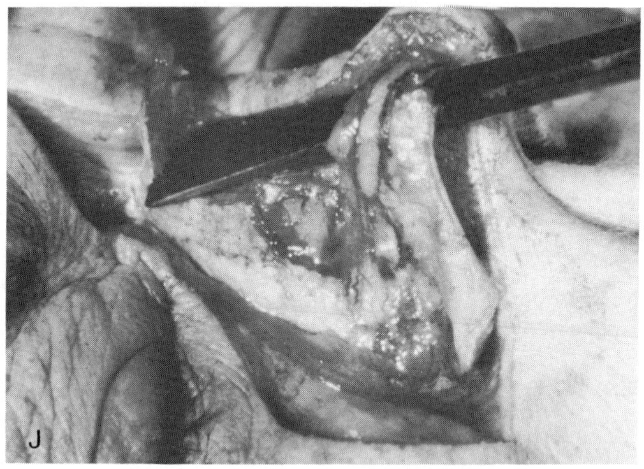

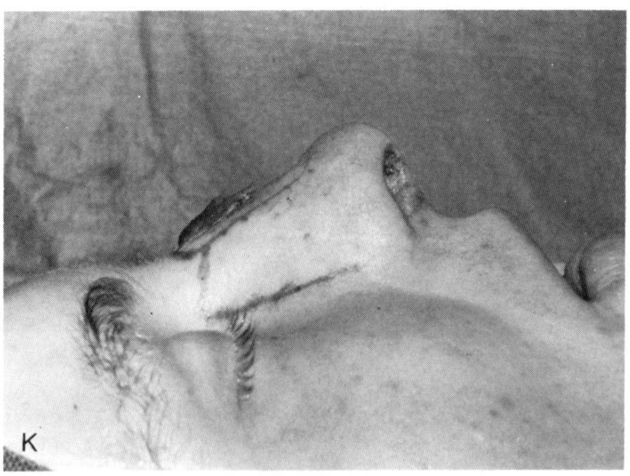

FIGURE 12–11 *continued.* (*I*) Initial cartilagenous lowering is begun with a no. 11 blade. (*J*) Final alignment of the cartilagenous dorsum is carried out with a no. 15 blade. (*K*) When the nasofrontal angle needs to be deepened, the osteotome can be directed into the region of the radix nasi. (*L1–4*) A sharp, flat osteotome engages the bony hump at the bony-cartilagenous junction.

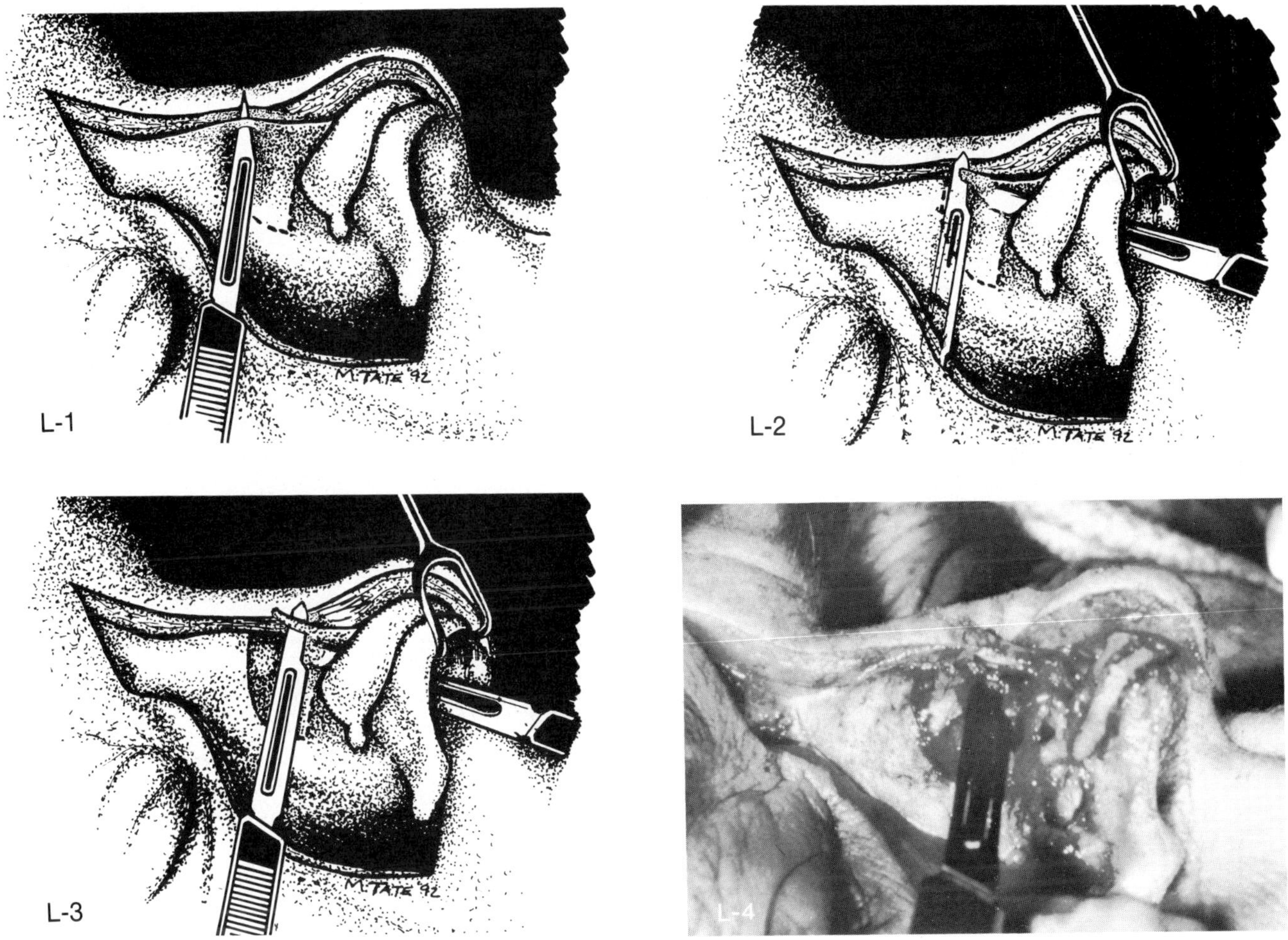

FIGURE 12–11 *See legend on preceding page*

Course rasps (no. 6 or no. 4) are preferred for the first few passes (Fig. 12–12). Honing can be completed with finer, diamond-type rasps (Figs. 12–13 and 12–14). Sharp rasps create less trauma and are, therefore, preferred.

Bone dust is created by rasping and should be totally removed. Residual osteocytes may survive and produce a postoperative deformity. Most debris can be removed by gently "sweeping" the undersurface of the dorsal nasal skin with a fine rasp.

OSTEOTOME TECHNIQUE

A sharp, wide osteotome may be used to remove larger humps. Initial subtotal removal is recommended with the osteotome. The remaining portion is removed with rasping.

Very large humps, particularly those that extend into the nasofrontal angle, can be removed as a single unit by incising the cartilagenous portion with a no. 11 blade and continuing the bony excision with an osteotome (Fig. 12–15). Rasps are preferred for removing the last millimeter or so of bone and for smoothing the bony dorsum.

It is risky to use an osteotome in a previously traumatized nose. The instrument usually follows the line of least resistance and may "dive" into an old fracture site, creating the need for reconstructive measures.

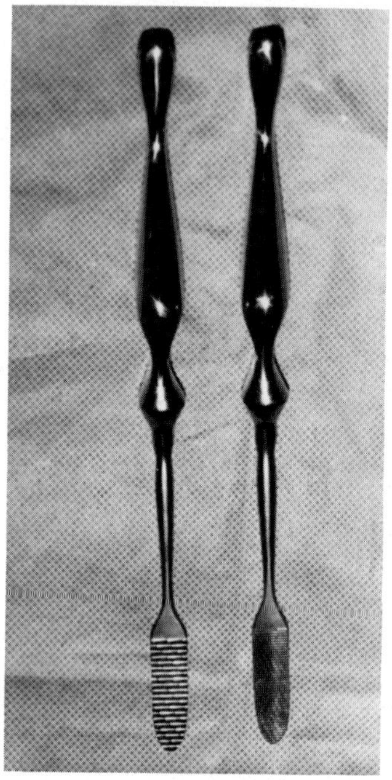

FIGURE 12–12. Nasal rasps should be sharp and designed for accuracy and control.

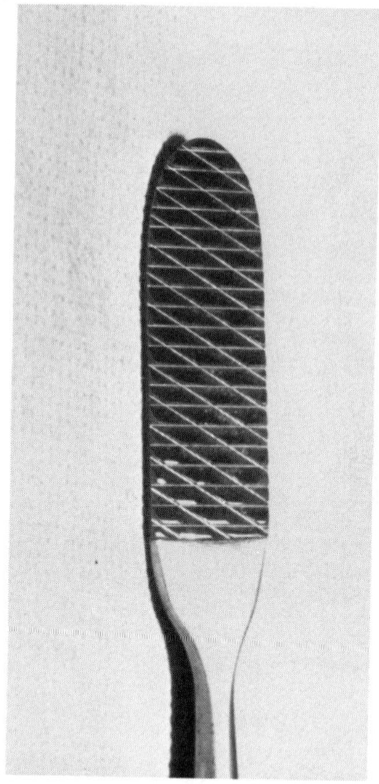

FIGURE 12–13. Coarser rasps are used on larger humps or for initial hump removal on smaller humps.

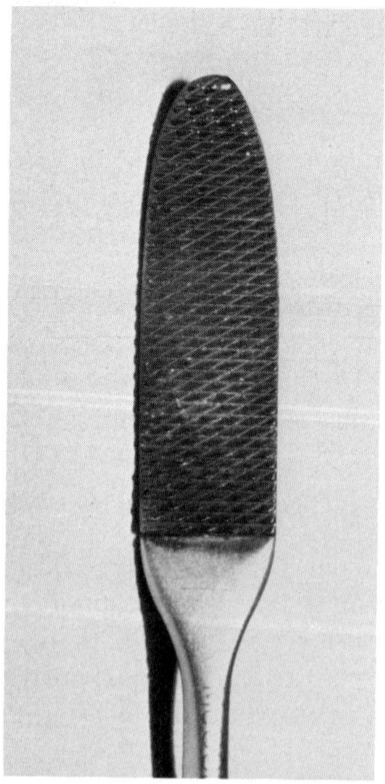

FIGURE 12–14. A more delicate rasp is used for providing the finishing touches and for rasping smaller bony irregularities.

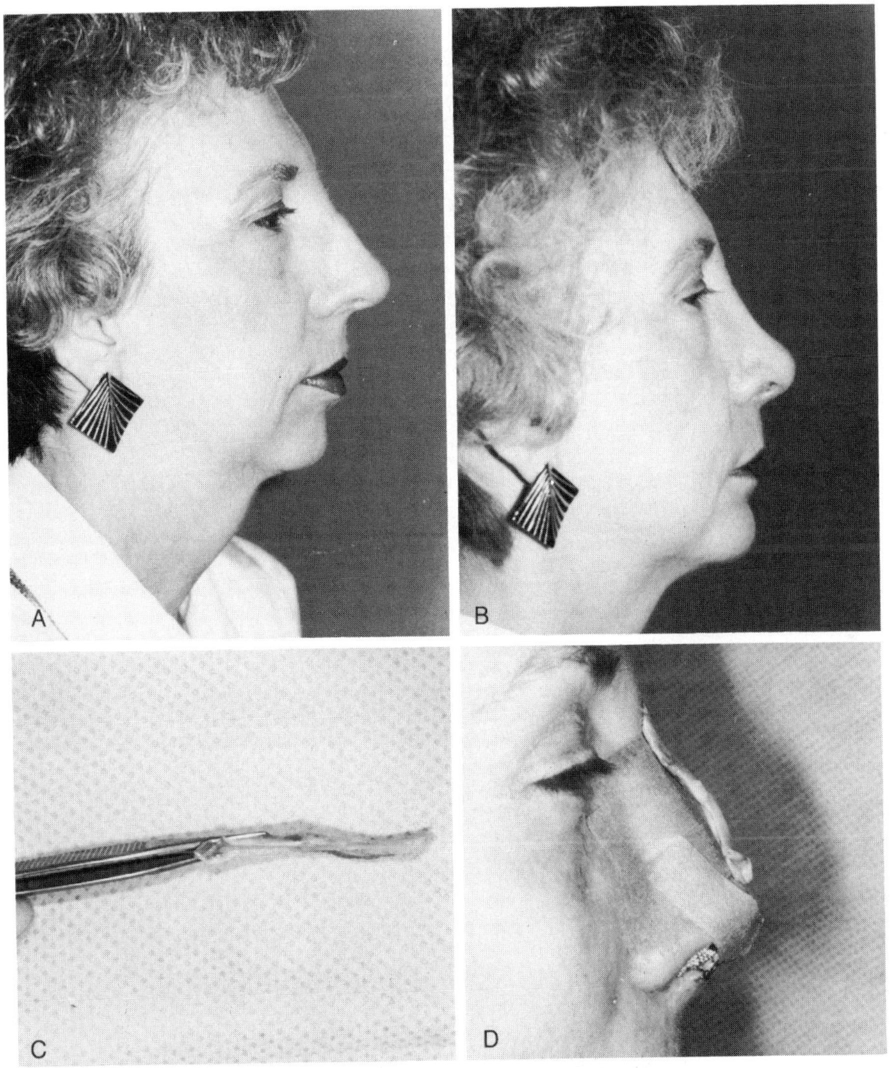

FIGURE 12–15. (*A* and *B*) Large bony humps that extend into the nasofrontal angle are best removed with an osteotome. (*C*) The bony and cartilagenous hump can be removed as a single unit. (*D*) All components of the hump are visible.

FLUSHING THE OPERATIVE FIELD

Visual inspection of the dorsum at the completion of hump removal is advisable. If rasping has been used in bony hump reduction, residual bone dust and debris should be removed. Although saline irrigations may be beneficial, this kind of debris usually can be removed by gently rasping the undersurface of the skin with a fine rasp.

If free osteocytes are left behind, they may survive, resulting in the appearance of an unexplained hump as postoperative swelling subsides. The same is true of loose fragments of cartilage or soft tissue, which can be identified at inspection.

FINAL NOTE

Final adjustments to the dorsum are best made toward the end of operation. Other steps in rhinoplasty might dictate some alterations in the dorsum (i.e., osteotomy, tip-plasty). Before the last sutures are placed and the dressings applied, a final inspection should be made.

Personal Communication

Simons, R.L. 1974–1992.

Suggested Reading

Denecke, H.J., Meyer, R. Rhinoplasty. New York: Springer-Verlag, 1976.
Rubin, F. F. The challenge of the nasal dorsum. Plastic and Reconstructive Surgery of the Head and Neck. Philadelphia: B. C. Decker, 1991, pp. 37–39.

CHAPTER 13

Mobilizing the Lateral Walls: Lateral and Medial Osteotomies

Numerous techniques have been described and myriad instruments developed to mobilize the lateral nasal walls. In this chapter, only the techniques I have used are described.

LATERAL OSTEOTOMIES

When a bony hump is removed, regardless of its size, lateral osteotomies should be performed. Otherwise, when swelling subsides, a flat, bony dorsum or an open-roof deformity will readily become apparent. Because I believe that elevating a periosteal tunnel reduces bleeding and minimizes postoperative edema and/or ecchymosis, this maneuver is always performed before lateral osteotomies (Fig. 13–1).

TECHNIQUE

A small incision is made perpendicular to the pyriform aperture at the anterior end of the right inferior turbinate with a no. 15 blade. The incision is carried through the mucosa and periosteum. Using a to-and-fro

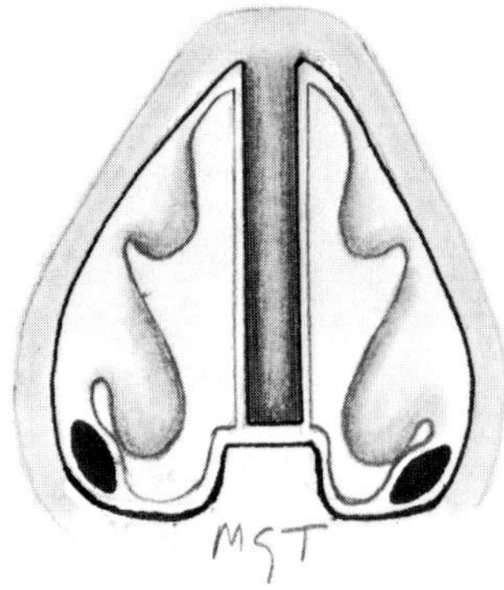

FIGURE 13–1. Subperiosteal tunnels are developed on the inner table of the bony vault for the osteotomy tract.

motion with the no. 15 blade, the periosteum on the undersurface of the frontal process of the maxilla is freed from the bones. A periosteal elevator (McCollough-Anderson) creates a subperiosteal tunnel on the medial surface of the frontal process of the maxilla and, more dorsally, the nasal bones (Fig. 13–2).

A guarded, straight Neivert osteotome is inserted into the pocket. An assistance gently strikes the blunt end of the osteotome with a surgical mallet while the surgeon directs the cutting end of the osteotome along the desired path. The surgeon's opposite hand palpates the edge of the osteotome as the assistant's mallet drives it cephalically (Fig. 13–3).

It is possible to create a desirable *curved osteotomy* with a straight osteotome. The surgeon must, however, steer the osteotome along the path of lesser resistance and direct it laterally as the instrument moves along its path toward the medial canthal region.

When the guarded end of the osteotome has reached the desired position (usually designated by a change in the resonance of the tapping sound), the surgeon then manually rotates the osteotome medially to create the desired back fracture, which should mobilize the lateral nasal walls. Manipulation with the thumb and index finger of the palpating hand can then "mold" the mobilized bones into their desired position.

It is essential that the lateral walls be completely mobile. Incomplete mobilization may lead to postoperative widening, resulting in either an open-roof deformity or, in the case of unilateral widening, a crooked nose.

After lateral osteotomies, if mobilization is not complete, a long, flattened instrument (no. 3 Bard-Parker surgical knife handle) can be placed inside the nose against the undersurface of the lateral walls and a force directed laterally (Fig. 13–4). Lateral displacement usually will complete the back fracture.

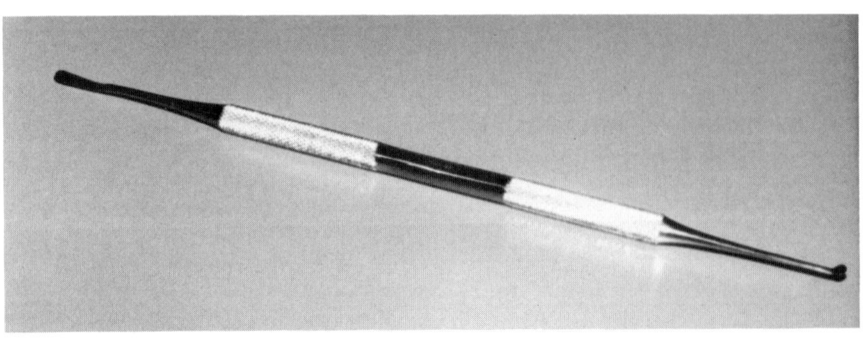

FIGURE 13–2. The McCollough-Anderson elevator has been designed to facilitate perichondrial-osteal elevation and to incise and remove septal cartilage.

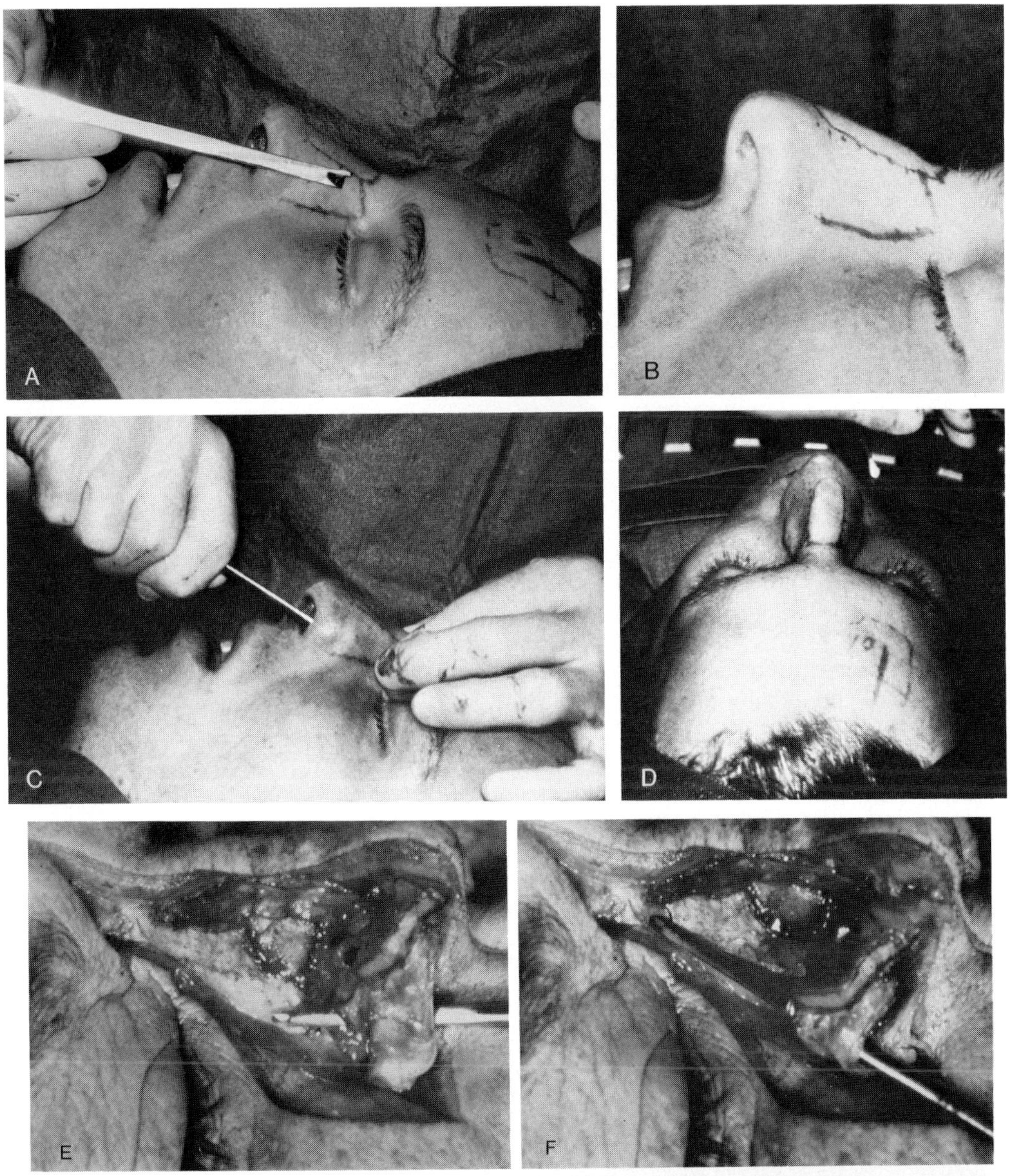

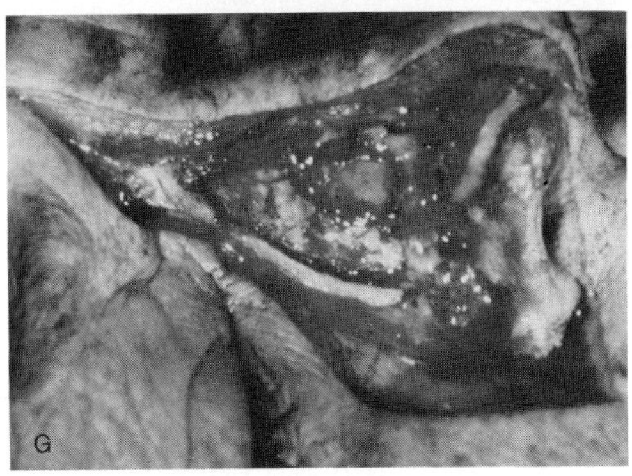

FIGURE 13–3. (*A*) A straight Neivert osteotome is used for lateral osteotomies. (*B*) The osteotome courses in the nasofacial groove until the solid bone of the radix nasi is encountered. (*C*) Rotation of the hand creates the back fracture. (*D*) The lateral wall must be mobilized and manipulated into its desired position. (*E*) Lateral osteotomy is begun at the pyriform aperture with a straight, guarded osteotome. The osteotome is carried dorsally to the solid bony portion of the radix nasi. (*F*) A natural medial osteotomy occurs from the lateral osteotomy's most cephalic extention to the superior extent of the bony hump removal. (*G*) The side walls of the nose are manipulated into their desired position with the thumb and index finger.

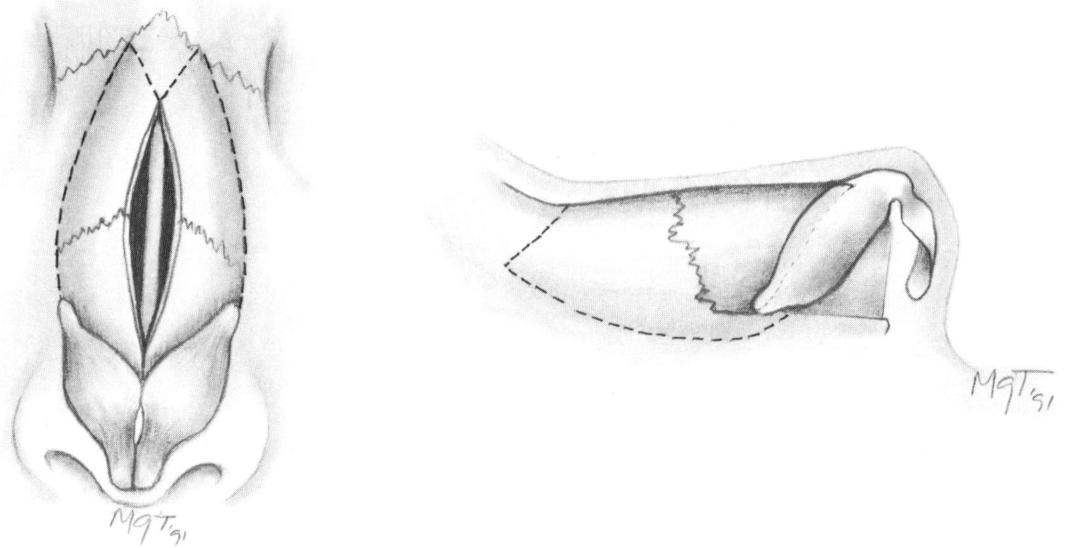

FIGURE 13–4. When lateral osteotomy is performed after hump removal, a back fracture (medial osteotomy) may be created by turning the osteotome medially or by directly creating the desired fracture line with a separate medial osteotomy maneuver.

It is imperative that initial greenstick fractures be completed; otherwise, the nasal bones tend to "float" laterally post operatively, resulting in an open-roof deformity (Fig. 13–5).

Excessive medially directed forces during mobilization of the lateral walls could inadvertently fracture the ethmoid bone or produce disarticulation at the ethmoid-quadrangular cartilage junction (rhinion). If this unfortunate event should occur, a saddle deformity would immediately appear. Reconstruction should take place at this time. If the closed technique is being used, the procedure should be converted to an external rhinoplasty, which provides panoramic visibility and ease of reconstruction (see sections on septal reconstruction and grafts and implants).

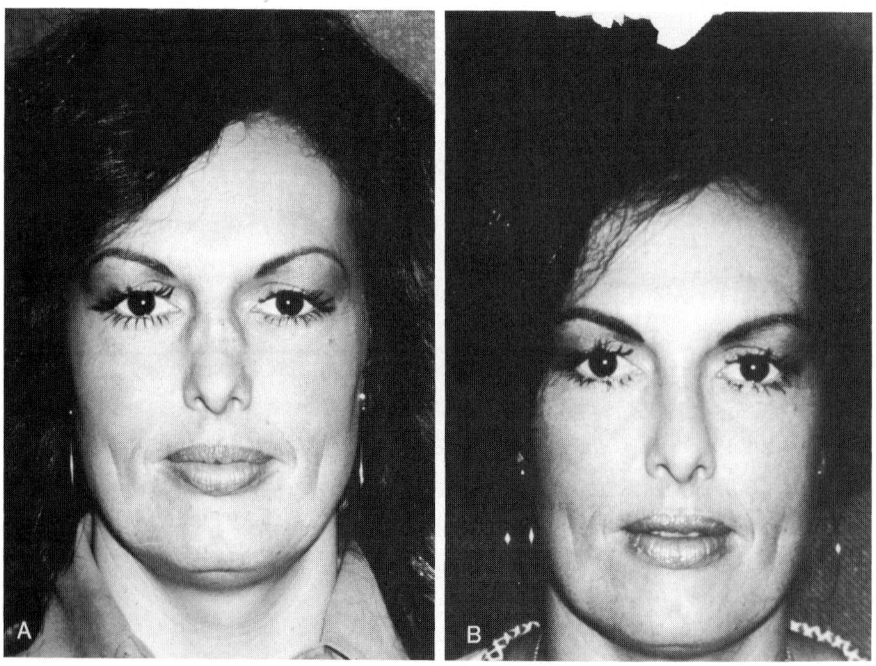

FIGURE 13–5. (*A*) Incomplete mobilization of the lateral walls can result in an open-roof deformity. (*B*) This is easily corrected by complete mobilization.

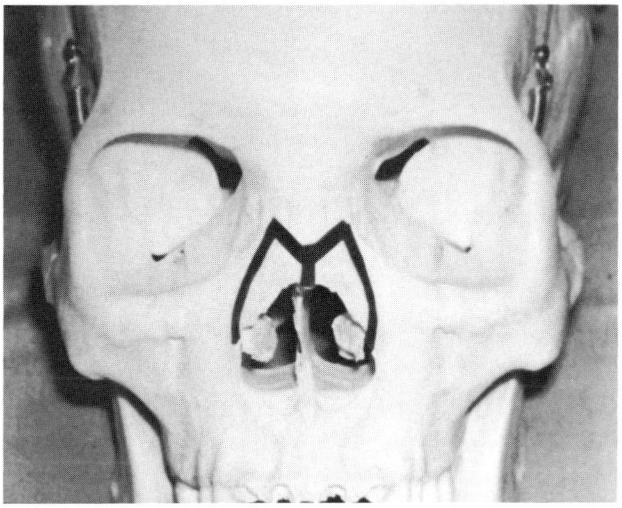

FIGURE 13–6. The lines of an ideal osteotomy are shown on the human skull.

MEDIAL OSTEOTOMIES

Medial osteotomies usually are not necessary—or desirable—when lateral osteotomies are performed as described above. When the bones are thick and not amenable to the techniques previously described, a "fading" medial osteotomy can be performed (Fig. 13–6). The tip of the osteotome is inserted into the nose adjacent to the dorsal aspect of the nasal septum on each side and then gently directed laterally toward, *but not to,* the medial canthus (Fig. 13–7).

A directed medial osteotomy might also be necessary in a nose that has previously received significant trauma resulting in comminution of the bony nasal complex. Like lateral osteotomy, the medial is performed with a straight, guarded Neivert osteotome. No additional periosteal or mucosal elevation is necessary.

TECHNIQUE

The osteotome is placed transmucosally at the junction of the ethmoid bone and the lateral bony wall. As an assistant taps the blunt end of the instrument, the surgeon directs the sharp end toward the medial canthus, but only for about 3 to 4 mm. It usually is not necessary to extend the

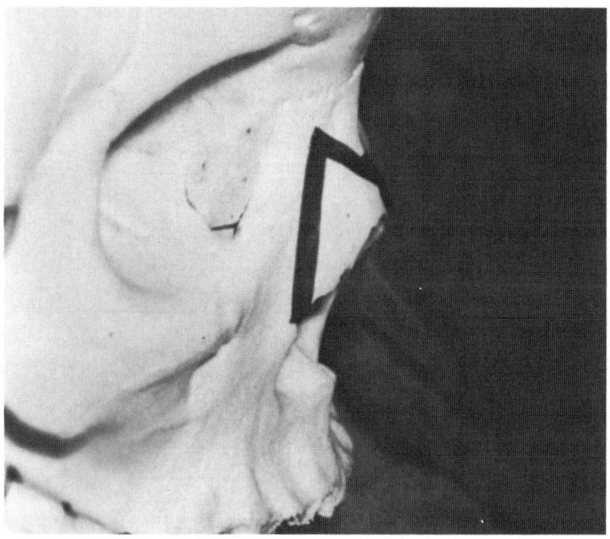

FIGURE 13–7. The osteotomy tract should be directed toward the medial canthus so as to intersect a real (or imaginary) line of the lateral osteotomy.

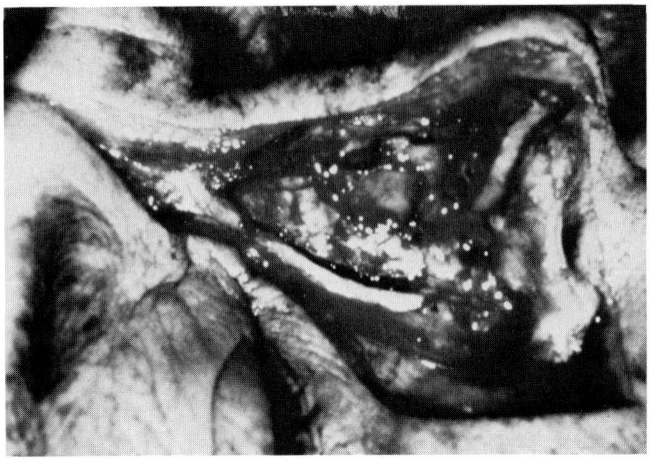

FIGURE 13–8. After osteotomy, the lateral nasal walls should be completely mobile and easily manipulated into their desired positions.

medial bone cut to join the lateral osteotomy (Figs. 13–8 and 13–9). Finger manipulation is less traumatic and should be effective once the medial track has been established.

Care must be taken to create identical radix angles as the osteotome travels laterally toward the medial canthus (Fig. 13–10). If an asymmetric radix is created with uneven cuts, the nose might appear crooked postoperatively. When an external or open technique is used, the medial osteotomy can be performed under direct vision.

In rare instances after medial and lateral osteotomy, the lateral walls still may not be completely mobilized. Special horseshoe-shaped instruments have been developed by Rubin and Quisling to help complete mobilization. A percutaneous osteotomy can also be performed with a 2-mm osteotome.

Inspection and palpation of the dorsum after mobilization is critical. Any irregularity must be addressed. After osteotomies and medial displacement of the lateral walls, the portion of the upper lateral cartilage that anatomically extends under the nasal bone usually springs upward. These portions can be trimmed with an angulated (Forman) scissors.

Dorsal irregularities of the central (ethmoid) complex can be gently rasped with a fine diamond-type rasp. Because they may provide an extra element of safety, rasps that cut on the forward stroke are recommended. The upward force tends to impact the mobilized elements against the more stable radix.

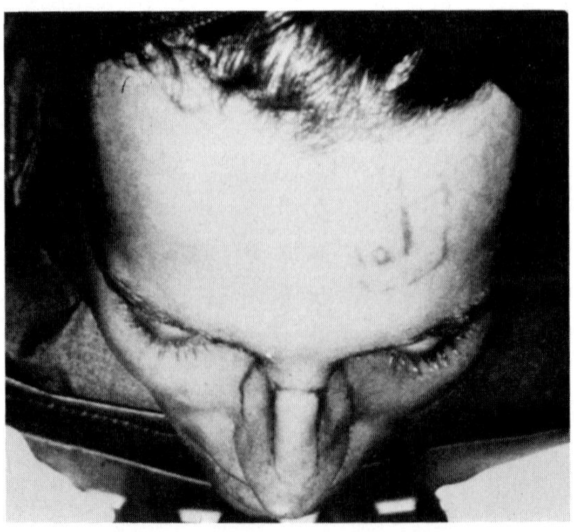

FIGURE 13–9. Both laterals are mobilized and placed in their desired positions.

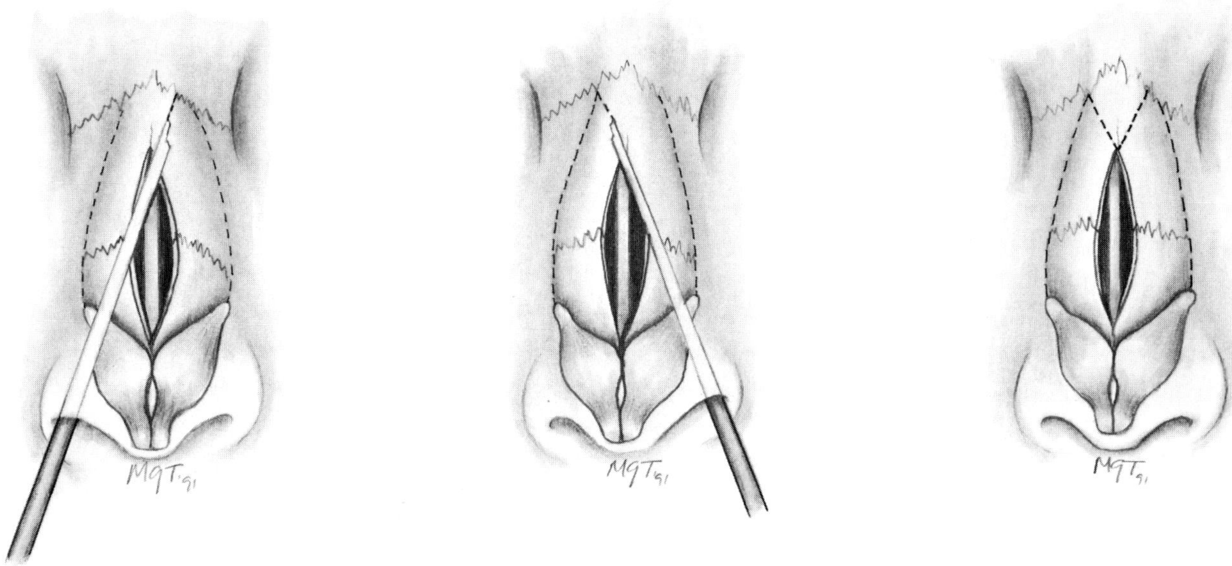

FIGURE 13–10. A directed medial osteotomy may be created with a straight Neivert osteotome.

Provided that the surgeon uses the thumb and index finger to temporarily stabilize them against the central (ethmoid) complex, small irregularities of the lateral walls can also be rasped. Unless performed cautiously and carefully, this maneuver could result in undue displacement (or avulsion) of the lateral walls. If the lateral bony wall inadvertently should become displaced, its position should be reestablished. Soft tissue fragments that are attached to the free elements can be sutured to surrounding tissues with 5-0 polyglycolic acid sutures. External rhinoplasty conversion might be necessary (see Ch. 15).

WHEN NO HUMP IS REMOVED

It is relatively easy to narrow a wide nose by mobilizing the lateral walls even when no hump has been removed or without medial osteotomies. If lateral osteotomies are performed as described, the back fracture seems to follow the desired path, eliminating the necessity of medial osteotomy (Fig. 13–11).

PERIOSTEAL ELEVATION

When periosteal elevation of the bony pyramid is carried out as previously described, an extra element of safety (against iatrogenic displacement) is built in.

For dorsal hump removal, the periosteum is elevated in continuity with the overlying skin and soft tissue, but only far enough laterally to allow for the introduction of rasps or osteotomies used to remove the bone (Fig. 13–12).

For lateral osteotomy, it is advisable to raise a periosteal tunnel on the medial surface of the lateral bony walls. By doing so, injury to the angular vessels may be avoided.

A significant periosteal attachment remains even when the lateral walls are mobilized; therefore, the possibility of undesirable and extreme medial displacement or collapse is minimized.

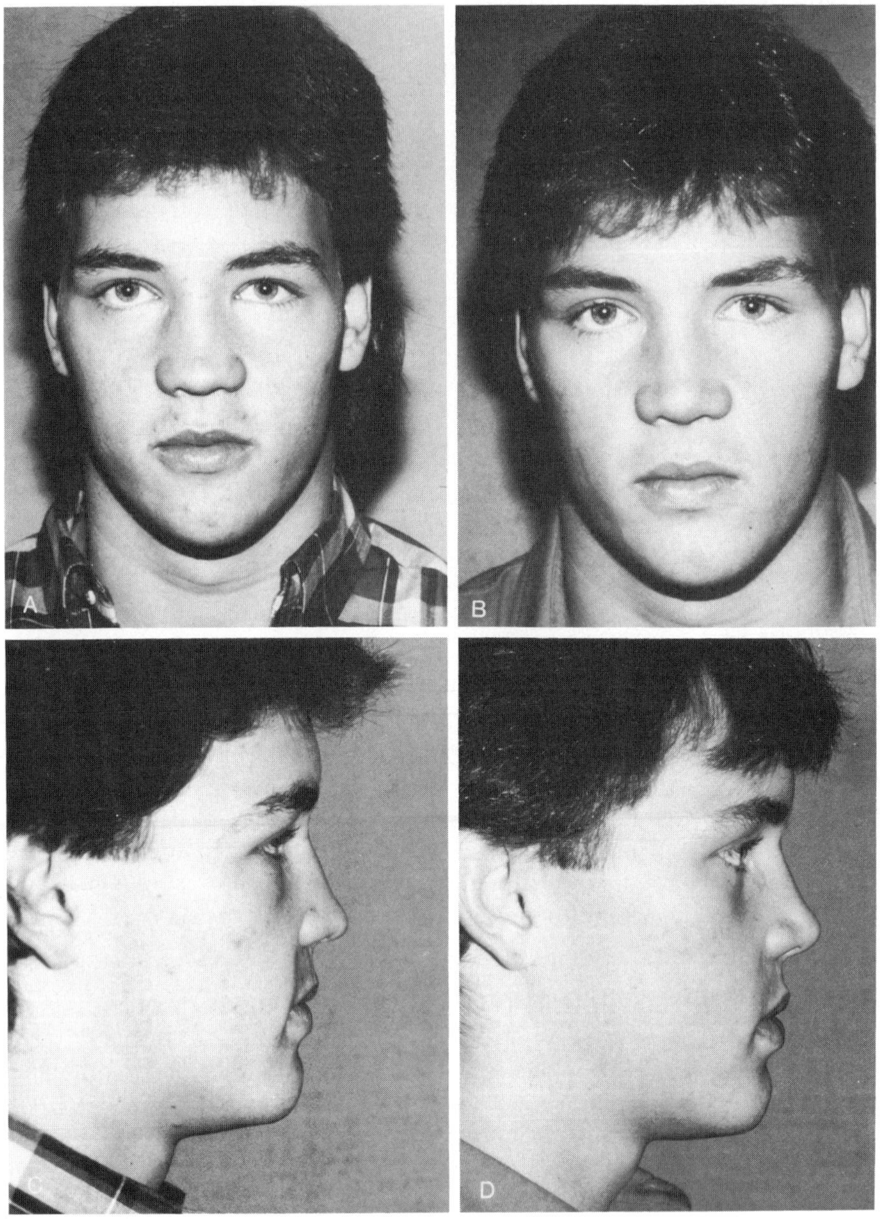

FIGURE 13–11. (*A* and *B*) In wide noses, it is desirable to narrow the pyramid with medial and lateral osteotomies. (*C* and *D*) Augmentation of the dorsum with morselized septal cartilage grafts may be necessary.

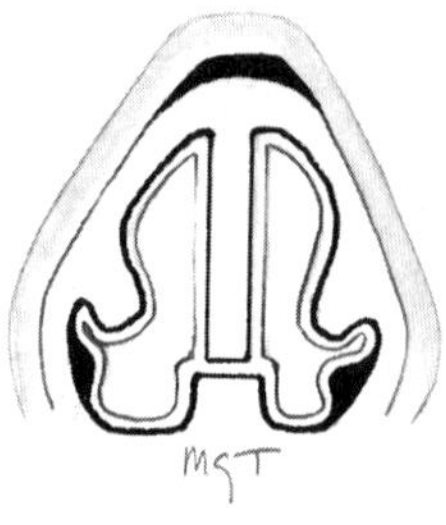

FIGURE 13–12. A periosteal tunnel is also elevated along the lateral osteotomy tract on the medial surface of the bony pyramid.

UPPER LATERAL CARTILAGES

Because the upper lateral cartilages constitute an integral portion of the cartilagenous pyramid, any significant cartilagenous hump removal detaches the cartilages from the septum. Unless the hump is extremely large, it usually is desirable to leave the mucosa intact at the septal–upper lateral cartilage junction. If redundant mucosa wells up in this space after hump removal and osteotomy mobilization of the lateral walls, the excessive mucosa can be removed with angulated (Forman) scissors (Fig. 13–13).

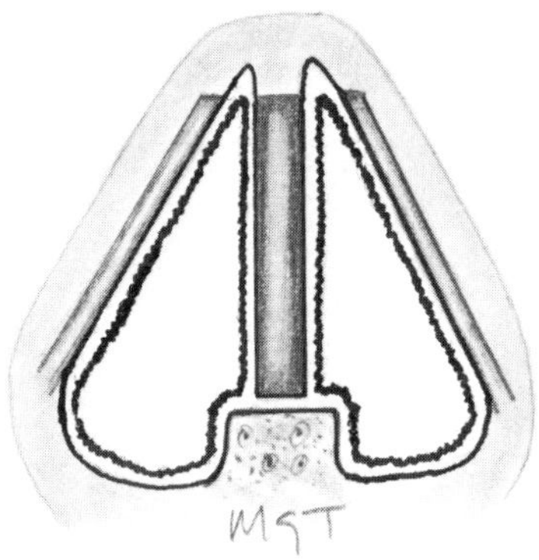

FIGURE 13–13. After hump removal, intranasal mucosa may herniate through the space between the septum and the upper lateral cartilages. If the herniation is excessive, the mucosa may be trimmed.

To help prevent scar tissue contraction and guard against valve incompetency, preservation of the mucosa is desirable in the valve area, even if some redundancy exists.

Junction tunnels usually are not necessary when the cartilagenous hump is removed as a composite (septum and both upper lateral components) with a no. 11 blade, as described in Chapter 9. Removing the cartilagenous hump in segments (i.e., septum first and upper lateral components independently) is not recommended.

When no hump is removed, it is desirable to narrow the cartilagenous vault; however, transmucosal separation of the upper lateral cartilage complex may be necessary. Even in these cases, the valve mucosa is preserved for the reasons previously stated. Transmucosal separation of upper lateral cartilages may be necessary in the platyrrhine-type nose when narrowing of the dorsum is desired.

Supratip definition may be enhanced by excising the prominent caudal "scroll" of the upper lateral cartilage. Preservation of the underlying mucosa is recommended (Fig. 13–14).

Except in long noses, when a significant amount of caudal septum must be excised, shortening of the upper lateral cartilages is not indicated. Only the amount of upper lateral cartilage that projects into the nasal vestibule after septal shortening should be excised. As a general rule, whenever cartilagenous removal of the upper lateral cartilage is carried out, mucous membrane is best preserved.

When final honing of the nasal dorsum is complete, the upper lateral cartilages should come to lie at the same height as the cartilagenous dorsum of the septum (Fig. 13–15). Excessive removal of upper lateral cartilages can lead to blunting of the intranasal angle created by the upper lateral cartilages and septum. Compromise of this angle can result in nasal valve incompetence.

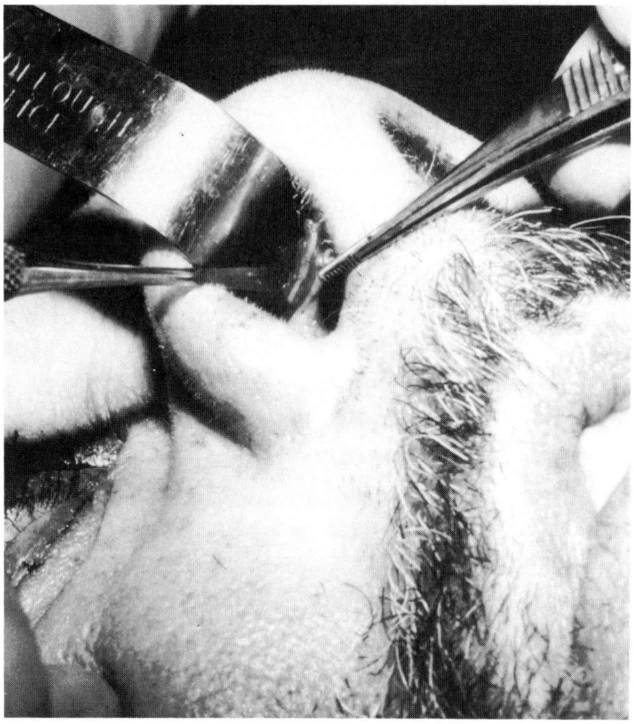

FIGURE 13–14. If excessively large, the scroll of the caudal border of the upper lateral cartilage may contribute to supratip fullness and may need to be excised.

If the upper lateral cartilages become introgenically separated from their attachment to the lateral nasal bony walls at any time during the operation, integrity should be established. Two small fenestrations can be bored in the nasal bones with an 18-gauge needle, so that the cartilage can be sutured to the bone (see Fig. 11–8). An external conversion might be necessary if this unfortunate event occurs.

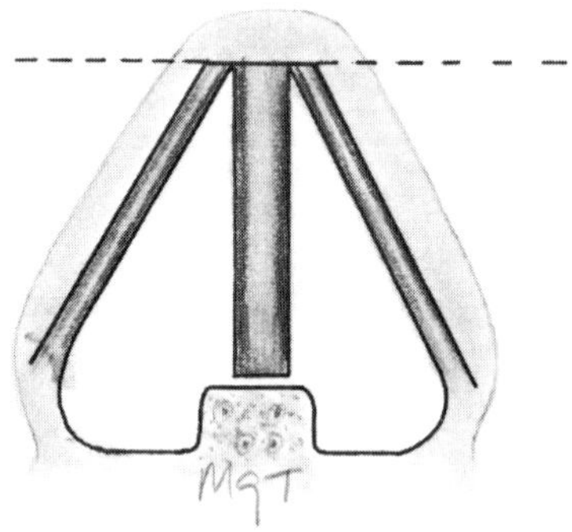

FIGURE 13–15. At the conclusion of operation the lateral walls of the nose should be in direct apposition to the perpendicular plate of the ethmoid, cephalically, and the cartilagenous septum, more caudally.

Suggested Readings

Denecke, H.J., Meyer, R. Rhinoplasty. New York: Springer-Verlag, 1976.

Rubin, F. F. Reconstruction of the bony nasal pyramid. Arch Otolaryngol 88:77–78, 1968.

Stucker, F. J. The nasal bony dorsum and cartilagenous, vault. Arch Otolaryngol 120:695–698, 1976.

CHAPTER 14

Surgery of the Nasal Tip

All great masters are chiefly distinguished by the power of adding a second, third, and perhaps a fourth step in a continuing line . . . with every additional step one enhances immensely the value of the first.

—Ralph Waldo Emerson

Most nasal plastic surgeons agree that surgery of the nasal tip is the most complex portion of rhinoplasty and the most difficult to master. Myriad factors, including the patient's age, sex, height, ethnic background, and skin quality, as well as strength of cartilages and asymmetry, dictate that each case be approached thoughtfully and systematically.

Each incision into (and excision of) nasal tissue results in an alteration in the structural framework of the nose that is countered by both an immediate and a delayed change in appearance. Failure to understand the effect each factor has on achieving the desired result leads to disappointment on the part of the patient and frustration on the part of the surgeon. Alterations to the nasal skeleton, when coupled with an understanding of anatomy, physiology, and the vagaries of healing, allow the surgeon-artist to achieve improved nasal tips not attainable by colleagues whose surgical armamentarium is limited (Figs. 14–1 and 14–2).

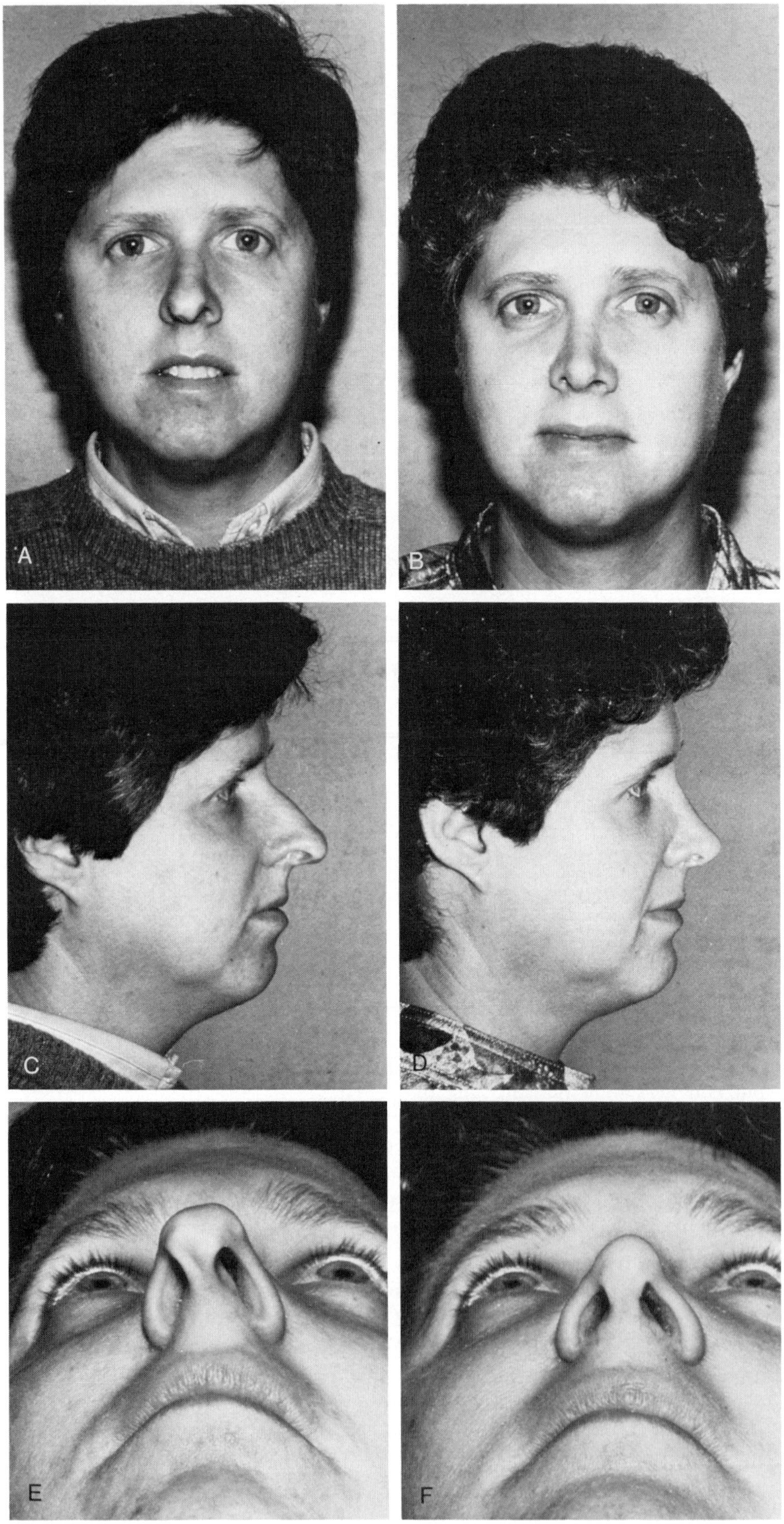

FIGURE 14–1. (*A* and *B*) Improvement in symmetry can be obtained by vertical dome division with suturing techniques. (*C* and *D*) An overly projected tip can be retrodisplaced by following the principles of the tripod concept. (*E* and *F*) Severely deformed, asymmetric tips may require aggressive treatment using most of the techniques in the surgeon's armanentarium. External rhinoplasty conversion is indicated.

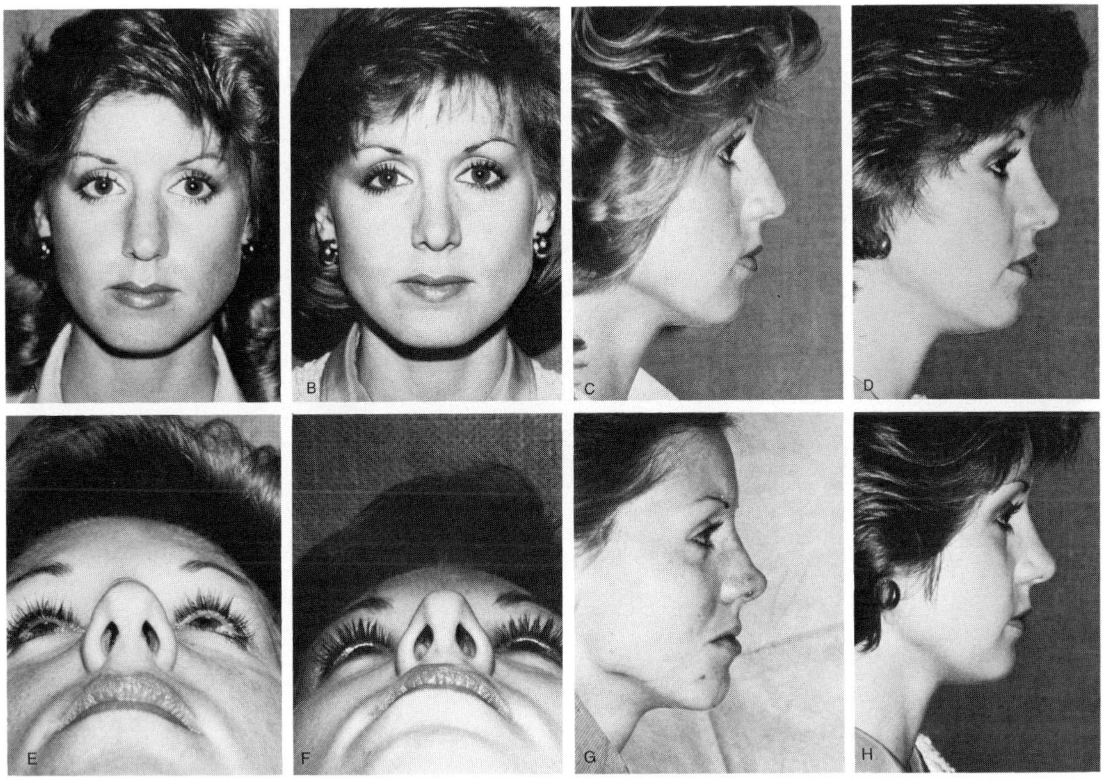

FIGURE 14–2. (*A* and *B*) When refinement is the surgical goal, the least amount of surgery that will produce the desired result should be performed. (*C* and *D*) Projection can be maintained when most of the elements of tip support are preserved. (*E* and *F*) A conservative complete strip with single dome suture fixation was all that was necessary in this patient. (*G*) At operation's end, the tip ought to appear overly projected and rotated. (*H*) As edema subsides and healing takes place over the subsequent 2 years, the tip settles into its final position.

The prudent surgeon recognizes when he has achieved the best result obtainable and then terminates the procedure. It has been said that "better is the enemy of good" (Morey L. Parkes, personal communication, 1974). In any operation, there exists a point of diminishing return; realizing when one has reached this point in a procedure comes with experience. And, in the critical eye of a perfectionist, "the ideal" is seldom achieved.

Knowing where to surgically place the nasal tip in relation to the dorsum at the conclusion of the operation is the key to obtaining predictable and acceptable results once healing has occurred. A number of factors, including swelling produced by local anesthetic injections and surgical insult generally, cause an artificial projection of the tip during surgery. Surgical maneuvers and suturing techniques also affect the operative appearance of the tip. Each surgeon must learn (in his hands) how much settling will take place within the ensuing months as healing occurs.

A good way to determine this is to take photographs at the end of the operation to accurately record the position of the tip in relation to the dorsum. Photographs also should be taken on follow-up visits at 3-month intervals for up to 24 months (Fig. 14–3).

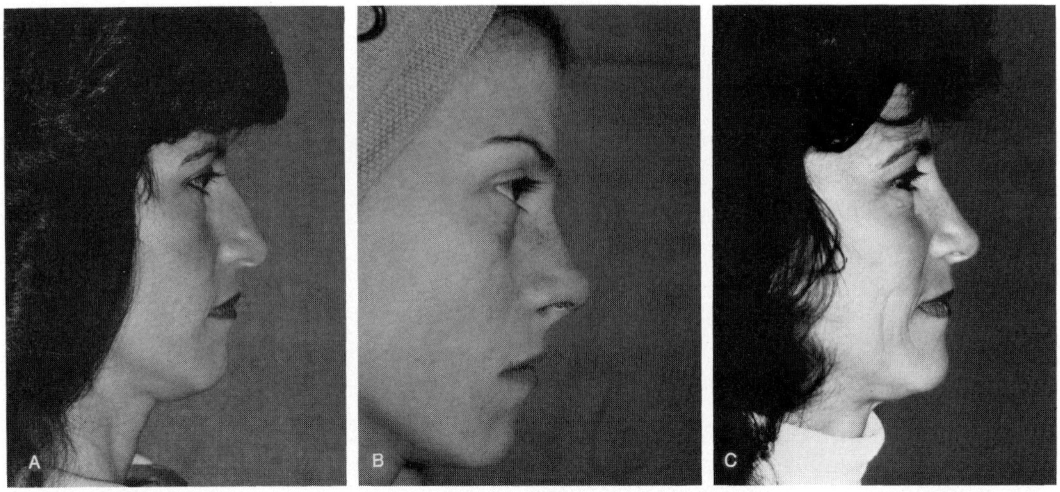

FIGURE 14–3. (*A*) Patient with tip ptosis. (*B*) At the end of the operation, the tip appears overly projected and rotated, partly because of swelling. (*C*) As healing progresses, the tip assumes its final position. The photo is taken 10 years postoperatively.

WHERE TO BEGIN

Conservative tip techniques are recommended for less-experienced surgeons and in noses that require minor modification. Geometric excisions and creative maneuvers are best avoided. I advocate a classic lower lateral cartilage delivery approach to tip-plasty.

After marginal and intracartilaginous incisions have been made, bipedical vestibulochondrial flaps can be developed with blunted scissors dissection. Cartilage delivery and inspection can then be achieved (Fig. 14–4).

The complete strip technique is the workhorse of conservative tip-plasty. Only the cephalic margins of the alar cartilages are excised. As the surgeon gains experience and comes to understand the complex dynamics of tip surgery, he might progress to more complex techniques. A comprehensive knowledge of anatomic variations in the alar cartilages and mastery of the various tip techniques could convert what might be considered a difficult tip-plasty to one that can be managed with relative ease and predictability.

Incisions should not limit or dictate which technique a surgeon might select. Most of the surgical maneuvers presented in this chapter can be performed through closed rhinoplasty.

SURGICAL PROGRESSION

Nasal tip surgery is a surgical progression (Fig. 14–5). This progressive concept affords the surgeon the opportunity to recognize when he has reached the peak of the plastic surgery risk-benefit curve (Fig. 14–6). A number of individual factors, however, may cause the surgeon to modify his plan. At any point in the progressive system when the desired result has been achieved, the tip-plasty should be terminated. Excessive strength or weakness of cartilage, skin thickness, and cartilaginous asymmetries may limit the success of appropriately performed classic technical maneuvers and dictate innovation.

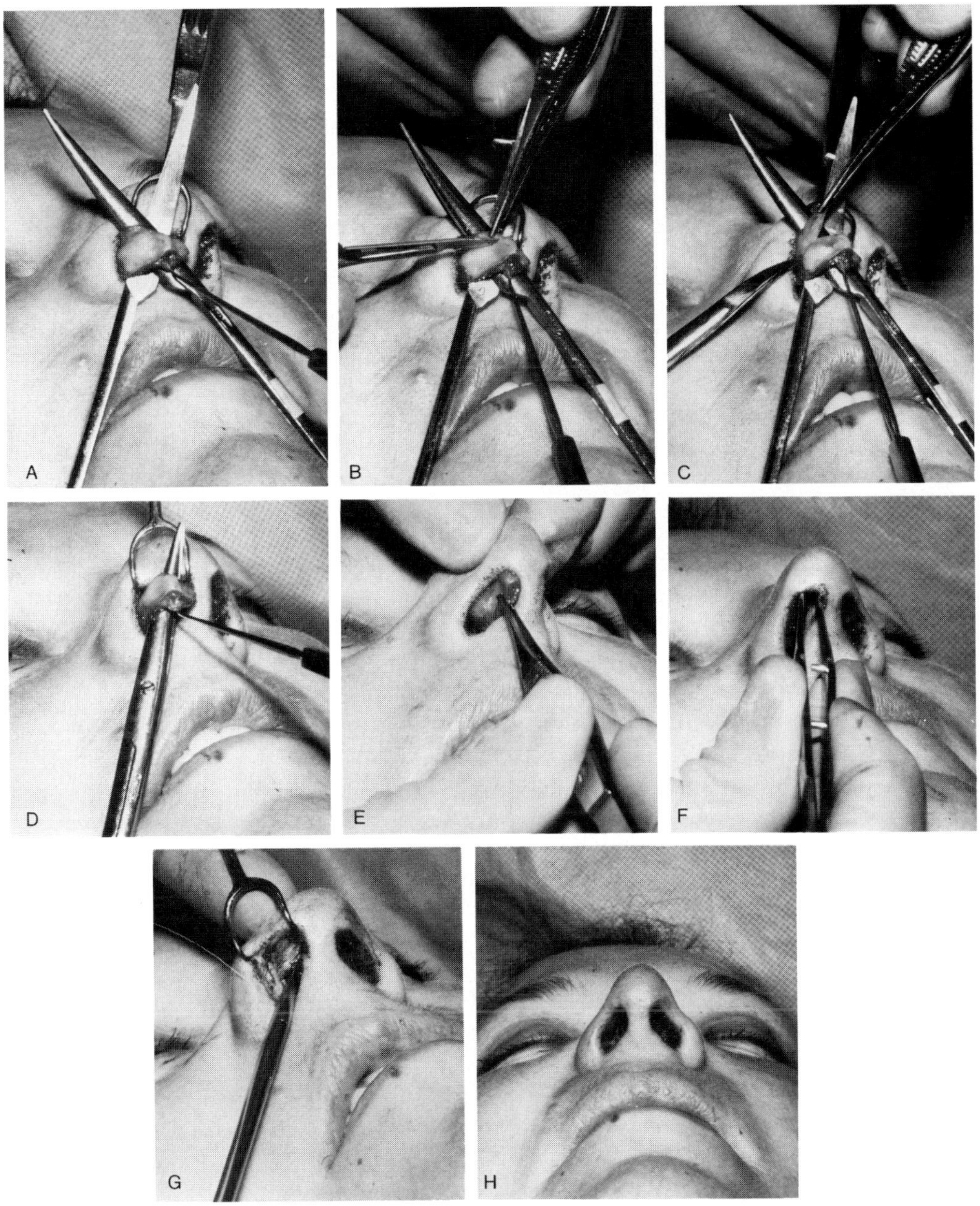

FIGURE 14–4. (*A*) After marginal and intercartilaginous incisions, the alar cartilage is delivered as a bipedical chondrocutaneous flap and the anatomic landmarks carefully and accurately identified. (*B* and *C*) Horizontal excision of the appropriate amount of lateral crus is performed, preserving the underlying vestibular skin. (*D*) It usually is advisable to leave at least a 4- to 6-mm wide complete or uninterrupted segment of lateral crus behind. (*E* and *F*) The remaining chondrocutaneous flap is placed back into its normal anatomic position and the degree of tip refinement is accessed. (*G*) Two 5-0 plain catgut sutures are used to close the marginal incisions. (*H*) When both alar cartilages have been modified, the lobule is inspected for symmetry. In many cases, nothing else need be done to the tip cartilages.

- Alar reconstruction (grafts)
- Dome division ("I" beam and sandwich grafting)
- Dome division
- Double dome scored unit
- Double dome intact unit
- Single dome intact unit
- Complete strip

FIGURE 14–5. Tip surgery progression.

Tommy Armour, a professional golfer, advised: "It's O.K. to scramble as long as one knows how to scramble." Armour's statement also applies to nasal plastic surgery. When more complex reconstructive techniques are indicated, an external approach might provide the additional exposure needed to facilitate correction. External rhinoplasty is particularly useful in noses with grossly asymmetric alar cartilages, augmentations, and revisions.

A fact often overlooked by surgeons debating open versus closed rhinoplasty is that the open approach is merely an extension of the closed approach. The classic "delivery" procedure can be converted to an external rhinoplasty at any time during the operation. The surgeon simply makes another incision in the surgical progression by connecting the two marginal incisions at or about mid-columella (Figs. 14–7 and 14–8). The transcolumellar incision, like the marginal, limen vestibuli, and septal incisions, provides additional exposure to the nasal skeleton.

Unlike other nasal incisions, however, the transcolumellar incision does nothing to alter the physical shape of the nose. An inverted V incision made at mid-columella where the skin is thin follows the aesthetic contours of the nasal tip and seems to produce the least conspicuous scar.

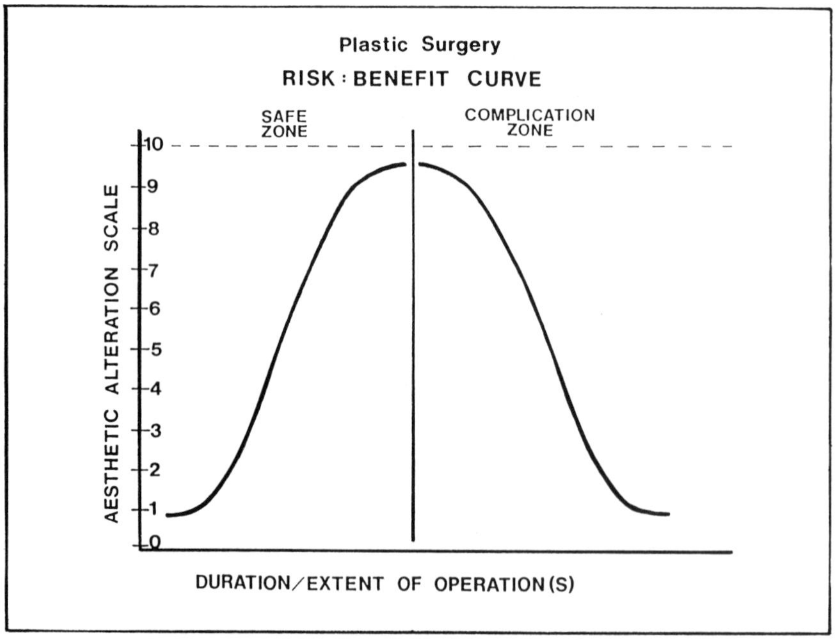

FIGURE 14–6. In any surgical adventure, one reaches a point at which one passes beyond the safe zone and into the complication zone.

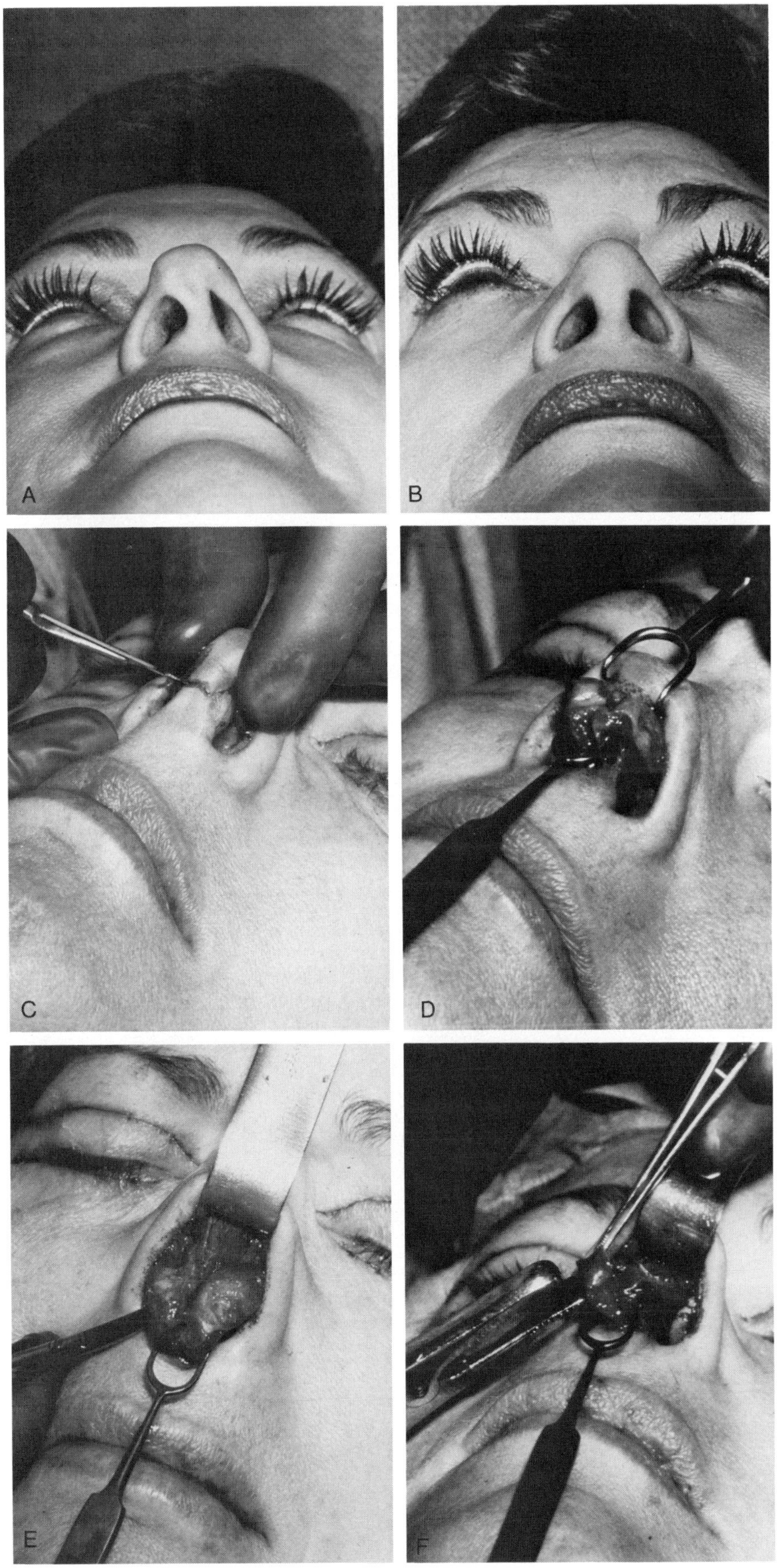

FIGURE 14–7. (*A* and *B*) When the tip cartilages are grossly asymmetric, an external conversion allows for more accurate assessment and correction. (*C*) External conversion can be achieved when previously made marginal incisions are connected with the inverted V transcolumellar incision. (*D*) A panoramic view of the tip cartilages often reveals irregularities and asymmetries not visible with more conventional techniques. After the transcolumellar incision, the tip skin can be lifted and retracted. (*E* and *F*) Abnormal configurations of the domes and the medial and lateral crura may be gently morselized and supported with cartilaginous grafts fashioned from the septum or from excised cephalic portions of the lateral crura. *Illustration continued on following page.*

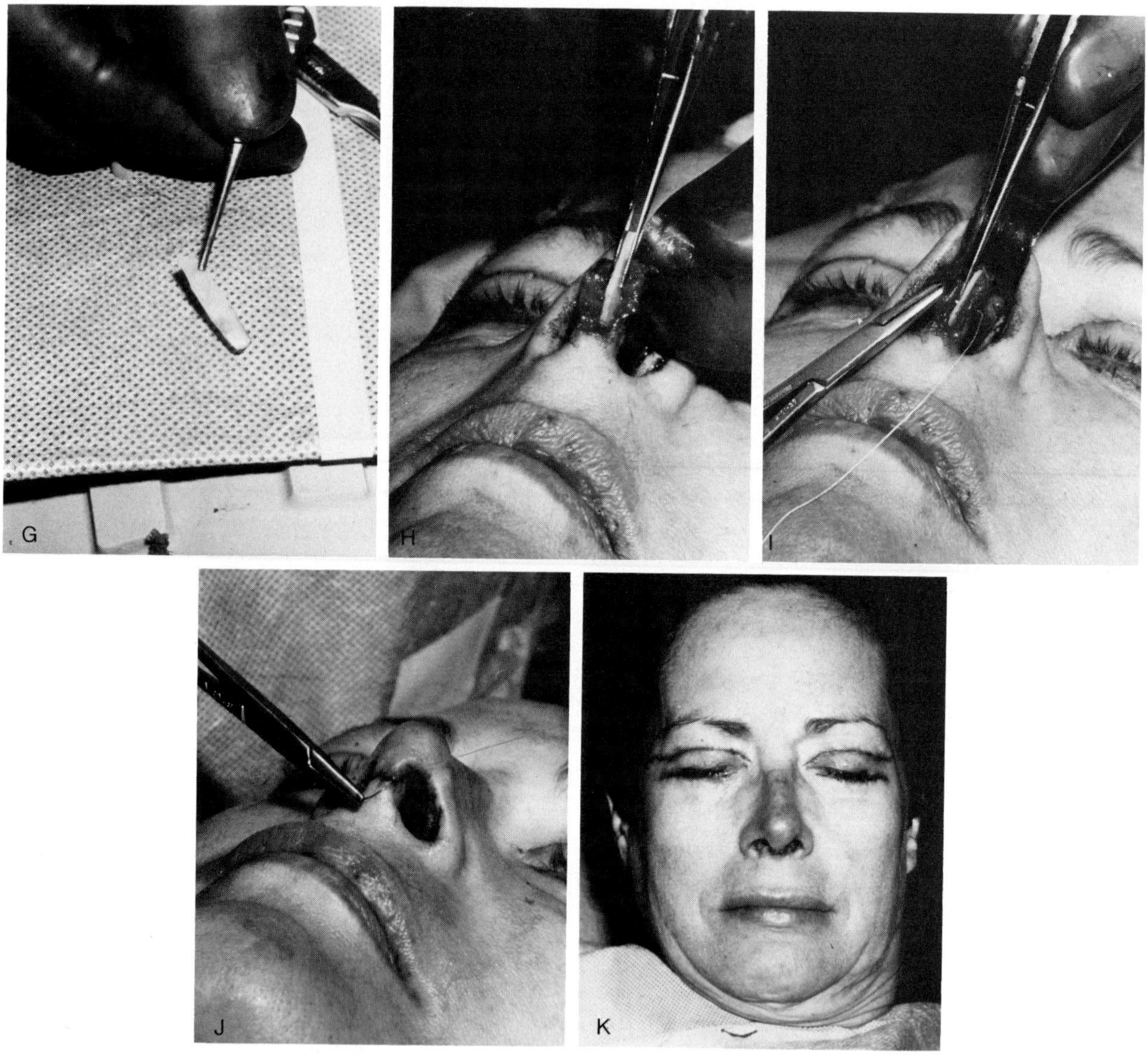

FIGURE 14–7 *continued.* (*G* and *H*) Cartilaginous grafts can be sutured to the morselized crura in a horizontal mattress manner with Vicryl sutures. (*I* and *J*) The transcolumellar incision is carefully closed (using magnification) with 6-0 fast-absorbing catgut sutures. (*K*) The result.

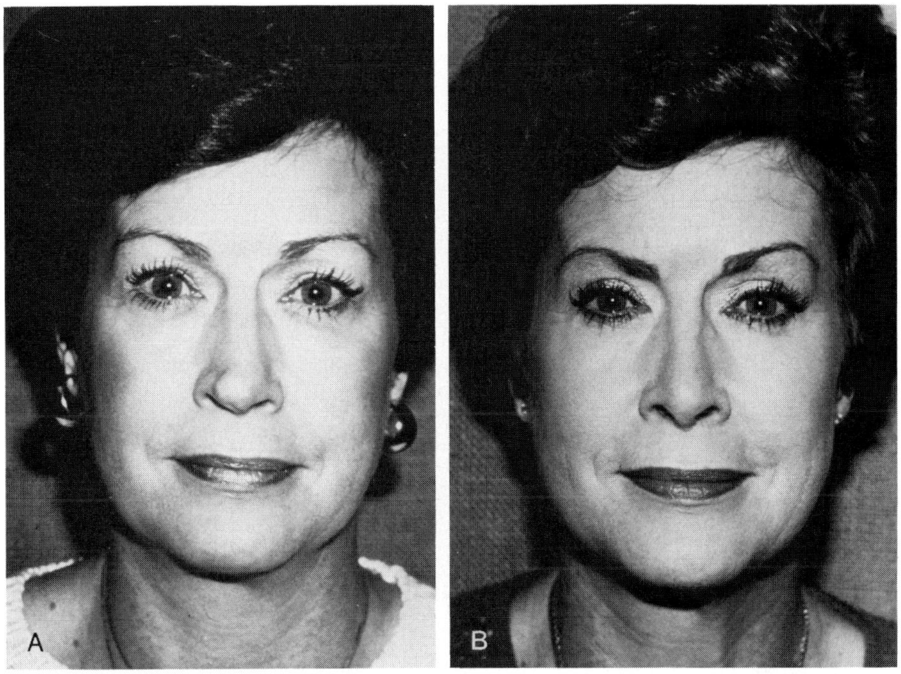

FIGURE 14–8. One year postoperatively the reconstructed tip cartilages have maintained the correction achieved intraoperatively. The transcolumellar scar can be seen in *B*.

ANATOMIC FACTORS

Understanding nasal architecture and the forces of dynamic and static anatomy are essential to predictable rhinoplasty. There are four principal factors that contribute to the position of the nonoperated nasal tip as it relates to other nasal and facial features (Fig. 14–9).

1. The attachment of the feet of the medial crura to the caudal margin of the nasal septum. Obtaining access to the nasal septum with incisions at the caudal end of the nasal septum may destroy one of the most important elements of tip support. If possible, the surgeon should avoid detaching the feet of the medial crura from the caudal border of the nasal septum.

Text continued on page 158

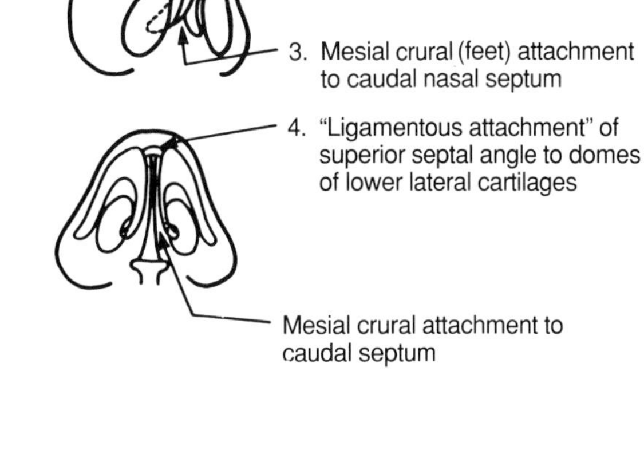

FIGURE 14–9. Principal anatomic factors of tip support.

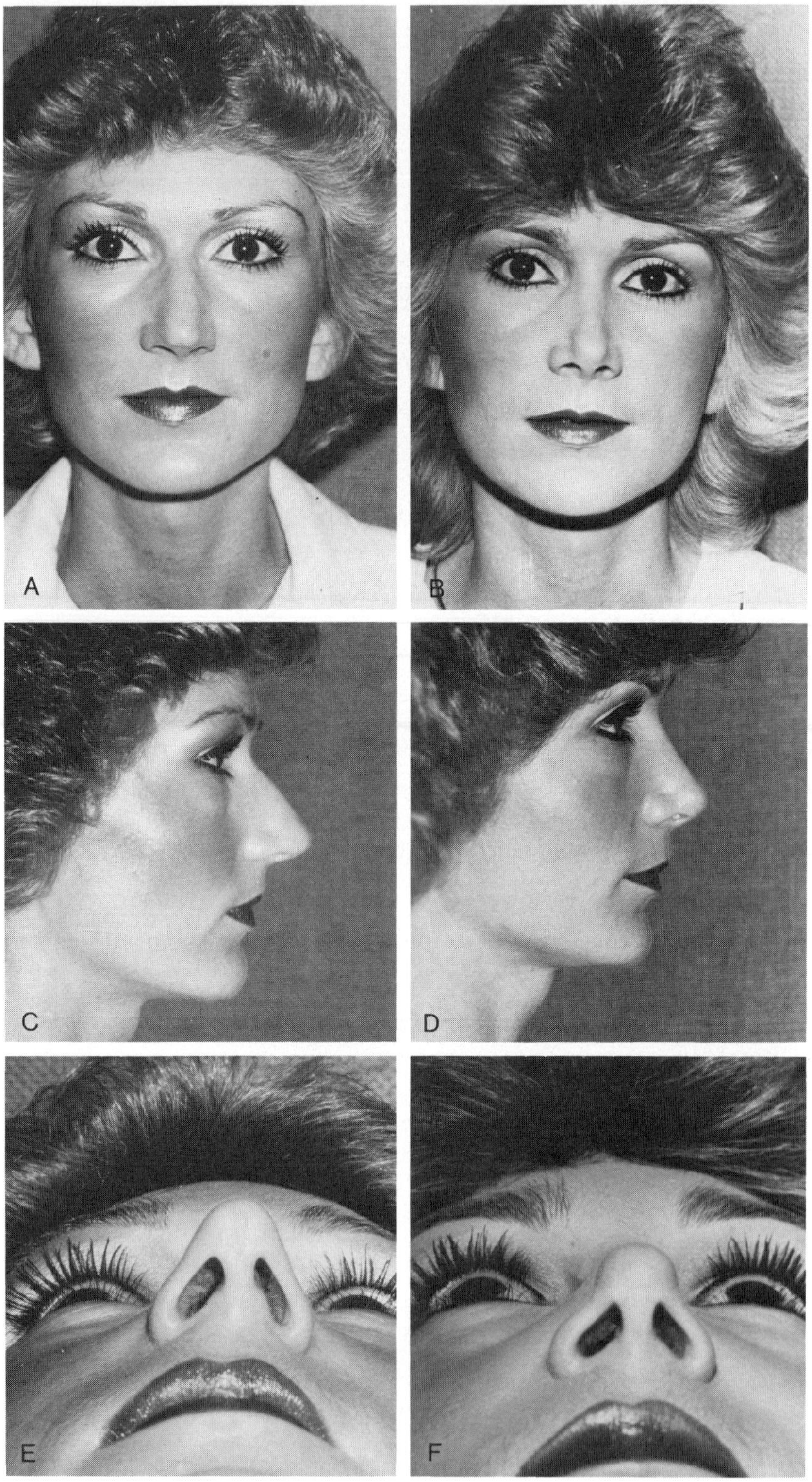

FIGURE 14–10. (*A* and *B*) Overly projecting tips may be retrodisplaced by shortening the cartilaginous legs of the tip tripod or interrupting their supporting mechanisms, or both. (*B* and *C*) When tip retrodisplacement maneuvers are carried out, the feet of the medial crura usually settle until they come to rest at the base of the columella. (*E* and *F*) No significant degree of alar flaring occurred in this patient.

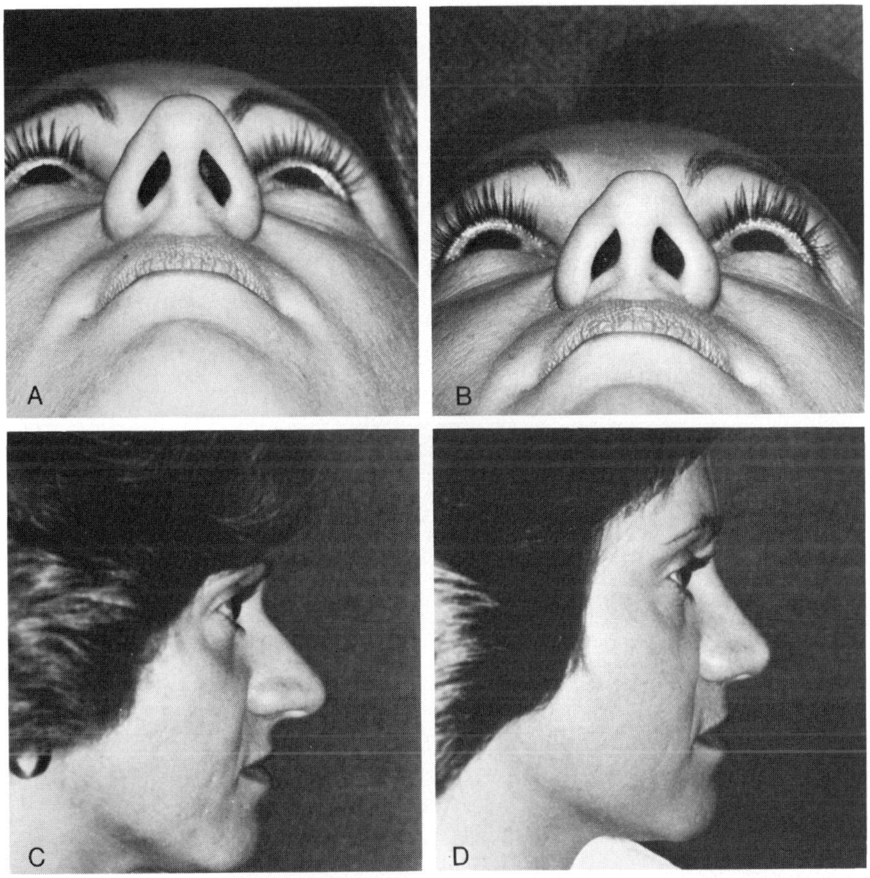

FIGURE 14—11. As is generally the case, when tip retrodisplacement occurs the alae flare, requiring alar sil resections. (Retrodisplacement at the overly projected tip was achieved by complete transfixion incision and rim strip tip technique.)

In the overly projected nose, the surgeon may want to reduce tip projection (Figs. 14–10 and 14–11). Incisions and/or excisions that disrupt the interlocking attachments of the skeleton of the nasal tip can be used to the surgeon's advantage in such cases. Tip retrodisplacement maneuvers are discussed in more detail in the next section.

2. The telescoping relation of the interlocking scrolls of the upper and lateral cartilages.

When a limen vestibuli incision is made and any portion of the cephalic border of the lateral crural component of the alar cartilage is removed, the interlocking relationship of the lower lateral cartilages to the upper lateral cartilages is disrupted.

3. The length, size, strength, and vector of the torque produced by the two lateral crura. The length, strength, and shape of each lateral crus produce forces that project the tip of the nose, both caudally and dorsally, away from the pyriform aperture. Removal of portions of the lateral crus weakens this anatomic girder and invites tip retrodisplacement and, to a lesser degree, tip ptosis.

4. The fibrous sling (Pitanguy's ligament) connecting the undersurface of the nasal skin and dorsal septum to the posterior margins of the domes of the lower lateral cartilages (Fig. 14–12). Dissection over the nasal dorsum and delivery of the alar cartilages interrupts the suspensory fibers of Pitanguy's ligament.

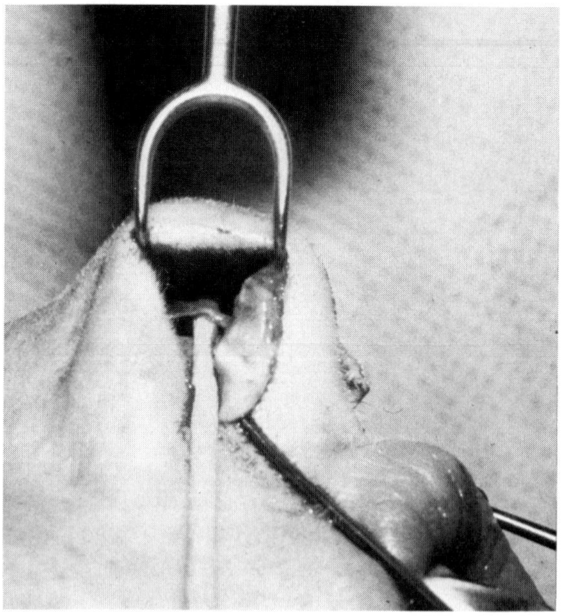

FIGURE 14–12. The ligamental attachment that connects the undersurface of the dorsal nasal skin with the cephalic border of the lower lateral cartilages is clearly identified in this patient.

TIP ROTATION AND PROJECTION: TRIPOD CONCEPT

In the early 1970s, Anderson popularized the tripod concept of tip rotation and projection.[1] It was a breakthrough in tip-plasty. Understanding the interactions of this anatomic tripod is a prerequisite to grasping the dynamics of tip modification.

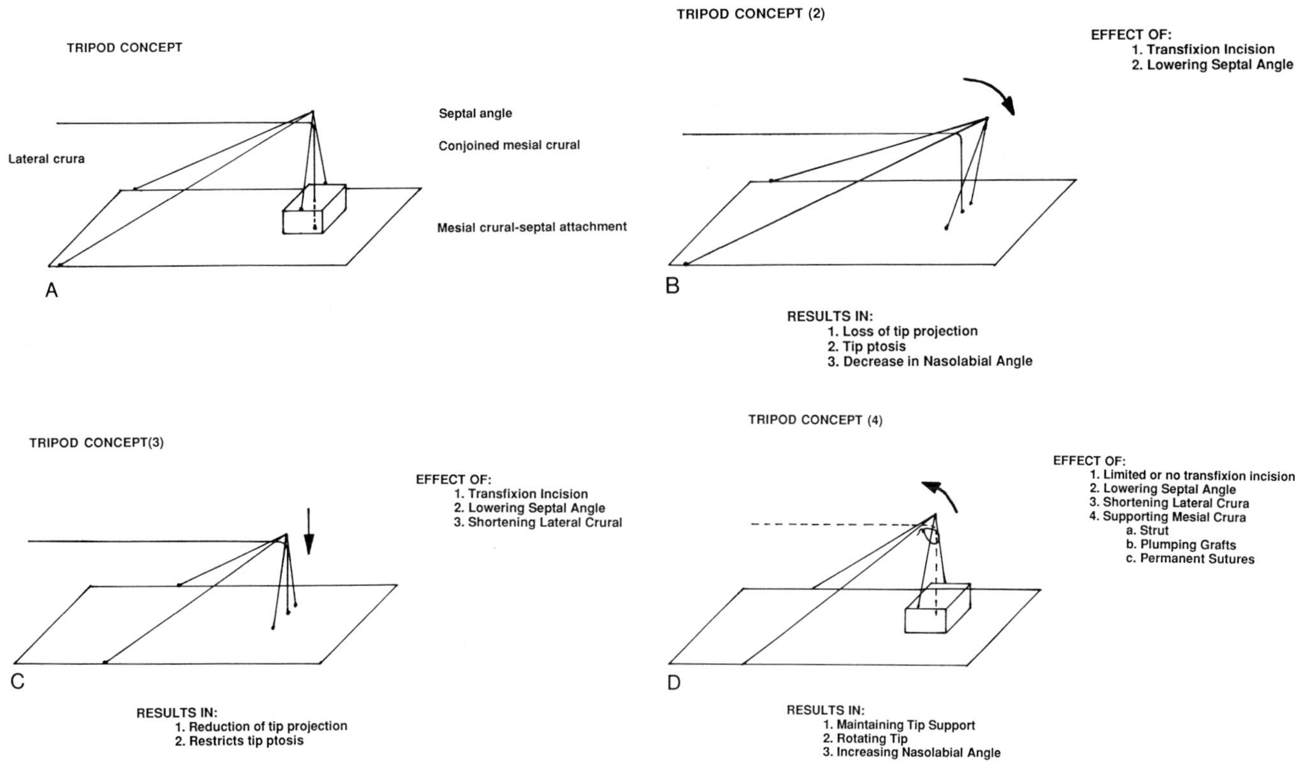

FIGURE 14–13. (*A*) Diagrammatic representation of the tripod concept of tip support. (*B*) Changes in the position of the tip are represented when the support of the medial leg of the tip is interrupted. (*C*) If all three legs are effectively shortened, tip retrodisplacement occurs. (*D*) The net effect of shortening the lateral legs and enhancing the medial leg is projection and rotation.

ANATOMIC TRIPOD

The combined anatomic configurations of the two alar cartilages constitute the legs of a tripod. The lateral crura make up two of its legs, and the conjoined medial crura make up the third leg (Fig. 14–13). Especially when their feet extend to the columellar base, the length and strength of the medial crura play a more crucial role in tip support than often is appreciated. In revisional rhinoplasty, this aspect of tip support may need to be reconstructed.

When upward rotation of the tip is desirable, cartilaginous columellar struts, plumping grafts, or permanent buried septocolumellar sutures can be used to support the medial crura central leg of the tripod. As its central component becomes the dominant leg, the tip rotates superiorly toward the forehead (Figs. 14–14 and 14–15).

TIP MODIFICATION TECHNIQUES

INTACT CRURAL TECHNIQUES

When the caudal margin of the alar cartilage is left intact, tip refinement can be enhanced by the horizontal excision of the bulky cephalic portion of

Text continued on page 162

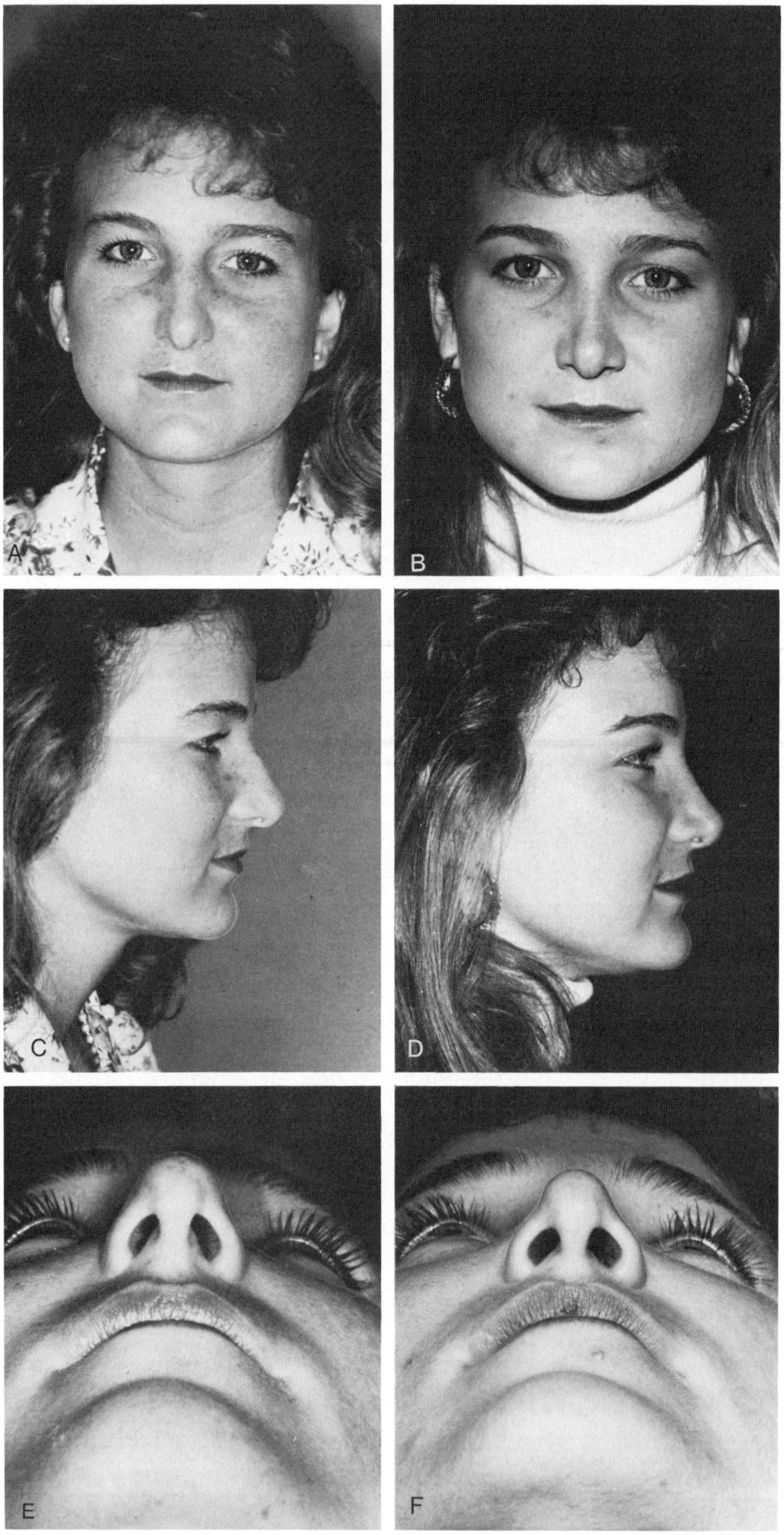

FIGURE 14–14. (*A* and *B*) Younger patients may require only minimal alteration of the nasolabial complex. (*C* and *D*) A small degree of tip rotation may be achieved by preserving the medial tripod support mechanism and complete strip excisions. (*E* and *F*) The position of the medial crura within the columella remains virtually unchanged.

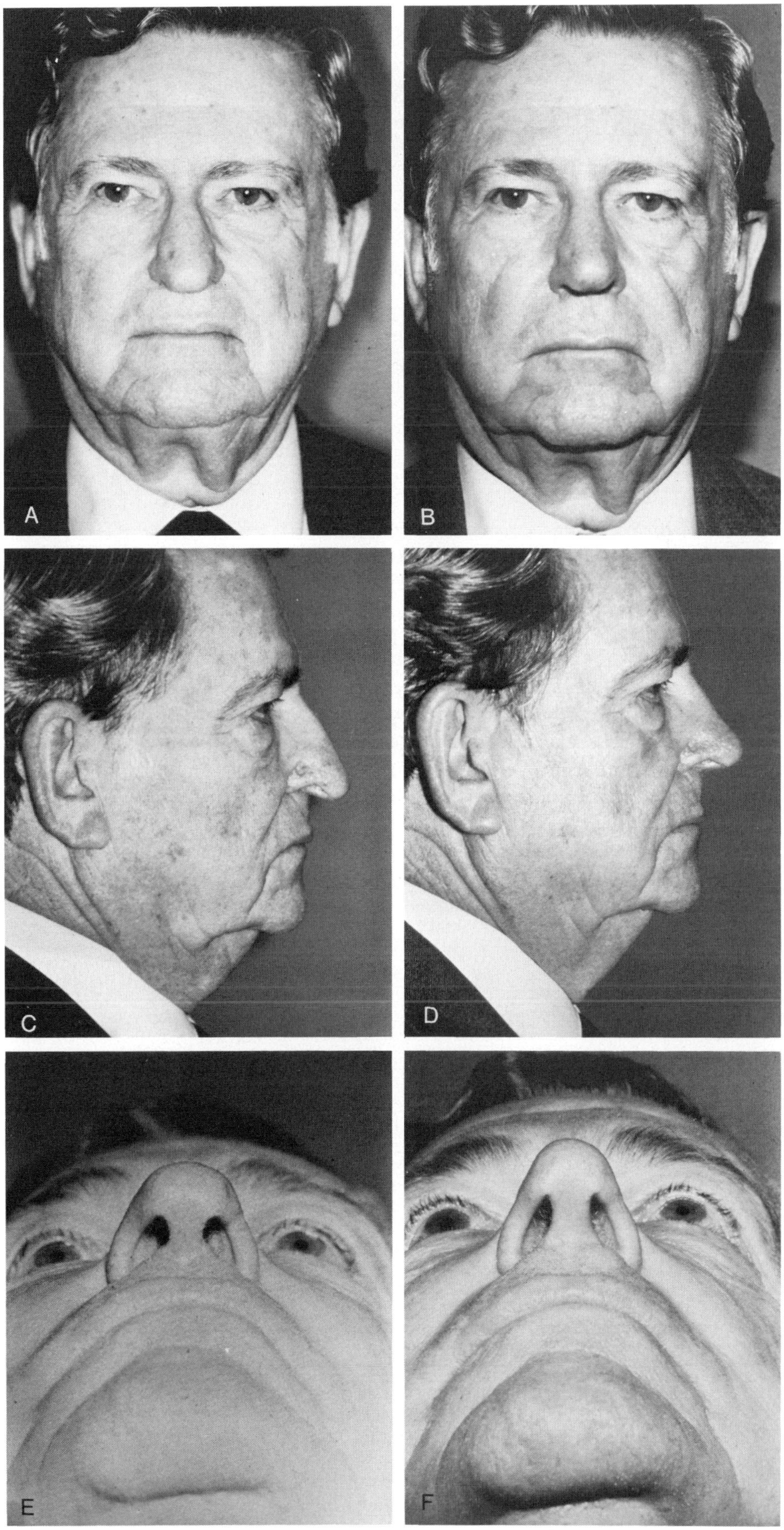

FIGURE 14–15. (*A* and *B*) More aggressive measures are required in the aging nose. (*C* and *D*) Rotation was achieved by dome division coupled with plumping grafts in the nasolabial angle and I-beam central cartilage graft. (*E* and *F*) In older patients, thicker skin covers any sharp edges that might result from vertical dome division.

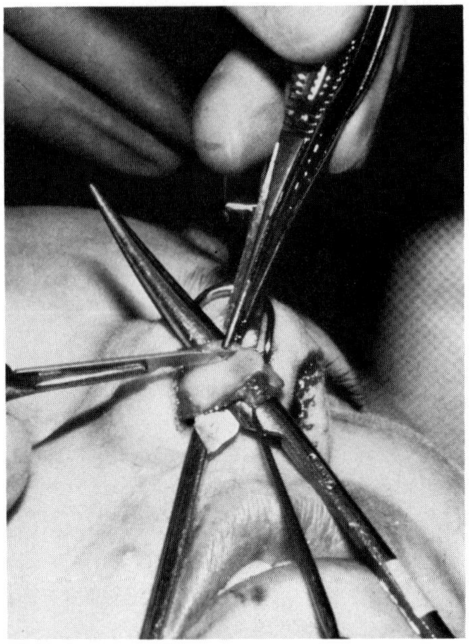

FIGURE 14–16. Excision of the horizontal segment of lateral crus usually begins at the internal soft triangle.

the lateral (and in some cases the medial) crus or by attempting to narrow the dome angle. The dome angle is created by the anatomic junction of the medial and lateral crura. It is bordered cephalically by the internal soft triangle and caudally by the external soft triangle (Fig. 14–16).

A more triangular lobule can be achieved by surgically creating a more acute dome angle. Narrowing of the angle between the external and internal soft triangles can be achieved by (1) horizontal mattress sutures, (2) careful scoring the cartilage at the dome angle, and (3) excising a triangular piece of cartilage posterior (or cephalic) to the margin of the alar cartilage at the dome (Figs. 14–17 and 14–18).

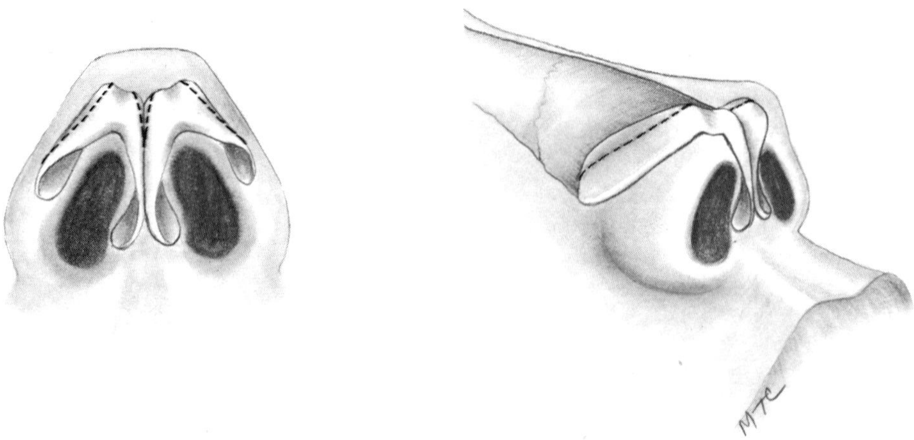

FIGURE 14–17. A wide or boxy tip may be caused by increased size and thickness of the lower lateral cartilages. The medial crural component just inferior to the dome may push the domes apart. A complete strip with appropriate cephalic excisions of the medial and lateral crura may allow the two dome angles to heal closer to each other and produce adequate lobular refinement. (Dotted lines depict the excision of unwanted cartilage.)

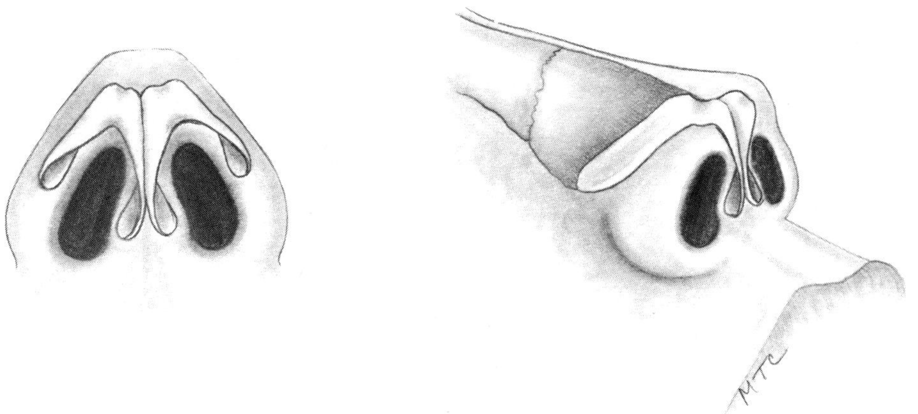

FIGURE 14–18. Excision of the excessive width of the lateral crura and reduction in the volume of the cephalic portion of the infradomas medial crus may be all that is required to allow the domes to heal in closer proximity. (Note that approximately 4–6 millimeters of the lower lateral cartilage is usually left behind to provide support.)

An isolated vertical incision into, but not through, the cartilage weakens the cartilage at the dome and helps to produce a more acute dome angle. The integrity of the medial and lateral crural components, however, may not need to be disrupted. Any incision into and/or through the cartilage of the dome carries with it the risks of visible or palpable sharp points in the lobule, as shown in Figure 14–19.

TRANSECTED CRURAL TECHNIQUES

Tip modification may also be accomplished by techniques in which an incision is made completely through the cartilage (and/or vestibular skin) at some juncture between the medial crural feet and the pyriform aperture connection of the lateral crus. These procedures constitute the second major category of tip-plasties (see Figs. 14–37 and 14–50).

Transected crural margin procedures can also be divided into three categories based on the point at which the transection occurs: (1) at the dome, (2) medial to the dome, and (3) lateral to the dome. Tip refinement procedures have been advocated in which the lower lateral cartilage is transected at or near the dome to create independent lateral and medial chondrovestibular flaps.[2]

These techniques, when performed as described, create a more triangular lobule (Fig. 14–20). The two medial crural flaps may be sutured to each other to create a central I beam on which the support of the lobule is dependent. The lateral crura must eventually come to rest against the apex of the central medial crural beam. The lobule may acquire a pinched look if a significant void is left by "borrowing" more than 3 mm of the lateral crus to obtain projection.

When vertical transection of the cartilage is carried out, the underlying vestibular skin may be left intact or it, too, can be transected. Entrapment of vestibular skin when it is transected and advanced superiorly with the medial crura does not appear to be a postoperative problem.

Tip-plasties have been described in which the lower lateral cartilages were transected medial to the dome. In these techniques, segments of the medial crus were excised and the lateral crura were advanced medially into

Text continued on page 166

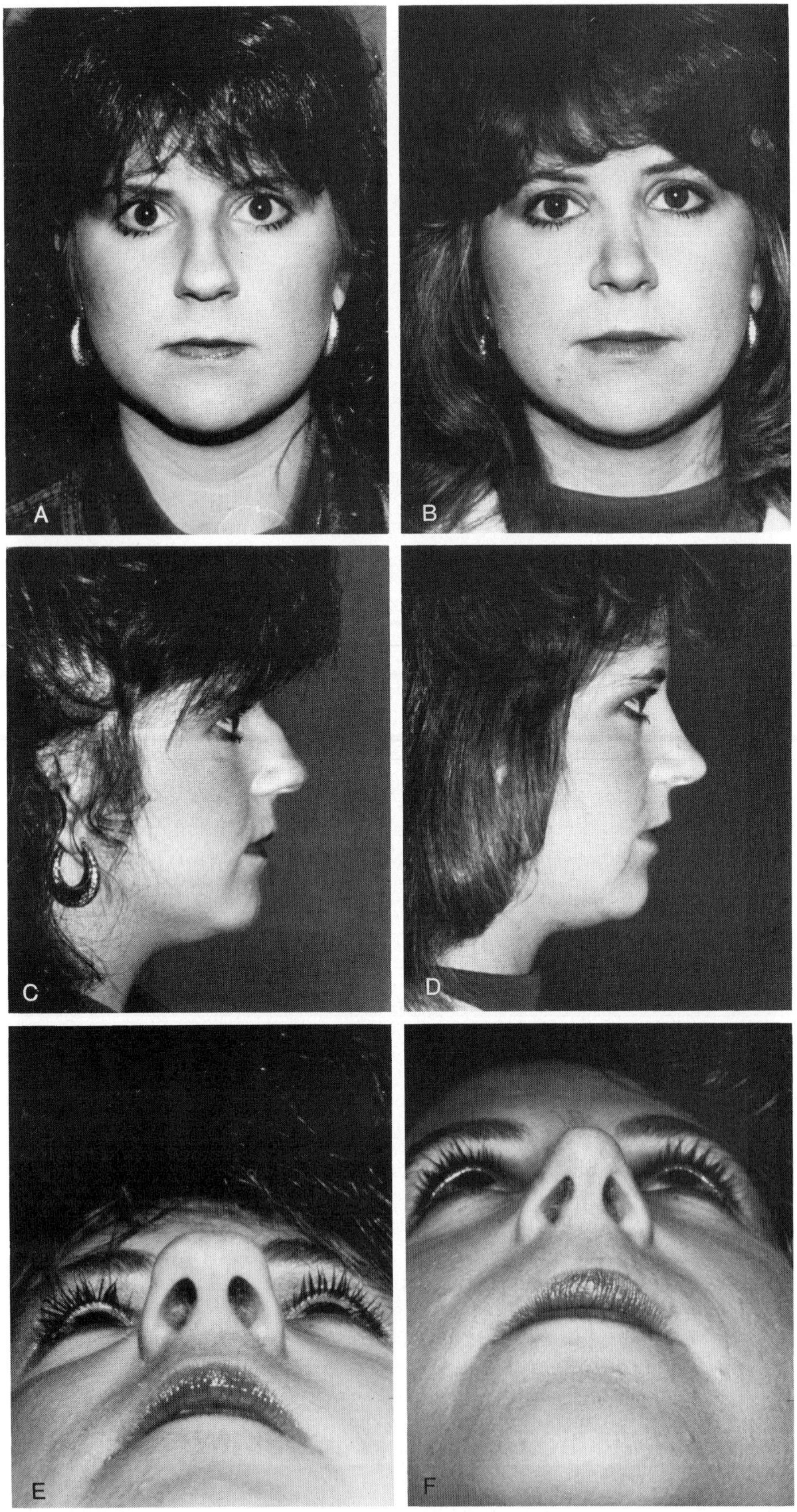

FIGURE 14–19. A patient with a boxy tip corrected by a double dome unit and division of the domes. Postoperatively, the right dome angle is visible.

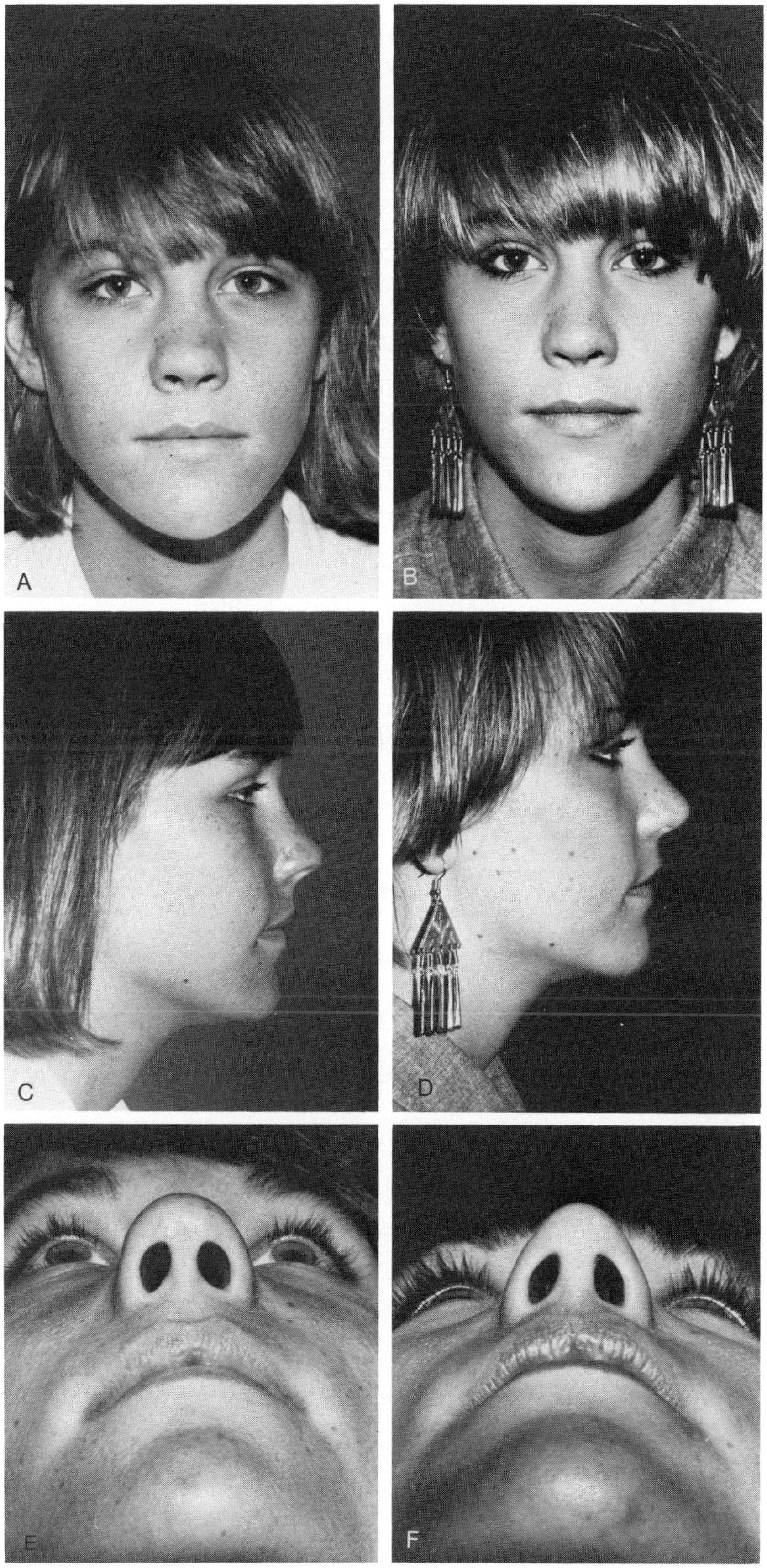

FIGURE 14–20. (*A* and *B*) An "operated" look can be avoided by conservative excision of lateral crura. (*C* and *D*) Maintaining tip projection is imperative in noses with a wide or boxy tip. (*E* and *F*) A more triangular lobule can be created in patients with thicker skin by vertical dome division with I-beam cartilage graft fixation.

the defects. Sutures were used to secure the advanced portion to the undisturbed sections of each medial crus. Vertical scoring of the lateral crura at the desired locations helped to create new dome angles.

Although the techniques had been used for quite some time, the terms "rim strip" and "lateral crural flap" were coined by Webster. In this maneuver, each lateral crus was transected lateral to its dome and portions beyond were excised.[3]

SYSTEMATIC TIP-PLASTY

Classification

Tip-plasty techniques can be classified into nine technical categories:

1. Complete strip
2. Single dome intact unit
3. Single dome transected unit
4. Double dome intact unit
5. Double dome transected unit
6. Independent crural flaps with I-beam fixation
   a. Medial crura I-beam fixation without cartilaginous strut
   b. Medial crura I-beam fixation with cartilaginous "sandwich" strut
7. Major tip reconstruction (with or without augmentation)
8. Rim strip
9. Lateral crural flap

Keeping in mind that improvement—not perfection—should be the primary objective in nasal plastic surgery, the more complicated and less predictable procedures are best reserved for more experienced surgeons. The risk-benefit curve shown in Figure 14–6 is particularly applicable in tip-plasty. Conservative techniques that preserve much of the normal anatomy are recommended for surgeons with limited experience. Although conservative measures might not always achieve the optimal degree of refinement, some improvement in the appearance of the lobule is achievable and, more important, no harm is done (Fig. 14–21).

Operative Considerations

Technical maneuvers that provide refinement to bulbous, wide, or boxy tips are described in the following sections. Both the advantages and the disadvantages of each technique are discussed. As the surgeon gains more experience, the incidence of unwanted sequelae with each technique can be lessened.

The operation usually begins as a closed rhinoplasty. The lower lateral cartilages are delivered and examined through marginal and intercartilaginous incisions (see Fig. 14–4*A* through *G*). Most tip-plasties can be accomplished without additional exposure. If additional exposure is required, it can be obtained by making an inverted V-shaped transcolumellar incision that connects the two previously made marginal incisions. The tip skin can then be reflected superiorly to expose the entire nasal skeleton (see Fig. 14–7*D*).

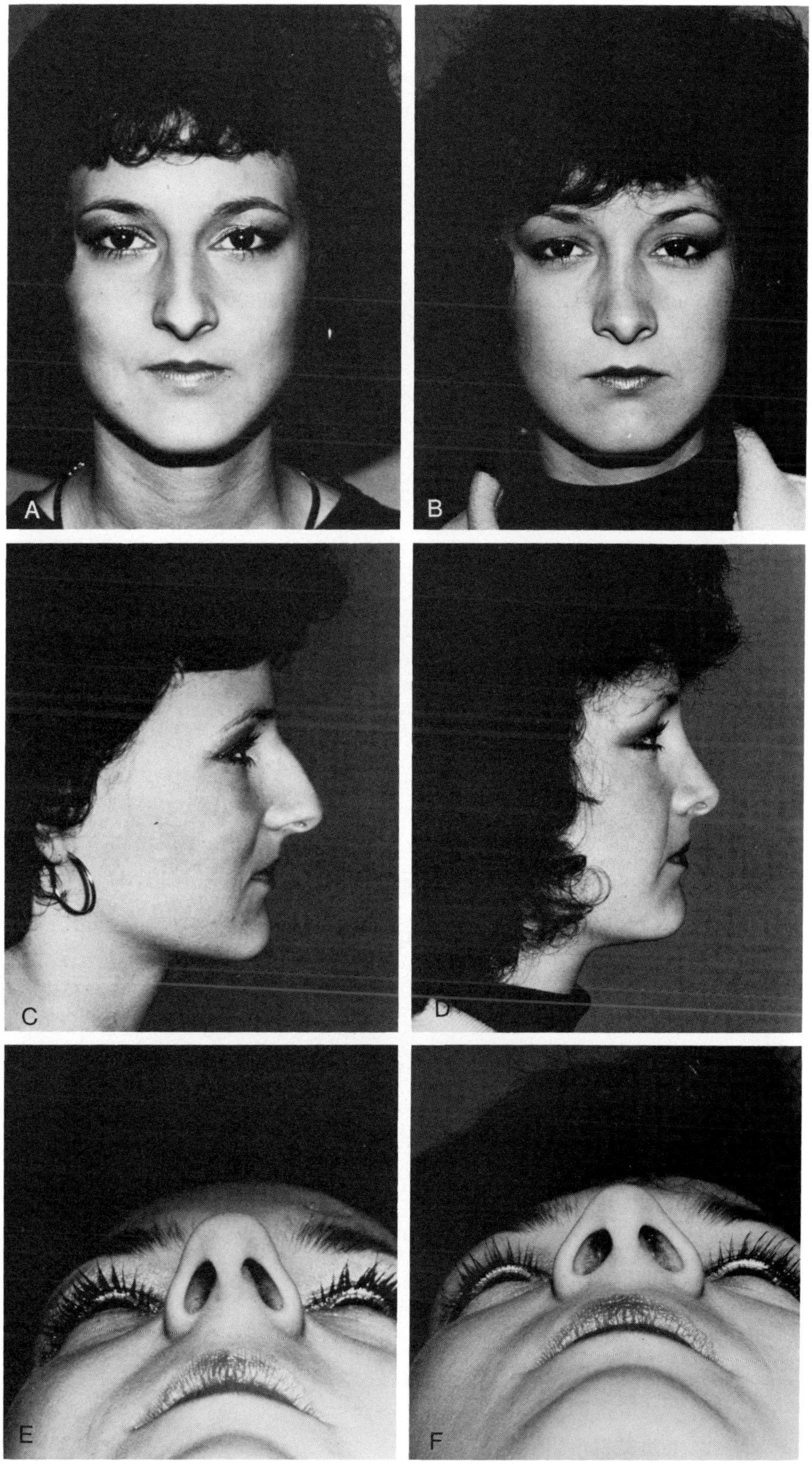

FIGURE 14–21. (*A* and *B*) Excision of only 4 mm of the cephalic portion of the lateral crus was required in this complete strip technique to produce tip refinement. (*C* and *D*) Supra-alar refinement is enhanced. (*E* and *F*) The little alteration that occurred in the lobule webbing of the nasolabial angle was corrected by excising the inferior septal angle.

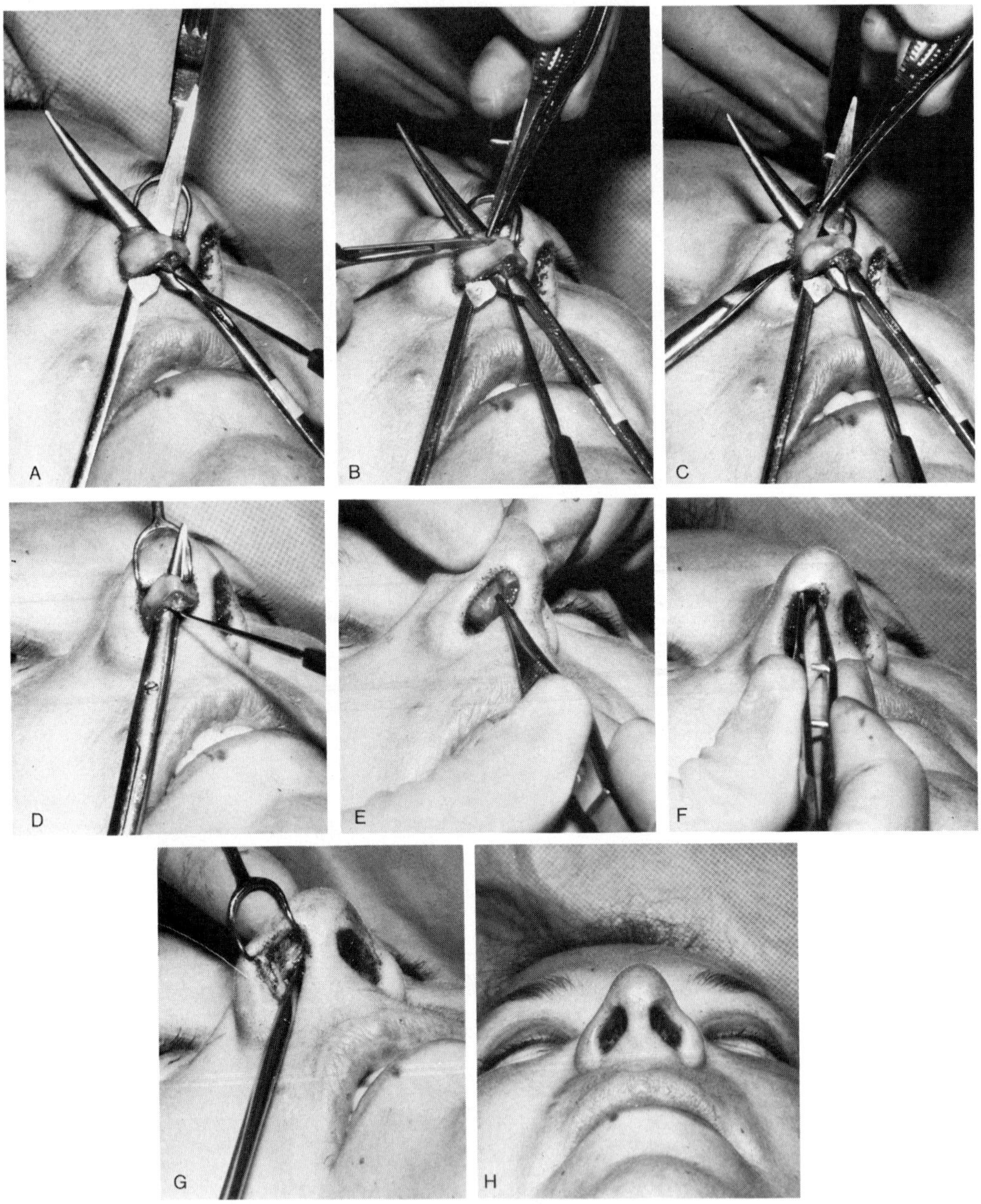

FIGURE 14–22. (*A*) Cephalic lateral crural excision begins at the internal soft triangle. (*B*) At least 4 to 6 mm of lateral crus should be left behind. (*C* and *D*) Underlying vestibular skin is preserved. (*E* and *F*) The remaining segment of the lower lateral cartilage is inspected and replaced into the nose. (*G*) The marginal incision is closed with two interrupted 5-0 plain catgut sutures. (*H*) When the procedure has been performed bilaterally, the appearance of the tip is inspected for symmetry. In the uncomplicated case, no additional tip maneuvers are necessary.

Complete Strip Technique

In the complete strip technique, the integrity of the inferior margin of each lower lateral cartilage is preserved from the foot of the medial crus to the most lateral extension of the lateral crus[3] (see Fig. 14–9). The technique is demonstrated in Figure 14–22.

Paramedian supratip refinement is created when the undesirable bulk of the cephalic portion of the lateral crus is excised. The incision into the cartilage should be made along a line parallel to its caudal or inferior margin, preserving the underlying vestibular skin. Only the necessary amount of the cephalic border of lateral crural cartilage is discarded. Such a reduction in the width of the lateral crus provides supra-alar definition and limits the amount of cephalic rotation.

A complete, or nontransected, lower lateral cartilage also minimizes alar notching and limits upward rotation in noses that are already short. In the vast majority of symmetric and nonplatyrrhine noses, the complete strip maneuver is all that is necessary to produce an aesthetically improved nasal tip. Projection and/or rotation can be effected by altering the position of the medial crural-septal relationship (Fig. 14–23).

Single-Dome Intact Unit Technique

A *single dome unit* can be created when the dome angle is left intact but narrowed by suture fixation of the medial crus to the lateral crus at the dome.[4] The technique is shown in Figures 14–24 and 14–25.

The more acute dome angle created by a horizontal mattress suture fixation provides additional lobular refinement and narrowing without surgical disruption of the integrity of the remaining complete strip of alar cartilage. The newly created dome angles are held in position by an absorbable 5-0 polyglactin (Vicryl) suture until a capsule of fibrous tissue replaces them.

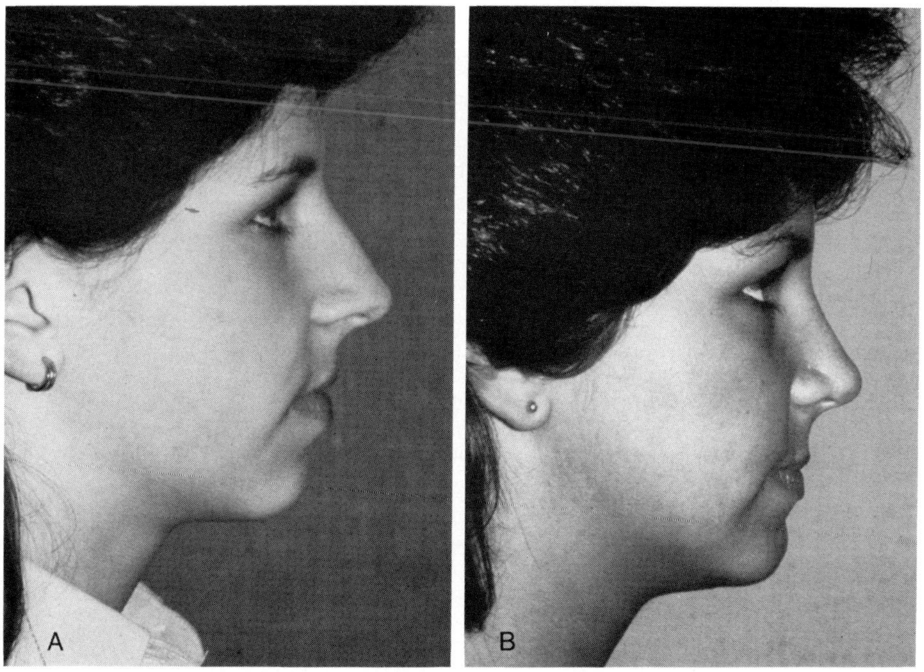

FIGURE 14–23. The overly projected "tension nose" appearance was corrected by allowing the medial leg of the tripod to settle after an extended complete transfixion incision. Chin augmentation was also performed.

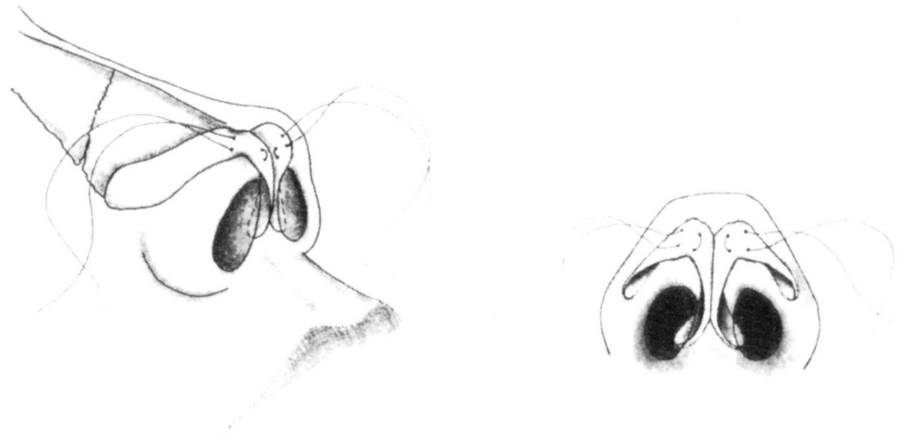

A B

FIGURE 14–24. If more narrowing of the lobule is desired, a single-dome procedure can be performed. The initial step involves precise identification of each new dome and the creation of a more acute angle between the medial and lateral crus with a 5-0 Vicryl horizontal mattress suture.

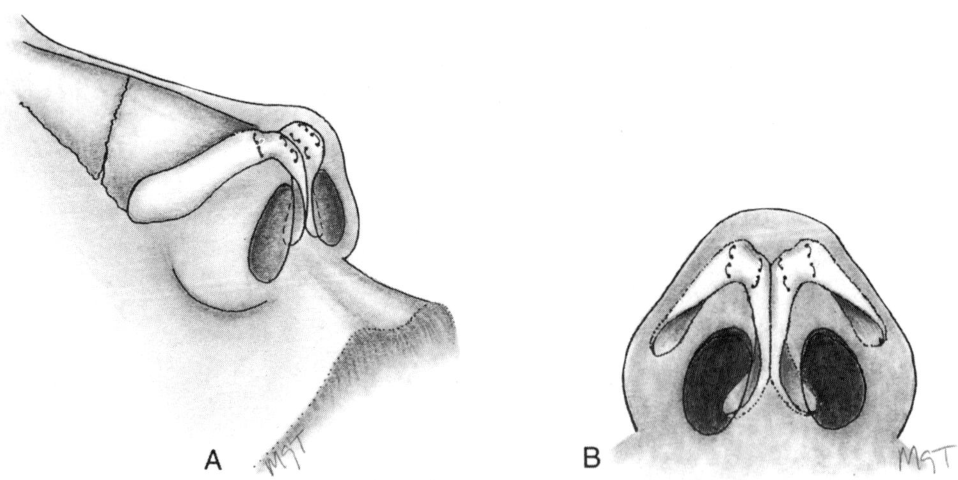

A B

FIGURE 14–25. When the horizontal mattress suture is tied, the dome angle is narrowed.

Investigators have demonstrated that (with respect to ear cartilage) controlled scar tissue elements can help to hold cartilage in a new, more desirable position after sutures have lost their tensile strength or have absorbed.

After the lower lateral cartilage has been delivered and the anatomic dome is identified, a complete strip maneuver is performed. Exact identification of the anatomic dome is an essential first step in tip-plasty, regardless of the technique to be used. By definition, the anatomic dome is that portion of the alar cartilage between the internal soft triangle superiorly and the external soft triangle (facet) inferiorly (see Fig. 14–22*D*).

A new dome angle can be surgically created by suture fixation when asymmetry is present. When the procedure is properly performed, the underlying vestibular skin is protected and preserved. A double horizontal mattress suture of 5-0 Vicryl suture creates a more acute dome angle.

This technique narrows the tip and, to a lesser degree, produces a minimum degree of tip projection because it increases the height of the lobule. Provided that adequate lobule narrowing has been obtained, each independently created single-dome unit may not need to be sutured to its counterpart (Figs. 14–26 and 14–27). The result is a more refined tip.

When the length of the lateral crural legs of the tripod are not excised or significantly shortened, upward rotation may be prevented in patients whose noses are already short.

With this technique, some of the sequelae that may be associated with vertical dome division techniques are avoided. Independent lower lateral flaps, which are created when the medial crus is completely separated from the lateral crus, can potentially produce sharp points that are visible through thinner skin. It stands to reason, however, that the ability to narrow and increase the height of the lobule that can be achieved when portions of the lateral crus are "borrowed" after dome division is not as great either.

Even though fibrous tissue elements hold cartilages in position,[5] the possibility exists that the "memory" of strong cartilages may return (at least partially) when sutures dissolve, either unilaterally or bilaterally. Therefore, the results of single-dome units may not theoretically be as predictable as transected techniques. When the cartilages are left intact, the capsule of fibrous tissue that holds the cartilages in their new position determines the final shape of the lobule—an imponderable that is beyond the surgeon's control once the dressing is applied.

Postoperative asymmetry could appear if unequal cartilage "memory" returns. Because it does not correct unilateral cartilage excess and/or deficiency, the single-dome unit usually is contraindicated in preoperatively asymmetric tips. In these cases, one often can find curvature of the medial crural components of the lower lateral cartilages, which may require special attention.

Single-Dome Transected Unit

After the new single dome has been created by suture fixation, a more permanently acute dome angle can be ensured with the following additional maneuver. Cutting into and/or through the cartilage can help to produce more narrowing of the nasal lobule (Fig. 14–28).[2] Both lobular narrowing and, to a lesser degree, projection can be assured because an even more acute dome angle exists (Fig. 14–29).

Text continued on page 174

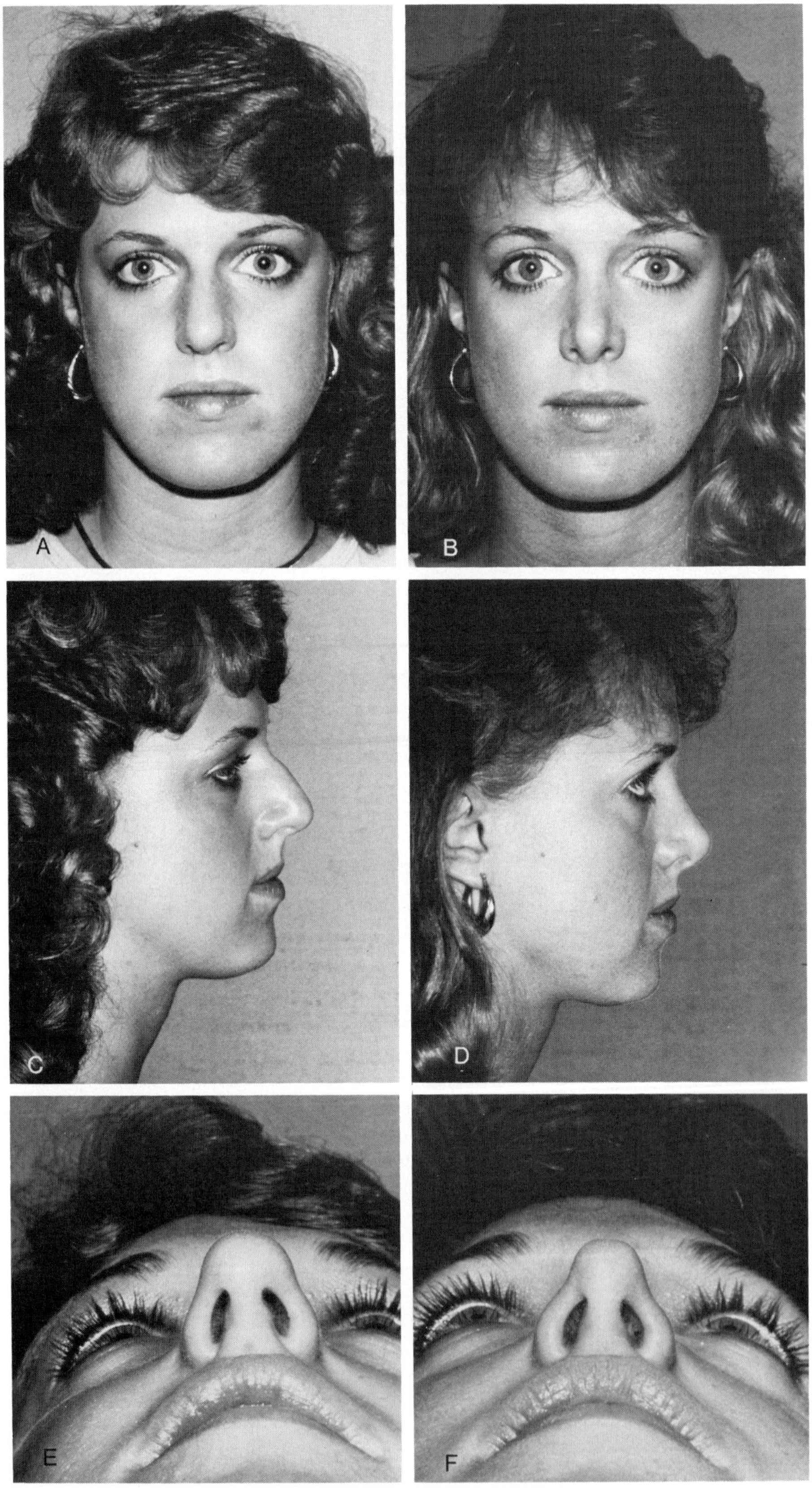

FIGURE 14–26. Patient shown before (*A*) and after (*B*) undergoing a single-dome unit procedure. Lobule narrowing is readily apparant. (*C* and *D*) The nasolabial angle remained essentially unchanged, but some of the webbing was corrected by extending the transfixion incision beyond the medial crura. (*E* and *F*) Lobular narrowing and "settling" of the medial crural foot plates are obvious.

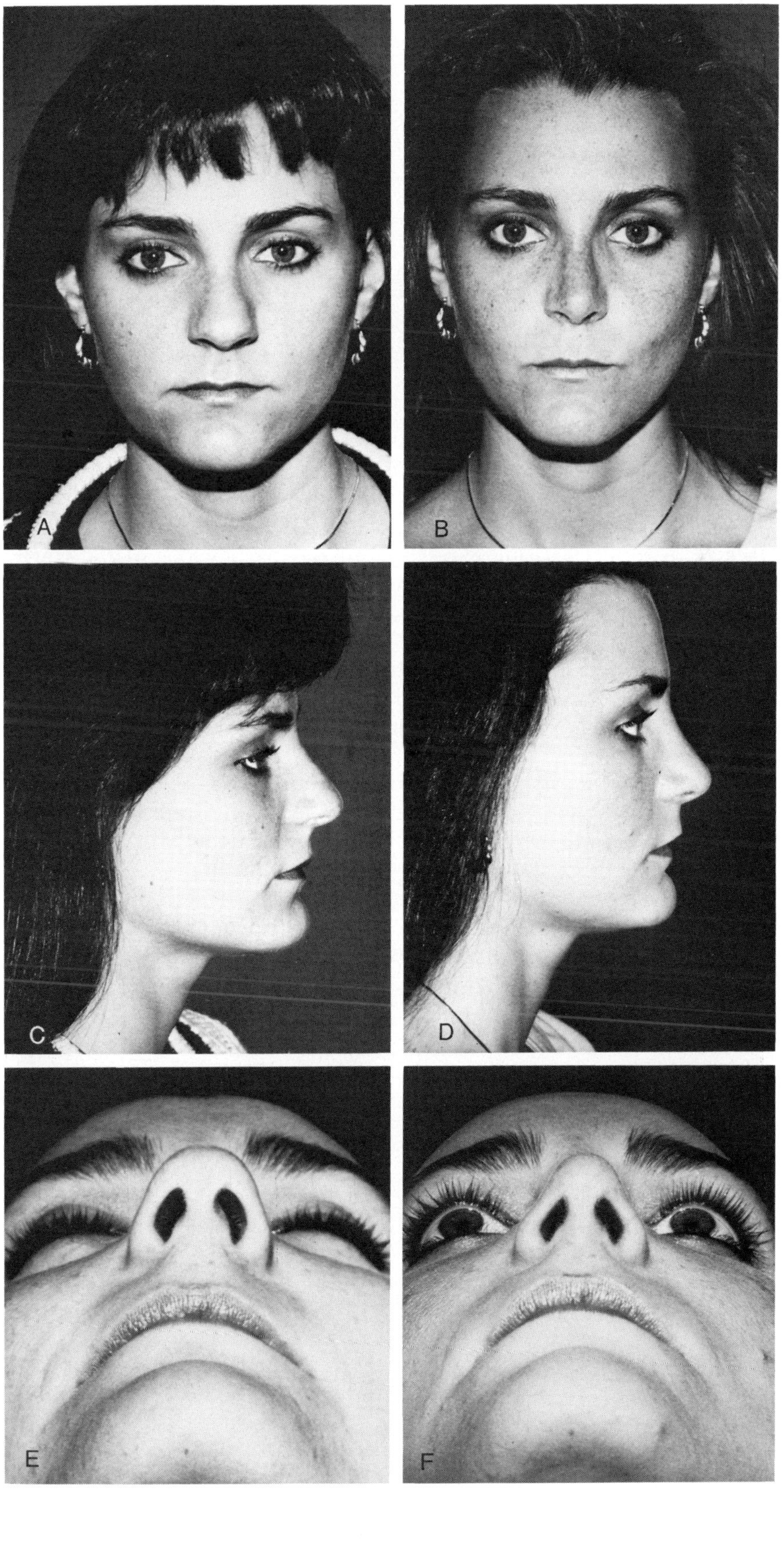

FIGURE 14–27. (*A* to *F*) Patient shown has had the nasal tip shaped with a single-dome intact procedure. Note the refinement of the lobule at 18 months after surgery.

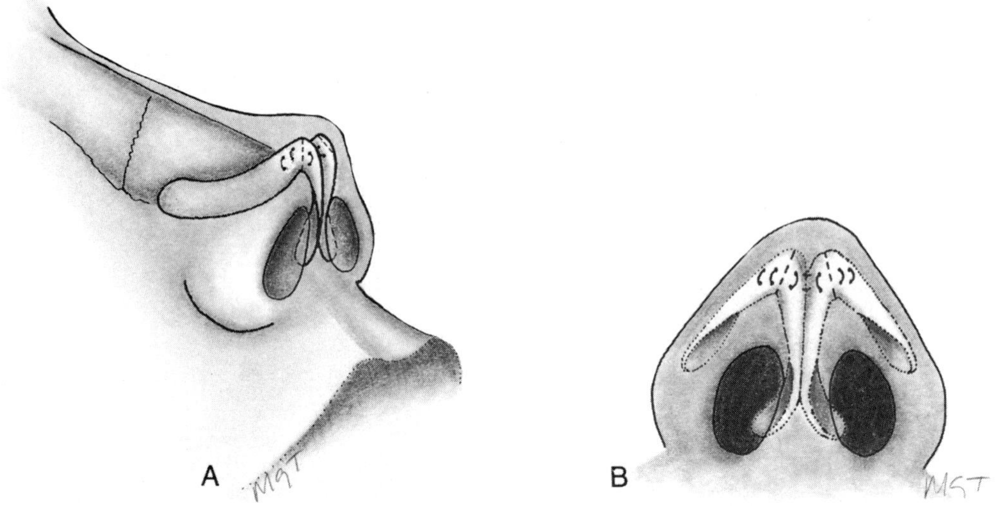

FIGURE 14–28. Technique used most often in a single-dome transected unit.

Sometimes the surgeon can correct dome asymmetries by carefully selecting the incision and/or division point. After complete transection, however, carefully excising excessively projecting portions of the transected medial and lateral components may be necessary, especially when asymmetry is present. The height of one or both domes can also be reduced in this manner.

Incomplete incision into, but not through, the cartilage can avoid some of the concerns stated above. A carefully placed single-dome mattress suture holds the newly altered domes in place until favorable fibrosis takes over.

Two independent single domes do not produce the degree of lobular narrowing that can be achieved if the two domes are sutured to each other to create a double-dome unit because some lateral curvature of the medial crural components of the tip cartilages may push the domes apart.

The *single-dome transected* technique is especially useful in patients with thick skin and/or a bulbous tip when no upward rotation is desirable.

Sharp points, a pinched nasal tip, alar notching, and excessive columellar show are possible sequelae of the single-dome transected technique, especially in patients with thin skin, as seen in Figure 14–30.

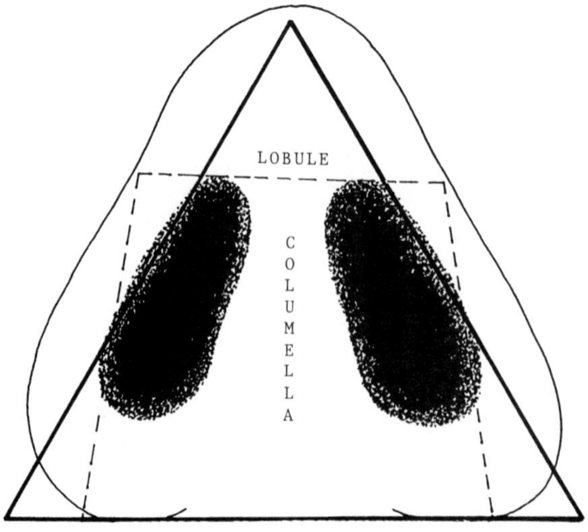

FIGURE 14–29. Ideal proportions of the nasal tip.

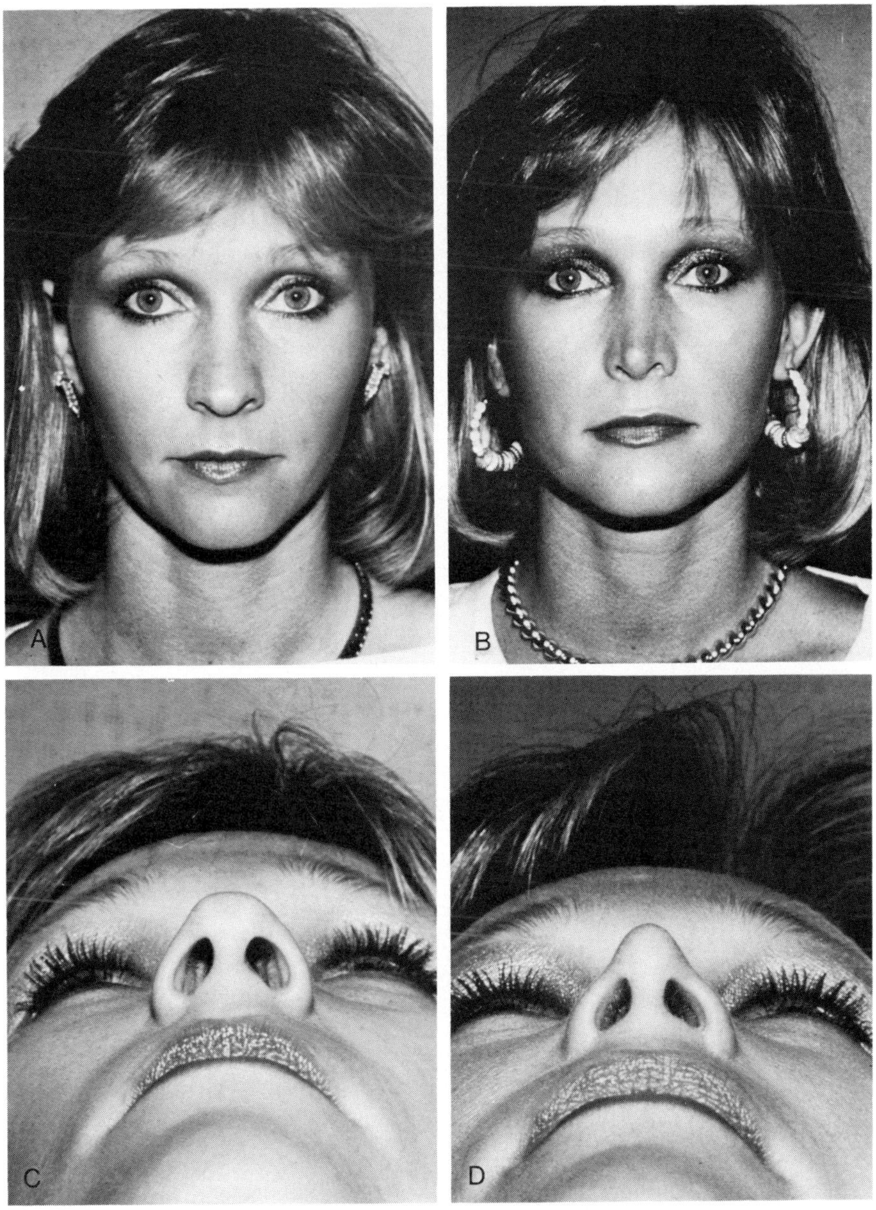

FIGURE 14–30. (*A* and *B*) In patients with thin skin and strong cartilage, interruption in the integrity of the cartilage at or near the dome may best be avoided. (*C* and *D*) Excessive narrowing of the lobule may occur. Although asymmetry was corrected, the exchange of one condition for another that may look "surgical" deserves thoughtful consideration.

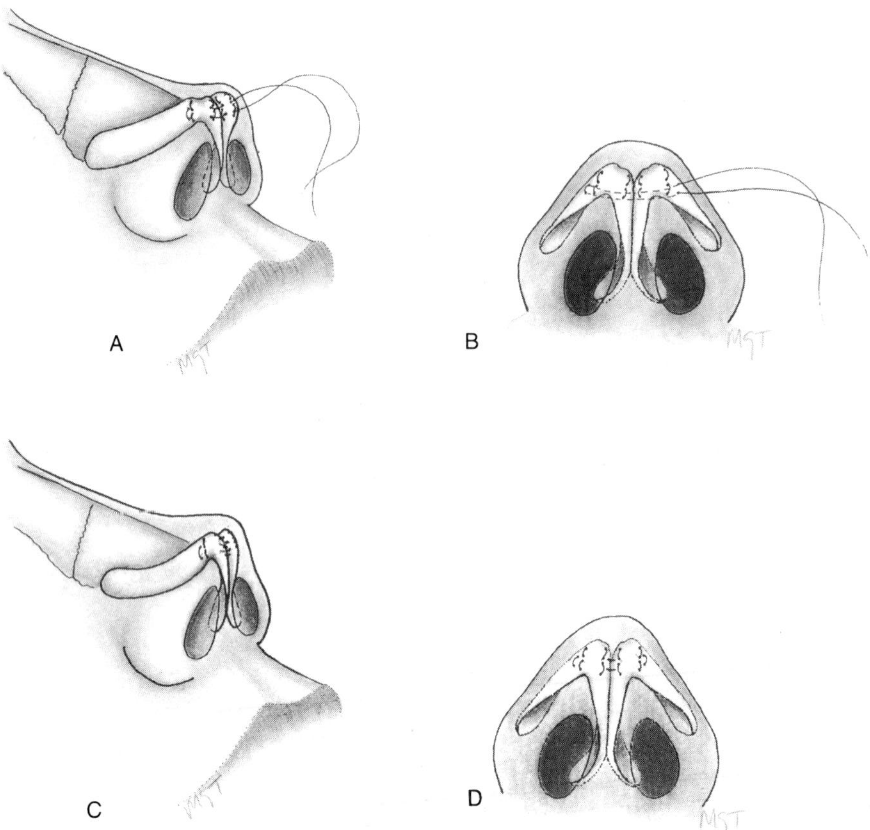

FIGURE 14–31. The double-dome unit is treated when the second mattress suture (placed in horizontal fat mattress fashion) binds the two new single domes to each other (*A* and *B*). A more triangular lobule is obtained when the suture is secured. Note that some degree of rotation and projection is also produced (*C* and *D*).

Double-Dome Intact Unit

The unpredictable vagaries of healing may potentially undo some of the result observed at the end of operation. Securing the position of the tip cartilages during the early stages of healing is crucial. In both the single and the double-dome units, suture fixation keeps the cartilages in their desired position until scar formation helps to stabilize them.

When the double-dome technique was first developed, I used morselization on each dome in an attempt to help create a weakened area at the junction of the internal and external soft triangles. The objective of morselization was to help produce a new dome angle.[6]

In the original technique, morselization of the cartilages was followed by suture fixation. With experience, I recognized that after morselization, the imponderables of healing may allow for cartilage to asymmetrically stiffen during the ensuing months. This fact coupled with the inability of morselized cartilages to accommodate suture fixation caused me to seek a more predictable dome division procedure. Morselization of the dome angle was abandoned.[7]

The desired relation of the two domes to each other is ensured by careful placement of an additional 5-0 Vicryl mattress suture that passes through *both* newly produced single-dome units. When this suture is tied, the *double-dome unit* is complete (Figs. 14–31 and 14–32). Not only is the intradorsal space eliminated, but some straightening of the subdomal medial crura occurs. The end result is an even more triangular and minimally projected lobule (Fig. 14–33).

As is the case with virtually all tip techniques, the addition of a cartilaginous strut inserted between the medial crura can help to maintain support and further enhances tip projection in the postoperative period.

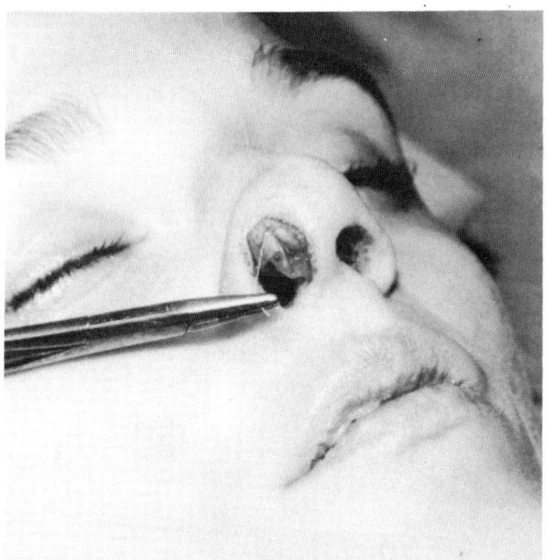

FIGURE 14—32. To produce even more narrowing and symmetry, a second suture secures the two newly created domes to each other.

Double-Dome Transected Unit

Once the double-dome unit complex is created, and to ensure against the possibility of the dome angle becoming less acute, it may be advisable to make an incision into and/or through the cartilage at the apex of each new dome (but not through vestibular skin), as described in the preceding section (Fig. 14–34). Trimming any sharp points at the transected edges of cartilages is also recommended.

The height of the lobule can also be reduced (should tip projection be excessive) by incremental and precise trimming of the new double-dome unit. If the tip cartilages are asymmetric, improvement may be achieved by either adding and securing appropriately fashioned cartilage grafts with sutures or trimming cartilage away from the deviant side. Care should be taken not to cut the horizontal mattress fixation sutures.

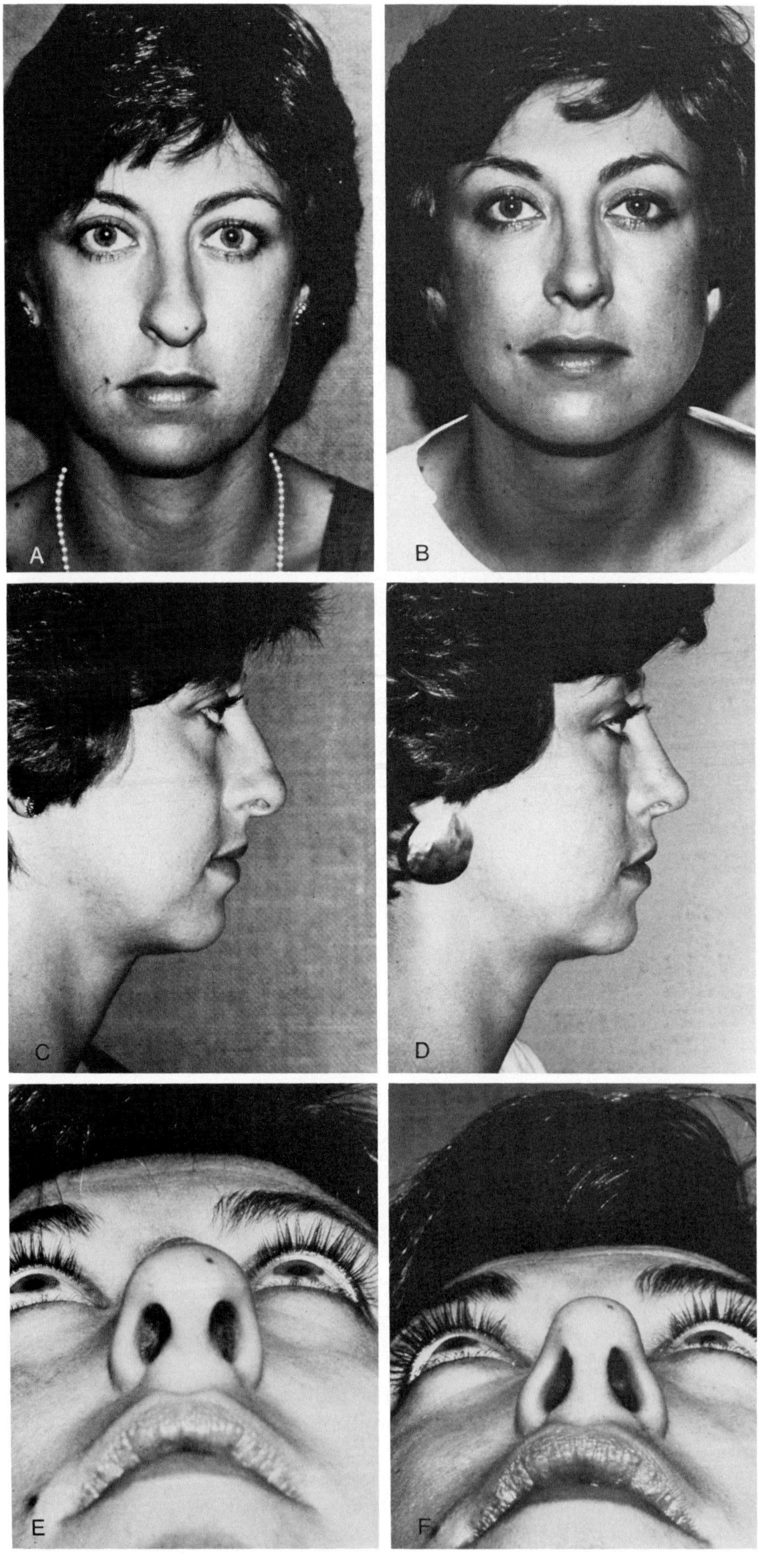

FIGURE 14–33. (*A* and *B*) A bulbous tip in a patient with relatively thin skin and strong cartilages lends itself to a double-dome intact unit technique. (*C* and *D*) As lobular narrowing occurs, some increased height of the lobule is also achieved. (*E* and *F*) About 1 year later, long after the polyglycolic sutures have dissolved, tip definition remains.

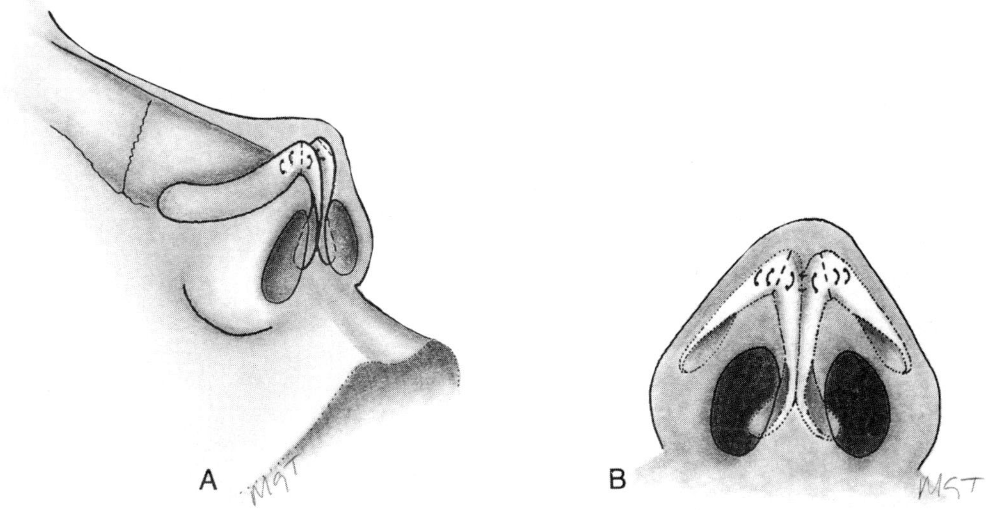

FIGURE 14–34. When the alar cartilages are thick, an incision can be made into the apex of the new domes to prevent postoperative widening, thereby extending the process to a double-dome *transected* unit.

Vestibular skin is left intact and unelevated in both the single-dome and the double-dome transected units. Even if the horizontal mattress suture should traverse it, the underlying vestibular skin assumes a physiologic position when the polyglactin sutures dissolve.

The *double-dome transected unit* offers the following advantages over many other tip techniques:

1. It produces predictable lobular refinement and at the same time prevents undesirable cephalic tip rotation in a person who needs no further shortening.
2. Because the medial and lateral crura are bound as a unit by a suture, some of the unwanted upward rotation that can occur with other vertical division techniques is averted.
3. Because the lateral crura are not permanently separated from the medial crura or shortened, the desirable torque factor based at the two pyriform apertures is preserved.

Figures 14–35 and 14–36 demonstrate suitable cases for this technique.

INDEPENDENT CRURAL FLAPS

Goldman described a tip-plasty in which he vertically divided both the lower lateral cartilage and the vestibular skin at or near the dome (Fig. 14–37). The two transected medial crural flaps were then sutured to each other to form a central support mechanism for the tip. The procedure was designed to achieve projection, rotation, and lobular refinement. Goldman attempted to ensure projection when he secured this medial crural complex to the caudal septum with two or three absorbable mattress sutures (Fig. 14–38).

When additional lobular height or narrowing is desired, a small portion of the lateral crus can be "borrowed" by making the vertical division 1 to 2 mm lateral to the dome. Projection and support may be limited by the length and strength of the medial crura (Figs. 14–39 and 14–40).

Text continued on page 185

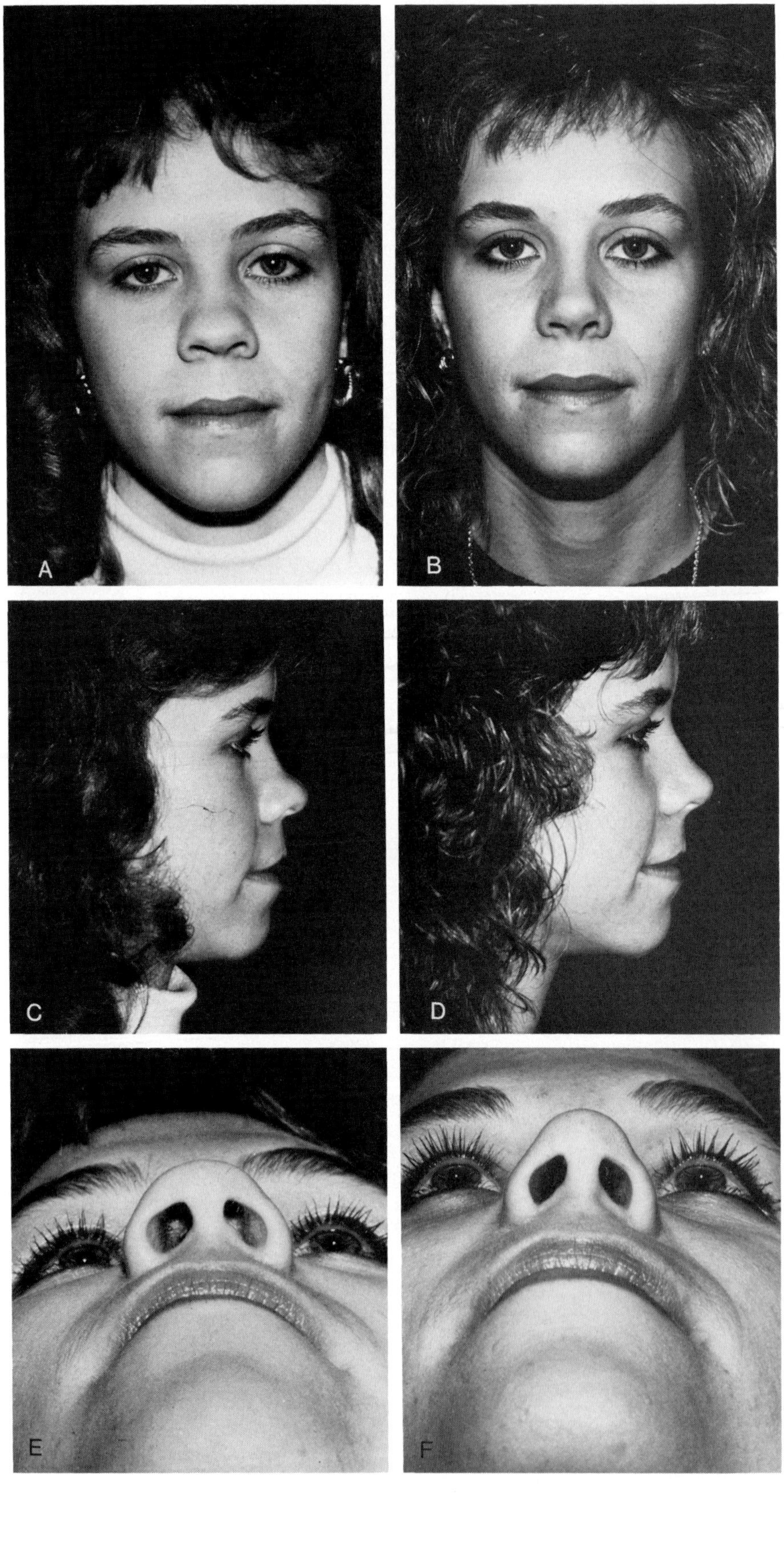

FIGURE 14–35. (*A* and *B*) Shorter and wider noses present a special challenge. The double-dome transected unit may be chosen as an alternative technique to dome division (Goldman-type). (*C* and *D*) Augmentation of the nasolabial angle and dorsum with septal cartilage grafts was necessary. (*E* and *F*) A more triangular lobule and improved nostril symmetry were achieved.

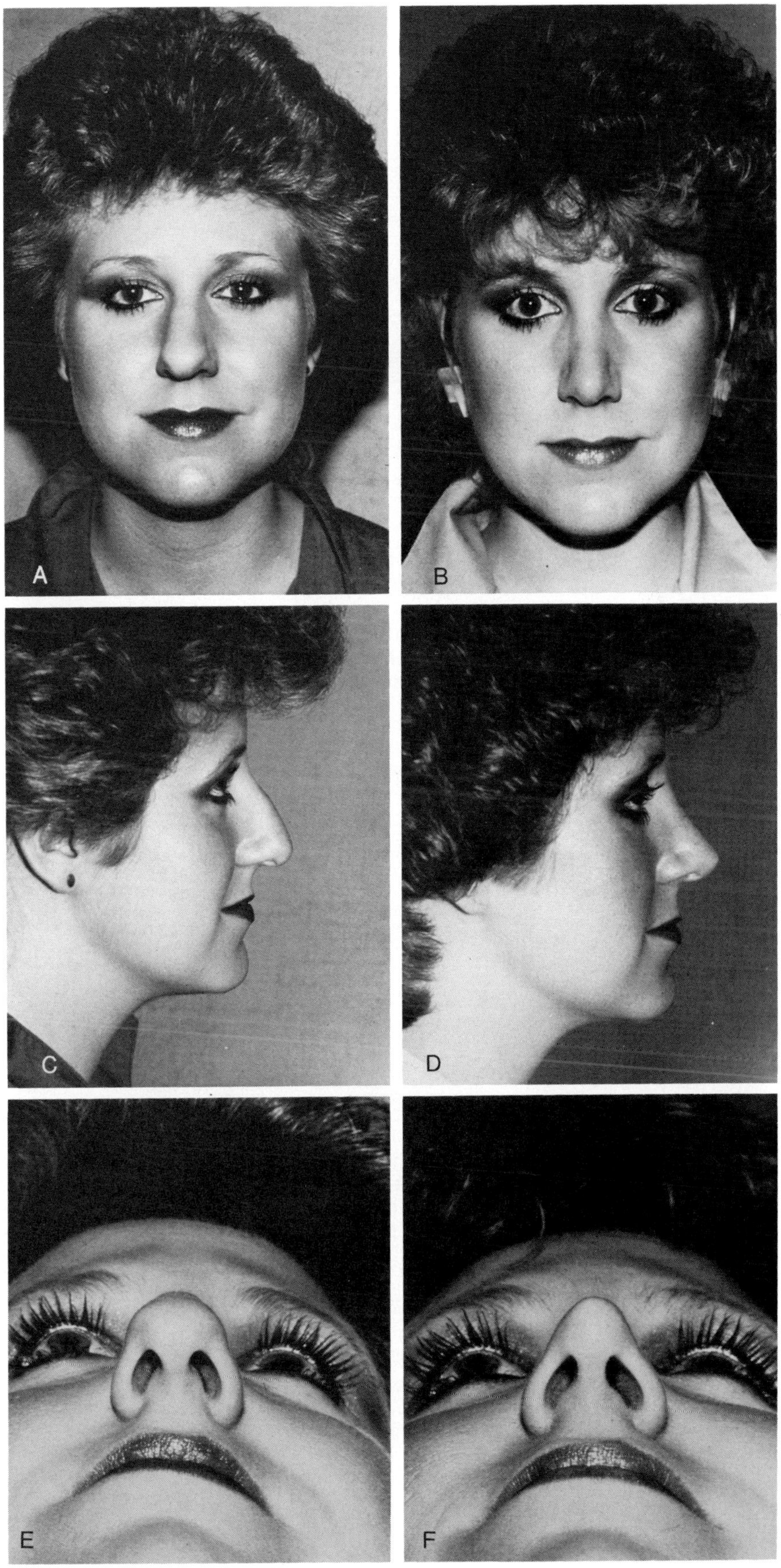

FIGURE 14–36. (*A* and *B*) When the tip cartilages are asymmetric, a double-dome transected unit may be indicated. (*C* and *D*) Projection and rotation can be enhanced with cartilage struts placed between the medial crura and into the nasolabial angle. (*E* and *F*) Tip symmetry can be established with sutures. An incision into and/or through the newly created dome angle helps to secure the shape of the reconstructed lobular architecture.

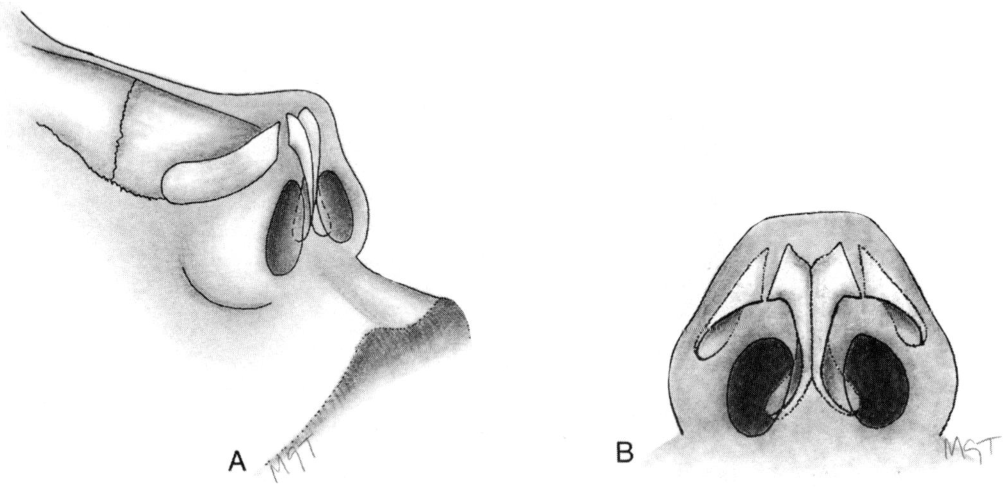

FIGURE 14–37. When it is desirable to increase the height of the lobule and obtain maximum narrowing, the lower lateral cartilage may be divided, including vestibular skin, 1 to 2 mm lateral to the dome.

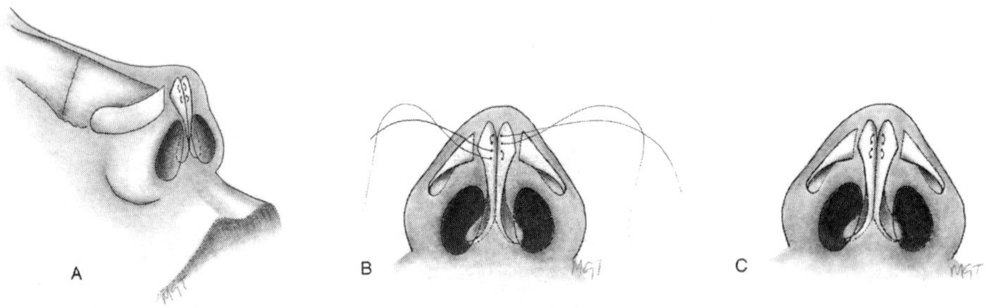

FIGURE 14–38. (*A* and *B*) If the cartilages are strong, the two medial crura are sutured together with two mattress sutures of 5-0 Vicryl suture. (*C*) A strong central support usually provides adequate projection and narrowing of the tip and lobule.

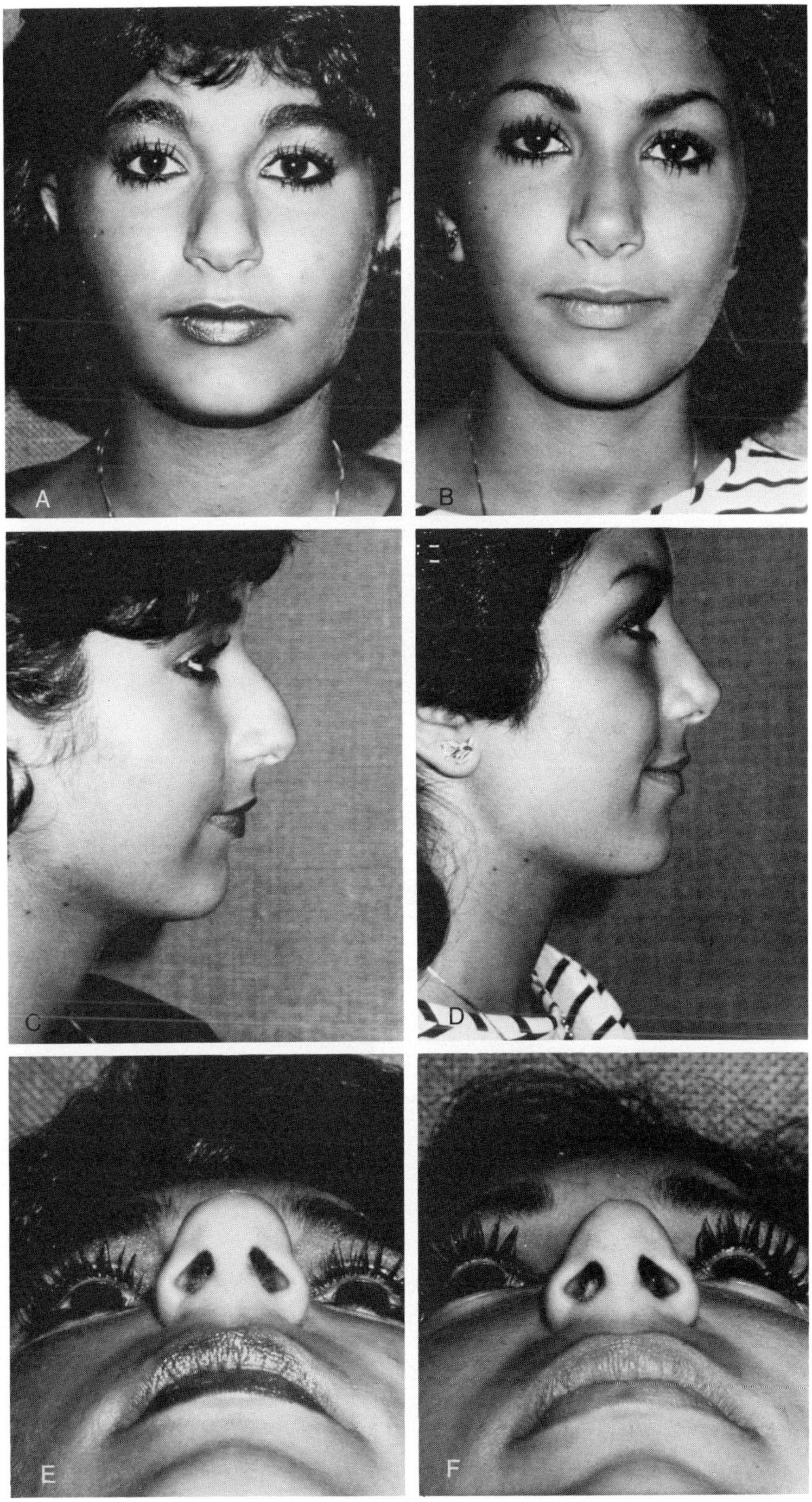

FIGURE 14–39. (*A* and *B*) When the skin of the tip is very thick, more aggressive narrowing techniques are necessary. (*C* and *D*) Tip projection may be maintained by limiting the transfixion incision and by suture fixation of the divided medial crural flaps. (*E* and *F*) Thicker skin camouflages the transected ends of the medial crura.

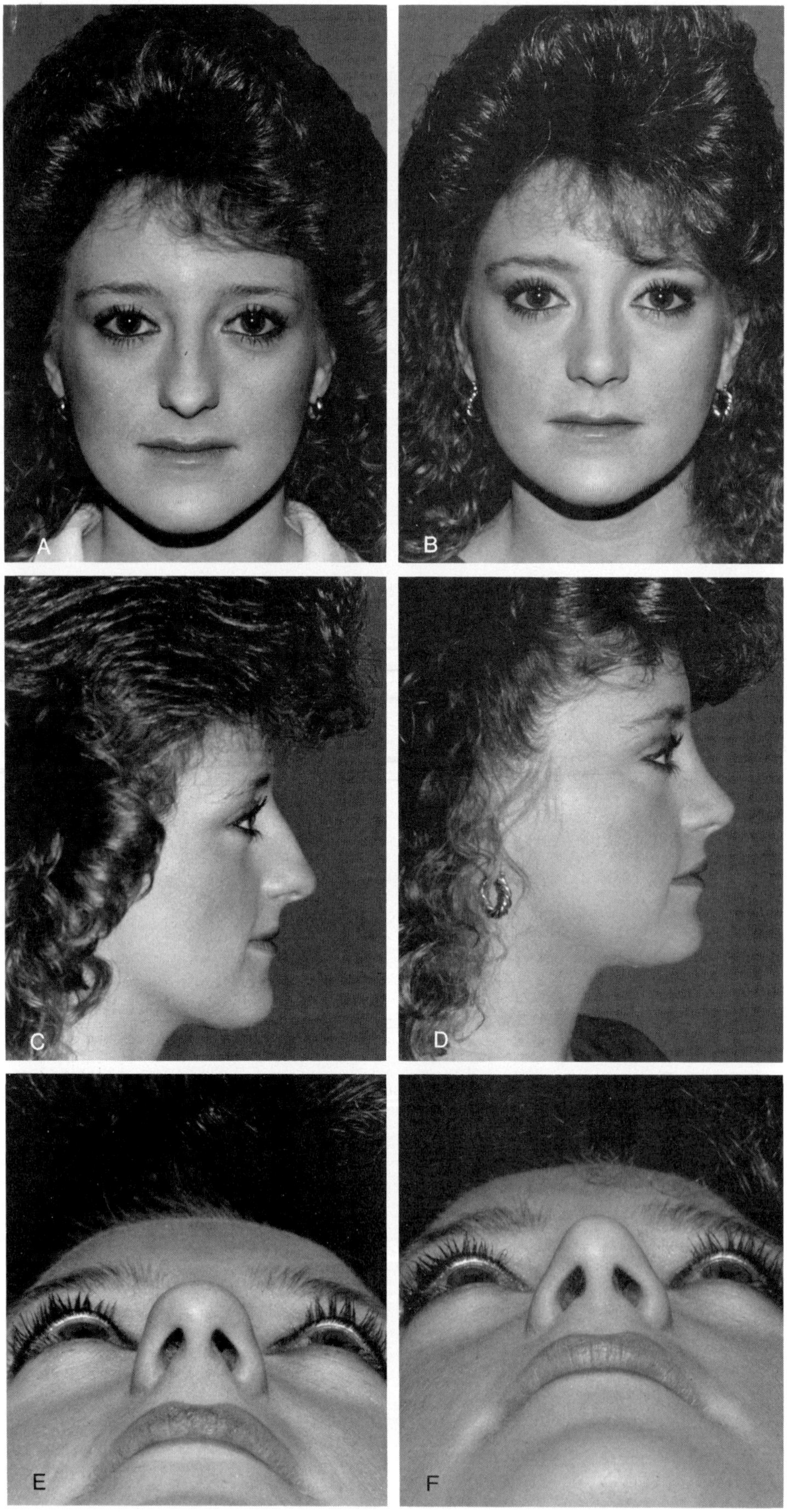

FIGURE 14–40. (*A* and *B*) In a patient with a small nose and a short columella, it is desirable to increase the height of the lobule by borrowing 2 to 3 mm from the lateral crus in a vertical dome division technique. (*C* and *D*) When tip projection can be obtained by increased lobular height, particularly when the alar cartilages are strong, columellar grafts that can produce unwanted nasolabial fullness in this patient can be avoided. (*E* and *F*) Even 1 mm of increased lobular height is helpful.

I-BEAM MEDIAL CRURAL FIXATION

In this modification of a classic technique, the key element of tip projection is based on the augmented central limb of the tripod. When the medial crura are short or weak, additional support to the complex can be obtained by accurately placing a long cartilage strut between them. A straight piece of septal cartilage is preferred. The graft is fixed with sutures in at least two points until favorable fibrosis occurs.

The medial crura are secured to the graft in a sandwich-like manner with two interrupted sutures of 5-0 Dexon polyglycolic acid. The "sandwiched graft" along with the two medial crura create a strong I-beam system. The graft ought to extend inferiorly past the base of the columellar and to within 3 mm of the premaxillary crest. The strut should extend superiorly at least to the transected ends of the medial crura.[8]

This technique is particularly helpful in platyrrhine noses, in those with infantile-like tips, and in revisional cases when large segments of alar cartilage have been removed. The technique is also useful in correcting the cleft lip nose. If additional projection is required in the patient with thick skin, the sandwiched tip graft can be extended about 1 mm higher than the two transected ends of the medial crura (Fig. 14–41).

By its nature, the I-beam sandwiched graft technique provides maximum structural support for tip projection and oftentimes helps to straighten deformed medial crura. The graft's intracrural permanent location is more predictable than onlay free shield grafts (Fig. 14–42).

POSSIBLE SEQUELAE

Excess columellar show, alar notching, and pinched lobules are rare but potential sequelae. With experience, these problems occur less frequently.

Even if complete transection of the domes is not indicated, a sandwiched lobulocolumellar tip graft may be placed between and secured to the medial crura and/or domes to strengthen the medial tripod leg. This can be helpful in single- and double-dome techniques as well.

ARCHITECTURAL TIP RECONSTRUCTION

Corrective rhinoplasties fall into two major categories, depending on iatrogenically produced faults: (1) errors of omission (not enough was done; Fig. 14–43) and (2) errors of commission (too much was done; Fig. 14–44).

Severely maimed noses resulting from either multiple unsuccessful surgeries, cancer extirpation, or major trauma with tissue loss may require total nasal reconstruction with regional and local flaps. Some of these issues are addressed in more detail in Chapters 23 and 24.

ERRORS OF OMISSION

For the *undercorrected* tip, the operation is approached with the same philosophy as in primary rhinoplasty, that is, remove, recontour, and/or reposition the excessive or malpositioned cartilage.

A postoperative pinched tip may be secondary to excessive excision of cartilage and/or vestibular skin at the time of the original surgery. If excessive cartilage has been removed from the lateral crural region, a carefully positioned convex cartilage graft may be secured with suture fixation over the deficient area.

Text continued on page 188

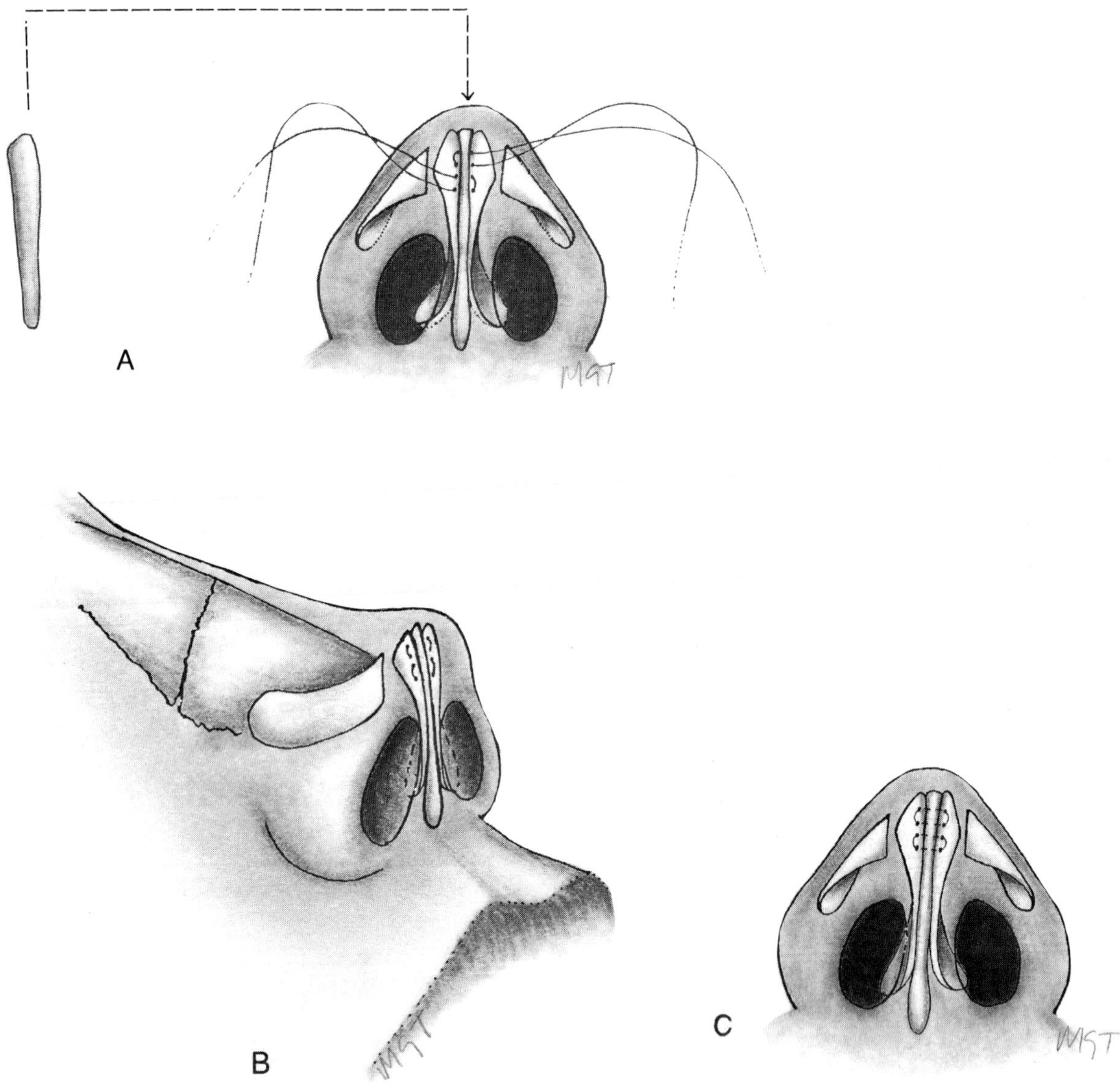

FIGURE 14–41. (*A*) When the medial crura are short or lack the necessary length or strength to support the tip, a piece of septal cartilage is placed between the medial crura and sutured in place. (*B* and *C*) The strut may extend inferiorly to within 2 mm of the nasal spine and may extend 1 to 2 mm above the transected medial crura in thick-skinned patients.

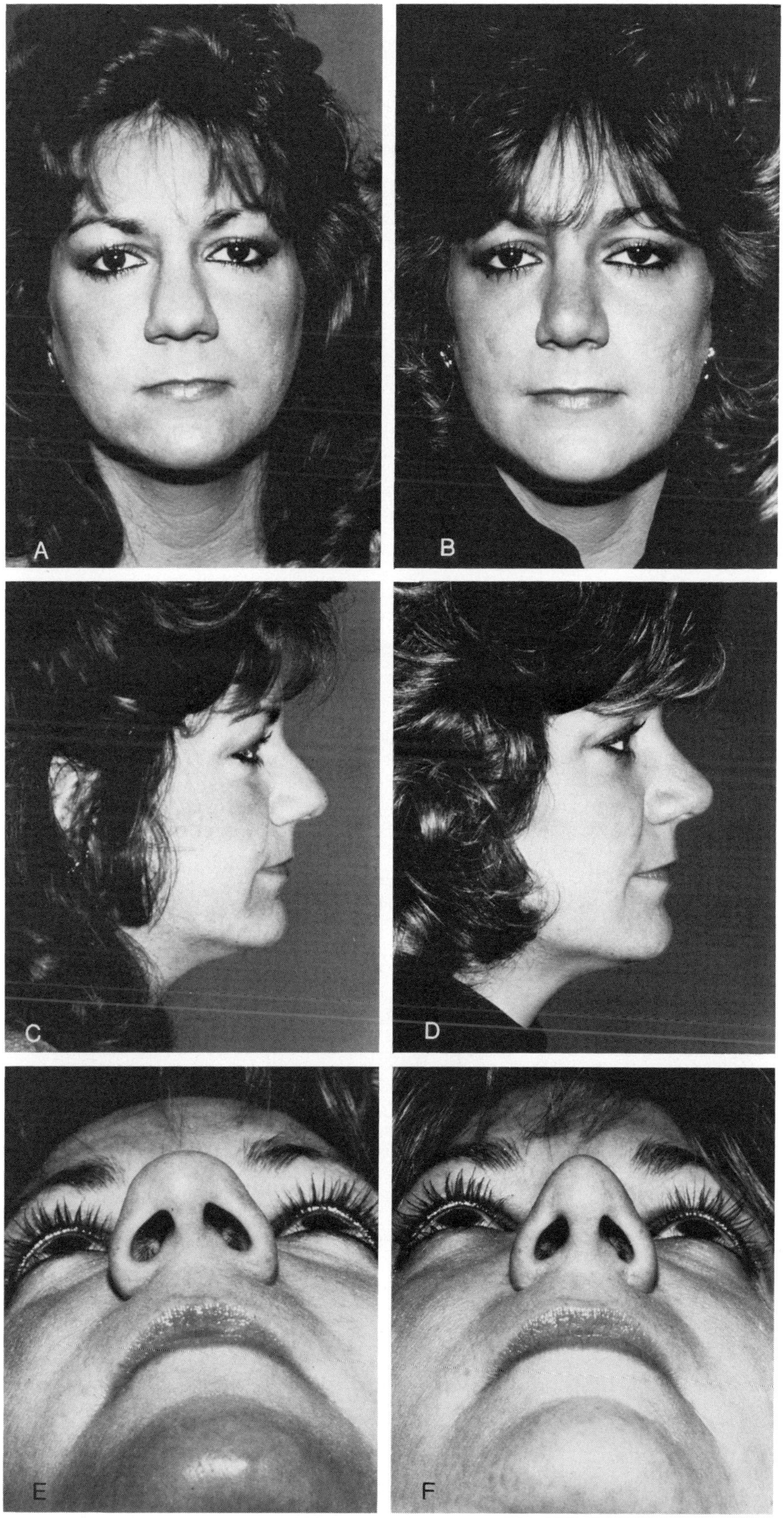

FIGURE 14–42. (*A* and *B*) When the nasal tip skin is thick and alar cartilages are frail, maximum narrowing and support may be provided by supporting the transected medial crural flaps with a large strut of septal cartilage. (*C* and *D*) The I-beam sandwich graft supports the central tip mechanism and may help to provide additional lobular height. (*E* and *F*) Narrowing of the nasal base typically occurs when projection is increased. The narrow lobule is indicative of the I-beam technique.

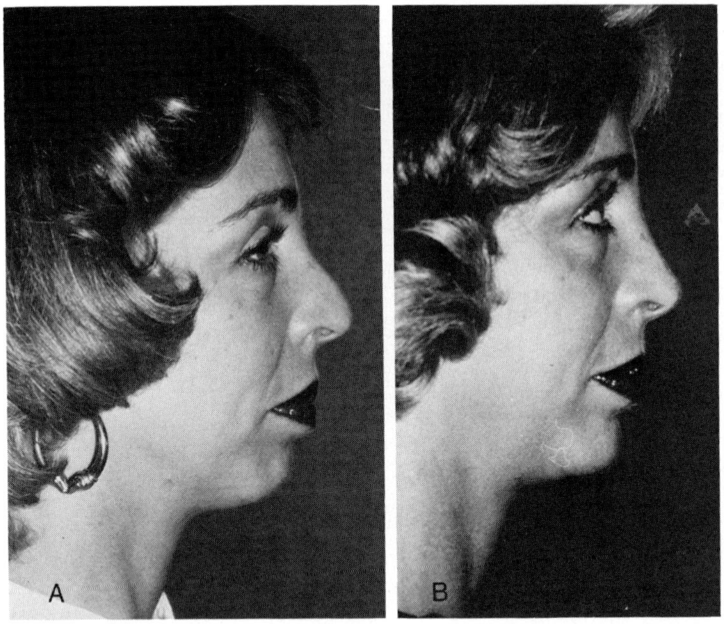

FIGURE 14–43. A polly-beak deformity may result from inadequate resection of the dorsal nasal septum, loss of tip support, or a combination of both. Correction can be obtained by completing dorsal cartilaginous resection and supporting the tip with a columellar strut. Chin augmentation was also performed in this patient.

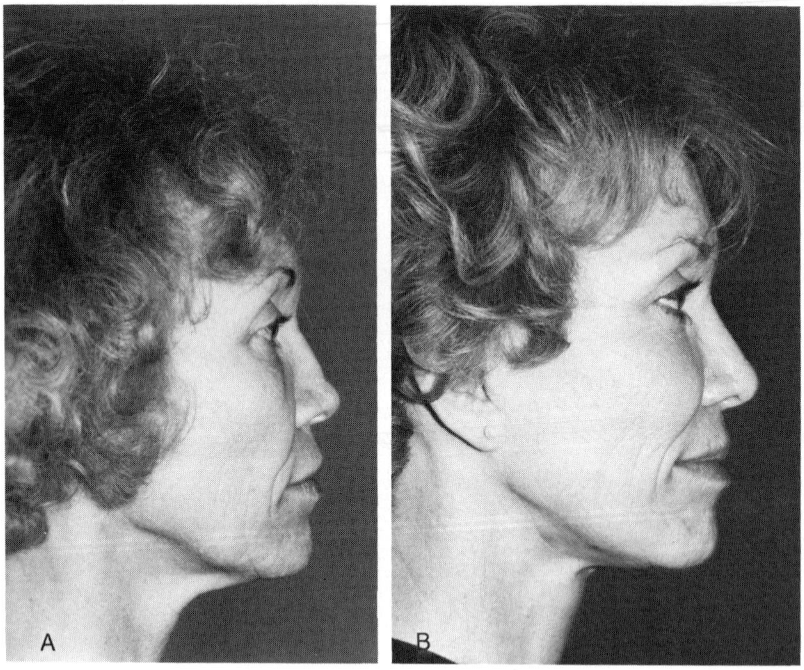

FIGURE 14–44. When much of the tip architecture has been destroyed or excised, reconstruction with multiple columellar, tip, and dorsal grafts is necessary.

When much of the alar cartilage is missing, a thin piece of auricular conchal cartilage usually is preferable to recreate the natural convex surface of the lateral crus (Fig. 14–45). A piece of septal cartilage, particularly if the patient's septum was deviated or crooked, also provides an excellent lateral crural graft. If an excess should exist on the opposite side, a strip of cephalic lateral crus can be transferred. These grafts usually are secured with 5-0 Dexon or Vicryl sutures. The knot is placed on the vestibular skin surface whenever possible.

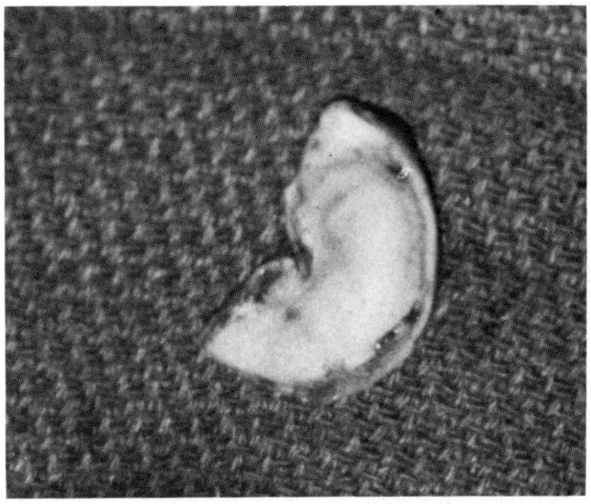

FIGURE 14–45. A piece of conchal cartilage obtained from the ear can be fashioned into curved grafts for tip reconstruction. A conchal bowl graft is shown.

If asymmetry is secondary to inaccurate or unequal tip cartilage transection, equivalent vertical divisions and precise suturing to the opposite crus may be all that are needed to achieve symmetry. Morselized or crushed onlay blanket cartilage grafts may help to camouflage irregularities (Fig. 14–46).

Sharp points, or "knuckles," in the region of one or both domes may be caused by sharp edges, particularly if cartilage transection, asymmetric suturing, or morselized dome techniques were performed in the original surgery (Fig. 14–47).

Buckling during healing after rim strip techniques or improper graft placement may also produce these undesirable irregularities known as "bossi." To correct the deformity, it might be necessary to shave a sharp edge of transected cartilage; divide and/or suture the knuckled domes to each other; shorten, reposition, or replace an improperly designed cartilagenous graft; or cover the deformities with blanket cartilage grafts.

ERRORS OF COMMISSION

When a complex reconstruction is anticipated, or when skeletal augmentation is necessary, an external (open) conversion may be helpful. The surgeon should not hesitate to connect the two marginal incisions with an inverted V transcolumellar incision at any time during the operation he thinks it is necessary. Converting a closed rhinoplasty to an external rhinoplasty often is helpful, particularly if the additional exposure would facilitate diagnosis and allow for excision of scar tissue as well as accurate suturing of grafts and implants (Figs. 14–48 and 14–49).

RIM STRIP PROCEDURE

As defined by Webster,[3] in the rim strip procedure all alar cartilage lateral to the transection point is excised and discarded (Fig. 14–50). If a significant degree of the tip rotation and/or tip retrodisplacement is desired in a nose with thicker skin and long lateral crura, transection and removal of cartilage at some point lateral to the dome may be desirable (Fig. 14–51).

When the two lateral legs of the tripod are shortened and central support is enhanced, significant tip rotation can be achieved. Paramedian supra-alar narrowing is also accomplished because a larger mass of cartilage has been removed.

Text continued on page 194

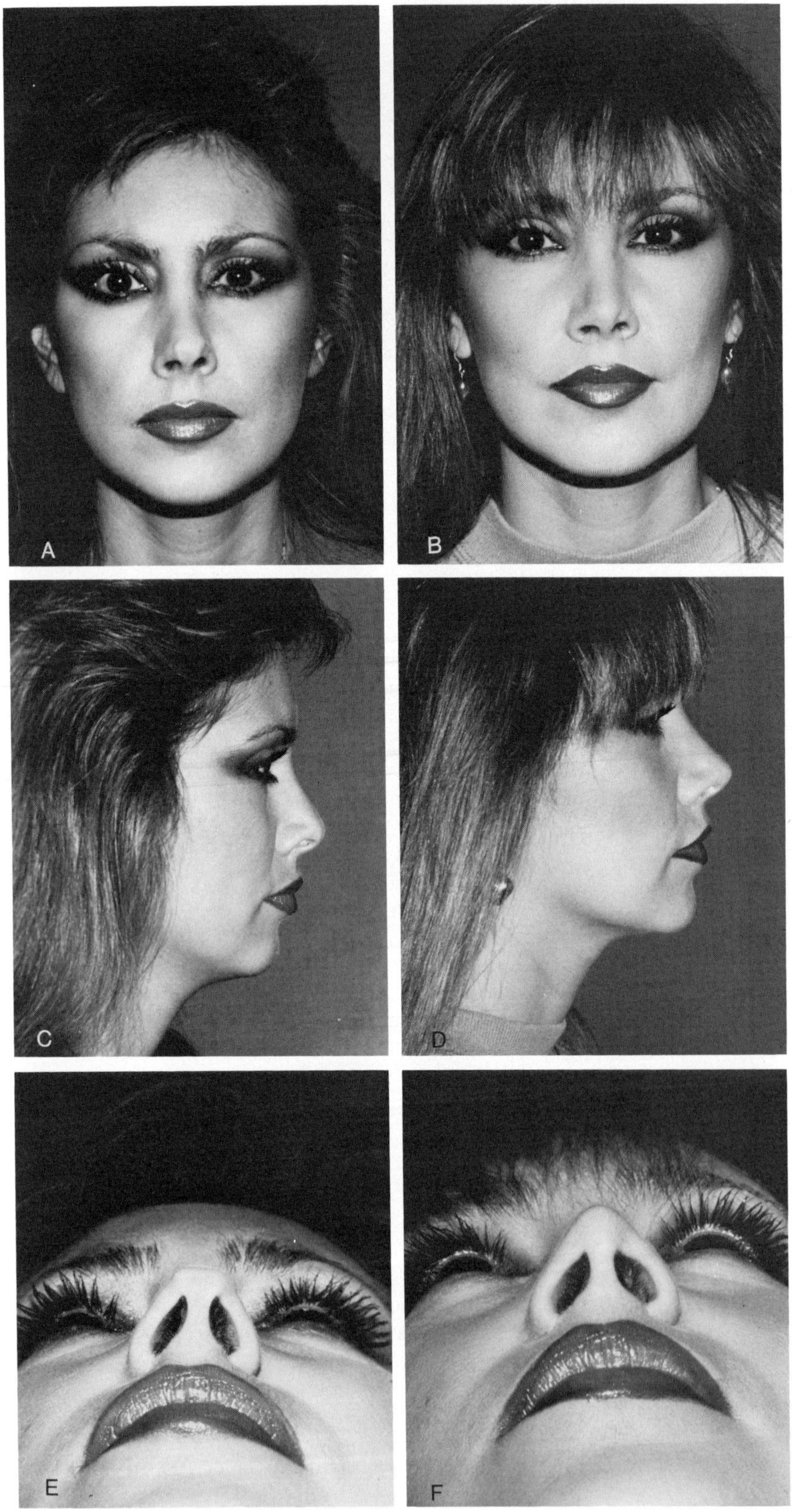

FIGURE 14–46. (*A* and *B*) A prior rhinoplasty left this patient with an asymmetric tip. (*C* and *D*) Because much of the support of the tip was not reestablished, ptosis occurred. (*E* and *F*) Failure to recognize and correct asymmetries in the dome areas resulted in bossi and intradomal widening. Medial crural fixation coupled with cartilaginous grafting to the lateral nasal walls provided support and symmetry.

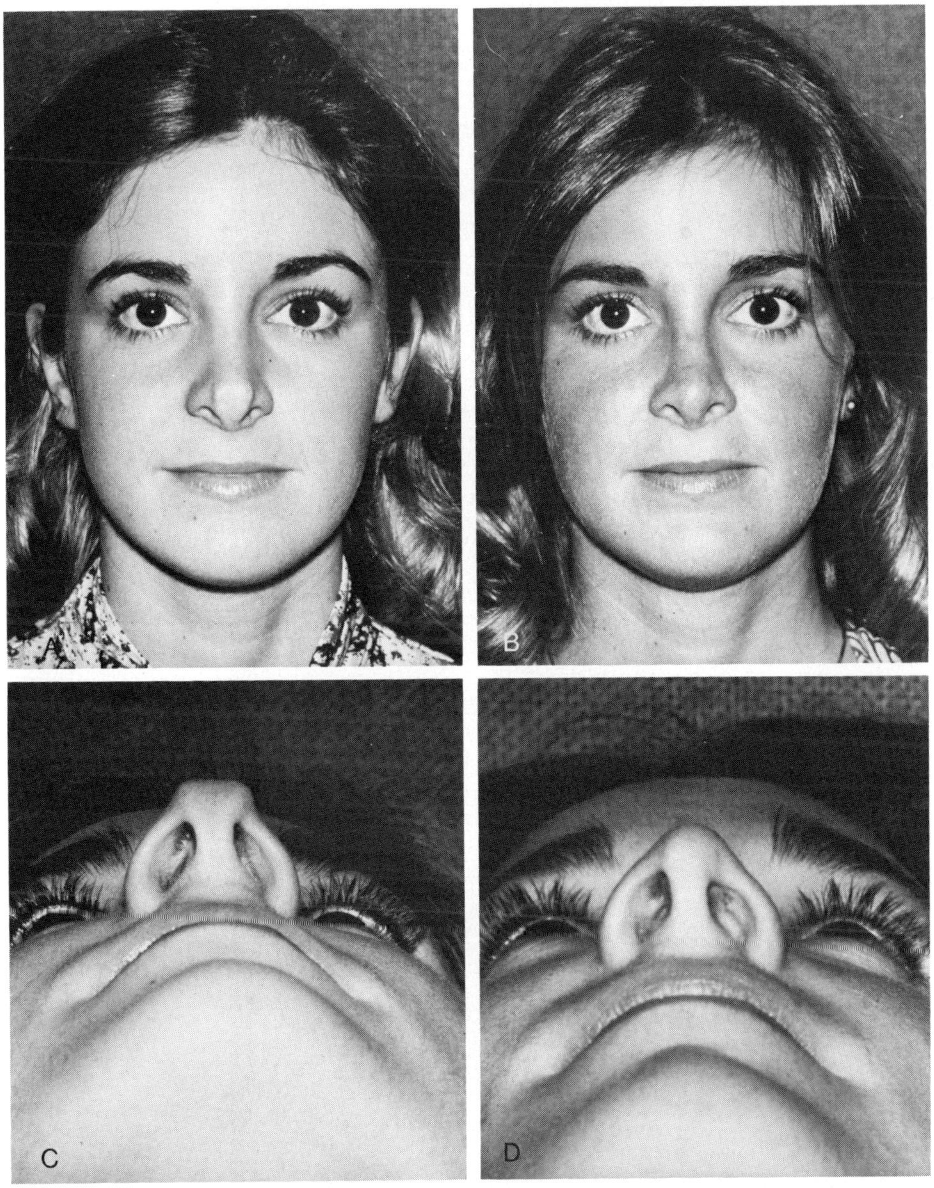

FIGURE 14–47. (*A* and *B*) Knuckling of the domes (bossi) may occur in patients who have thin skin and intradomal bifidity and whose surgery is performed through nondelivery techniques. (*C* and *D*) After delivery, the two domes may be sutured to each other to eliminate the intradomal defect. Nostril asymmetry still exists.

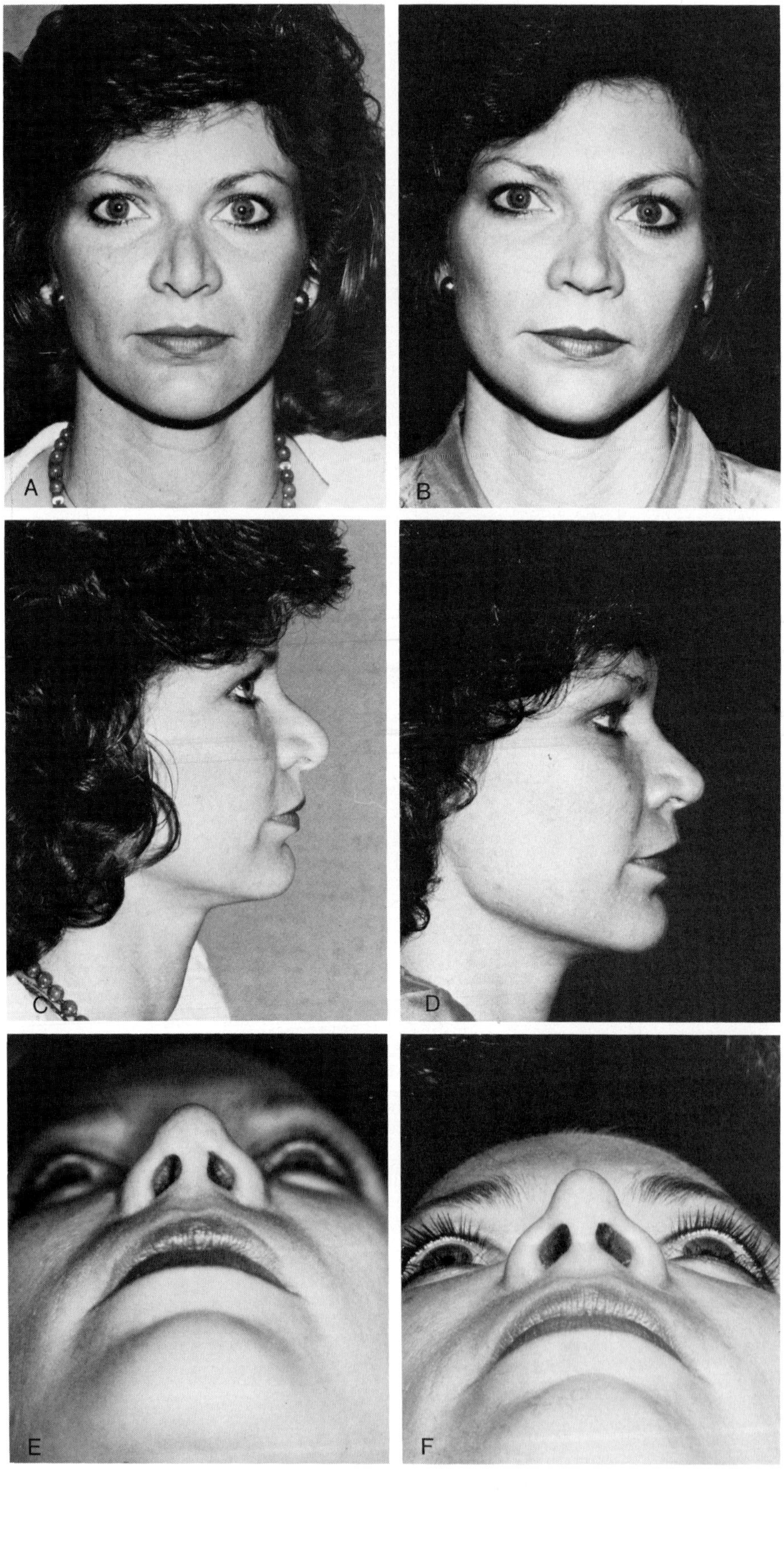

FIGURE 14–48. (*A* and *B*) A previously performed rhinoplasty resulted in numerous unwanted sequelae in this patient. (*C* and *D*) Revision required excision of a large scar mass in the supratip region (see intraoperative photographs), dorsal augmentation, and an I-beam tip-plasty. (*E* and *F*) The procedure was performed through an external, or open, approach.

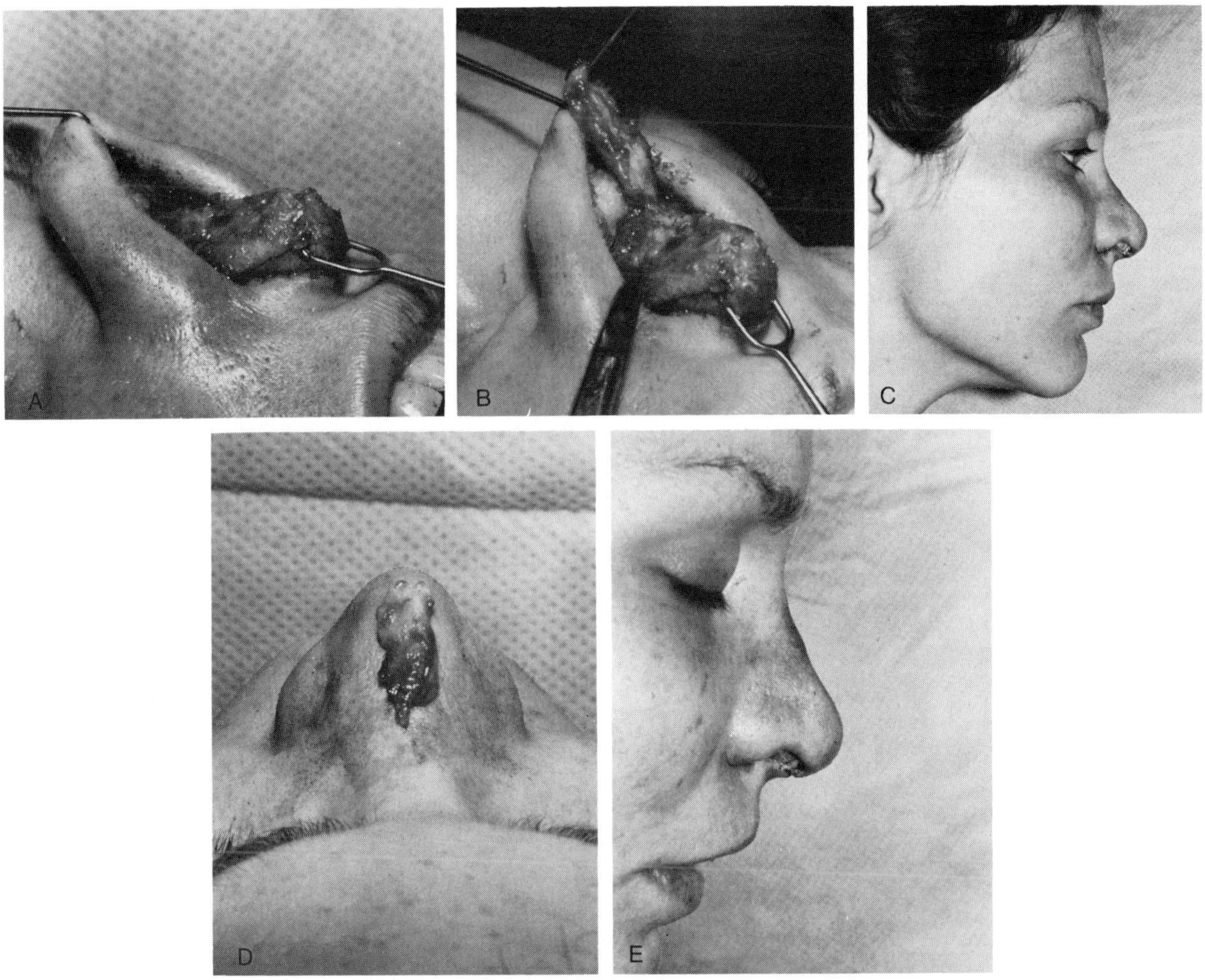

FIGURE 14–49. (*A*) The dorsal nasal skin is retracted, revealing a large mass of scar in the supratip region. (*B*) The remaining segments of alar cartilage are identified, and dissection is begun. (*C* and *D*) The mass of scar is removed. (*E*) After an I-beam tip-plasty and cartilaginous graft augmentation over the bony dorsum, the intraoperative appearance of the nose is improved in 2-year postoperative photograph shown in *D*.

Definition: Rim Strip Procedure Leaving a Triangular Portion of Lateral Crura at the Pyriform Aperture

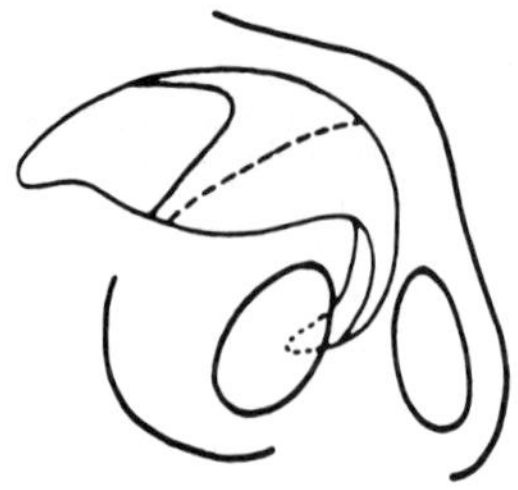

Advantages

1. Allows for Maximum Tip Rotation
2. Prevents Retraction of Alar Margin
3. Prevents Pinching of Lateral Supra-alar Area in Thin-Skinned Patients

Disadvantages

1. Limits Supra-alar Definition of Tip in Thick-Skinned Patients

FIGURE 14–50. The rim strip technique is accomplished as shown in this drawing. All cartilage lateral to the transection point is removed.

The rim strip technique may be helpful in the rare cases in which dome division may not be indicated yet maximum rotation is desired.

If the medial crural and lateral crural components of the dome are pulled together during healing with scar tissue contraction (either symmetrically or asymmetrically) these unwanted sequelae can occur. They are more common, however, in patients with thin skin. When a cleft is visible between the lobular portions of the medial crura, "bossi" or "knuckles" are virtually assured (Figs. 14–46, 14–47 and 14–52).

Negative factors associated with rim strips are the loss of lateral crural skeletal support, tip retrodisplacement and supra-alar pinching. Because the two lateral tripod legs have been significantly shortened, the strip settles toward the pyriform aperature and can often collapse inward toward the vestibule.

If the procedure is performed through an intracartilaginous or retrograde approach, asymmetric excision of cartilage occurs more frequently than when the alar cartilage is delivered.

Failure to recognize existing cartilagenous deformities is also possible unless both the caudal and the cephalic borders are visualized. Asymmetry of the medial crura often goes undetected.

Additional tip-supporting maneuvers are required when the rim strip technique is used, except in patients who have overly projecting tips (Fig. 14–53). Cartilaginous struts, plumping grafts, or batons may be used to provide tip support and rotation. Additional central support is required, since the element of tip projection afforded by an intact lateral crus is removed.

LATERAL CRURAL FLAP

Even when the surgeon believes that he is using the rim strip procedure, some portion of the lateral crus in the region of the pyriform aperature usually is left behind. The lateral crural flap technique[9] (also described by Webster) is similar to the rim strip, except that some portion of the lateral crus attached to the bony pyriform aperture is preserved (Fig. 14–54). Theoretically, this technique may avoid some of the sequelae encountered in the overzealous removal of alar cartilage, but it, too, is seldom indicated.

Text continued on page 198

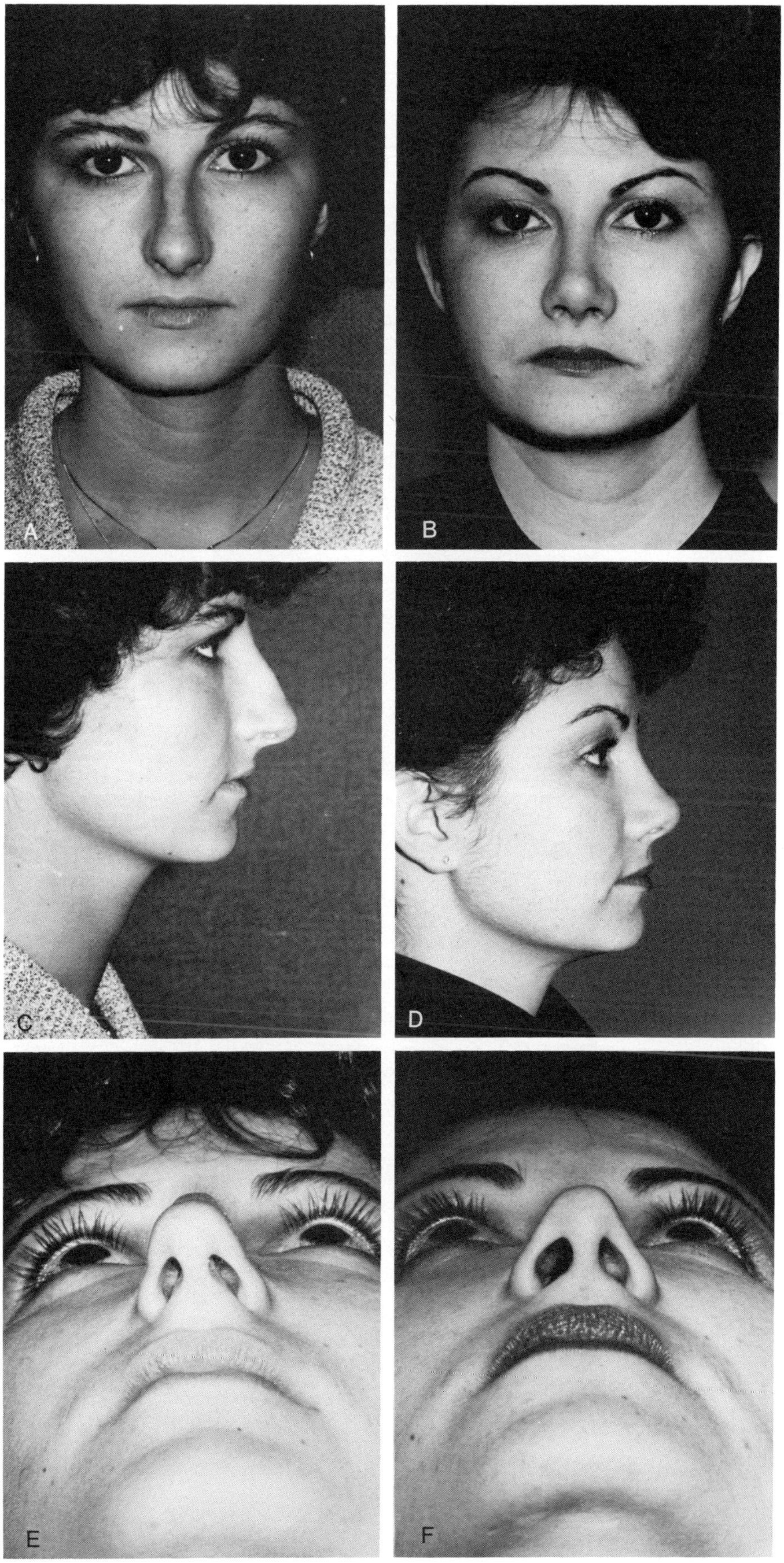

FIGURE 14–51. (*A* and *B*) A rim strip procedure was performed through an intracartilaginous incision in this patient. The postoperative photograph demonstrates a 10-year result. (*C* and *D*) Retrodisplacement and rotation were obtained by shortening the lateral legs of the tip tripod and strengthening the central leg with a cartilaginous strut. (*E* and *F*) The preoperative asymmetry of the alae was not corrected.

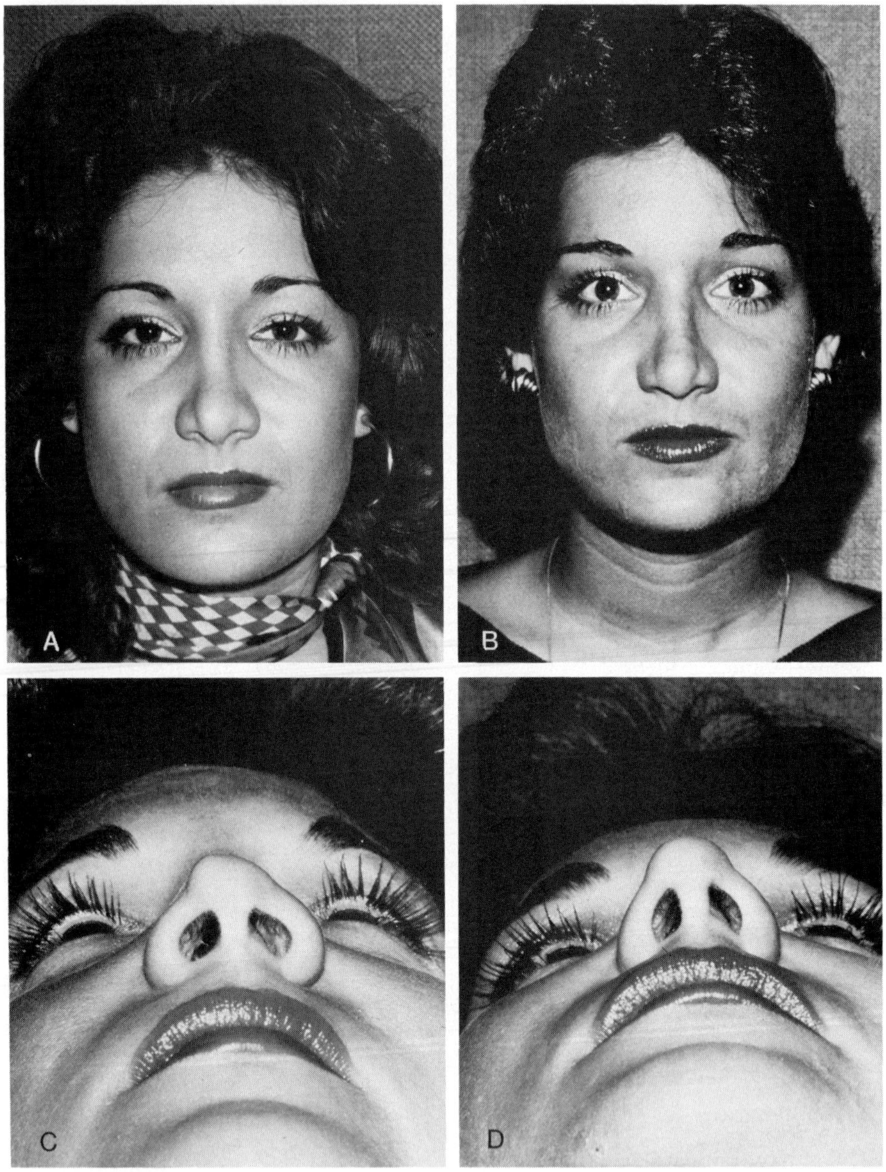

FIGURE 14–52. (*A* and *B*) This patient had a previous rhinoplasty performed through a cartilage-splitting (intracartilaginous) approach. A rim strip procedure had been performed. Knuckling of the right dome occurred postoperatively. (*C* and *D*) At revision, asymmetric excision of the cartilages was found and corrected. The domes were sutured to each other and an onlay graft was placed along the border to the lateral crura.

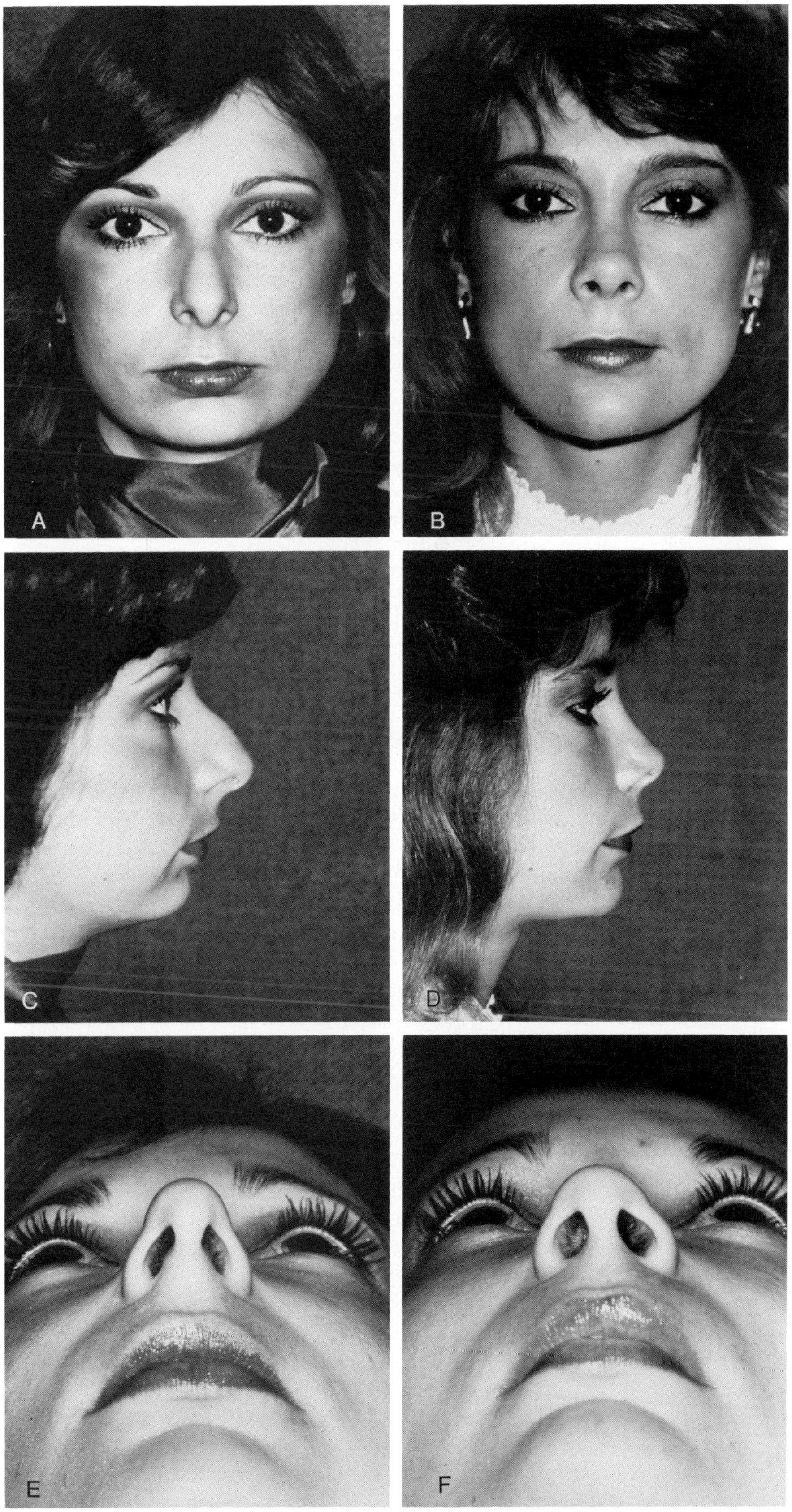

FIGURE 14–53. (*A* and *B*) A rim strip procedure was performed in this patient. The postoperative photograph represents a 4-year result. (*C* and *D*) The overly projecting tip was retrodisplaced by shortening the lateral tripod legs (rim strip) and excising the caudal septum and nasal spine. Chin augmentation was also performed. (*E* and *F*) Webbing of the nasolabial angle was corrected.

Definition: The Anterior Border of the Lower Lateral Cartilage Has Been Interrupted Lateral to the Dome and Proximal to the Pyriform Aperture

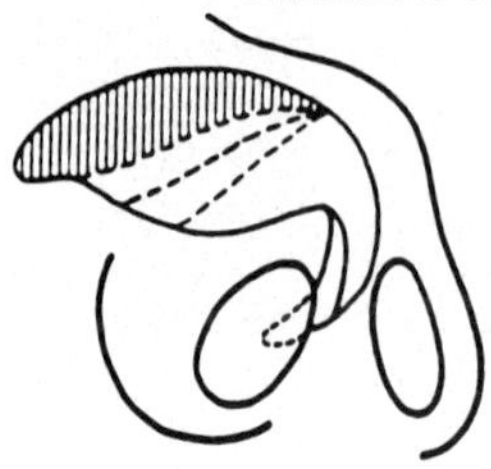

Advantages

1. Provides Maximum Tip Rotation
2. Allows Greater Supra-alar Definition in Thick-Skinned Individuals

Disadvantages

1. Loss of Tip Support
2. Pinching of Lateral Supra-alar Region in Thin-Skinned Patients
3. Retraction or Pinching of Alar Margin in Thin-Skinned Patients
4. Accentuation of Nostril Flaring

FIGURE 14–54. A lateral crural flap is achieved when a portion of the lateral crus past the point of transection is preserved.

LATERAL CRURAL TURNOVER GRAFT

When the lateral crura are concave rather than convex after excision of the cephalic portion, that segment may be turned over and sutured to the remaining concave segment (Figs. 14–55, 14–56, and 14–57). The opposing vectors of force tend to straighten the lateral crus and produce a more natural-looking tip.[10] In my experience, other techniques, such as a thinner complete strip with the incorporation of supporting maneuvers (i.e., struts, plumping graft) of the medial crural leg of the tripod, along with grafting over the lateral crural concavity can achieve much of the definition the surgeon might attempt to obtain with a lateral crural flap or rim strip (Fig. 14–58).

ALAR CONSIDERATIONS

Da Vinci's criteria of facial proportions dictated that the base of the nose be no wider than the distance between the medial canthi. When the alae are too wide (or asymmetric), the excision of appropriate amounts of the alar sils allows the surgeon to narrow the base of the nose and achieve better symmetry (see Fig. 18–4). In some cases, an alar sil resection may be required only on one side. If both sides are wide and asymmetric, different amounts of the alar sil may be removed (Fig. 14–59).

COLUMELLAR-SEPTAL CONSIDERATION

A crooked columella or asymmetric tip might be caused by a severely deviated or dislocated septum (Fig. 14–60). If the columella is crooked as a result of asymmetric medial crura, partial or complete division and/or

Text continued on page 205

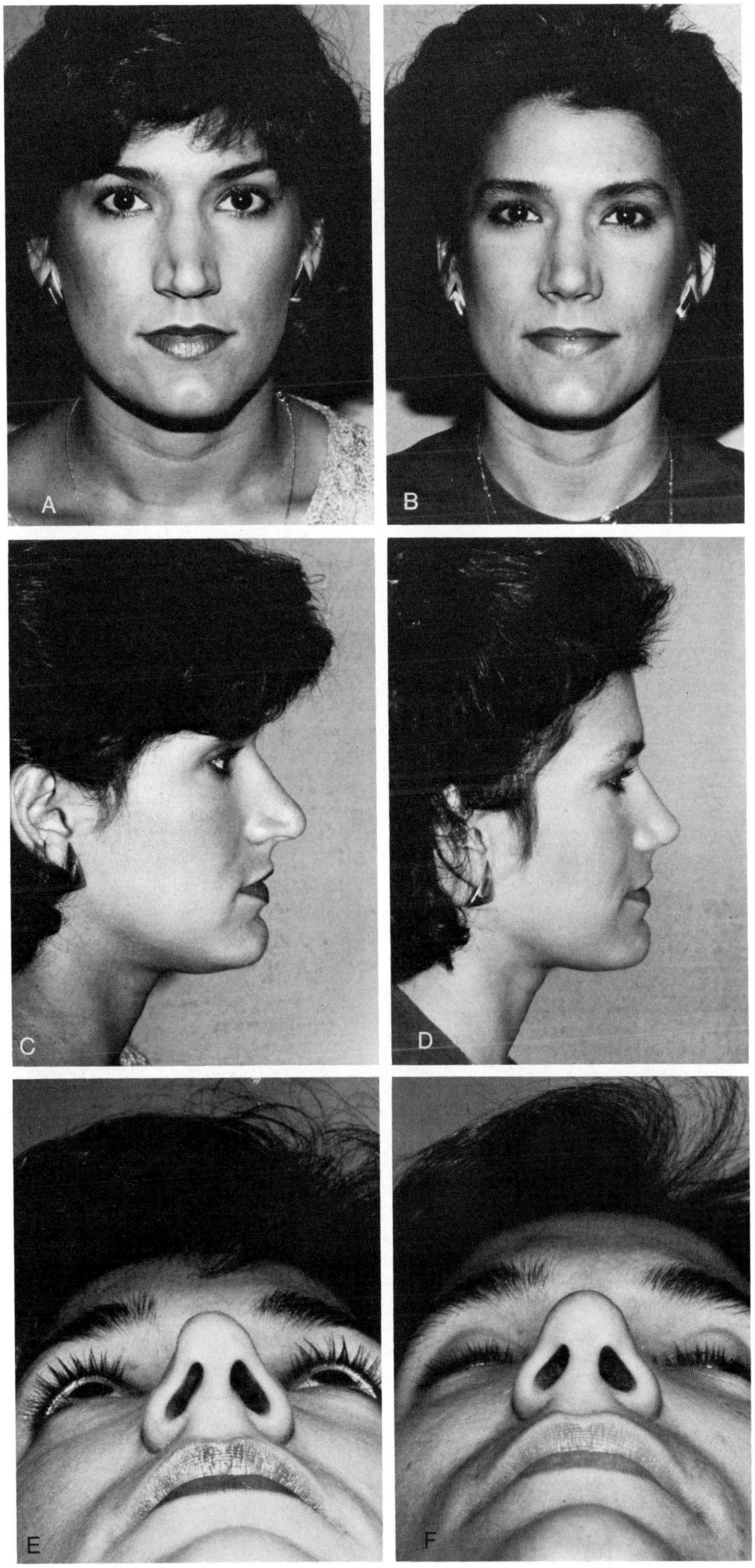

FIGURE 14–55. (*A* and *B*) This patient was an excellent candidate for the lateral crural turnover graft. The concavity of the lateral crura were corrected by the technique described in Figure 14–57. (*C* and *D*) Although the tip looked as though she had undergone an overly aggressive tip-plasty, she had never had surgery. (*E* and *F*) The procedure may be performed through a closed or an open approach. The transcolumellar scar is barely visible.

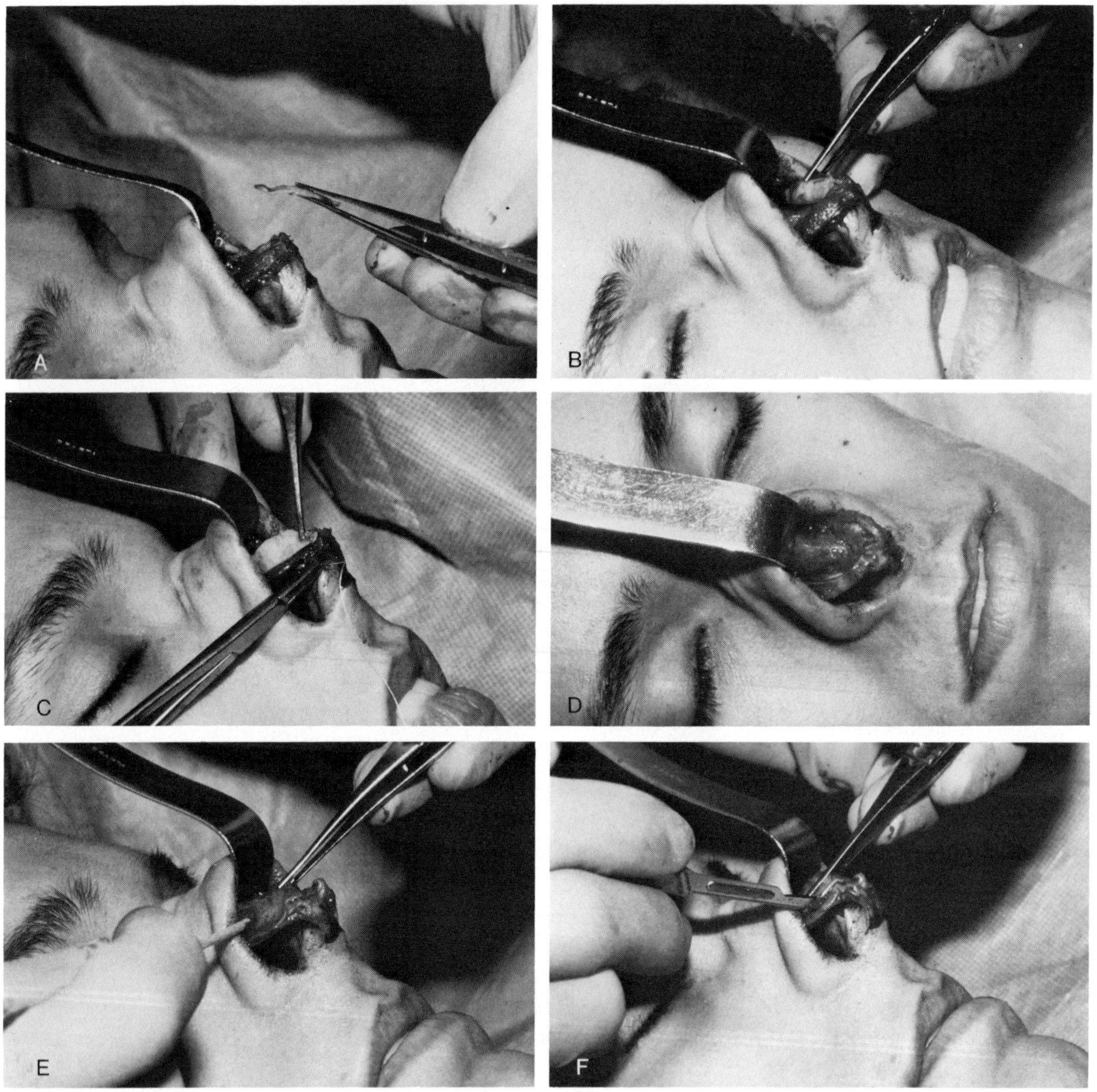

FIGURE 14–56. The lateral crural turnover graft technique is demonstrated in this sequence of intraoperative photographs. A portion of the concave superior lateral crus is excised, turned over, and sutured to the remaining complete strip with interrupted 5-0 Vicryl fixation sutures. See Figure 14–57 for a schematic demonstration of the turnover graft technique.

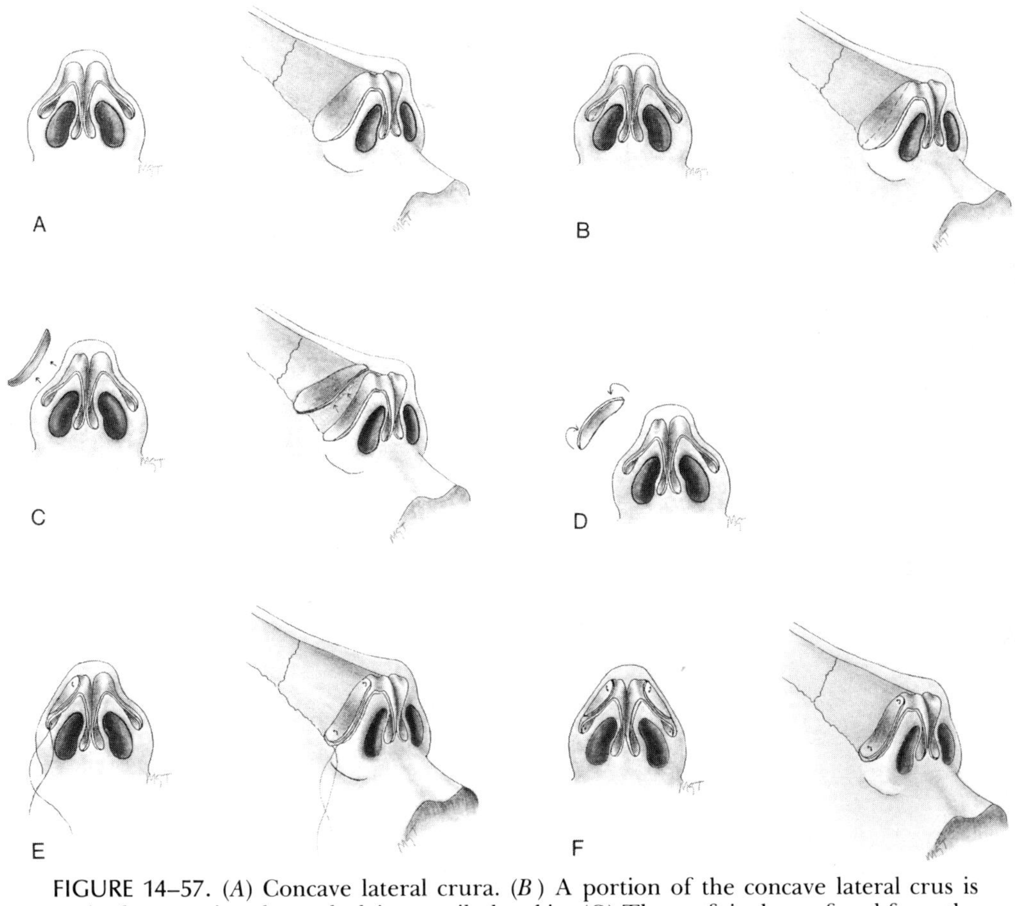

FIGURE 14–57. (*A*) Concave lateral crura. (*B*) A portion of the concave lateral crus is excised preserving the underlying vestibular skin. (*C*) The graft is shown freed from the underlying tissues. (*D*) The graft is turned over so that it becomes a convex piece of cartilage. (*E*) The convex graft is sutured to the remaining concave portion of the lateral crus with mattress-type sutures (5-0 Vicryl). (*F*) The convex-concave vectors cancel each other, resulting in a straightened and bulkier lateral crus.

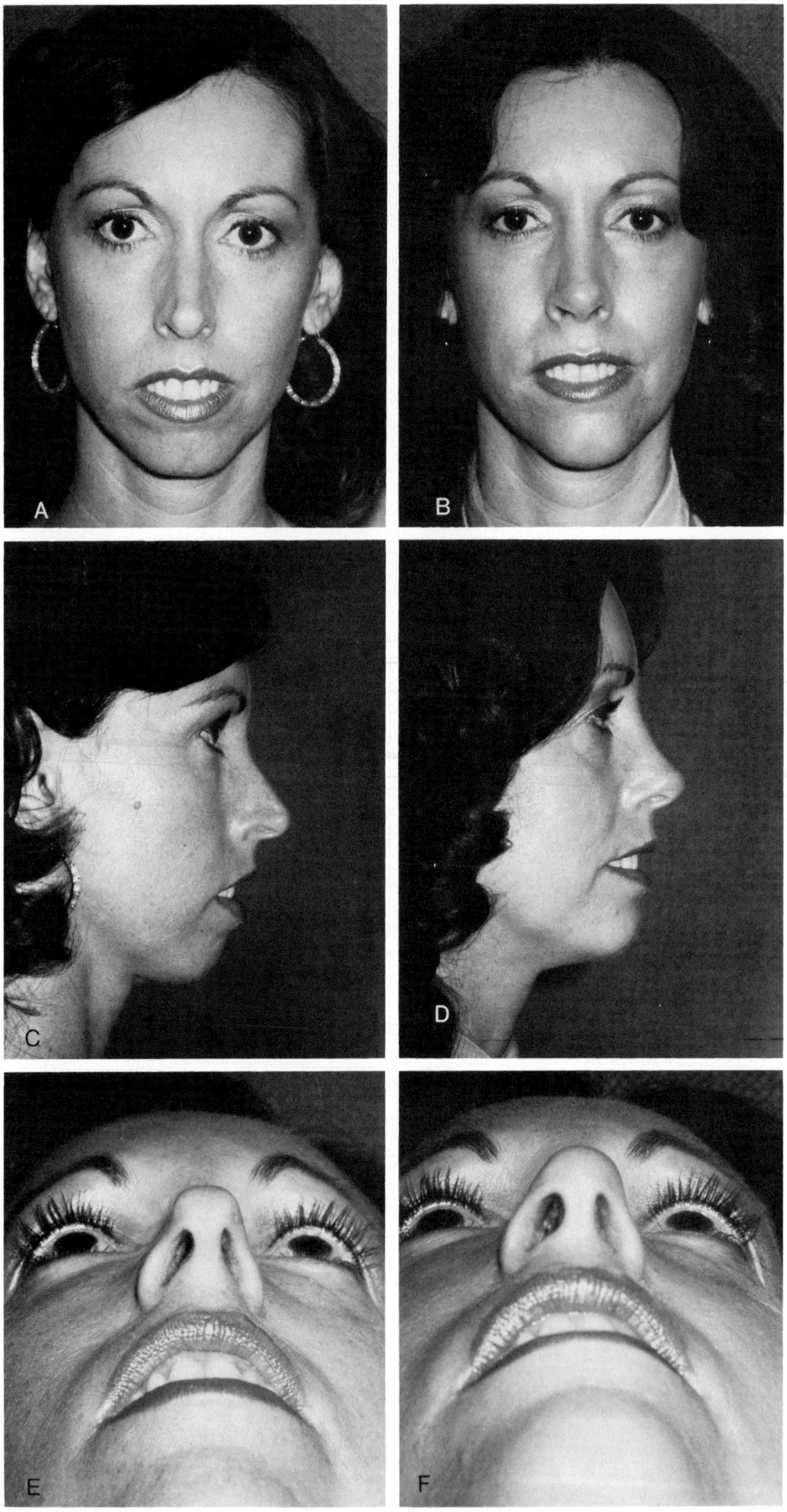

FIGURE 14–58. (*A* and *B*) Before the turnover graft technique was available and external rhinoplasty had found its place in contemporary surgery, I used the lateral crural flap (1976) through a cartilage-splitting incision whenever tip retrodisplacement, rotation, and prevention of lateral alar collapse was desired. (*C* and *D*) The desired result was achieved in the nose. Chin augmentation was also performed. (*E* and *F*) The preoperative asymmetry was not corrected.

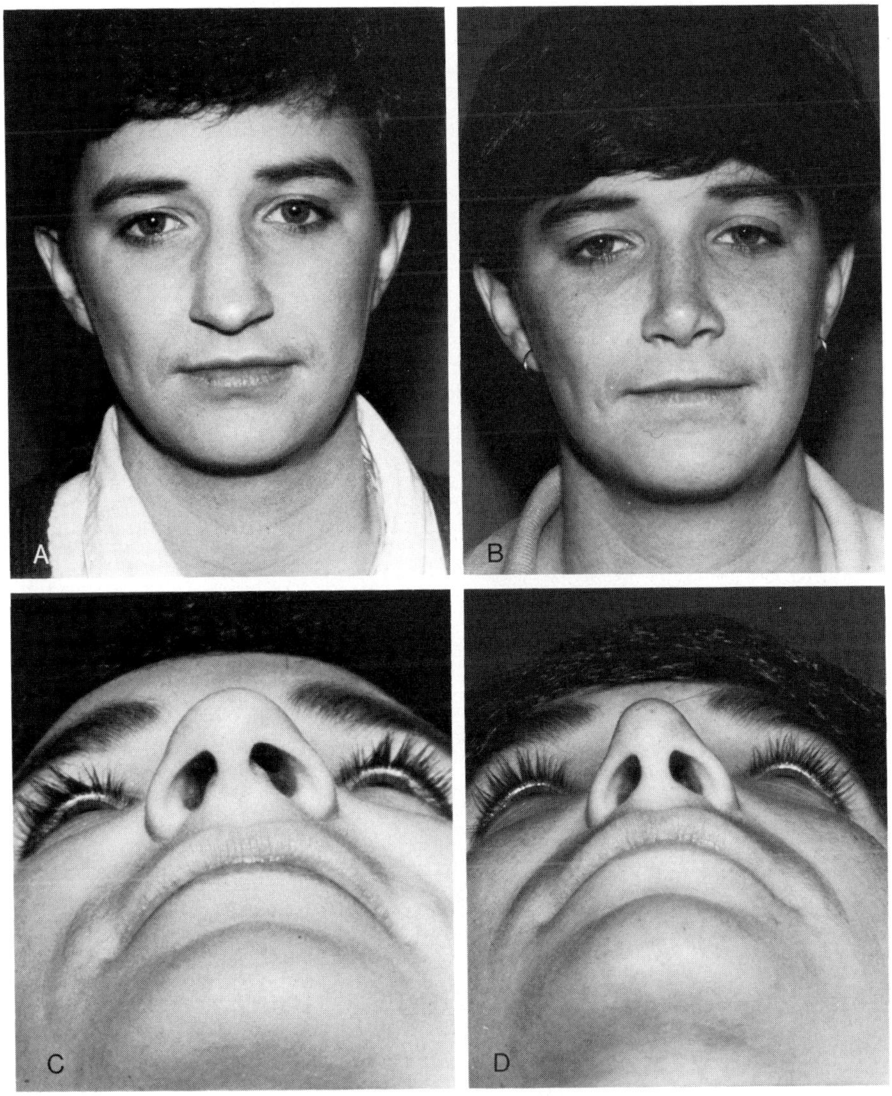

FIGURE 14–59. A wide alar base can be narrowed by carefully planned alar sil excisions (see Figure 18–4 *A–C*).

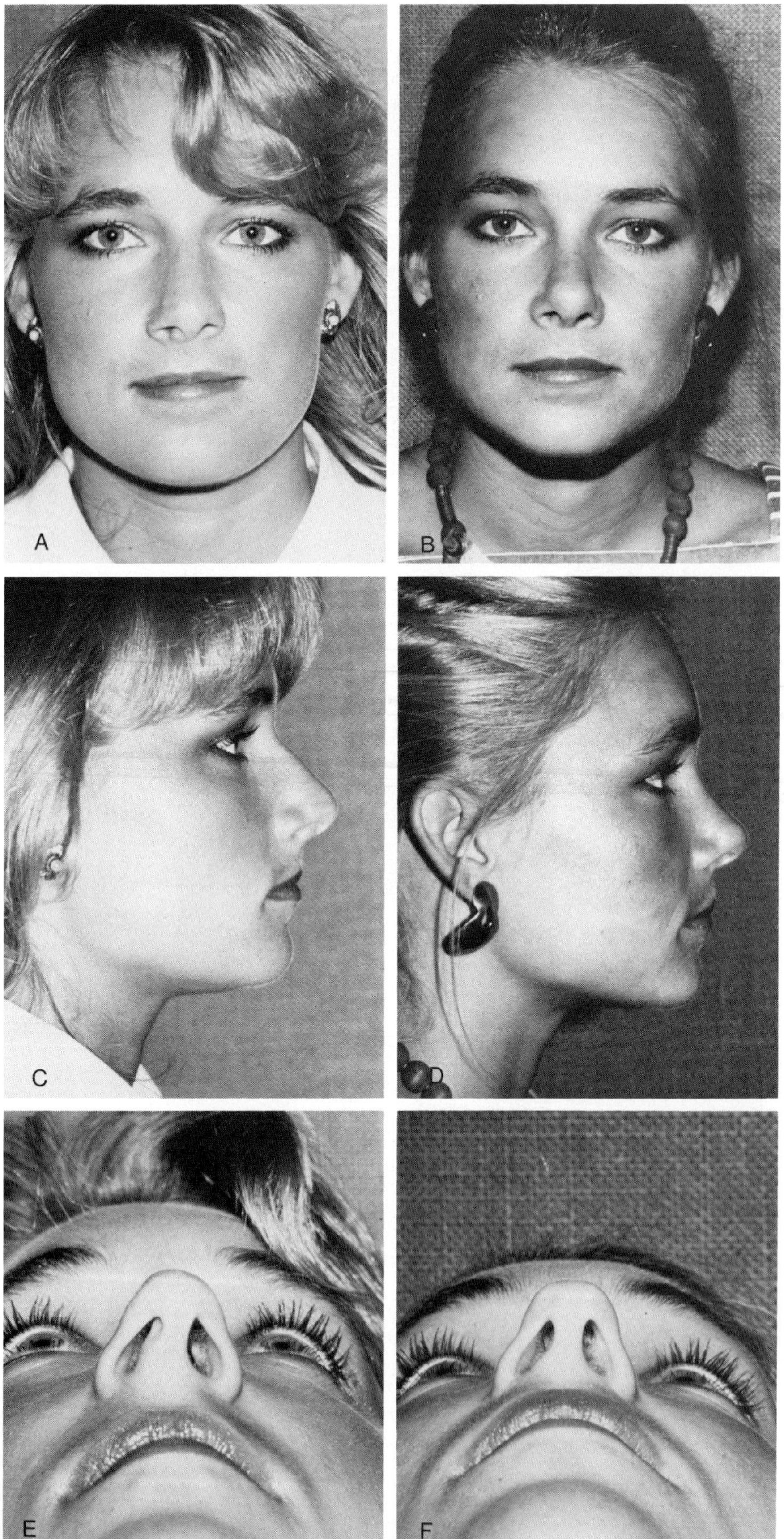

FIGURE 14–60. Columellar deformity caused by a deviated nasal septum. Correction of the septal deformity improved the appearance of the columella. (*A*) The columella is pulled to the right of midline. (*B*) Connecting the septal deformity straightened the columella. (*C*) Excessive columella show is noted. (*D*) Shortening the septum created a more pleasing nasolabial angle. (*E*) Nostril asymmetry and unequal dome heights are obvious. (*F*) Septoplasty (swing-door type) and conservative tip-plasty corrected the problems.

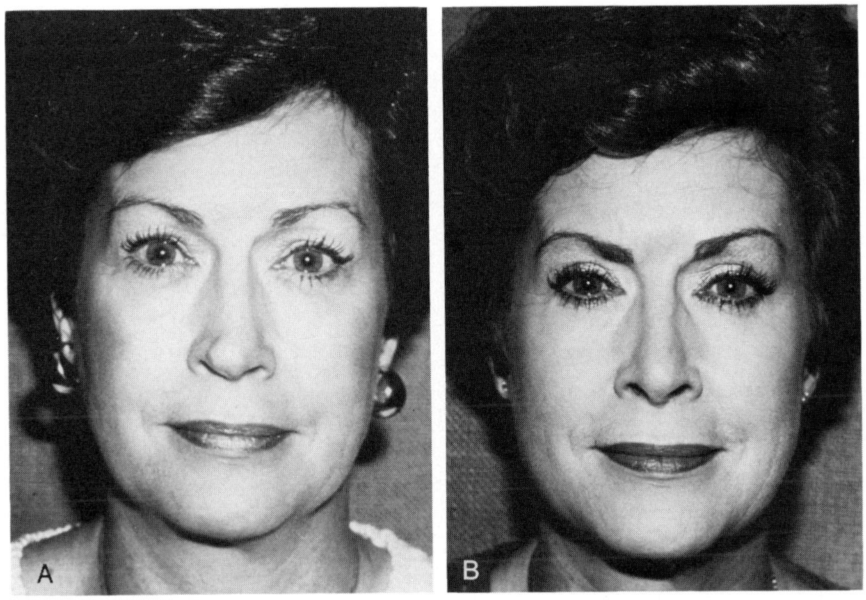

FIGURE 14–61. (*A*) Columellar deformities may be secondary to asymmetries of the medial crural portions of the lower lateral cartilages. (*B*) In this patient, the caudal septum was straight. Correction involved morselization and intracrural splinting with a cartilage graft.

careful morselization of the abnormal cartilage may "break" the memory of the deviant cartilage (see Figs. 14–7 and 14–8). A straight sandwich cartilage graft from the nasal septum secured with an absorbable 3-0 chromic mattress suture can be used to achieve the desired correction (Fig. 14–61).

If the base of the columella is excessively wide, soft tissue removal between the medial crura may produce narrowing. Until fibrosis sets in, it is best to suture the medial crura together with two 3-0 chromic mattress sutures.

EXTERNAL TIP-PLASTY

Any tip procedure can be performed accurately and precisely under the direct visualization provided by the open approach. It may be advisable for inexperienced surgeons to do their first several cases through this approach. Once the surgical dynamics and anatomic relations of the nasal components are more thoroughly understood, the surgeon can then select the appropriate method for the case at hand, realizing that he can always convert the operation to an external approach.

External rhinoplasty conversion is extremely helpful in difficult revisional cases and complicated primary procedures (see Fig. 14–7*A* through *E*). Maximum visibility for diagnosis and correction can be obtained when the dorsal skin flap is reflected. In an experienced surgeon's hands, this approach is not required for most primary nasal plastic operations.

As is the case in primary rhinoplasty, the operation may be begun by carrying out the classic delivery technique. If it is desirable, the marginal incisions may be connected with an inverted V transcolumellar incision.

The postoperative scar on the columellar usually is inconspicuous. Placing the incision at mid-columella, where the skin is thin, and using good plastic surgical principles for skin closure and wound care help to ensure acceptable scar magnification (Fig. 14–62). The scar may be more prominent if the incision is placed in the thicker skin toward the base of the columella.

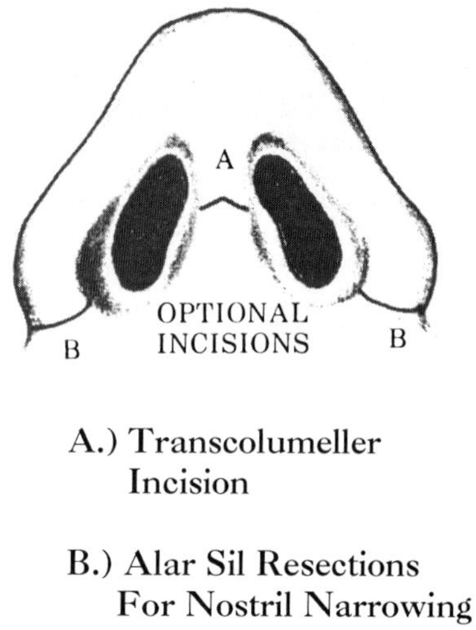

FIGURE 14–62. (*A*) The columellar incision is made in certain difficult cases. (*B*) The alar incision is made when nostril width is reduced.

Most nasal plastic surgeons agree that reflection of the dorsal nasal skin flap provides a panoramic exposure not obtainable with any of the closed techniques. The external conversion usually facilitates the diagnosis and correction of complex deformities.

A columellar scar is the only predictable disadvantage of external rhinoplasty. Nasal plastic surgeons should not hesitate to add the transcolumellar incision to their armamentarium.

PARTIAL RHINOPLASTY

Some modification or refinement of the nasal tip cartilages ought to be performed in the vast majority of rhinoplasties. Minor modifications in the size and shape of the lower lateral cartilages often result in some tip definition. When the cartilages are freed from the overlying skin and internal nasal tissues, they can be repositioned, supported and/or molded into a better position and secured with a properly applied tip dressing (Figs. 14–63 and 14–64).

POLLY BEAK

Supratip rounding, or polly beak, may result from (1) insufficient removal of superior septal angle cartilage; (2) incomplete removal of Pitanguy's suspensory ligament; (3) loss of tip support; (4) soft tissue buildup during healing, or (5) all of the above.

Loss of tip projection usually accompanies a polly beak (Fig. 14–65). When it is determined that an inadequate amount of cartilaginous dorsum

Text continued on page 211

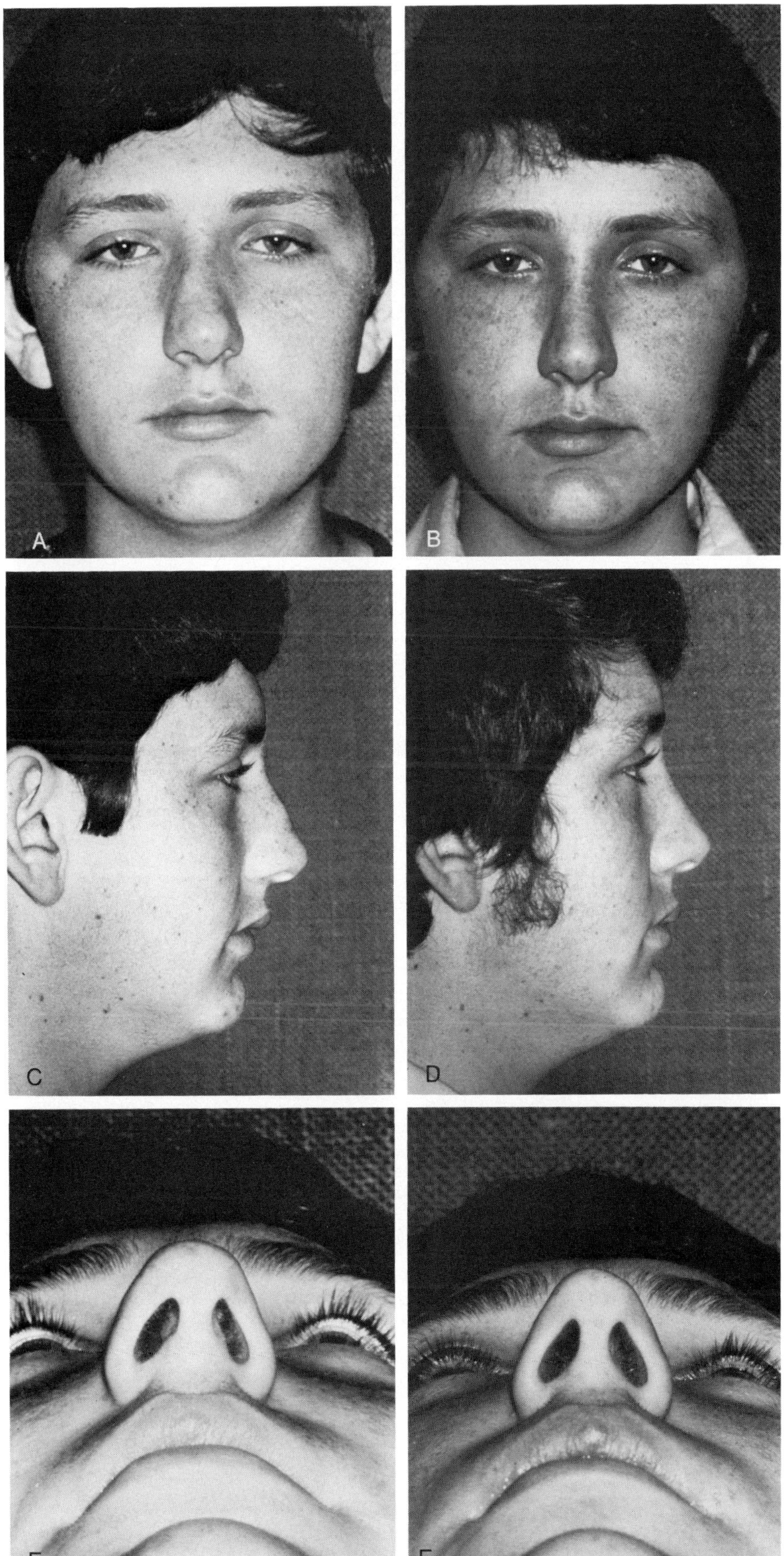

FIGURE 14–63. (*A* and *B*) In patients who were pleased with the appearance of their nose before trauma, partial corrective rhinoplasty may be indicated. (*C* and *D*) A small dorsal hump was removed. (*E* and *F*) The septal deviation was corrected, but no tip surgery was performed.

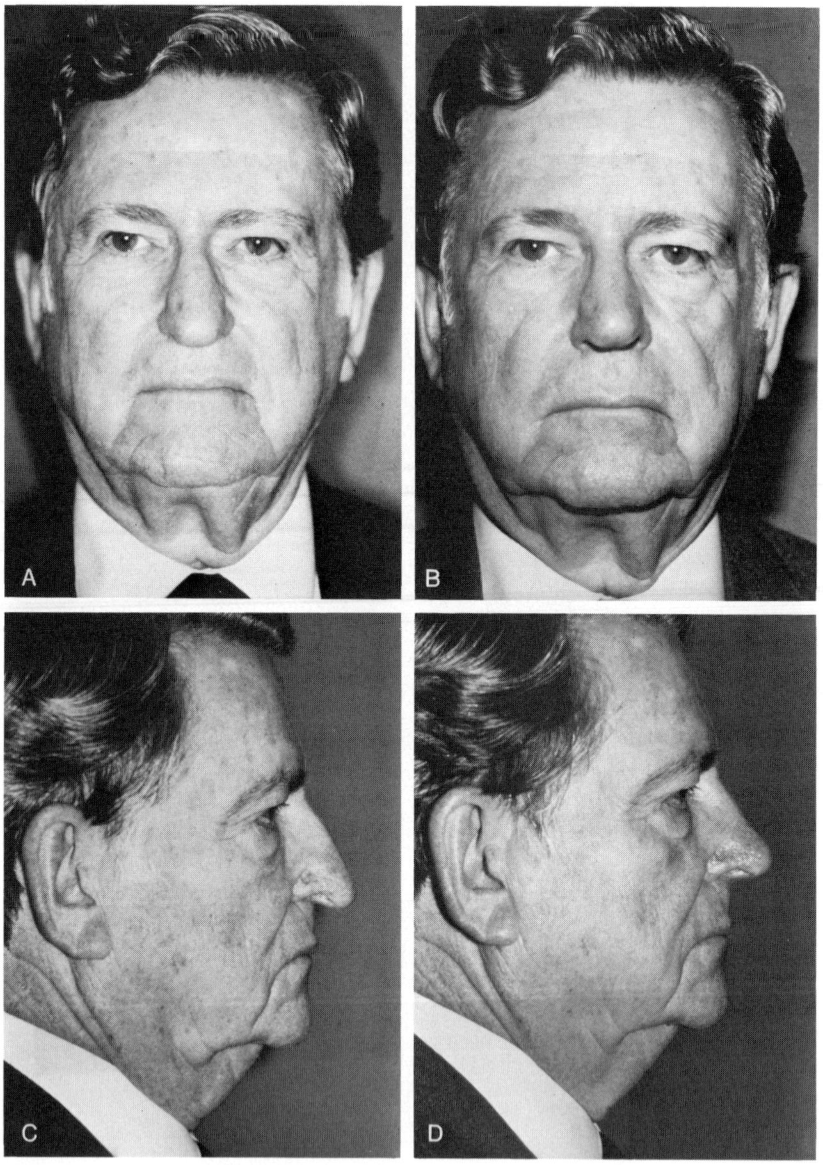

FIGURE 14–64. (*A* and *B*) Some patients whose noses were straight in youth develop ptosis as aging occurs. (*C* and *D*) A relative hump develops as the tip descends. Tip-plasty alone may be all that is required for aesthetic and functional improvement. I-beam fixation or plumping or strut grafting is generally necessary in these cases.

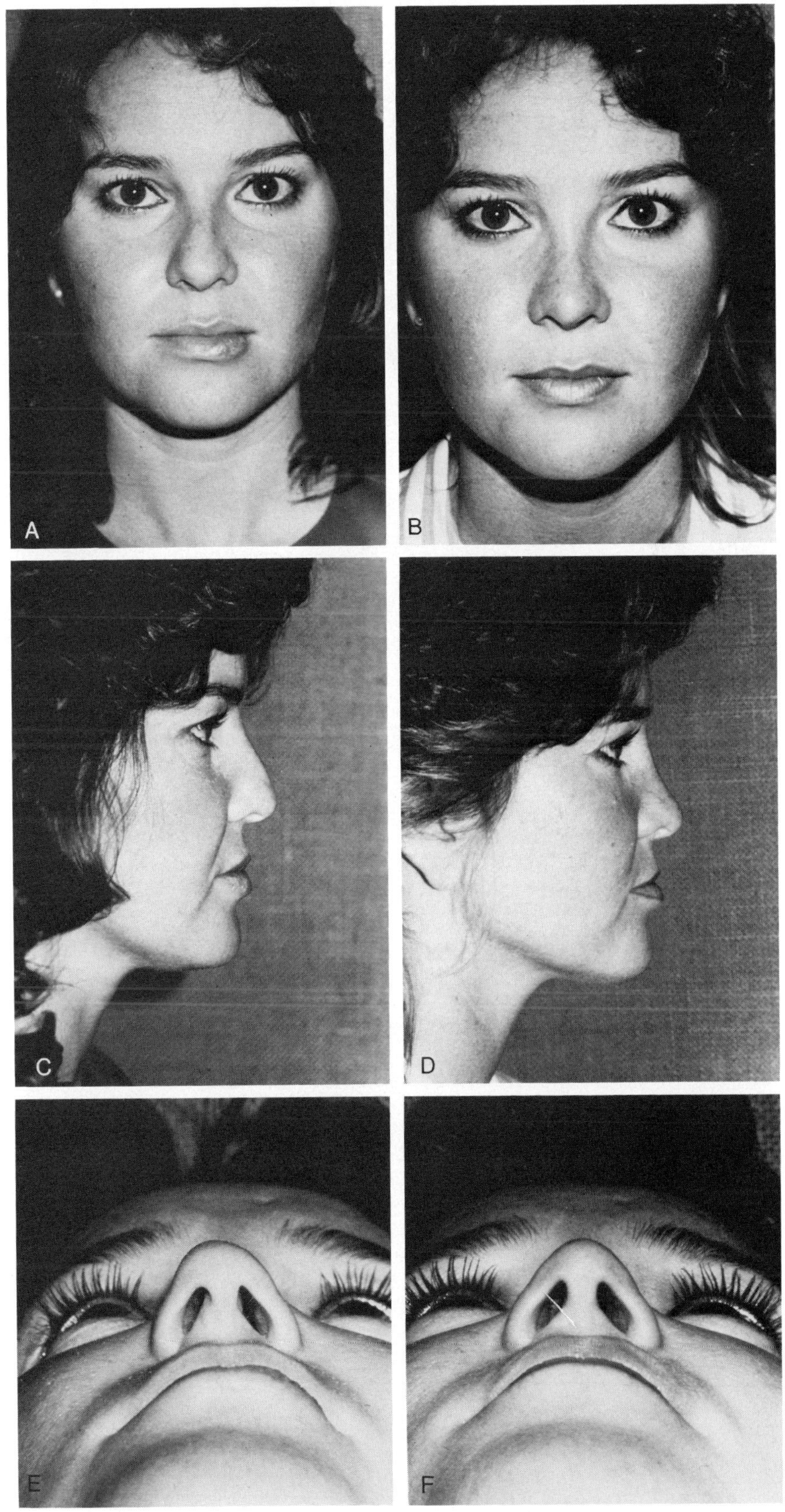

FIGURE 14–65. (*A* and *B*) This patient presented with telltale sequelae of unsuccessful rhinoplasty. (*C* and *D*) A short columella and loss of tip support coupled with inadequate resection of the superior septal angle resulted in a classic polly beak. (*E* and *F*) No tip-plasty had been performed. A complete strip was carried out at revision. Additional support was provided by an intracrural cartilaginous strut.

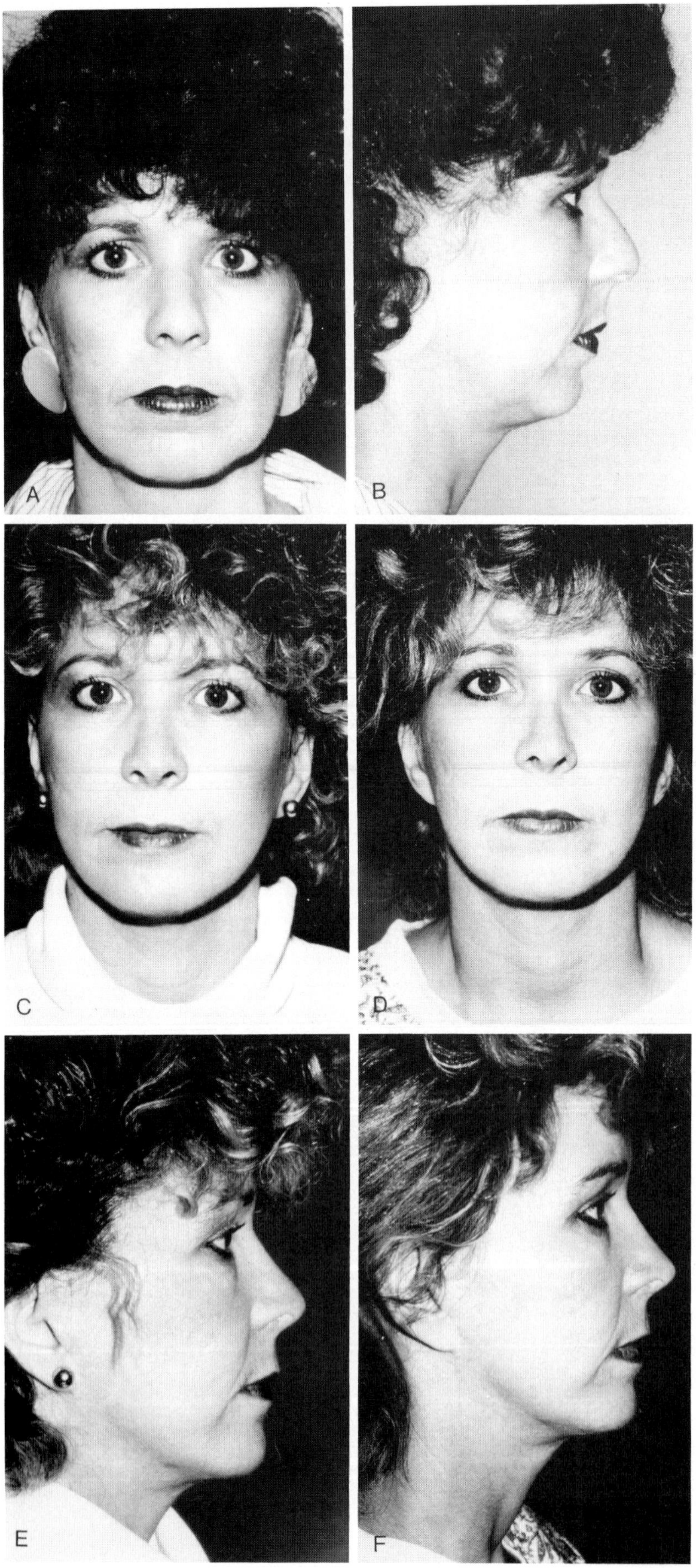

FIGURE 14–66. (*A* and *B*) In patients who tend to form excessive scar tissue, every attempt to provide maximum tip support and projection must be used (e.g., I-beam techniques, shield or tip grafts). (*C* and *D*) Postoperative supratip soft tissue fullness may be controlled by intra-lesional steroids (Kenalog, 20 mg/ml, injected as often as every 3 to 4 weeks) until the problem resolves (*E* and *F*).

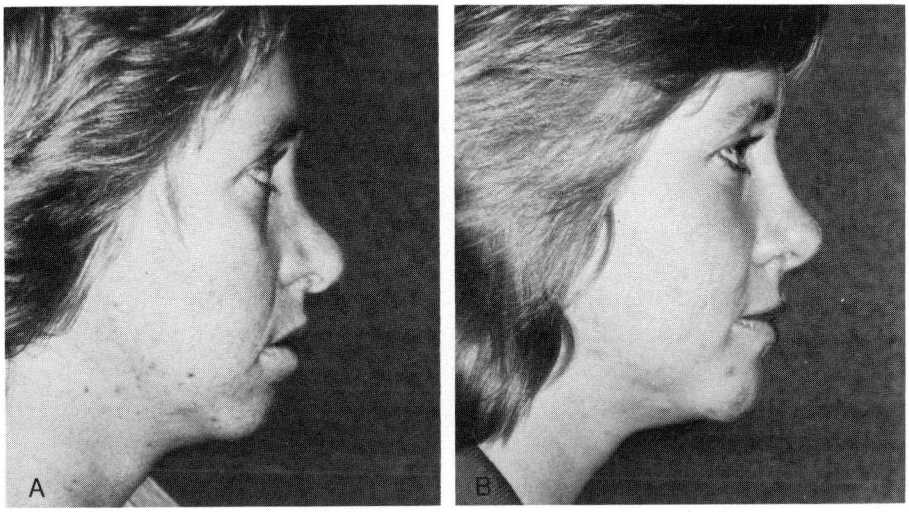

FIGURE 14–67. (*A*) Excessive columellar show may result from retraction of the alae, excessive and uncorrected length of the caudal septum, or bowed medial crura. (*B*) Shortening the nasal septum, releasing scar tissue contracture at the alar margin, and adding a cartilaginous graft corrected many of the problems in this patient.

has been excised, the revisional surgeon need only complete the operation that was prematurely terminated by the initial surgeon. More often, however, a polly beak is associated with overaggressive removal of tip cartilage, loss of tip support, and retrodisplacement. Increasing tip projection, coupled with freeing and excising supratip scar tissue, can achieve a more desirable result (Fig. 14–66).

The ptotic or inadequately rotated tip may also need (1) further shortening of a portion of the caudal nasal septum; (2) excision of the caudal ends of the upper lateral cartilages; (3) removal of the cephalic portions of inadequately trimmed lower lateral cartilages; and (4) augmentation of the medial crural legs of the tripod. Septal shortening should be carried out only if, after pressing the tip toward the root of the nose, it is determined that the septum is pushing the infratip lobule inferiorly (see Fig. 14–64).

In most cases, reconstruction of the domes with an I-beam system technique, coupled with sandwiched grafts, struts, and plumping grafts, is also required. By utilizing this technique, the revisional surgeon may effectively lengthen and strengthen the medial crural leg of the tip tripod and achieve the desired tip projection.

Sometimes excessive columellar show ("hanging" columella) can be corrected by removing the projecting and excessive portions of the caudal septum (Fig. 14–67). In rare instances, excision of a portion of the membranous septum may also be necessary. More often, the hanging-columella deformity is a result of bowed medial crura. Correction may require the shaving of the anterior (caudal) edge of the involved medial crus.

A retracted columella, on the other hand, commonly is caused by a tissue deficiency or a dislocated caudal septum. Correction must include the addition of autogenous cartilage or a composite graft and/or correction of the dislocated caudal septum (Fig. 14–68).

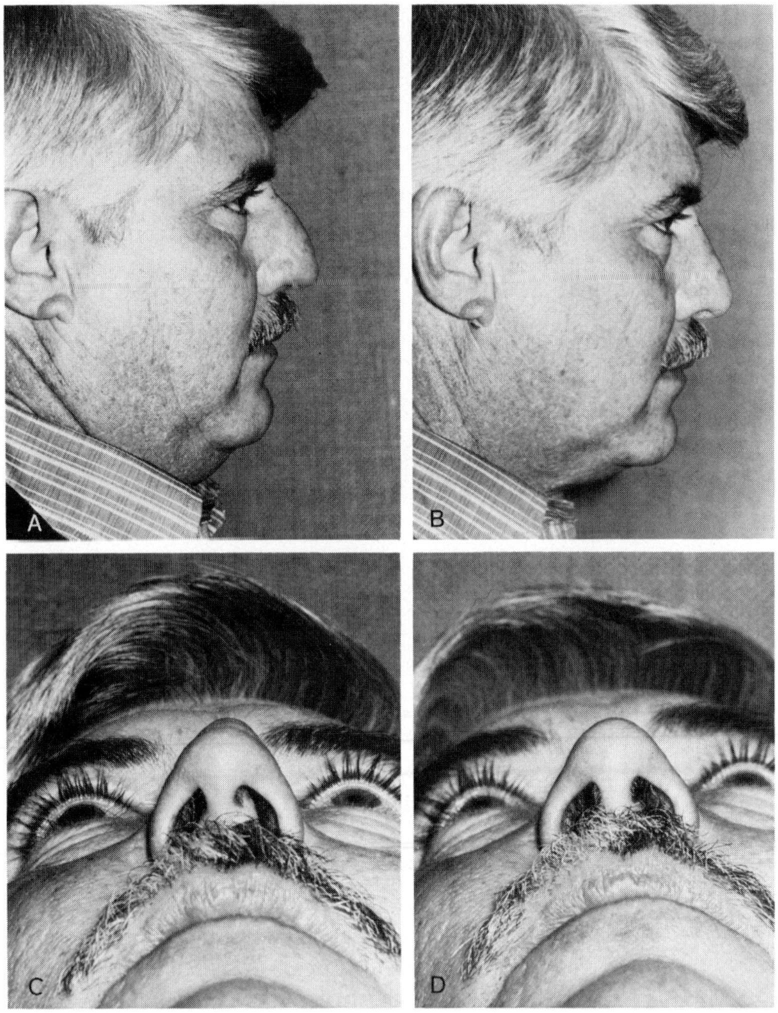

FIGURE 14–68. (*A* and *B*) A retracted columella may occur if the caudal septum is dislocated. Septoplasty and a cartilaginous strut corrected the problem in this man. (*C* and *D*) A straighter septum prevents retraction of the columella.

References

1. Anderson, J.R.: The Dynamics of Rhinoplasty, in Proceedings of the Ninth International Congress in Orthrhinolaryngology. Excerpta Medica International Congress Series 206, Amsterdam, Excerpta Medica, 1969.
2. McCollough, E.G., Gilbert, S.E., Langsdon, P.R.: The difficult nasal tip, *Current Therapy in Otolaryngology-Head and Neck Surgery,* Toronto, B.C. Decker, 1987, pp. 118–123.
3. Webster, R.C.: Advance in surgery of the tip. Otolaryngol Clin North Am 10:615–644,
4. McCollough, E.G.: Surgery of the nasal tip. Otolaryngol Clin North Am 20:769–784, 1987.
5. Feuerstein, S.S., and Adams, J.B.: Surgery of the protruding ears, Chapter 24, Instructional Courses of AAOHNS, Vol. 1, 275–281, 1988.
6. Goldman, I.B.: Surgical tips on the nasal tip. Ear Nose Throat J 33:583, 1954.
7. McCollough, E.G., and English, J.L.: A new twist in nasal tip surgery: An alternative to the Goldman tip for the wide or bulbous lobule. Arch Otolaryngol 111:524–529, 1985.
8. McCollough, E.G.: Surgery of the nasal tip. In Daniel, R. (ed.): Rhinoplasty: Aesthetic Plastic Surgery. 1993.
9. McCollough, E.G., and Mangat, D.: Systemic approach to correction of the nasal tip in rhinoplasty. Arch Otolaryngol 107:12–16, 1981.
10. McCollough, E. G., and Fedok, F. G.: The interal crura turnover graft: Correction on the concave internal crus. Laryngoscope 103:463–469, 1993.

CHAPTER 15

External Rhinoplasty

Although the external, or open, approach to nasal surgery has been used for many years by Goodman in Canada, its popularity in the United States has only recently increased. It is neither a new technique nor an operation unto itself. Open rhinoplasty is a natural extension of the classic operation, closed rhinoplasty.

When conditions found preoperatively (or encountered intraoperatively) dictate, the surgeon should consider connecting the marginal incisions by making an incision across the columella and reflecting the nasal skin dorsally (Fig. 15–1). The transcolumellar incision is an extension of the marginal incision used to expose the tip cartilages. When the dorsal nasal skin flap is reflected, exposure is intensified, allowing for more accurate diagnosis and correction of some nasal deformities.

The decision to connect the marginal incisions may be made at the beginning of operation, when tip-plasty is performed, or at any time it is determined that additional exposure is desirable.

When the alar cartilages are grossly asymmetric or, in revisional cases, require total or subtotal reconstruction of the alar cartilage complex with grafting, both the exposure obtained by reflecting the dorsal nasal flap and the proficiency of correction are unparalleled (Fig. 15–2).

In severely twisted noses that require disarticulation and/or morselization of the dorsal septal strut, the external approach enables the surgeon to reestablish the relation of the cartilaginous and bony pyramid with ease (Fig. 15–3). If dorsal augmentation is required, this approach allows grafts and/or implants to be accurately and adroitly secured.

Text continued on page 219

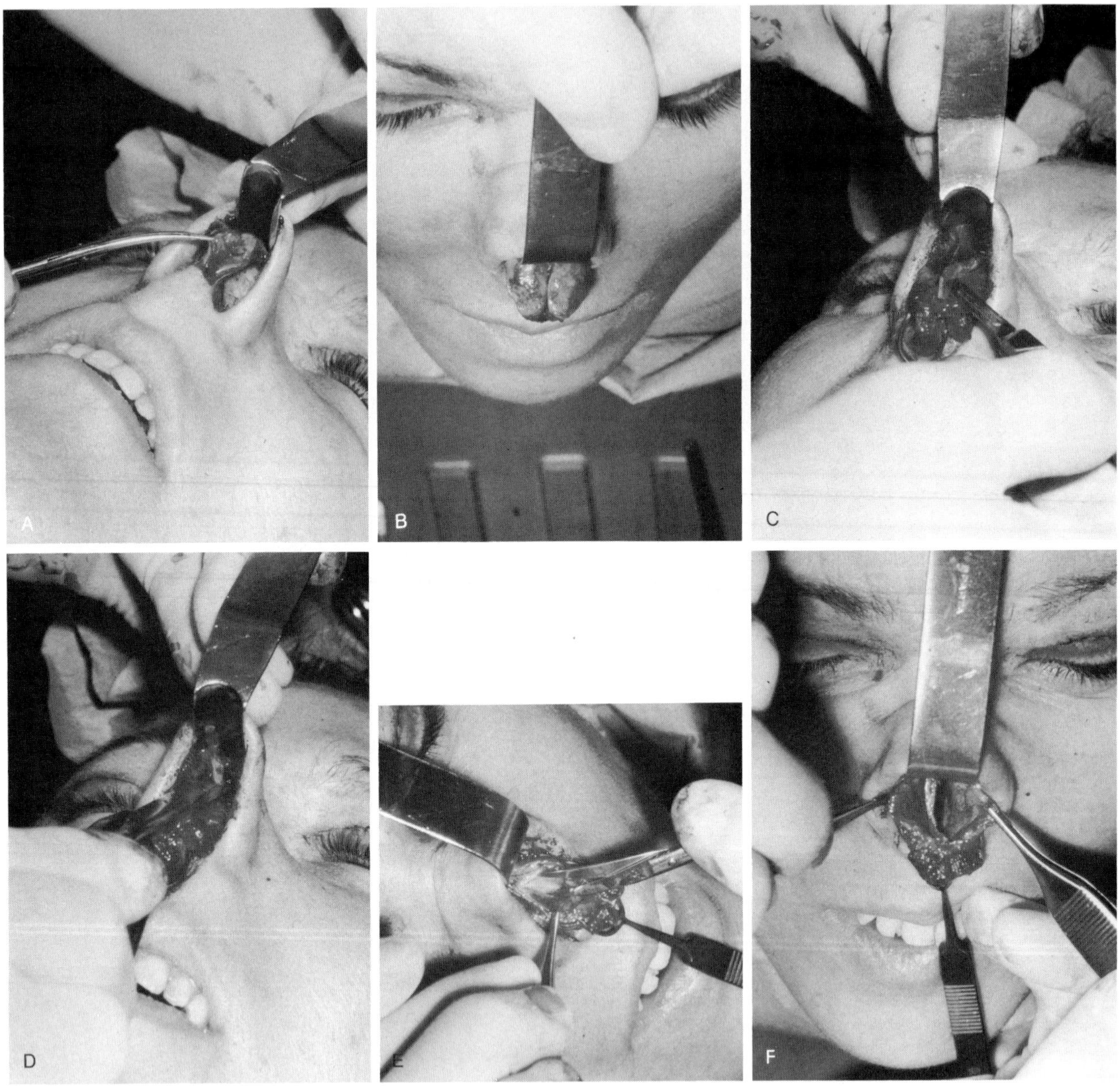

FIGURE 15–1. (*A*) Deformities of the medial crura are accurately identified. (*B*) Both domes and lateral crura are inspected for symmetry. (*C*) A cartilaginous hump is incised with a No. 11 blade. (*D*) Amputation of the cartilaginous component of the hump is carried out with an angulated scissor. (*E*) Mucoperichondrial flap elevation and/or separation of upper lateral cartilages begins at the superior septal angle. (*F*) When necessary, bilateral flap–upper lateral separation can be accomplished. *Illustration continued on following page*

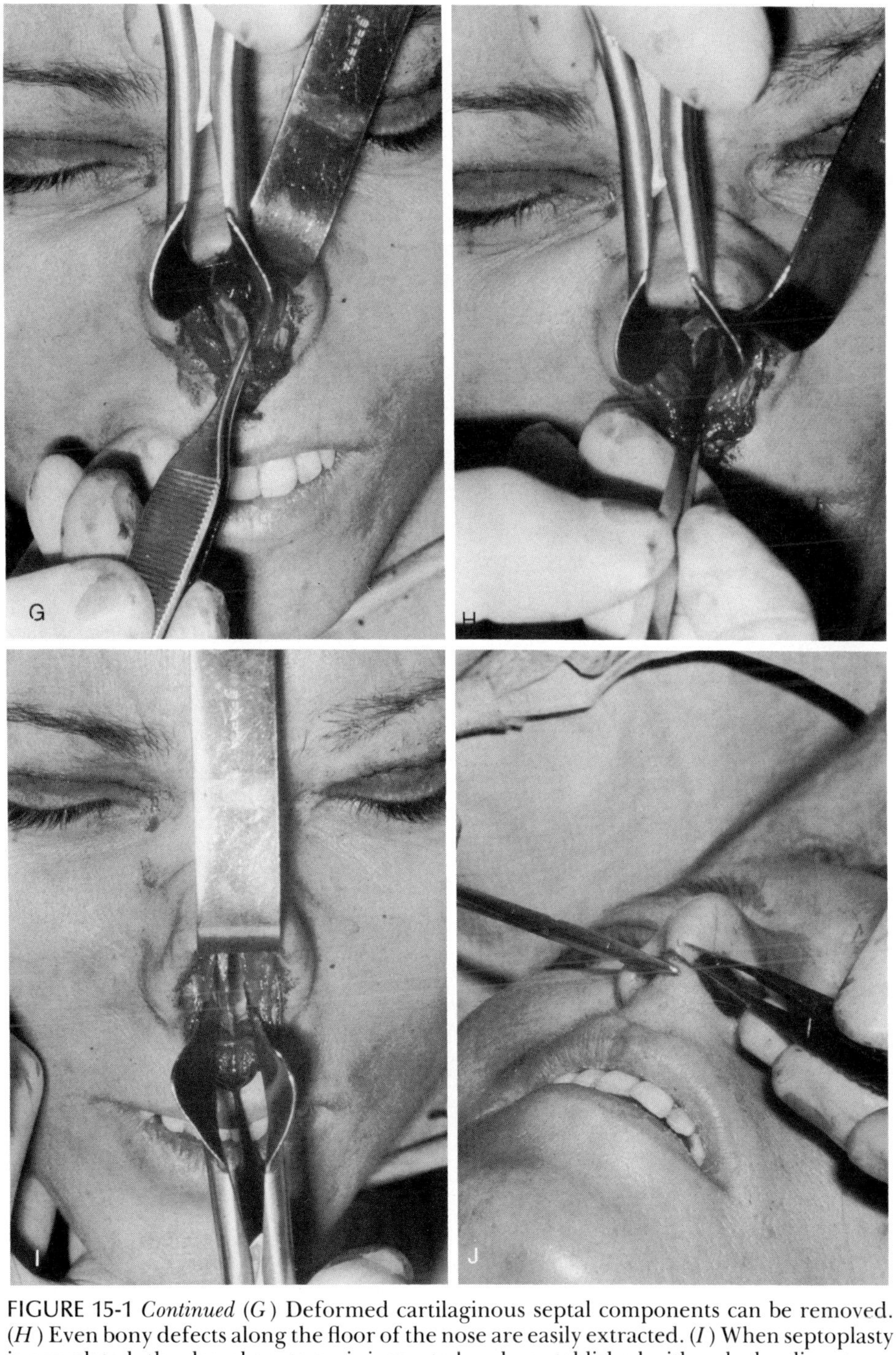

FIGURE 15-1 *Continued* (*G*) Deformed cartilaginous septal components can be removed. (*H*) Even bony defects along the floor of the nose are easily extracted. (*I*) When septoplasty is completed, the dorsal anatomy is inspected and reestablished with polyglycolic sutures (5-0). (*J*) The transcolumellar incision is closed under magnification with 6-0 fast-absorbing catgut.

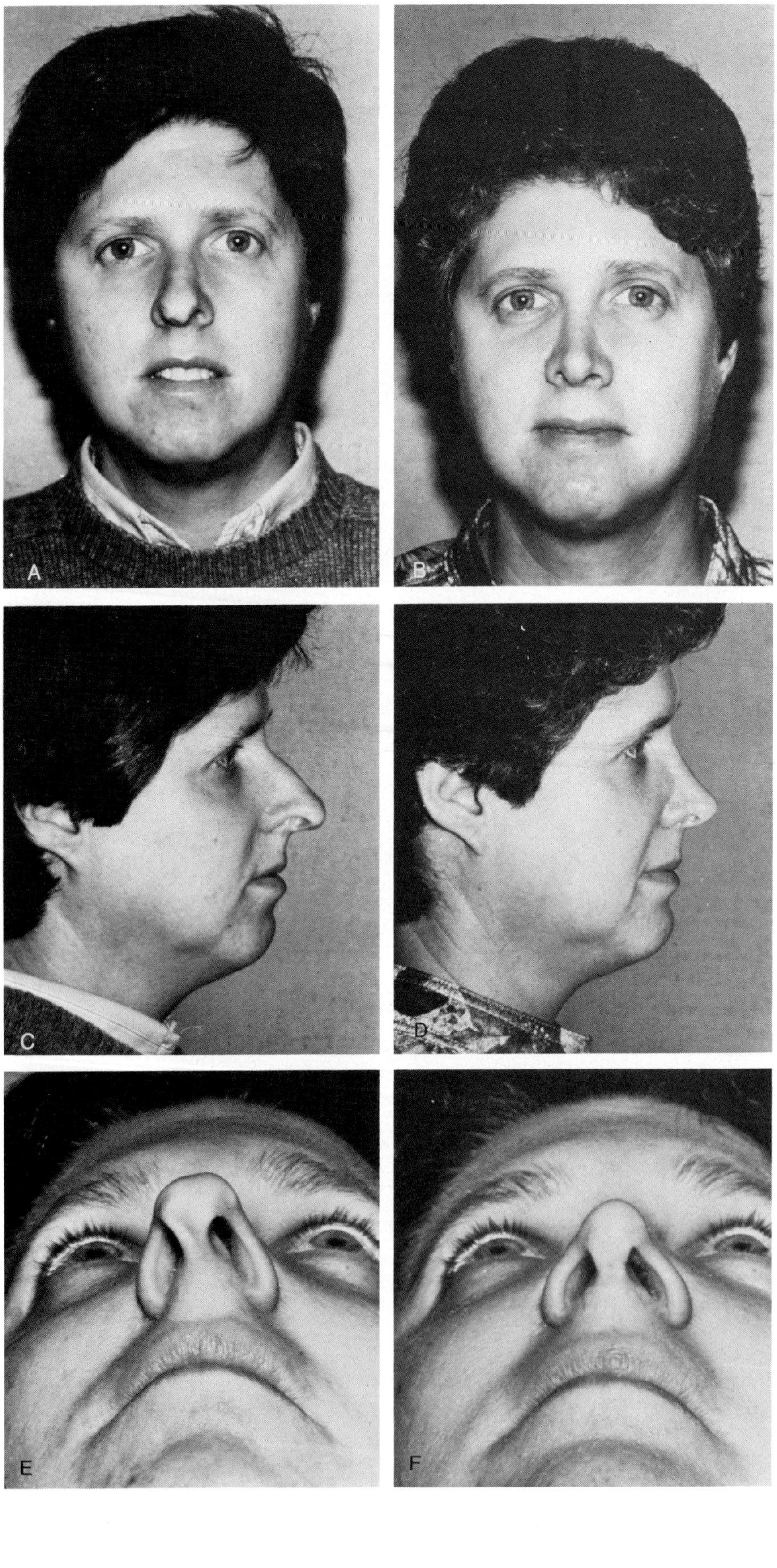

FIGURE 15–2. Severe tip distortion caused by twisted and gnarled alar cartilages. Difficult problems may be more easily corrected through an external approach. The transcolumellar scar is barely visible (*F*).

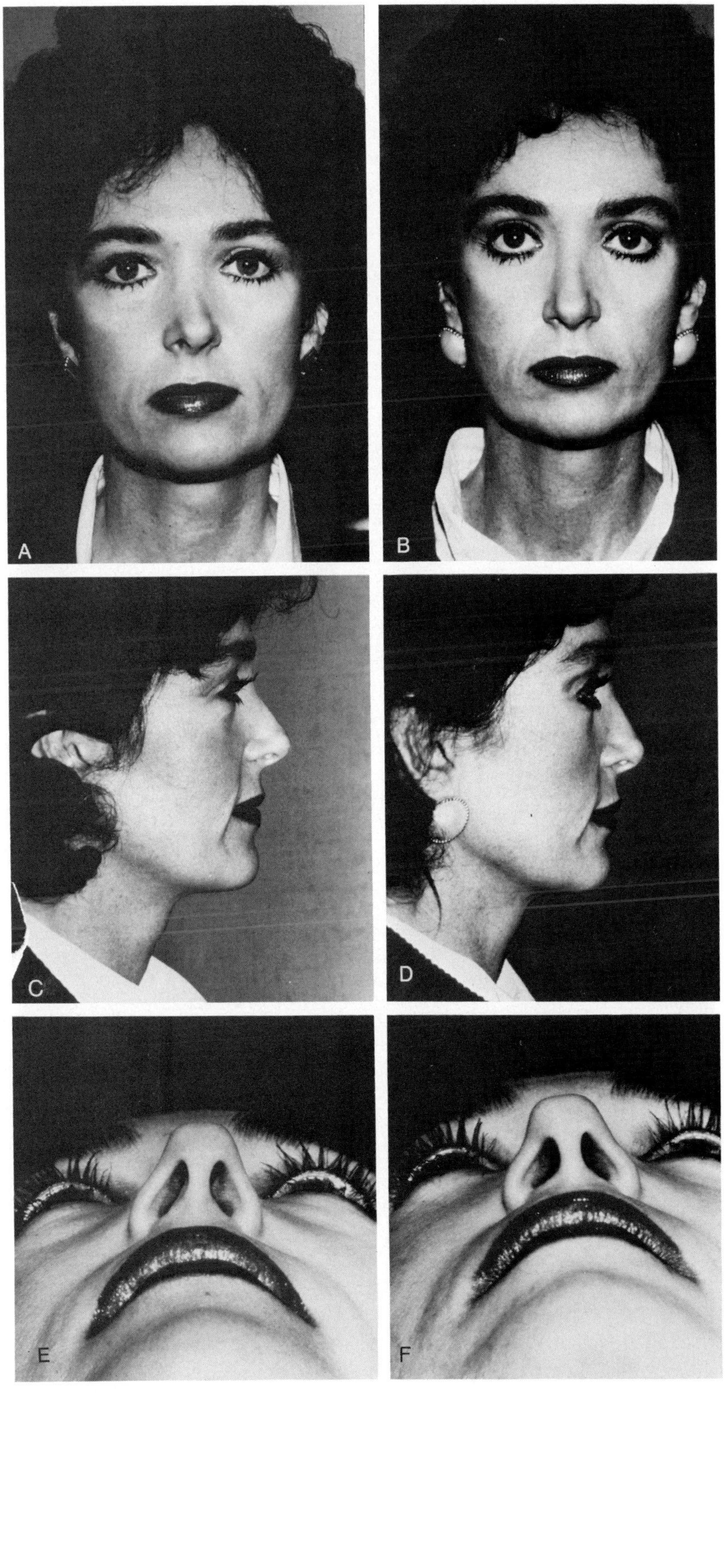

FIGURE 15–3. (*A* and *B*) When the cartilaginous dorsum is crooked, especially in revisional cases, external rhinoplasty assists the surgeon in identifying and correcting the deformities. (*C* and *D*) Minimal alteration to the dorsum was requested. (*E* and *F*) No additional surgery was required on the tip cartilages. Septal straightening created better symmetry.

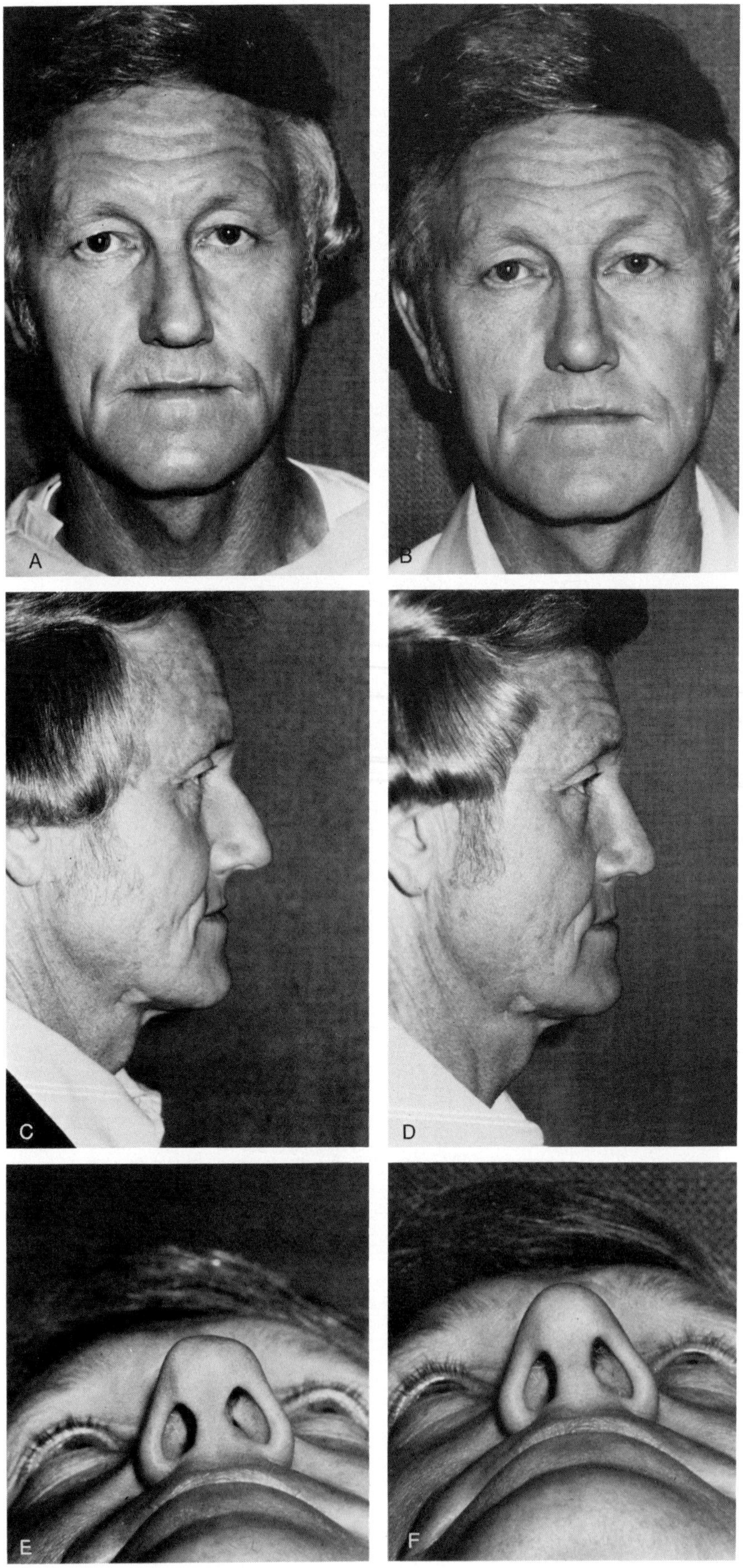

FIGURE 15–4. (*A* and *B*) Because of the severity of the septal deformity and asymmetry of tip cartilages, external rhinoplasty conversion was elected. (*C* and *D*) A strong nasal dorsum is desirable in men. (*E* and *F*) The transcolumellar scar usually heals well and, in most cases, is imperceptible.

A strong argument could be made for encouraging the novice to perform several rhinoplasties through the external conversion approach before attempting a closed rhinoplasty. It might be unnecessary, however, for any surgeon to become totally dependent on this approach.

Even though the transcolumellar incision usually heals well and the scar is virtually imperceptible, the existence of the transcolumellar scar can be avoided as the surgeon gains experience.

Although rare, there is an increased risk of tissue loss if the blood supply of the superior portion of the columellar flap should be compromised.

SHAPE OF THE INCISION

Scar camouflaging is practiced by plastic surgeons of various specialties. Good camouflaging principles dictate that scars not only be narrow and flat but also follow natural anatomic lines. Because the base of the nose is pyramidal, logic prescribes that the transcolumellar scar follow similar lines. The inverted V seems to be the most logical pattern to mimic (Fig. 15–4).

At the conclusion of operation, the transcolumellar incision is closed with 6-0 fast-absorbing catgut (Ethicon #1916). Interrupted sutures that *evert* the skin edges are recommended. Magnification is helpful when high-priority suturing is carried out.

The wound is splinted with a strip of tan Micropore paper tape, which also serves as a covered dressing and traps some moisture so that most sutures dissolve during the first postoperative week. Catgut suture reactions have not been observed when this modus operandi is used. The tape and any residual suture material are removed at 1 week.

Suggested Readings

McCollough, E. G., Gilbert, S. E., Langsdon, P. R.: The difficult nasal tip. In Gates, G. A., ed. Current Therapy in Otolaryngology—Head and Neck Surgery. Toronto: B. C. Decker, 1987, pp. 118–123.

McCollough, E. G., and Mangat, D.: Systematic approach to correction of the nasal tip in rhinoplasty. Arch Otolaryngol 107:12–16, 1981.

CHAPTER 16

Acutely Deviated Nose: Nasal Fractures

CLASSIFICATION

For the purposes of this discussion, nasal fractures are classified as follows:

1. Simple fracture—interruption and/or displacement of integrity of bony or cartilaginous components of the nose (Fig. 16–1)
2. Comminuted fracture—multiple fracture sites of the bone and/or cartilaginous components, usually associated with displacement and disfiguration (Fig. 16–2)
3. Compound fracture—a simple or comminuted fracture along with disruption in the integrity of the nasal skin or the internal mucosal or vestibular lining (Fig. 16–3)

EVALUATION

The surgeon may examine the patient shortly after injury or may not have an opportunity to do so until many years later. Noses may be acutely twisted from recent trauma or may be crooked as a result of events that occurred previously. Sometimes both situations exist.

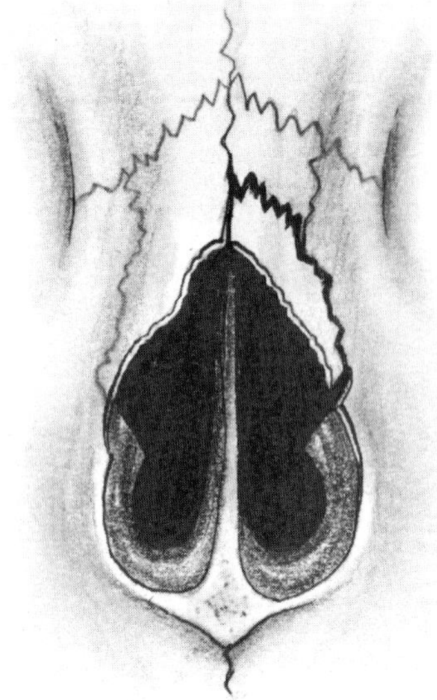

FIGURE 16–1. Depression of only a segment of the bony pyramid is noted.

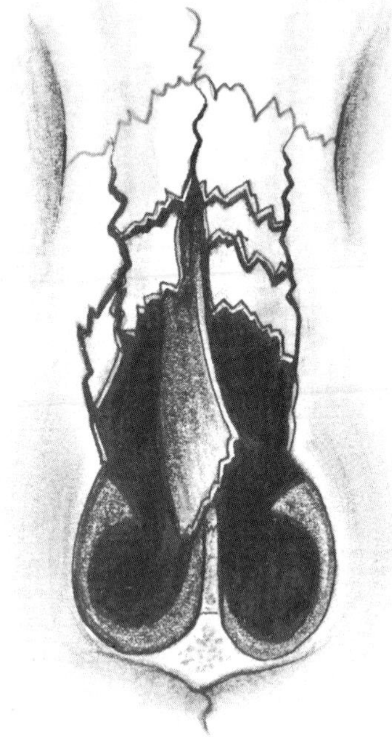

FIGURE 16–2. Multiple fracture sites result in free segments of bone and a compromised airway.

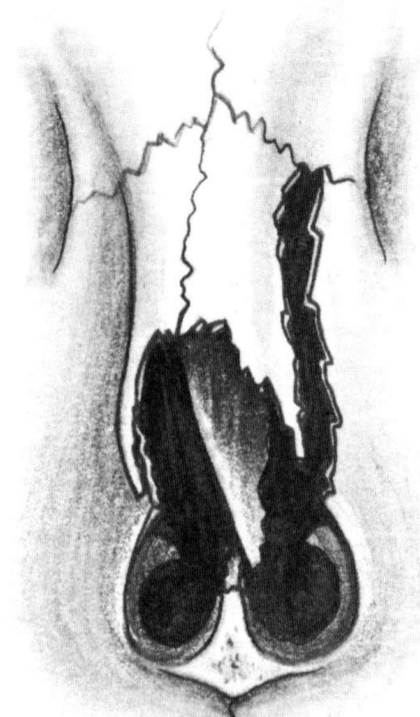

FIGURE 16–3. A dislocated pyramid commonly is associated with bony and cartilaginous septal fractures.

Certain conditions dictate the manner in which the surgeon treats the nasal injury. Two conditions that require immediate attention are septal hematoma and lacerations to the nasal skin (Figs. 16–4 through 16–7).

When a nasal injury is part of a multiple traumatic episode, especially that of a life-threatening nature, nasal reconstruction should be set aside until the other injuries are stabilized.

Evaluation of the patient is dictated by the history and physical findings. Consideration should be given to whether the blow to the nose was severe enough to have caused concomitant internal head injuries or cervical spine injuries or to have jeopardized the patient's airway.

The injured nose should be inspected, palpated, and, in some cases, evaluated radiologically. Inspection and palpation are more easily carried out when the patient is seen shortly after injury and swelling is minimal. Trained eyes and fingers often are more valuable than radiographs because cartilaginous injuries are not visible in x-ray studies. Radiological studies and photographs may provide some help in documenting the condition of the nose before treatment.

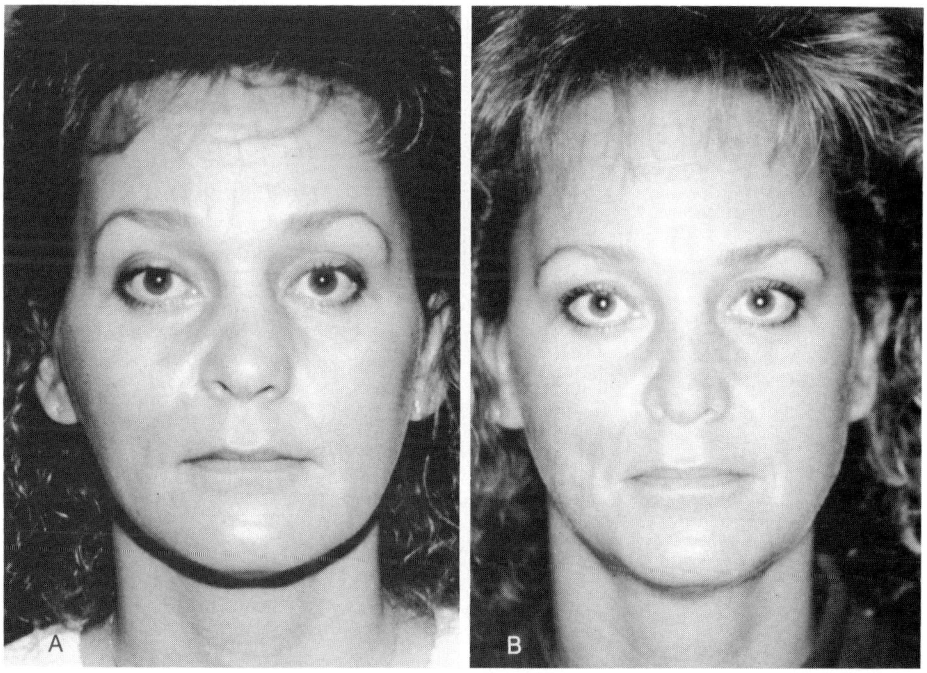

FIGURE 16–4. (*A* and *B*) Because of the nature of this injury, treatment was carried out in multiple stages. Initially, the wounds were cleaned and debrided and closed reduction was performed. Wood fragments extruded from the nose, and antibiotic therapy was continued for several weeks. Definitive treatment was delayed for 2 months.

If the nose is bleeding at the time of examination, appropriate measures must be taken to control epistaxis. Restoring the patient's blood pressure and pulse rate to the normal range for that patient is essential. Sometimes finger pressure applied over the vessels in the nasolabial and nasofacial regions is helpful. Topical and, in some instances, injectable anesthetics combined with topical and injectable vasoconstrictors are useful both in reducing blood flow and in diminishing discomfort (Fig. 16–8).

Suction and illumination often reveal an internal laceration, which can then be cauterized with electrical or chemical agents and devices. If these more conservative measures fail, Surgicel can be applied to the bleeding sites once they have been identified. Bleeding is controlled both by the hemostatic makeup of the Surgicel and by the pressure exerted against the wound. Seldom are more radical techniques of nasal packing required to control nasal bleeding.

Text continued on page 227

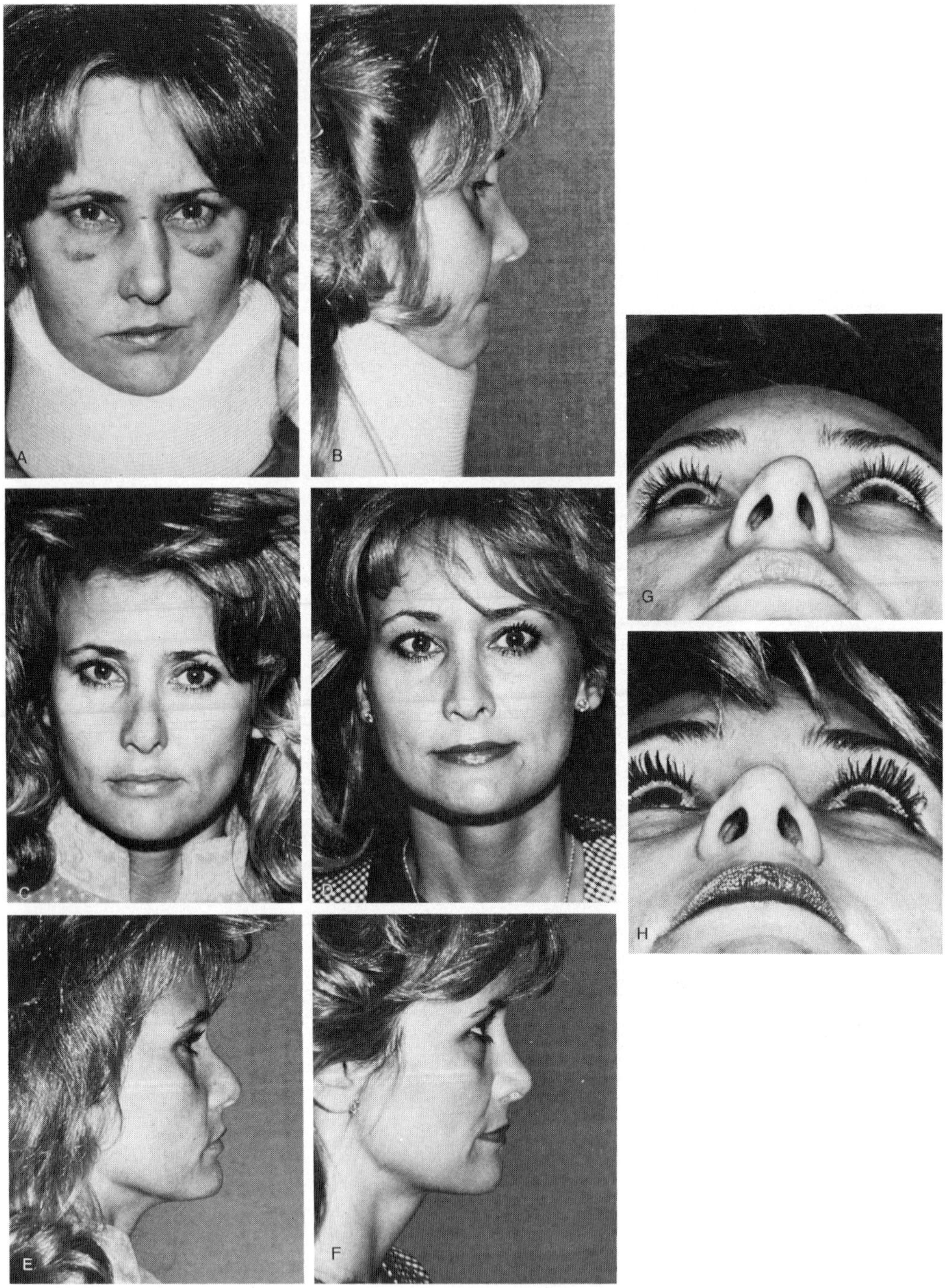

FIGURE 16–5. (*A* and *B*) Associated injuries may dictate when definitive treatment of a nasal injury is performed. (*C* and *D*) Nasal surgery was performed shortly after the injury occurred, while the patient was hospitalized. The patient later returned for revisional rhinoplasty. (*E* and *F*) Dorsal augmentation with cartilaginous grafts and an I beam–type tip-plasty was performed. (*G* and *H*) Septoplasty helped to create better tip symmetry.

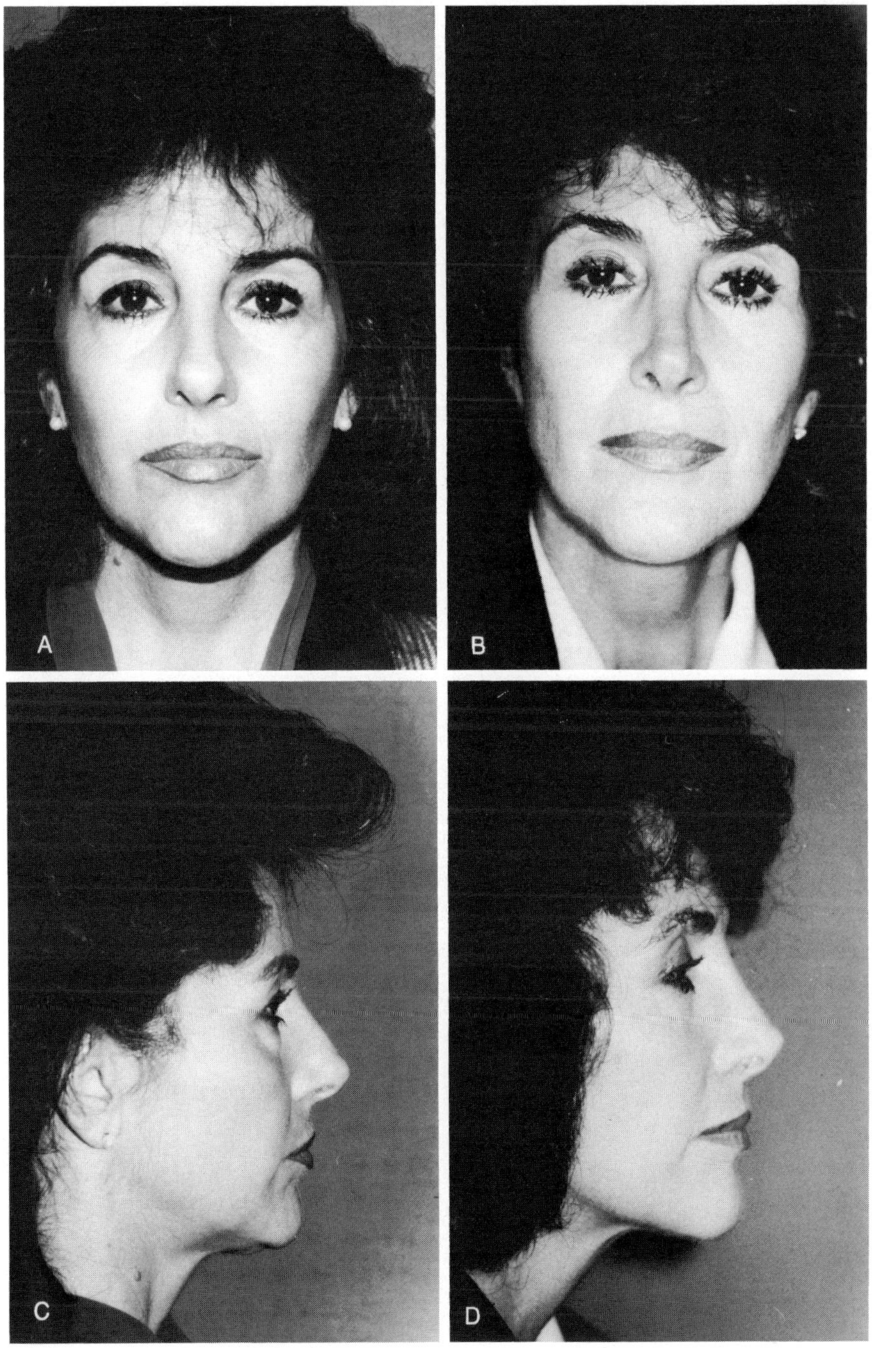

FIGURE 16–6. (*A* and *B*) This patient previously had undergone rhinoplasty and later sustained a compound, comminuted nasal and septal fracture. Immediate repair was performed. (*C* and *D*) Mobilization and manipulation of the nasal architecture and wound closure was all that was required.

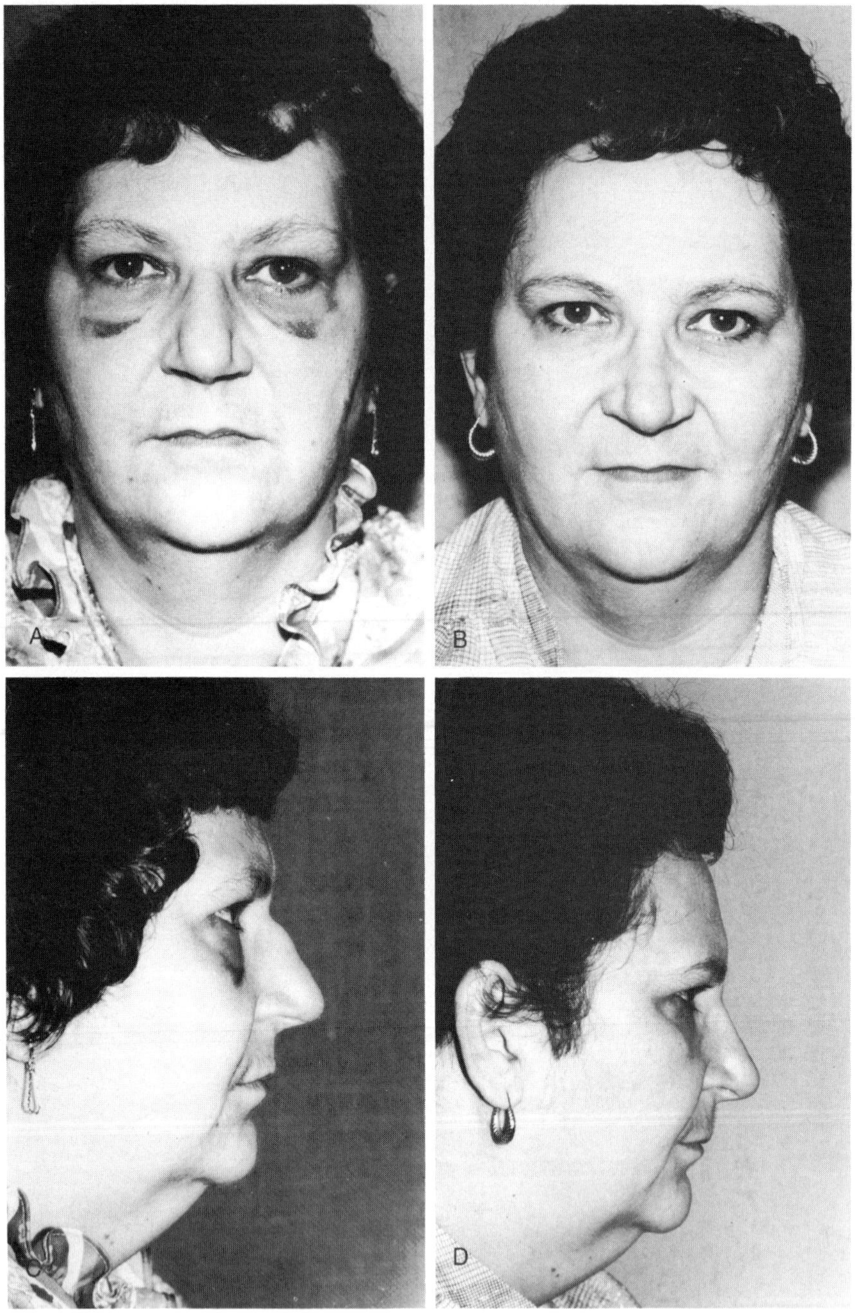

FIGURE 16–7. (*A* and *B*) Many patients have wanted to have rhinoplasty performed since adolescence, but circumstances prevented them from having surgery. (*C* and *D*) The necessity of having an injury repaired provides the stimulus to have the size and shape of their noses changed at the same time. Rhinoplasty and fracture repair were performed about 10 weeks after injury.

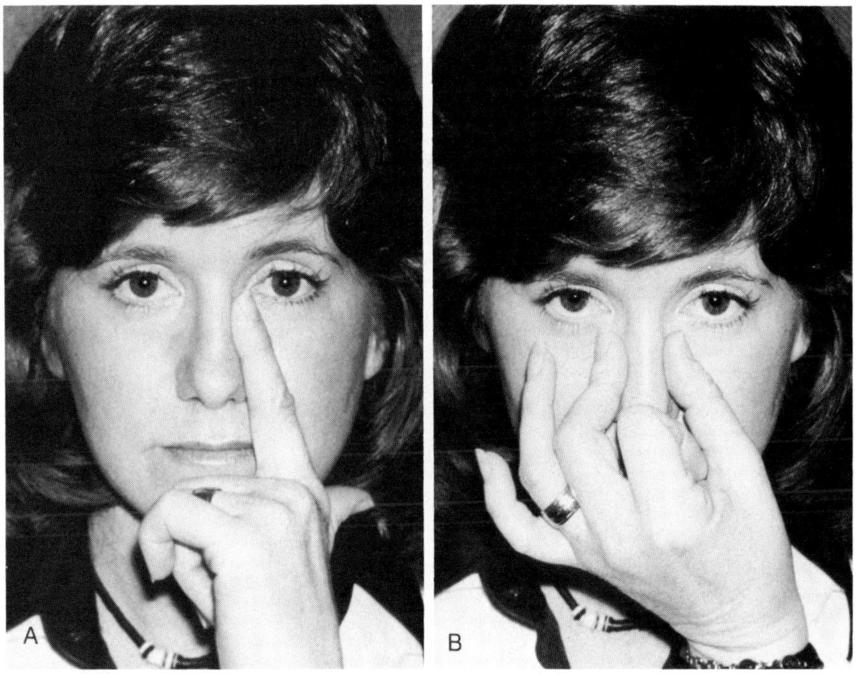

FIGURE 16–8. Unilateral or bilateral pressure applied with a finger over the vessels that course along the nasolabial and nasofacial grooves can reduce the blood flow to portions of the nose and may help to stop the bleeding.

When bleeding has been controlled, the standard nasal photographic documentation (i.e., frontal, lateral, oblique, and base views) should be obtained for the medical record. External lacerations are cleaned and inspected. Suture repair usually is carried out at the time of initial treatment even though bony and cartilaginous injuries might be deferred to a later date.

A septal hematoma, if identified, must be evacuated, bleeding controlled, and mucoperichondrial flaps repositioned with basting sutures (see Ch. 10) or appropriate packing. If left untreated, the pressure of a septal hematoma could destroy septal cartilage. A hematoma might also become infected and lead to the development of a septal abscess with destruction of the cartilaginous support of the nose and/or a septal perforation (Fig. 16–9).

After appropriate evaluation and emergency measures have been carried out and after consultation with the patient (or the patient's family in the case of a minor), the surgeon must devise a conclusive treatment plan.

Depending on the situation at hand, definitive correction may be recommended immediately or deferred to a more opportune time. The time of day, day of the week, work or school schedules, amount of swelling, associated injuries, and the patient's desire to have aesthetic changes made to the nose are factors that deserve consideration.

Ideally, a nasal fracture should be repaired within 7 to 14 days; otherwise, the fragments begin to heal in a nondesirable location and make correction more difficult. Only in extreme circumstances should correction be delayed for longer than 6 weeks (Fig. 16–10).

ADDITIONAL PROCEDURES

Before treatment, it is advisable to inform patients who have sustained nasal trauma that more than one operation might be required. Even if a definitive operation is attempted in the initial treatment, the vagaries of healing might dictate that subsequent procedures be performed.

Text continued on page 230

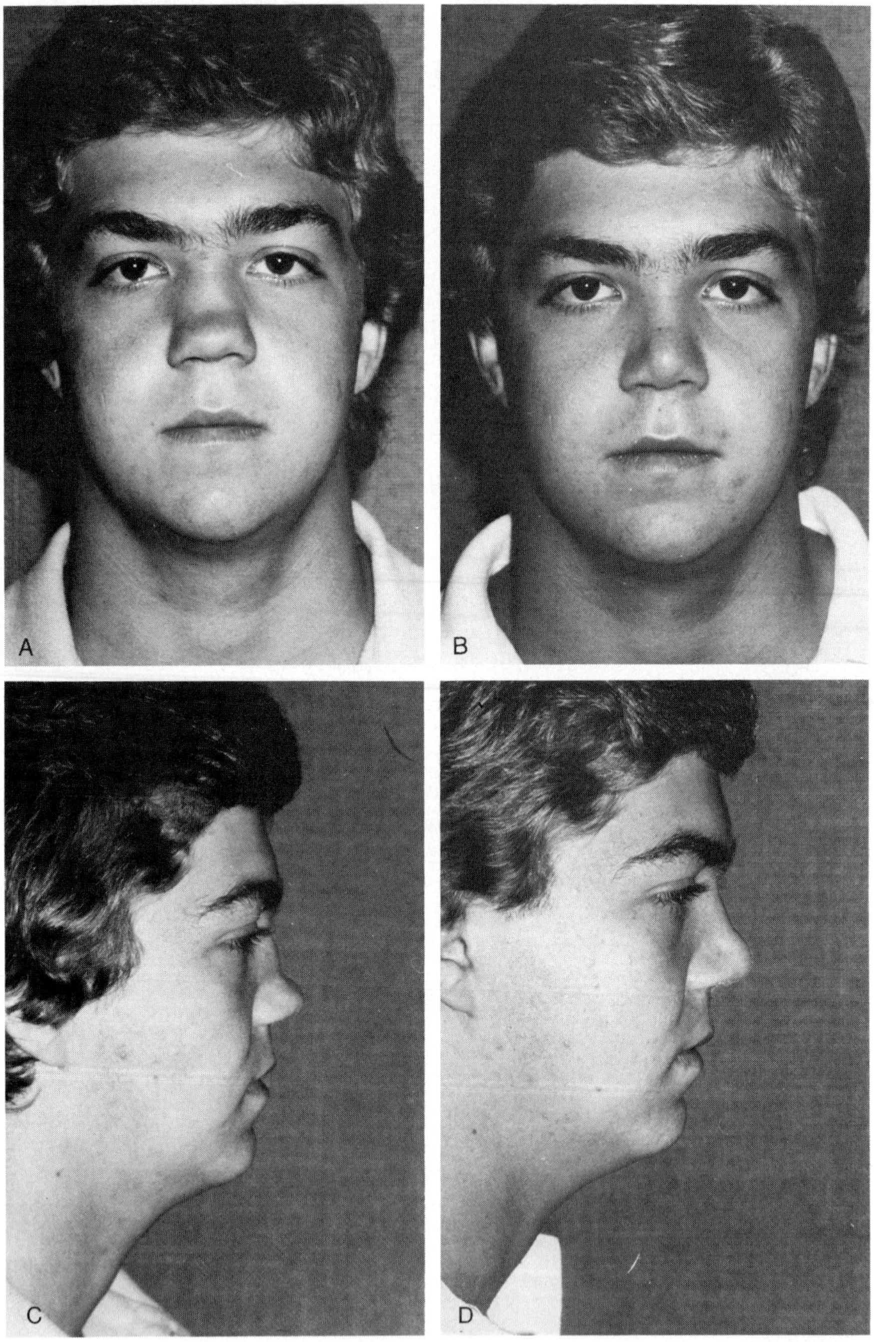

FIGURE 16–9. (*A* and *B*) An unrecognized or untreated septal hematoma may result in dissolution of most or all of the septal cartilages. (*C* and *D*) Dorsal saddle deformity and columellar retraction are sequelae of failure to treat septal hematoma. Reconstruction required auricular cartilage augmentation osteotomies and tip-plasty. Vertical dome division with I-beam grafting was used for tip-plasty.

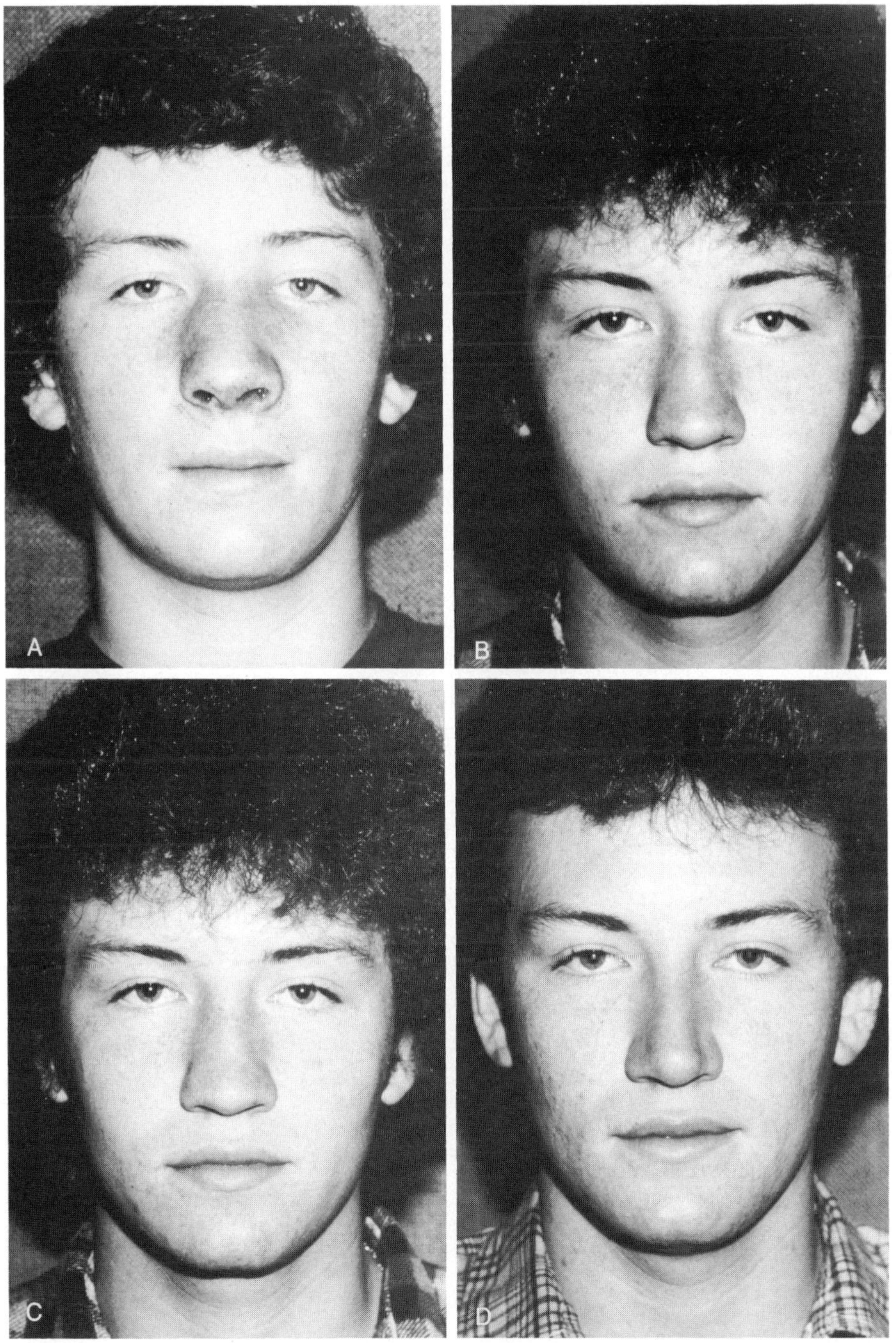

FIGURE 16–10. (*A* and *B*) Severely malpositioned bony and cartilaginous components of the nasal architecture should be corrected with conservative methods within 7 to 14 days, even in younger patients. (*C* and *D*) Definitive treatment can be delayed until the patient has achieved physical maturity (2 years after injury in this patient).

SURGICAL CORRECTION

Repair of a nasal fracture is approached in the same manner as described in previous chapters dealing with the methods of nasal surgery. Provided no other major injuries have occurred, local anesthesia with monitored sedation (twilight anesthesia) is preferred (see Ch. 7).

After the patient is put at ease, the nose should be completely anesthetized to ensure the patient's comfort. Depending on the extent of injuries and the amount of aesthetic improvement planned, the operation proceeds in the same manner as for elective septorhinoplasty. The appropriate septal surgery is performed to establish or maintain the nasal airway. Dislocated septal elements are placed in their appropriate positions and secured as described in Chapter 10. Cartilaginous hump removal in the case of delayed repair (if it is desired or indicated) is carried as described in Chapter 12.

Small bony humps can be reduced with gentle rasping. Care should be taken to secure the lateral walls with the thumb and index finger of the assisting hand. Fine, sharp rasps can be used to gingerly remove unwanted bone.

Even though a fracture might involve only one lateral wall of the nose, bilateral osteotomies are recommended. Conservative fracture reduction in which fragments are manipulated, lifted, and packed into position often proves to be unsatisfactory after the swelling subsides.

The lateral walls of an untraumatized nose typically are convex. A depressed fracture rarely can be lateralized to its original and undisturbed position. If medial displacement occurs during healing, the side walls of the nose will be uneven and the nose will appear crooked (Fig. 16–11).

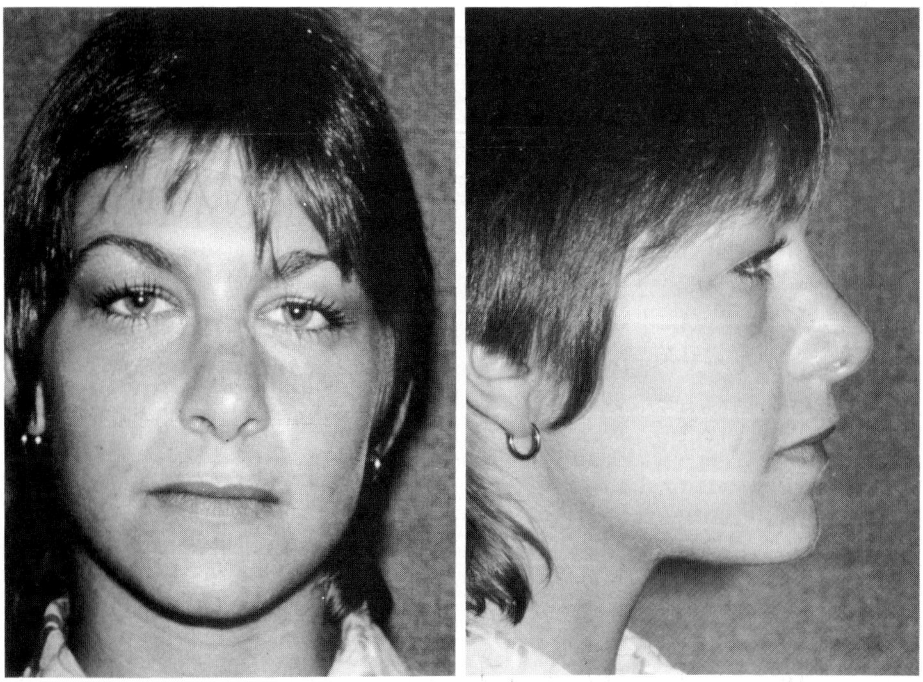

FIGURE 16–11. This patient underwent repair of a nasal fracture, but because the septal deviation was not corrected, the nasal bones healed asymmetrically, resulting in a crooked nose.

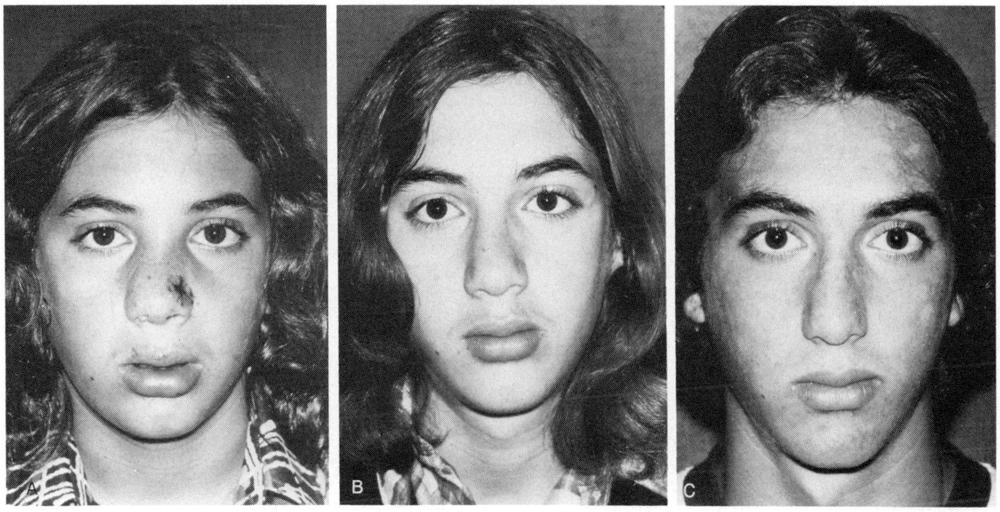

FIGURE 16–12. (*A*) The patient sustained nasal and septal fractures at an early age. (*B*) Only enough surgery was performed initially to improve the airway. (*C*) The patient returned at maturity to pursue additional correction.

Incorporating the principles of elective rhinoplasty, bilateral osteotomies can be performed in the nasofacial groove and below the extent of most fracture sites. Both lateral walls are mobilized and manipulated into their desired position. Some might consider this surgical approach to the acutely injured nose too radical for most nasal fracture corrections, but in the long run, the results are more predictable and more acceptable. In children and younger adolescents, however, the least amount of surgery is recommended to provide an adequate airway and reestablish the integrity of the nasal skeleton. Definitive correction is deferred until the nasal structures are more mature (Fig. 16–12).

In adults, when multiple deformities such as subluxation, loss of dorsal support, and collapse of the lateral walls exist, the operation becomes one of reconstruction. Suture fixation, splinting, and grafting may be required. Open (external) exposure often is helpful, especially when extensive grafting or fragment fixation is required (Fig. 16–13).

Septal cartilage is preferred when support is needed; the excised cephalic portion of the lower lateral cartilages can be used when small depressions exist. Auricular conchal cartilage from one or both ears can correct most saddle deformities. Bank or irradiated cartilage, although readily available, is less predictable than autogenous cartilage (Fig. 16–14).

Silastic or mesh implants seldom are recommended in the management of acute nasal trauma.

POSTOPERATIVE CARE

Management of the patient after nasal fracture correction is essentially identical to that after elective rhinoplasty (see Ch. 6).

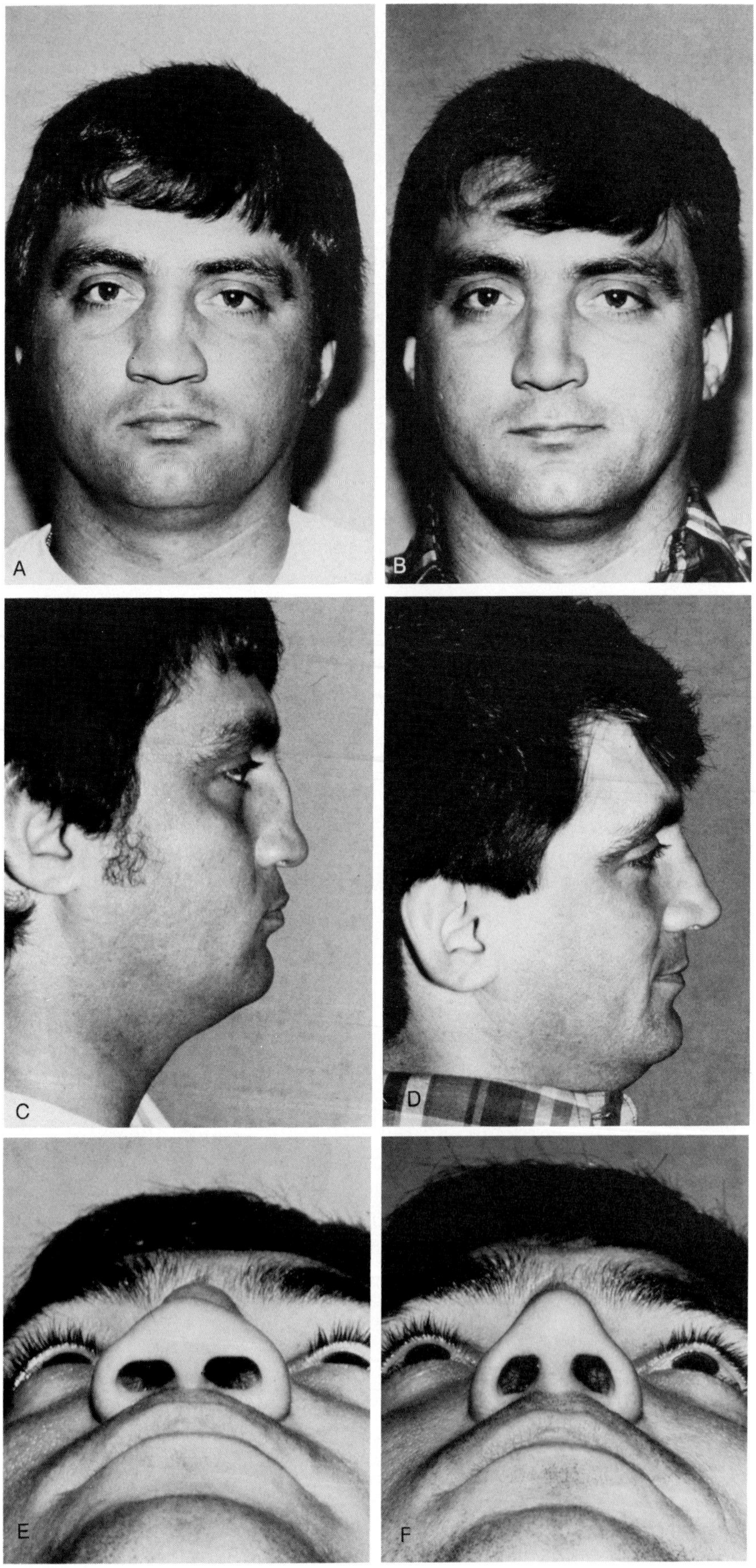

FIGURE 16–13. (*A* and *B*) Untreated injuries may result in multiple deformities that require complex reconstructive techniques later. (*C* and *D*) Augmentation with cartilage grafts and Mersilene mesh corrected the saddle and columellar refraction. (*E* and *F*) An I beam–type tip-plasty corrected the tip deformity.

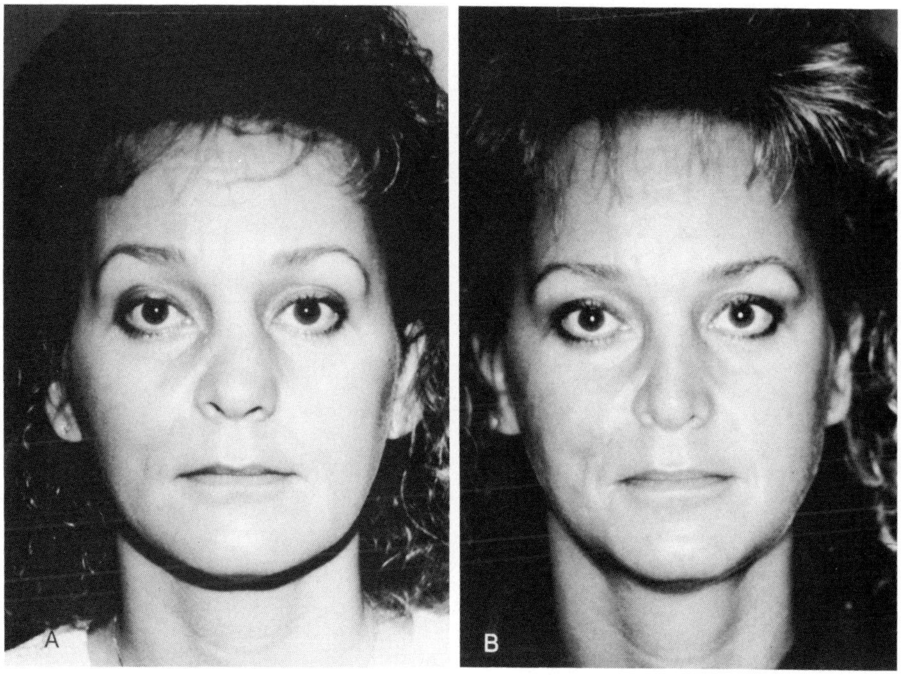

FIGURE 16–14. Camouflage grafting on the concave side of a deviated nose, coupled with mobilization, manipulation, and fixation of the nasal architecture, may help to straighten longstanding traumatic deformities.

Suggested Reading

Thomas, J. R.: The crooked nose. In Gates, G. A., ed. Current Therapy in Otolaryngology—Head and Neck Surgery. Toronto: B. C. Decker, 1987, pp. 123–125.

CHAPTER 17

The Crooked Nose

The vast majority of twisted noses result from trauma. As the head passes through the birth canal, the nose is subjected to the most intense continuous compression that it normally should experience. Septal dislocations caused by the birth event may go undetected until the nasal bridge develops at puberty.

Injuries sustained early in childhood may not produce an immediate visible deformity (Fig. 17–1). During childhood, the nose is putty-like and lacks a distinct bridge. With the approach of adolescence, the nasal dorsum develops and the septum grows. Deviations may then become more apparent.

For these reasons, the history of a memorable traumatic episode may be difficult to elicit; nevertheless, trained eyes and fingers usually can uncover information not otherwise obtainable. When nasal injuries are evaluated by untrained practitioners, deformities often are overlooked. As a rule, radiologic examination is inadequate in diagnosing one of the most common deformities—dislocation or fracture of the cartilaginous septum.

IATROGENIC DEFORMITIES

Factors that lead to postoperative asymmetry include asymmetric hump removal, poorly performed osteotomies, disarticulation of the upper lateral cartilages from their attachment of the nasal bones, failure to correct an underlying deviation of the bony and cartilaginous septum, faulty tip surgery, malpositioned sutures, and improperly applied nasal dressings (Fig. 17–2).

Text continued on page 238

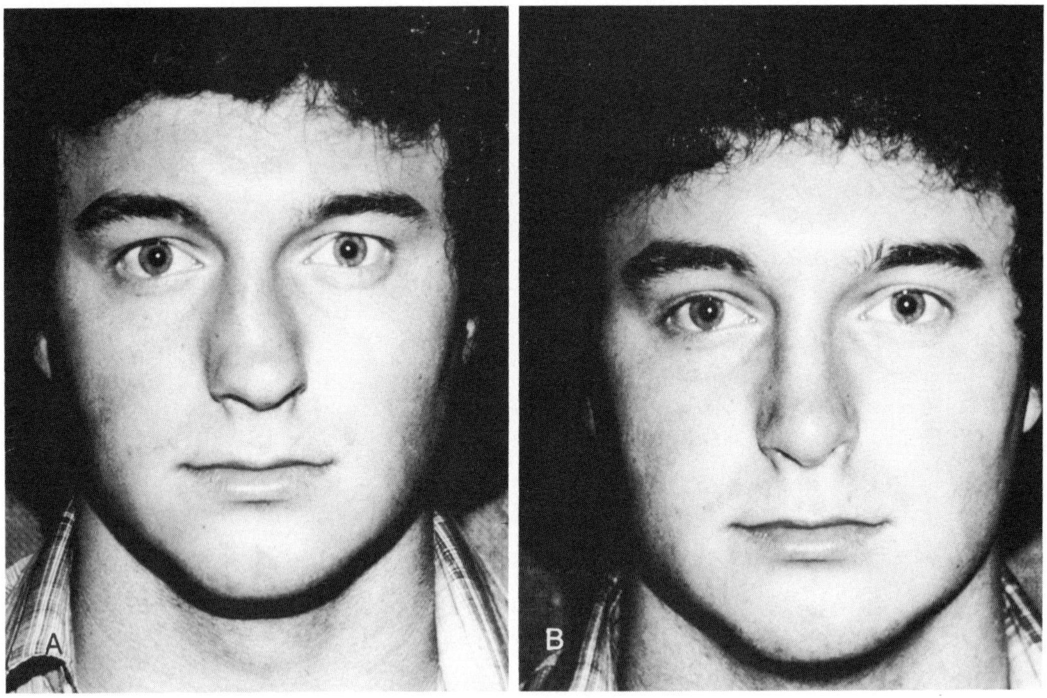

FIGURE 17–1. (*A*) A childhood injury did not produce a visible deformity in this young man's nose until he reached adolescence. (*B*) Correction involved complex reconstructive rhinoplasty to straighten the dorsal septum.

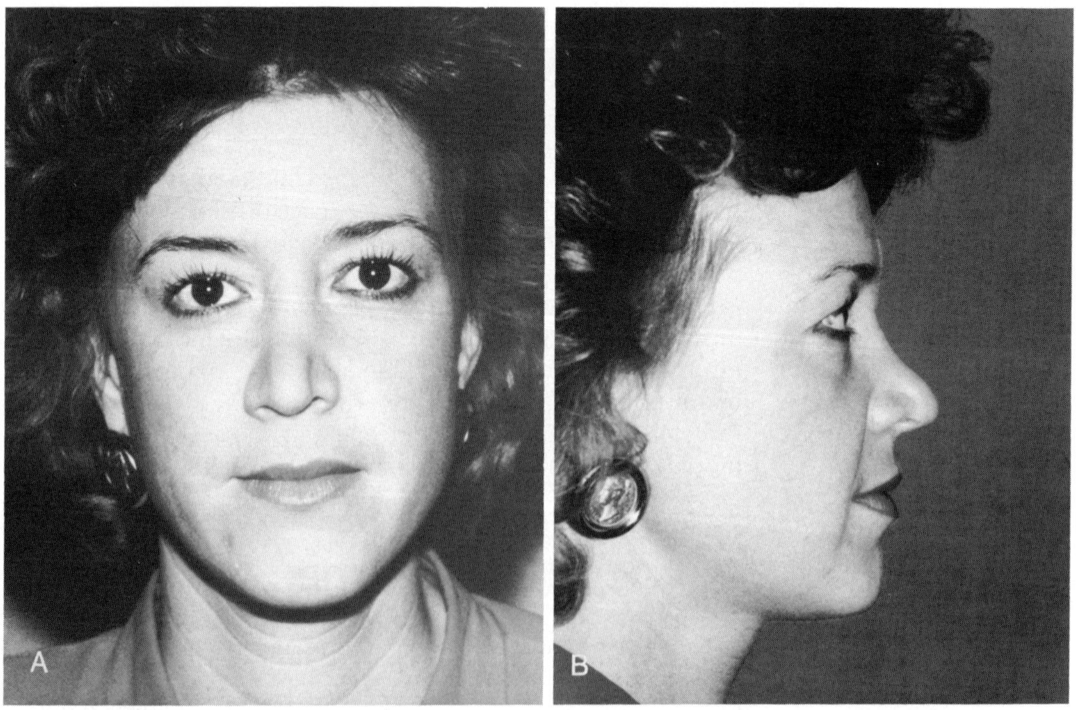

FIGURE 17–2. This patient was left with a crooked nose as a result of septorhinoplasty. Overly aggressive removal of bone coupled with disarticulation of the upper lateral cartilages from the nasal bones was responsible for the telltale signs of unsuccessful surgery.

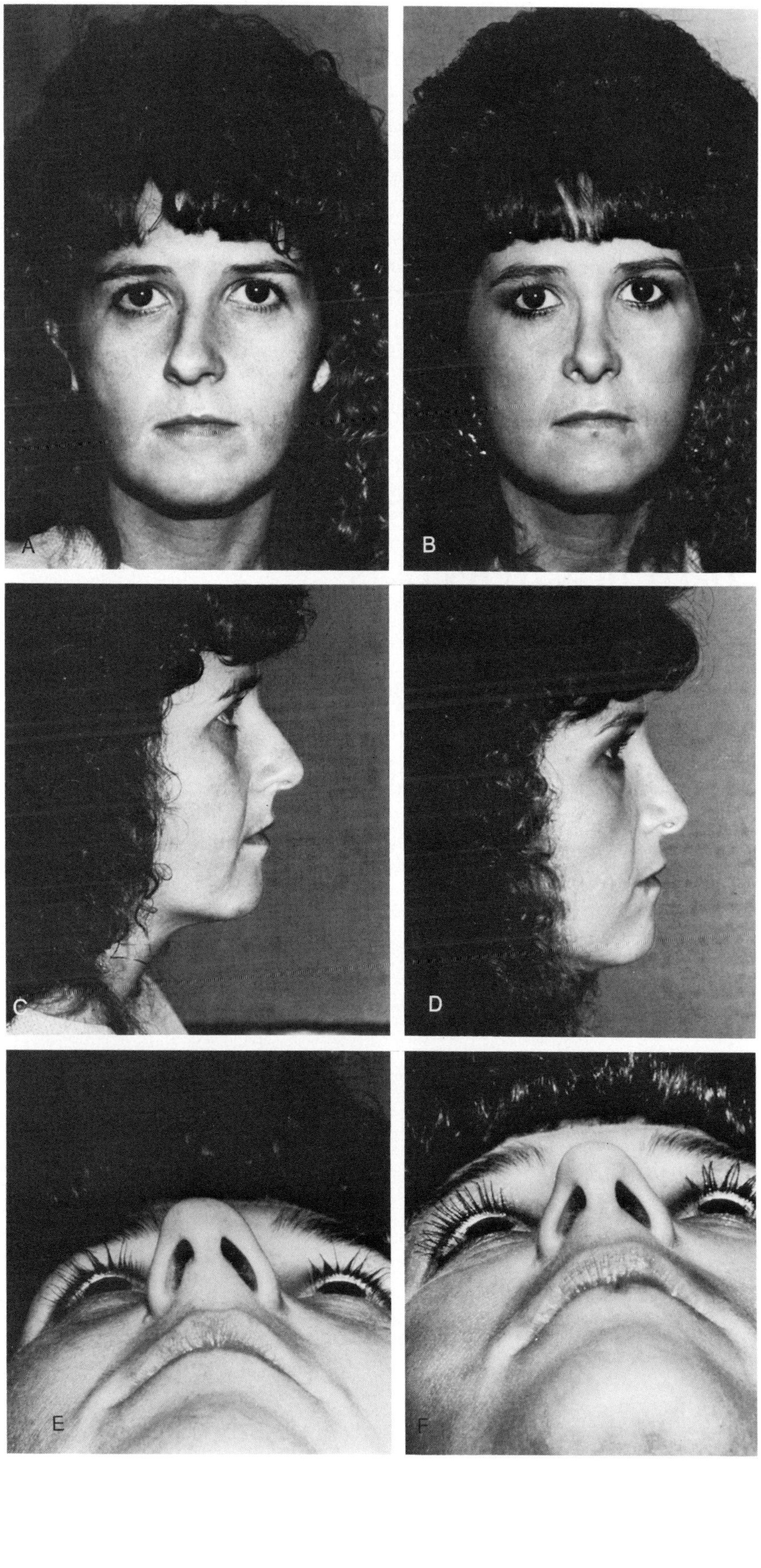

FIGURE 17–3. (*A* and *B*). When the injury extends into and beyond the bony cartilage junction cephalically and dorsally and to the floor of the nose, aggressive measures must be considered. It may not be possible to totally straighten a twisted nose. (*C* and *D*) Care must be taken to preserve the integrity of the dorsal cantilever whenever possible. (*E* and *F*) A swing-door procedure was performed to help straighten this caudal septal deformity.

If the surgeon can determine which of these factors is responsible for the deformity, he should attempt the appropriate correction. It is advisable to wait until 6 to 12 months have passed before attempting revisional surgery.

Because surgery of the twisted nose is one of the most complex and difficult corrections in nasal plastic surgery, consultation with a colleague experienced in revisional or reconstructive surgery is advisable. It is imperative that the surgeon be prepared to perform extensive septal surgery when faced with correcting a twisted nose deformity. These techniques are described in Chapter 10. The nasal plastic surgeon must also be prepared to reconstruct the alar cartilage framework and to use grafts and implants to replace and/or support missing or damaged elements.

Prudence must prevail when the risk-benefit ratio is questionable. Sometimes it is better to accept some persistent deformity than to risk nasal collapse or another mishap by continuing to incise, displace, or remove structural components (Fig. 17–3).

If the patient who has sustained nasal trauma is not seen by the operating surgeon until several days have passed, management proceeds as for a semielective twisted nose or revisional rhinoplasty (see Ch. 26).

CORRECTION TECHNIQUES

Grafts

CAMOUFLAGE GRAFTING

Minor deviations can be camouflaged by overlaying straighter cartilaginous grafts along the dorsum or by filling in concavities to correspond with a convexity on the opposite side of the nose (Fig. 17–4). Morselized cartilage is preferred for camouflaging techniques. Although septal or alar cartilage is best, auricular cartilage may be used for larger defects.

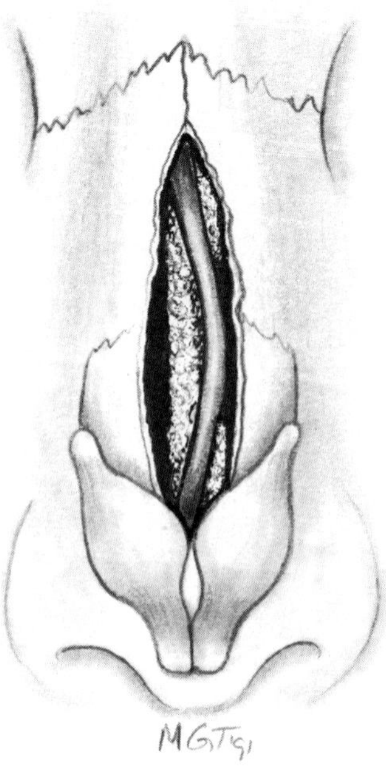

FIGURE 17–4. Crushed cartilage can be placed over concave or depressed areas.

Crushed cartilage is less likely to become displaced, and the edges of the graft are less visible and palpable after postoperative swelling subsides (Fig. 17–5). Some investigators have suggested that survival rates may be higher if the cartilage is gently morselized.

FRAMEWORK GRAFTING

If the dorsal strut of cartilage is crooked, the upper lateral cartilage complex is separated from the septum through an external approach. Gentle morselization of the dorsal septal cartilage can be carried out and then supported by a straight piece of unmorselized septal cartilage (see Ch. 10).

In a similar manner, a caudal deviation may be straightened with an adjacent cartilage graft (Figs. 17–6 and 17–7).

COLUMELLAR GRAFTING

Columellar strut grafts may be helpful in providing tip support or in helping to straighten deformed medial crura. Gentle morselization of the medial crura followed by transcolumellar sutures help to fix the medial crura to the nonmorselized graft and may achieve the desired result (Figs. 17–8 and 17–9). Smaller morselized grafts can help to fill an infratip bifidity or a columellar depression.

INJECTABLE GRAFTS

Collagen and fibril-like materials are effective for the short term, but they eventually are destroyed by the body's immune system. Fat cells transferred from one part of the body to another, especially when injected, seldom survive the transfer. Although Fibril contains some of the patient's own tissues, the initial improvement seen after injection seems to be short lived.

THE FATE OF GRAFTS

When grafting is required at the initial procedure, all, none, or any portion of the graft might survive. Patients should be advised that additional grafting might be required within 12 to 18 months.

Silicone

Medical-grade liquid silicone is probably the ideal material to use to correct small depressions of the nose. When silicone is injected at the correct depth and in small amounts, migration and granuloma formation seldom are reported. No hard evidence exists that, when used judiciously, silicone causes autoimmune, neoplastic, or neurologic afflictions. Even so, it is not available for use.

Virtually all needles and syringes are coated with medical-grade silicone, which serves as a lubricant. Dr. Norman Orentreich, considered by many to be the leading expert on silicone, estimates that a patient with insulin-dependent diabetes deposits several cubic centimeters of silicone in his or her body each year.

Text continued on page 244

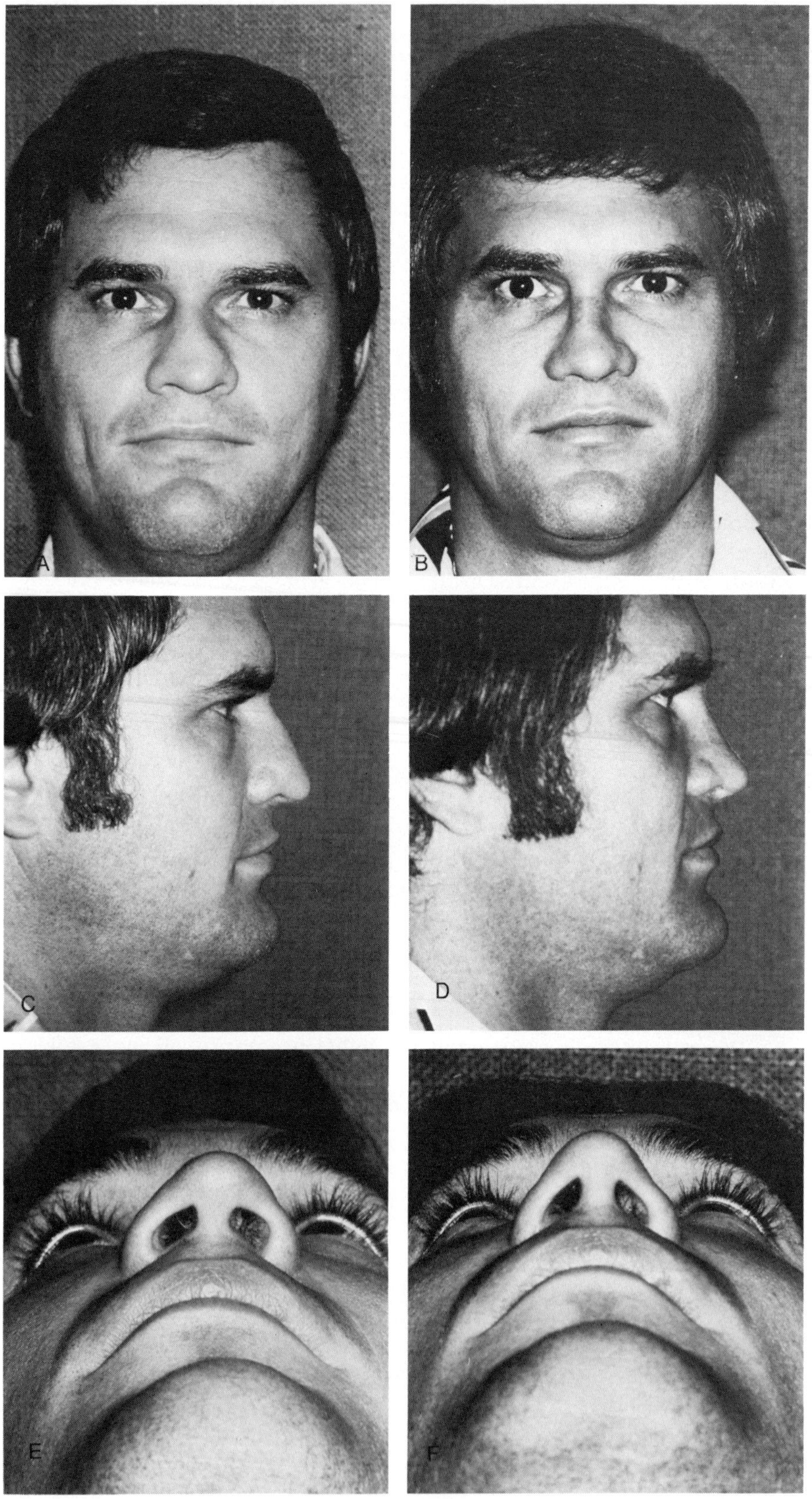

FIGURE 17–5. (*A* and *B*) Deformities that involve both bony and cartilaginous components may require disarticulation at the bony-cartilaginous septal junction and suture fixation of the dorsal cantilever as well as osteotomy mobilization of the lateral bony walls. Camouflage onlay grafts were placed on the concave side. (*C* and *D*) Dorsal height can be maintained with suture fixation and internal splinting. Columellar refraction was corrected with cartilage plumping grafts. (*E* and *F*) The deviation of the septum seen in (*E*) has been corrected. Conservative complete strip tip-plasty was performed.

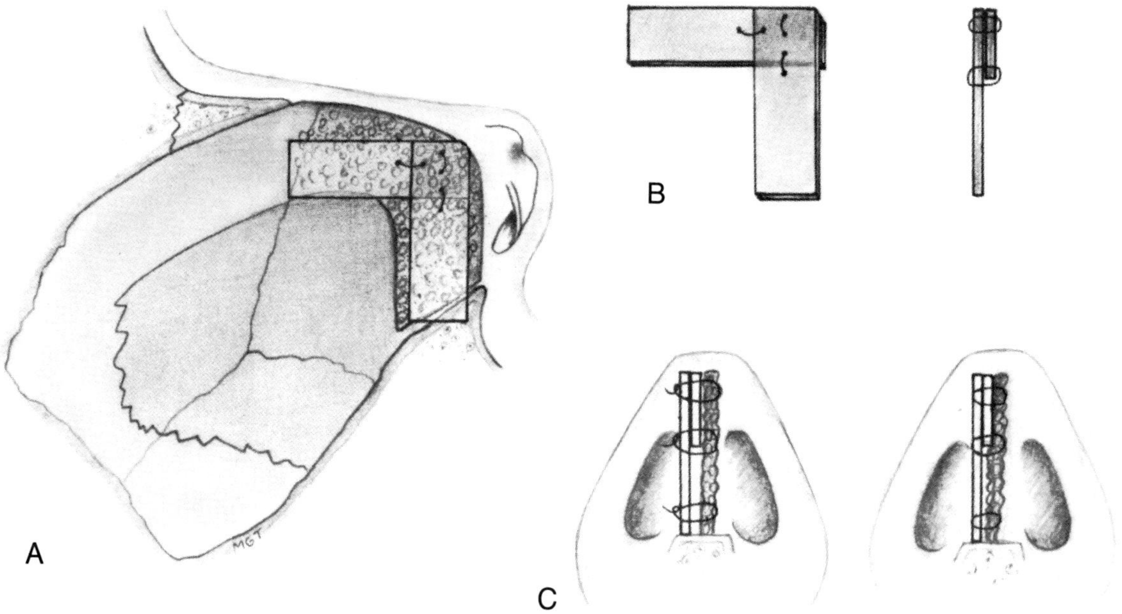

FIGURE 17–6. (*A*) A crooked cartilaginous cantilever may be gently morselized (after bilateral mucoperichondrial flap elevation and separation of both upper lateral cartilages from the septum through an open or external approach). Autogenous splinting and reconstruction may be carried out with septal cartilage grafts sutured into position. (*B*) Two pieces of septal cartilage may be used to create an L-shaped graft. (*C*) The graft is then sutured to the morselized cantilever.

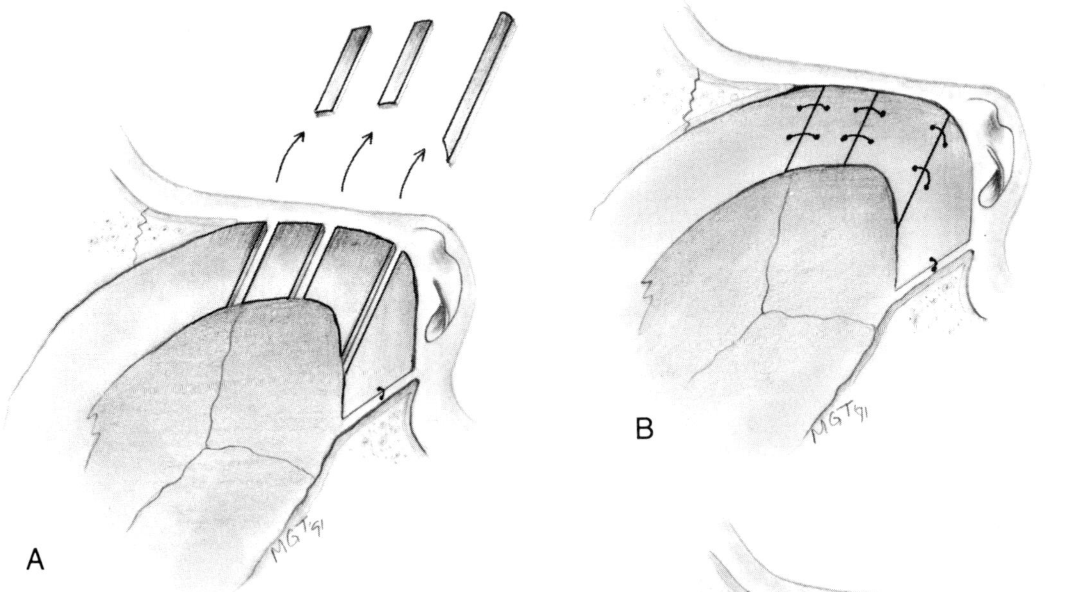

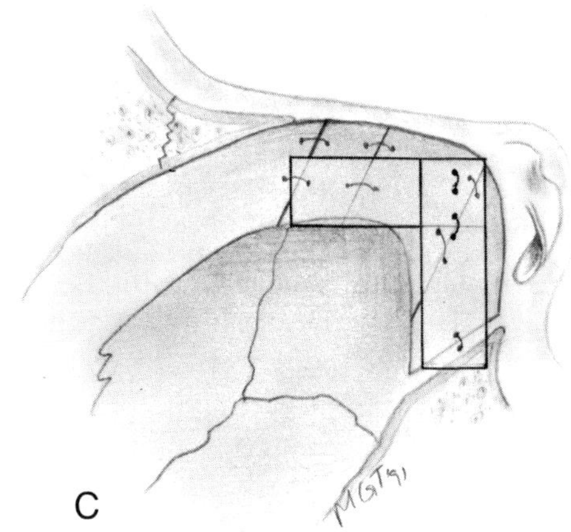

FIGURE 17–7. (*A*) The dorsal and caudal cantilever may also be divided into independent segments, which are then sutured together (*B*) and supported by an L-shaped cartilaginous graft (*C*). Internal splints are recommended for additional support during the early stages of healing.

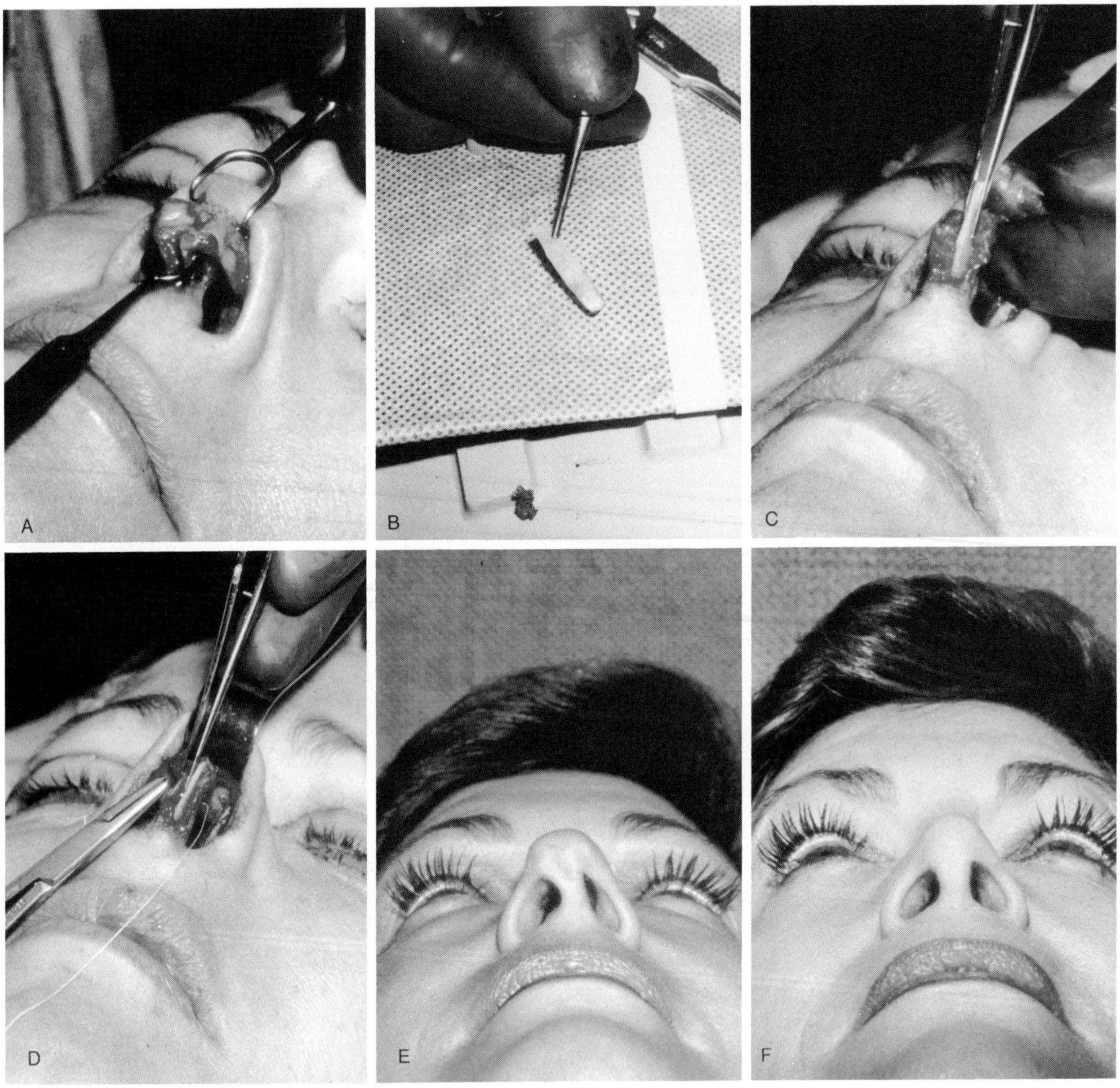

FIGURE 17–8. (*A*) Columellar grafts may be more accurately sutured in place through an external approach. (*B*) A straight piece of septal cartilage is preferred. Edges are tailored for easier insertion. (*C*) The graft is placed in a pocket between the medial crura. (*D*) Horizontal mattress sutures (5-0 polyglycolic acid) are placed to secure the medial crura to the graft. (*E*) Preoperative documentation of the patient's deformities. (*F*) Six months postoperatively, the inverted V transcolumellar scar is undetectable.

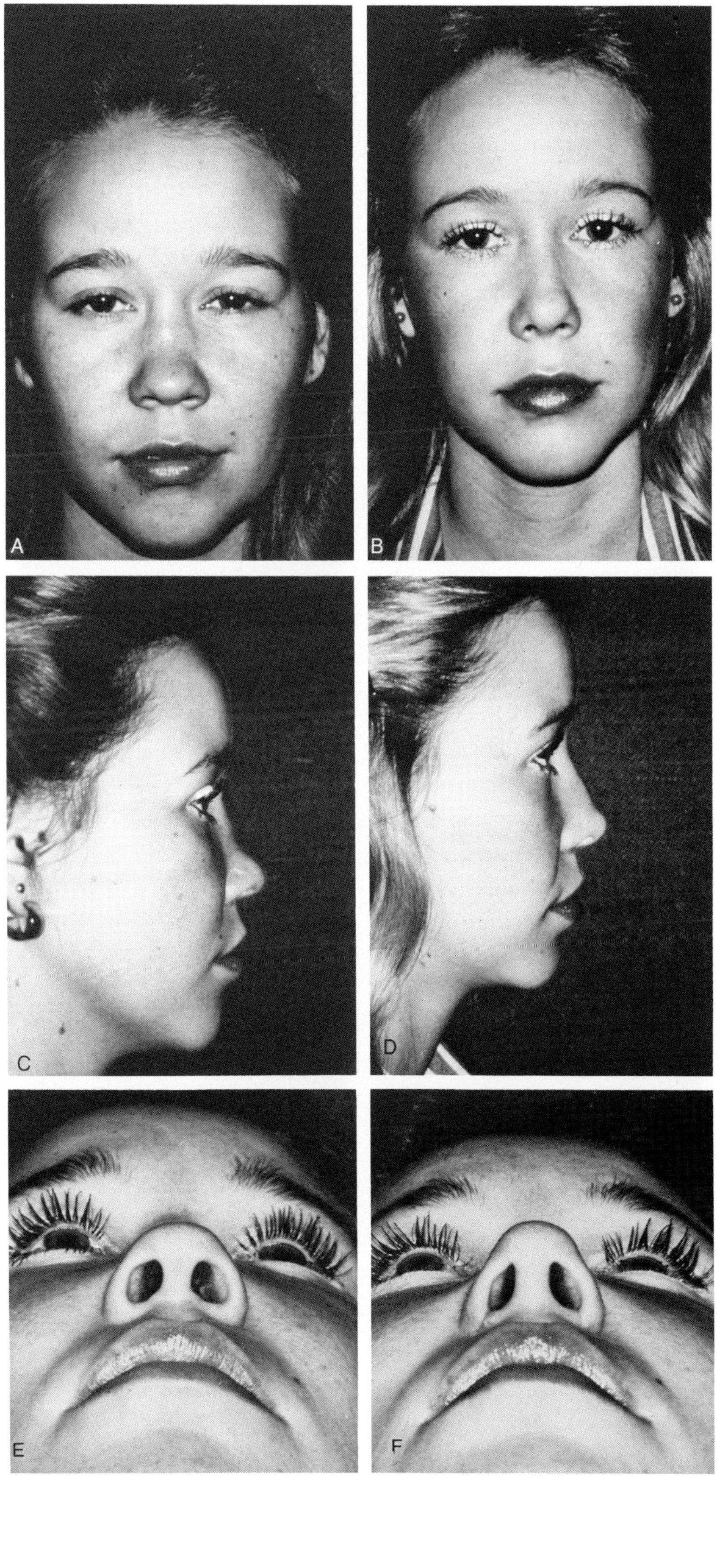

FIGURE 17–9. (*A* and *B*) Trauma at an early age resulted in an untreated septal hematoma. Correction of the sequelae involved reconstructive rhinoplasty. (*C* and *D*) Columellar retraction and dorsal augmentation were corrected with auricular cartilage grafts. (*E* and *F*) Vertical dome division with medial crural suture fixation (Goldman type) was used for tip-plasty.

Synthetic Implants

Experience with man-made implantation materials varies from surgeon to surgeon. Infection, dislocation, and extrusion are some of the dreaded sequelae that can occur when an implantation procedure is unsuccessful; however, around the world, myriad materials are used with great success (Figs. 17–10 and 17–11).

Antiseptic handling of implantation materials, limiting incisions, and instituting antibiotic therapy (regional and systemic) may reduce the incidence of infection. Porous or mesh implants are saturated with antibiotics (gentamicin) before insertion.

Minimizing the dissection to create a pocket just large enough to accommodate an implant may help to reduce displacement. It is also imperative that incisions be closed adequately to minimize postoperative contamination.

Frequent or severe trauma to the nose may also cause an implant to extrude.

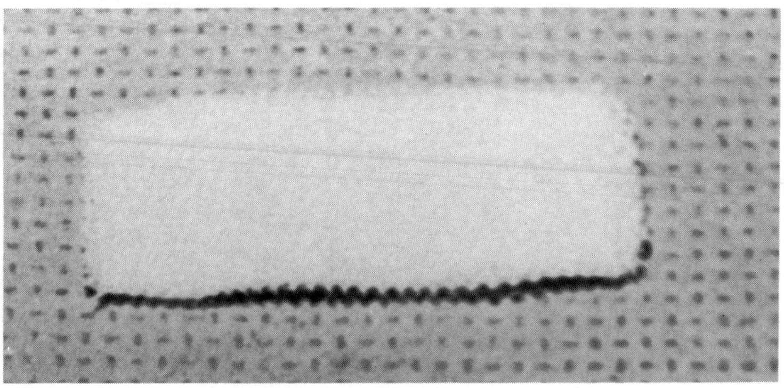

FIGURE 17–10. Mersilene mesh may be folded and sutured to create an acceptable dorsal nasal implant.

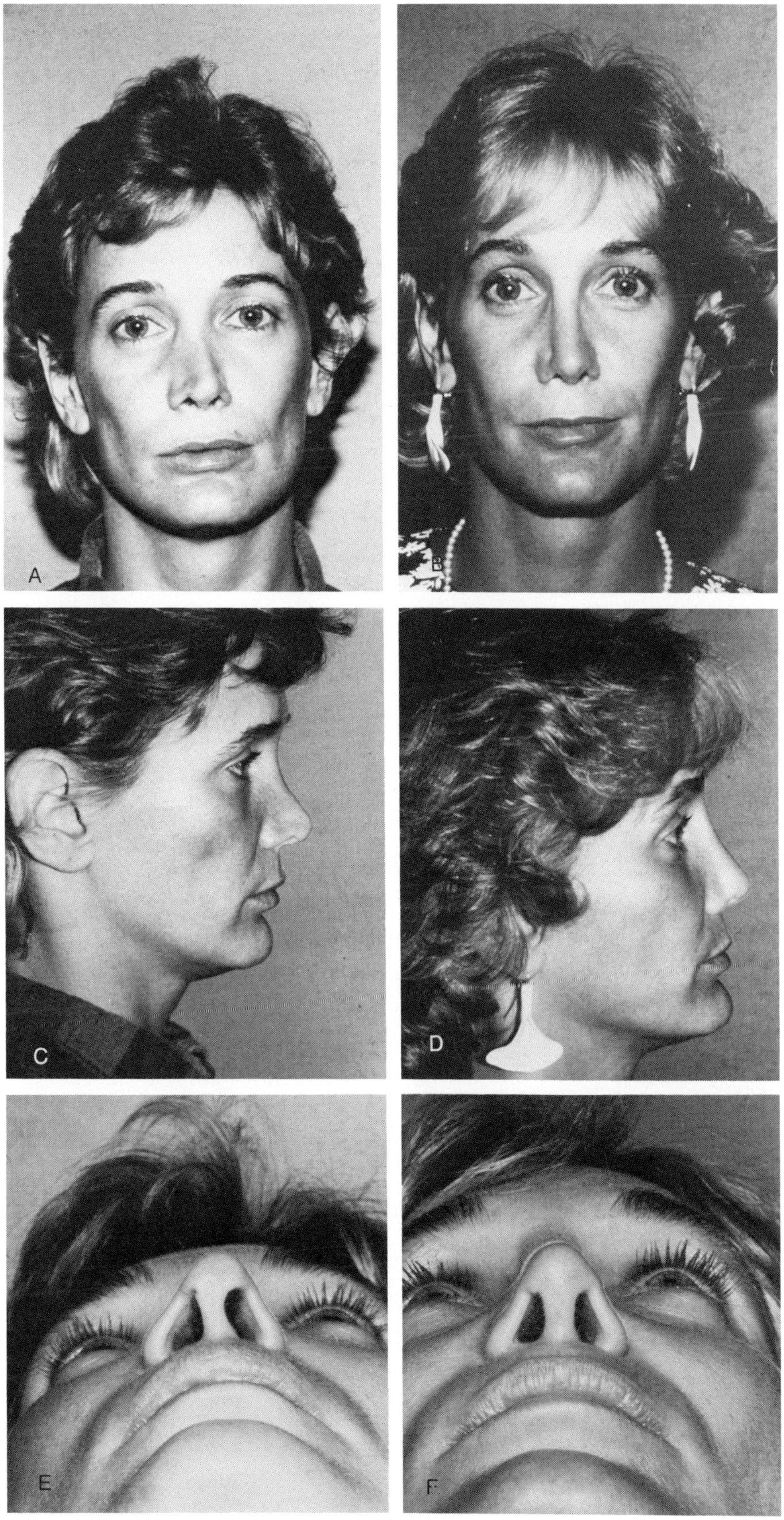

FIGURE 17–11. (*A* and *B*) When multiple surgeries have resulted in the loss of nasal architecture, alloplastic camouflaging implants are an acceptable alternative for correction. (*C* and *D*) Dorsal height may be reestablished. (*E* and *F*) Cartilage grafts may be used to reestablish the architectural integrity of the tip.

Suggested Readings

Rees, T.: Surgical correction of the severely deviated nose by extramucoral excision of the osseocartilaginous septum and replacement as a free graft. Plast Reconstructive Surg 78:320–330, 1986.

Stucker, F., Shockley, W., Briarly, R.: Management of nasal trauma in children. Arch Otolaryngol 110:190–192, 1984.

Thomas, J.R.: The crooked nose. In Gates, G.A., ed. Current Therapy in Otolaryngology—Head and Neck Surgery. Toronto: B. C. Decker, 1987, pp. 123–125.

CHAPTER 18

Altering the Alar Base

In Leonardo da Vinci's ideal face, the width of the nose should not extend laterally beyond an imaginary line dropped vertically from each medial canthus. After all other steps have been performed, attention should be directed to the width and shape of the alar base.

Function should not be sacrificed for appearance. The competency of the nasal introitus must not be unduly compromised. A wide columella might be a relative contraindication to alar sil resection.

When a caudal dislocation or deviation of the septum contributes to asymmetry, septoplasty should be performed before alar sil surgery. In some overly projected noses, setting the widened medial crural footplates back closer to the face can also help (Fig. 18–1). As in other aspects of rhinoplasty, it is essential that the surgeon recognize how much narrowing can be achieved without jeopardizing function.

Alae that are flared at rest may be refined, but flaring that occurs with smiling cannot be corrected (Fig. 18–2). Alae that are wide and implanted into the face more laterally cannot be permanently narrowed by conventional techniques (Fig. 18–3).

TECHNIQUE

If possible, incisions or excisions should be restricted to the sil region. The incision should be planned to preserve a portion of the natural curvature of the alae (Figs. 18–4 and 18–5*A*).

Text continued on page 251

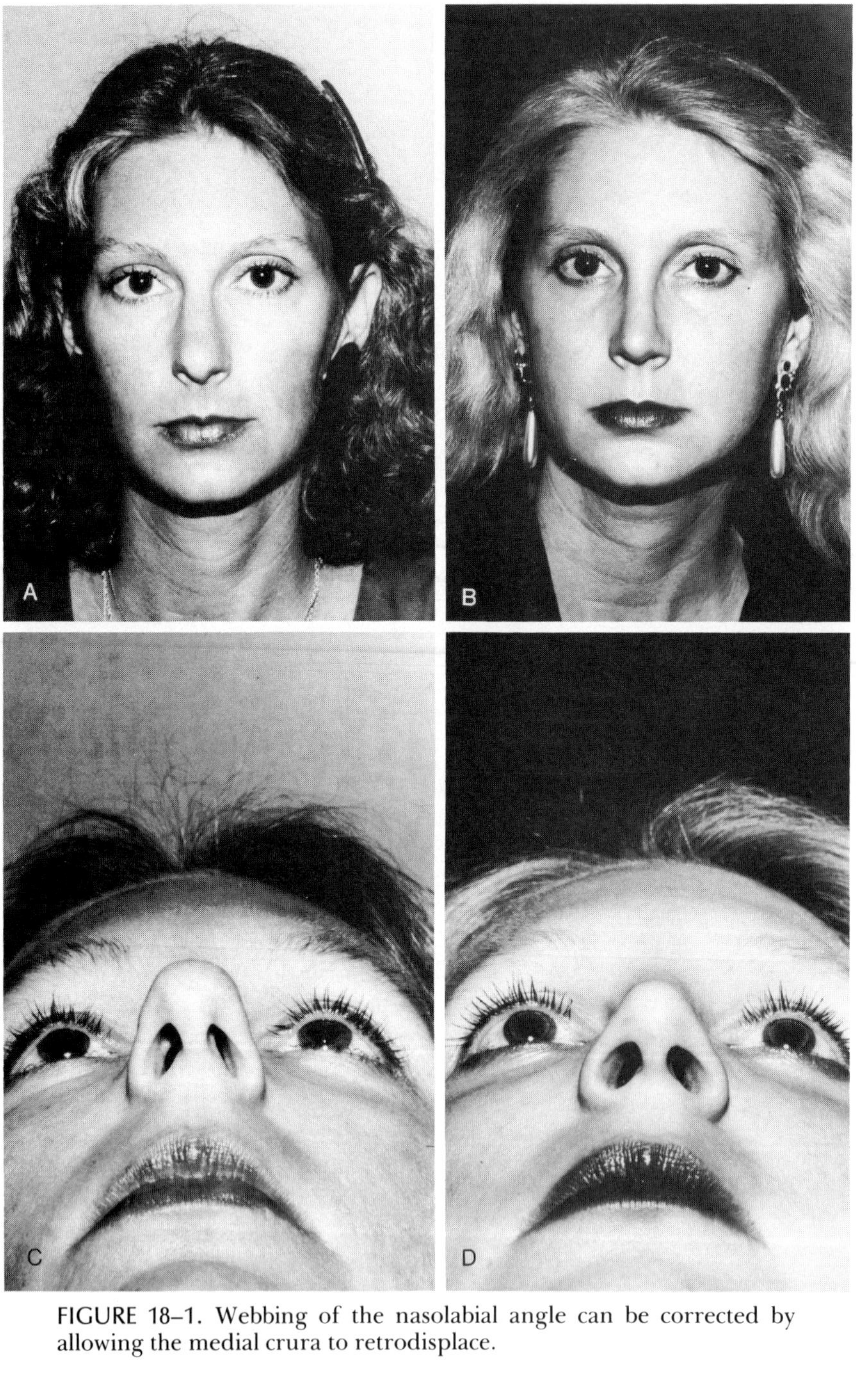

FIGURE 18–1. Webbing of the nasolabial angle can be corrected by allowing the medial crura to retrodisplace.

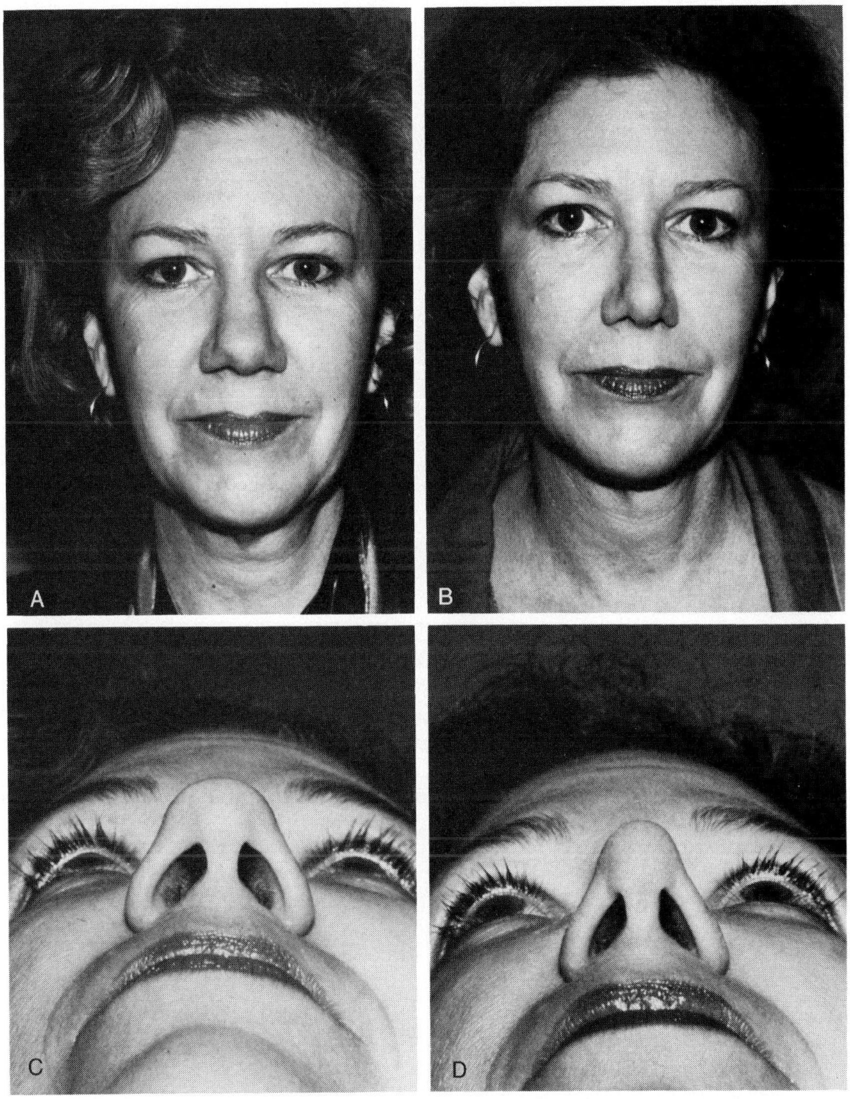

FIGURE 18–2. (*A* and *B*) Anteroposterior views before and after alar base narrowing. (*C* and *D*) Base views demonstrate the appearance of the nose after sil resections.

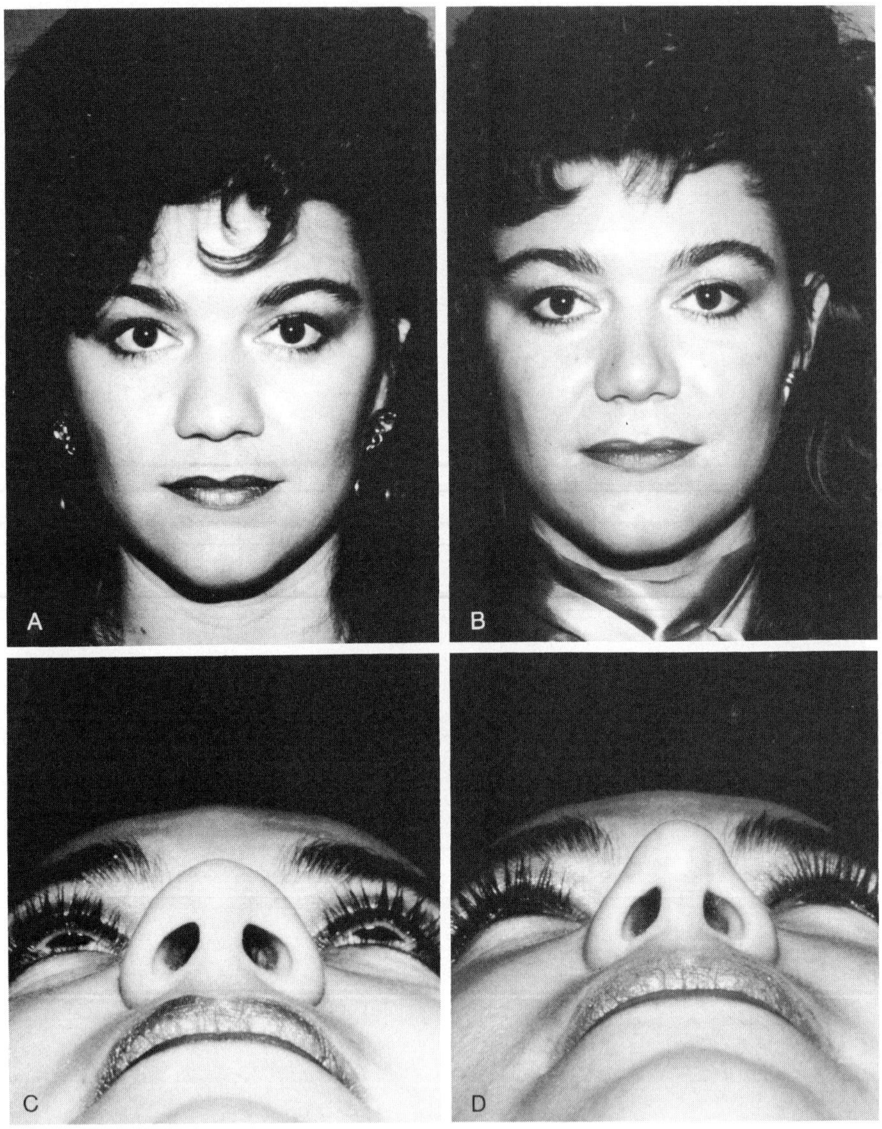

FIGURE 18–3. (*A* and *B*) When the width of the nose extends beyond an imaginary line dropped vertically from each medial canthus, alar-plasty should be performed. (*C* and *D*) When well designed and carefully sutured, the scars are imperceptible.

An effective and efficient method of resecting the unwanted portion of tissue can be carried out with Adson-Brown or Griffis-Brown forceps and a No. 11 blade (Fig. 18–5*B*). Soft tissue resection should be carried into the floor of the vestibule and tapered to an angle (Fig. 18–5*C*). Only when a relatively large amount of tissue has been removed is an incision carried into the nasofacial crease. This extended maneuver can create an advancement-rotation flap and may help to prevent postoperative widening (Fig. 18–6).

Excision of a crescent-shaped portion of alae (as described by Weir) seldom is indicated. Serious complications can result when this type of excision is carried to the extreme (Fig. 18–7).

Closure of the wound is crucial to obtaining pleasing scars. Deep or buried sutures are not necessary. Accurate wound edge approximation and eversion can be accomplished with 5-0 plain catgut sutures. In the postoperative period, if the sutures are saturated with hydrogen peroxide six to eight times daily and kept moist with a mild ointment, most suture material disintegrates during the first 5 to 6 days.

Alar sil resections are generally indicated in the non-Caucasian nose. When loss of tip support occurs during rhinoplasty, alar base narrowing may be needed in the patient of any race.

When tip projection is either maintained or increased, the necessity to perform alar base resection is lessened. Conversely, as tip retrodisplacement occurs, the alae flare (Fig. 18–8).

Text continued on page 255

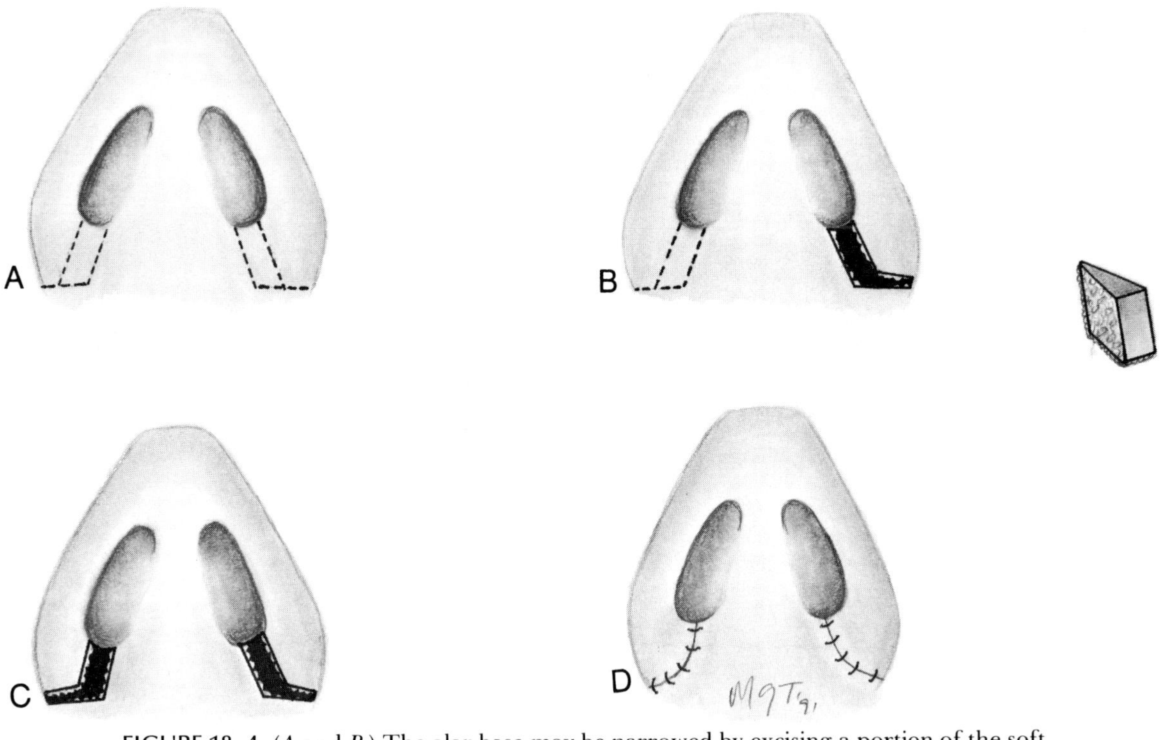

FIGURE 18–4. (*A* and *B*) The alar base may be narrowed by excising a portion of the soft tissue of the alar sil. In extremely wide noses, the incision (excision) may be extended into the nasolabial crease to create an advancement flap. (*C*) It is desirable to preserve some of the natural curvature of the nostril. (*D*) Accurate suture closure with 5-0 plain sutures usually is adequate.

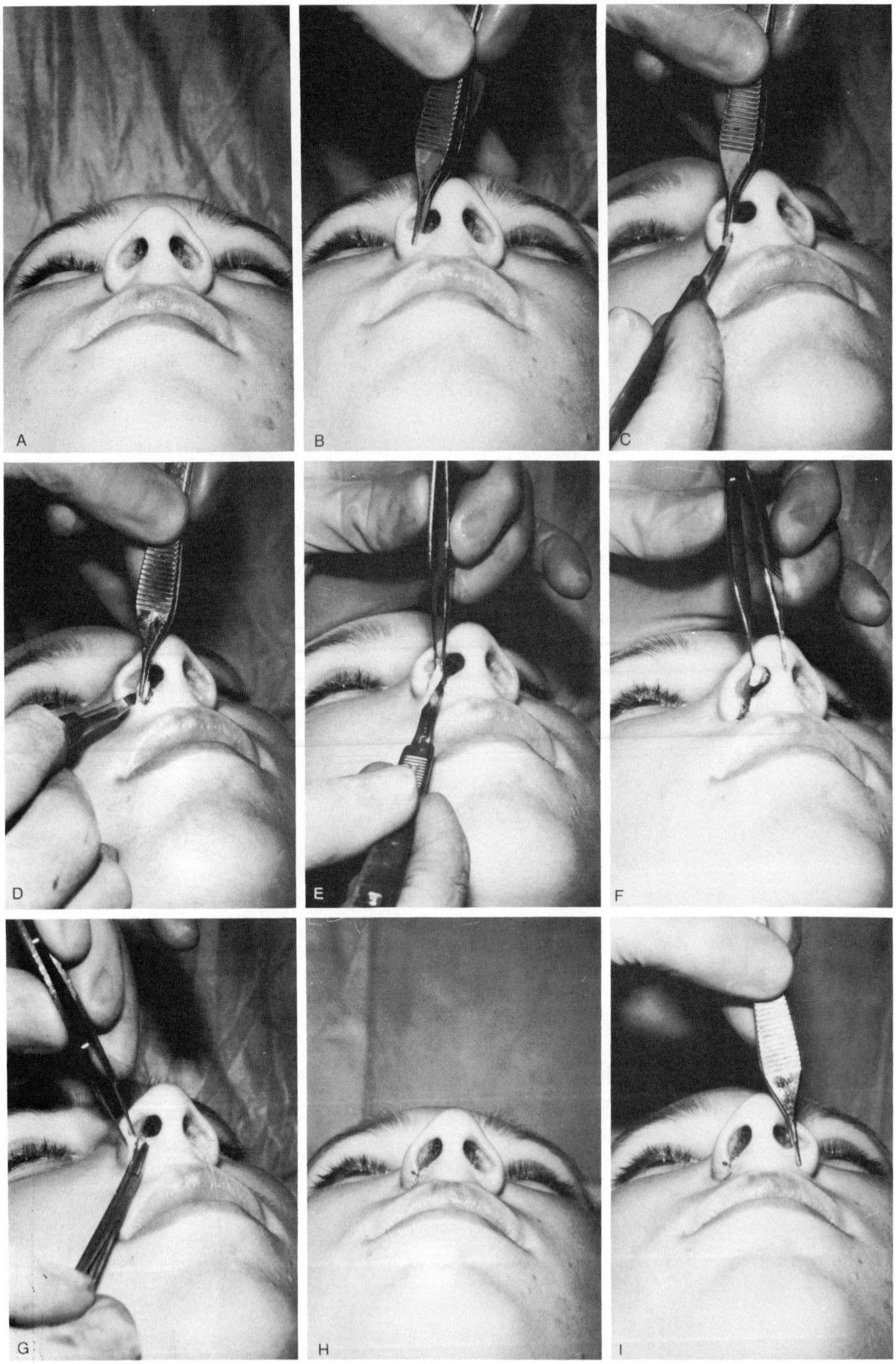

FIGURE 18–5. Intraoperative demonstration of the method of alar base narrowing I prefer. (*A*) Patient with wide alar base and well-developed sils. (*B*) Adson-Brown forceps grasp the sil to secure its position. (*C*) A No. 11 blade (edge up) is passed adjacent to the medial edge of the forceps. (*D*) The procedure is repeated along the forceps' lateral edge. (*E*) The section of tissue is freed from the floor. (*F*) The defect and bloc of tissue are shown. (*G*) The wound is closed (under magnification) with 5-0 plain catgut suture. (*H*) Note the new shape of the nostril when the defect is repaired. (*I*) A similar procedure is repeated on the opposite side.

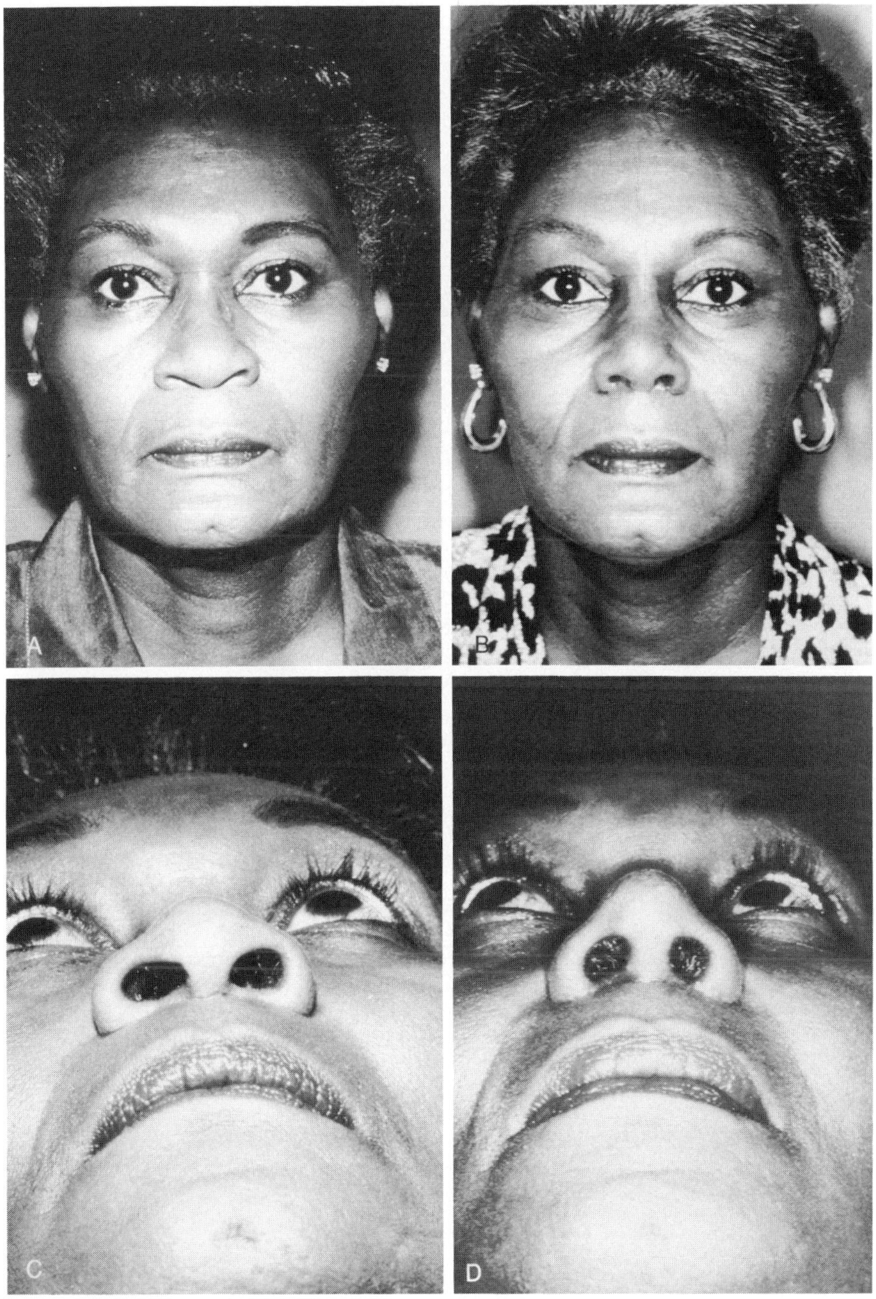

FIGURE 18–6. (*A* and *B*) Alar base resections can provide additional refinement in the platyrrhine nose. (*C* and *D*) After the wound has healed, the scars are barely perceptible.

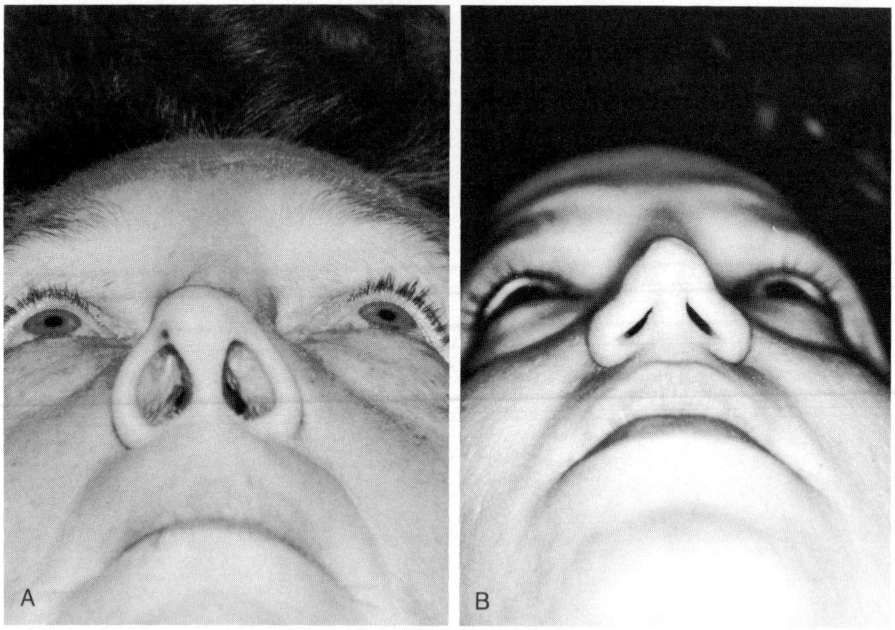

FIGURE 18–7. Scarring and removal of soft tissue elements at the base of the nose may compromise the introitus. (*A*) This patient, who had previously undergone nine nasal operations, has a widely patent introitus but a non-functional valve area. (*B*) Excessively thick skin and a small introitus in this patient who presented for a postoperative complication combine to set the stage for problems, especially if the lateral crura are interrupted.

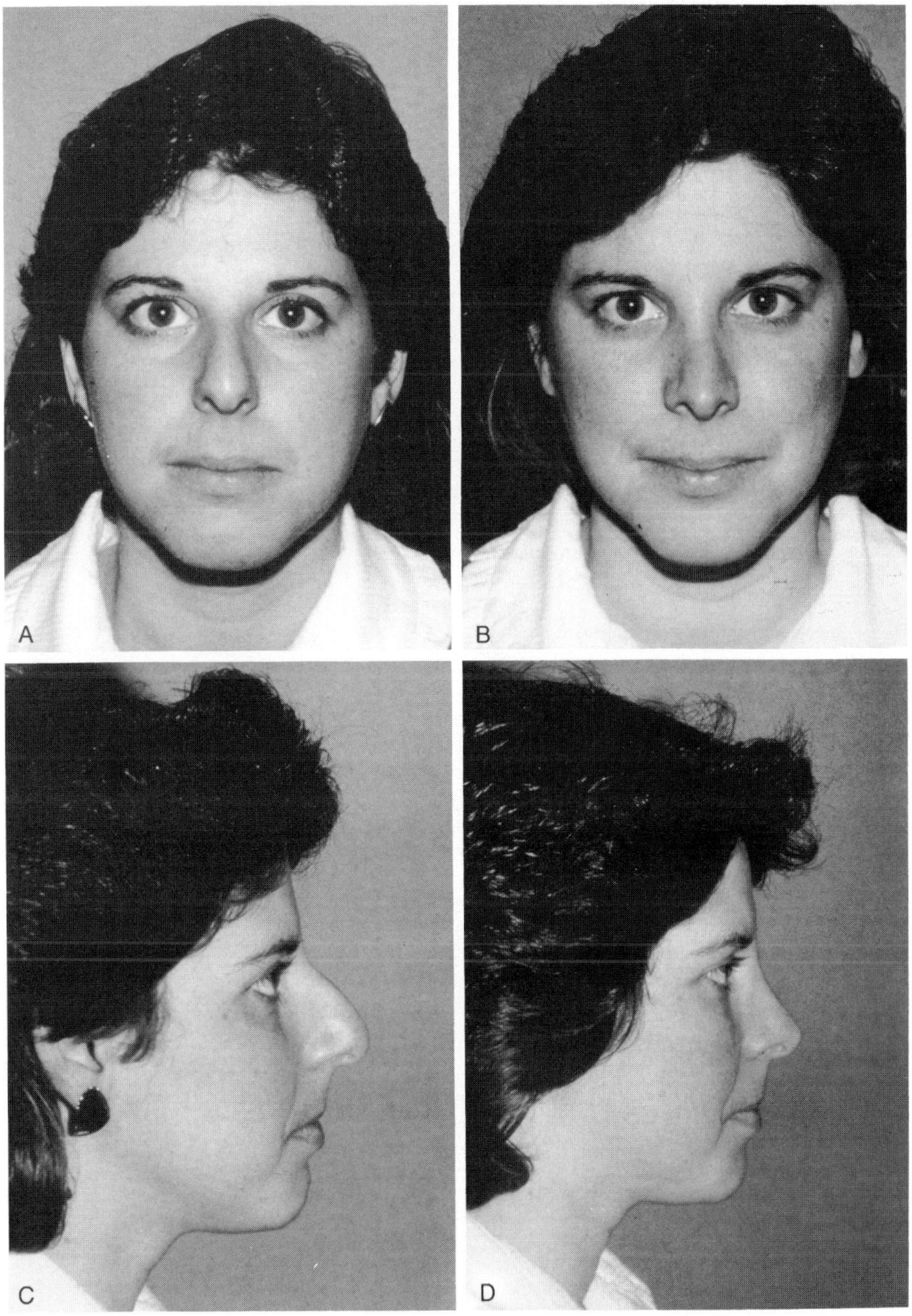

FIGURE 18–8. (*A* and *B*) As surgical retrodisplacement occurs in an overly projected or tension nose, some flaring of the alae may take place and be desirable. (*C* and *D*) As tip retrodisplacement occurs, the desired aesthetic curvature of the alae ensues. Webbing of the nasolabial angle is also alleviated.

Suggested Reading

Joseph, J.: Rhinoplasty and Facial Plastic Surgery. 1931. Reprint. Phoenix, Ariz.: Columella Press, 1987, p. 111.

CHAPTER 19

Finishing Touches: Little Things That Count

It has been said that 90 per cent of tasks can be completed in 10 per cent of the time they actually take. This statement might be slightly exaggerated when applied to rhinoplasty, but there is little question that a few additional percentage points of improvement can be obtained by a thoughtful assessment of the intraoperative result and "fine tuning."

It is important for a surgeon to know when to stop operating and to accept what he or she believes is the best result possible in a given case. In any procedure, there is a point of diminishing return beyond which the bell-shaped curve of aesthetic improvement begins to move downward (Fig. 19–1).

A few fine points deserve consideration. Ideally, at the end of the operation:

1. the septum should be in a midline position;
2. the operated areas should be free of debris;
3. the upper lateral cartilage should be at the same height as the cartilaginous dorsum;

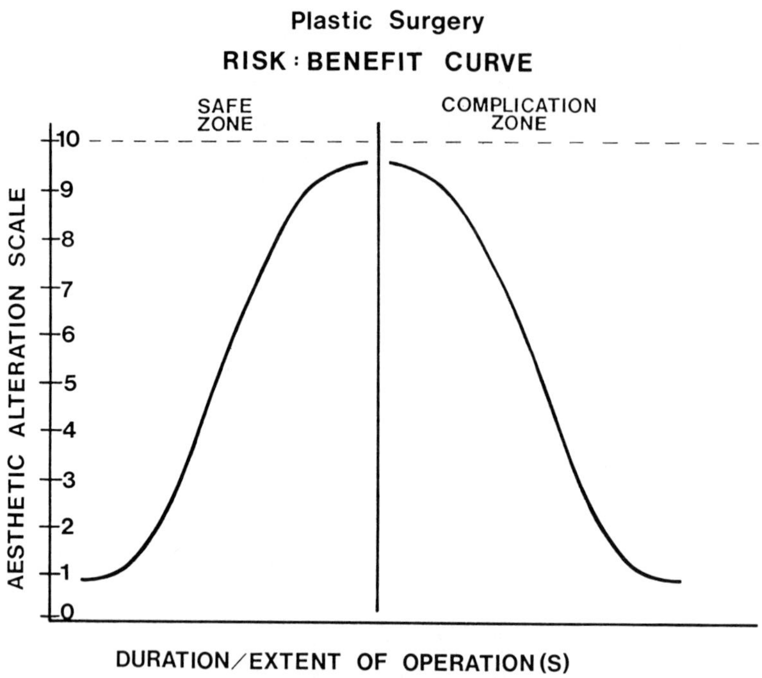

FIGURE 19–1. At the point in the operation when the surgeon believes that the best result possible has been obtained—even if perfection has not been achieved—the next prudent step is to close the incisions and apply the dressings.

4. the superior septal angle should be the lowest point of the nasal dorsum and the rhinion should be the highest;
5. the lateral nasal walls should be mobile and free of greenstick fractures;
6. the lower lateral cartilages are inspected for symmetry;
7. intranasal incisions are closed with 5-0 plain catgut sutures;
8. the nose is molded to express collected blood and tissue fluids; and
9. a dressing is carefully applied to secure all elements for healing.

NASAL DRESSINGS

Properly applied nasal dressings play a more important role in good rhinoplasty results than many surgeons realize (Fig. 19–2).

TAPING

Tan-colored Micropore paper tape secures the dorsal soft tissues to the new skeleton. Extra pressure in the supratip obliterates dead space and may help to prevent soft tissue polly-beak. Tip cartilages can be molded with a carefully applied "sling" strip that can secure tip projection and bring the dome angles together to help ensure definition of the lobule.

SPLINTS

A metal splint is fashioned from a round disk and backed with Elastoplast tape, which helps to prevent oxidation. The splint is molded over the

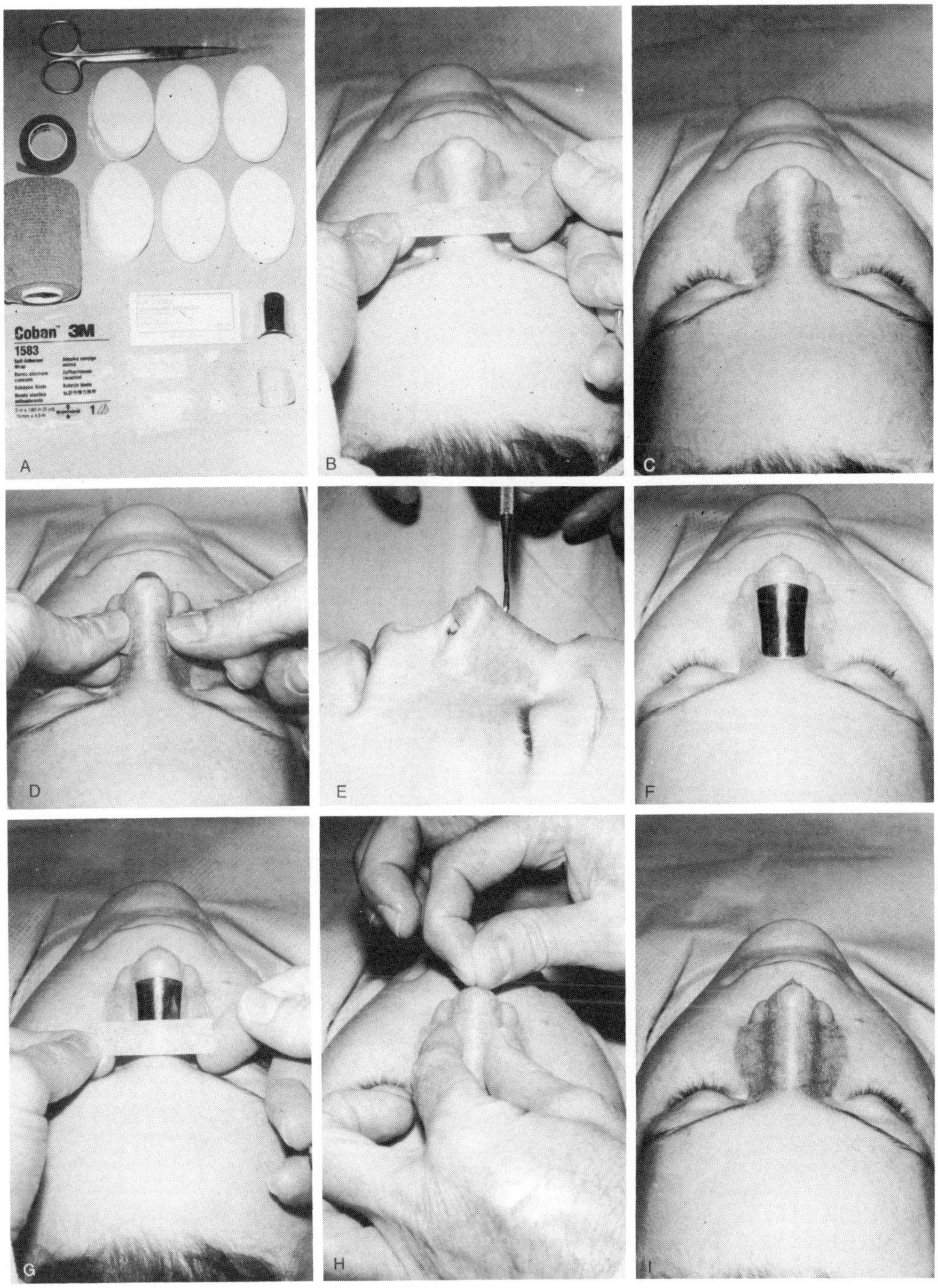

FIGURE 19–2. (*A*) Supplies needed for nasal dressing. (*B*) Strips of Micropore tape are cut into the desired lengths. (*C*) Tape is applied over the nasal dorsum to secure the skin to the newly constructed skeleton. (*D*) A tip "sling" is created using a strip of Micropore tape. (*E*) Additional pressure is applied over the supratip region to obliterate dead space. (*F*) A metal splint backed with Elastoplast tape is applied over the initial layer of tape. (*G*) The splint is secured with another layer of Micropore tape. (*H* and *I*) After the splint is secured along the dorsum, another strip of tape is placed around the tip as a sling. *Illustration continued on following page*

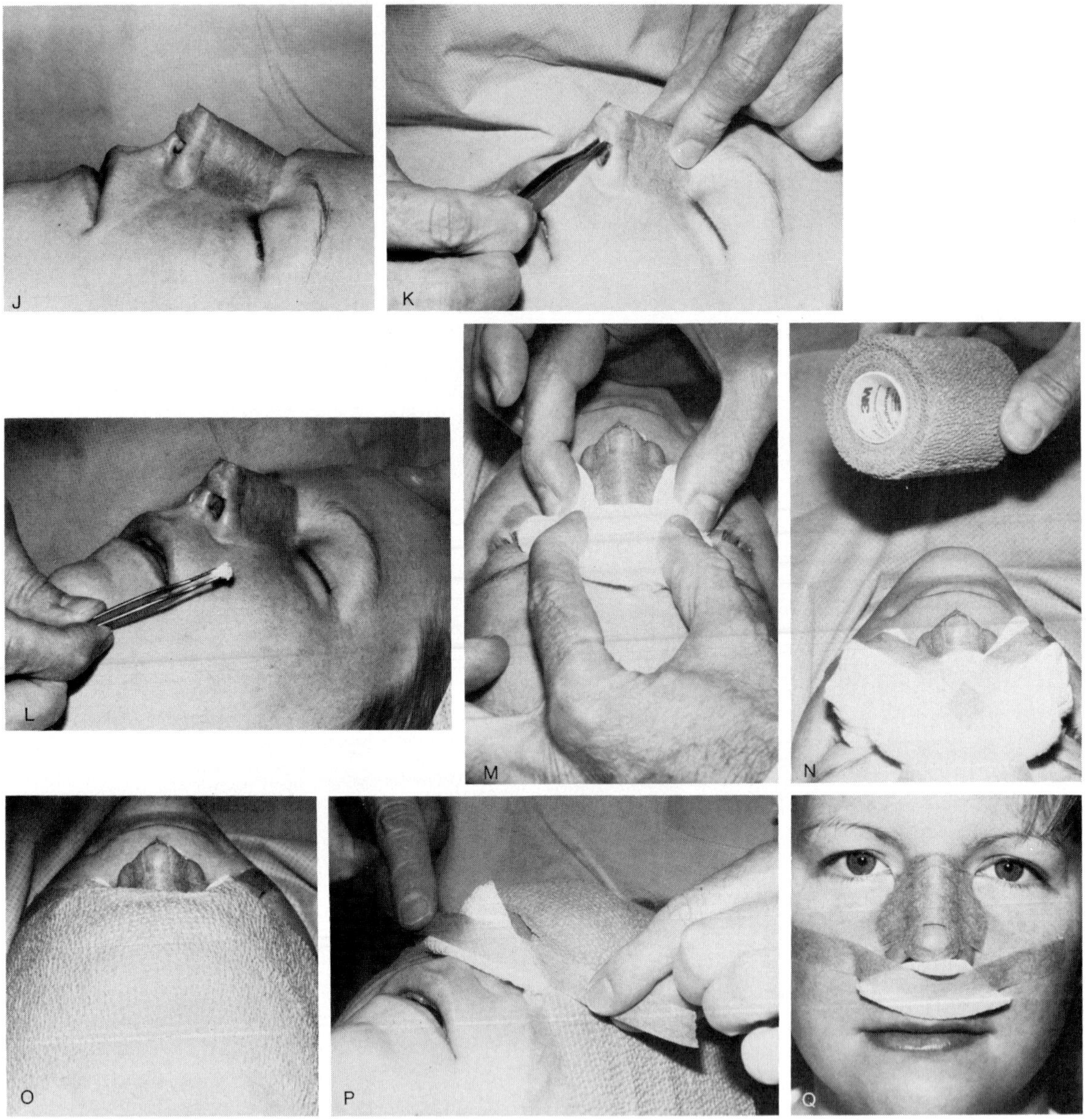

FIGURE 19–2 *Continued* (*J*) The dressing applied at the end of the operation remains in place for 1 week. (*K*) Two small pieces of Surgicel are placed in the domes of the nasal vestibule for support for 1 week. (*L*) Two larger pieces of Surgicel are placed at the introitus on each side to prevent sniffing, but no internal packing is used. The Surgicel is removed the morning after surgery. (*M*) Folded eyepads are placed into the medial canthal and glabellar regions. (*N*) The eyepads are secured with strips of Micropore tape and circumferential Coban dressings. (*O*) The eyepad compression dressings are removed after 4 hours. (*P* and *Q*) A "drip" dressing may be worn for several days if nasal drainage occurs.

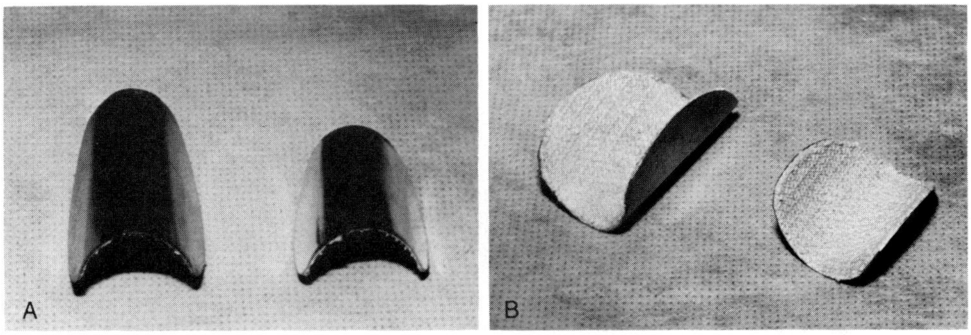

FIGURE 19–3. External splints. (*A*) Splints can be fashioned into different sizes and preshaped. Final adjustments can be made with finger-molding on the patient. (*B*) The splint is backed with Elastoplast tape.

tapered end of an I.V. pole. The final molding can be accomplished with the fingertips once the splint is placed over the initial tape dressing (Fig. 19–3).

The splint is secured in position with another layer of Micropore tape. Pressure from a splint or taping (especially as postoperative swelling occurs) could compromise blood supply and lead to postoperative scarring.

PACKING

Internal packing is not required after septorhinoplasty because the dead space between the mucoperichondrial flaps has been obliterated with a running mattress suture of 4-0 plain catgut.

Internal splints are used only when a swinging door septal procedure has been performed or when nasal synechiae were lysed in revisional or reconstructive cases. The splints prevent reanastomosis of the severed ends of the cicatrix during the first postoperative week.

Two small pieces of Surgicel are placed in the dome of the vestibule to help support and secure the position of the domes of the lower lateral cartilages. These two pieces of Surgicel remain in place until the 1-week postoperative visit.

A larger piece of Surgicel is placed in each nostril to prevent sniffing and serves as a drip dressing during the first 12 to 16 hours postoperatively. The larger Surgicel dressings are removed the morning after surgery. Most patients are able to breathe gently through their noses on the first operative day. Some congestion, similar to that which exists when one has a cold, persists for several days.

Postoperative edema and ecchymosis may be reduced with properly applied pressure dressings. The concept of applying pressure over a venipuncture site to help prevent ecchymosis is carried over to rhinoplasty surgery.

Provided no ecchymosis is present when the operation is completed, much of the potential edema can be prevented if, after the eyelids are taped with a strip of Micropore tape, six eyepads are applied over the osteotomy tracts and nasofrontal angle. The eyepads are secured with a circumferential Coban dressing for 4 hours. When the circumferential dressings are removed, cold compresses should be applied during the next 12 to 24 hours, the head of the bed should be kept elevated for approximately 2 weeks, and physical activity must be kept to a minimum to diminish bleeding from and into the perinasal tissues (Fig. 19–4).

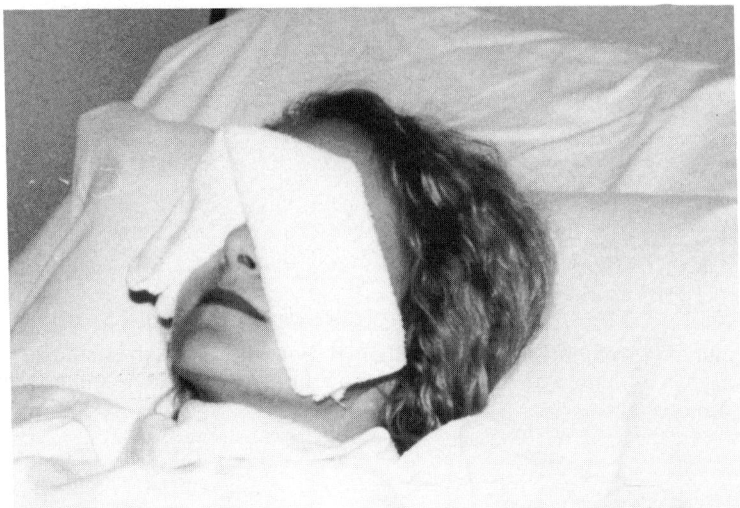

FIGURE 19–4. Cold compresses placed over the eyes and nose after surgery may minimize postoperative edema and ecchymosis.

MANAGING EARLY SOFT TISSUE POLLY-BEAK

In patients whose nasal skin is thick or oily and in some revisional cases, even if the previously described methods of taping the supratip region are used, some supratip fullness may appear within 1 to 2 weeks of operation. Triamcinolone (Kenalog), 10 to 20 mg/mL, can be injected into the subdermal layers of the supratip region with a one-piece tuberculin syringe at 2- to 3-week intervals. Intralesional steroids soften the area and, in many cases, prevent the long-term formation of supratip scarring. If the surgeon does not become aware of this condition until several weeks (or months) have passed, triamcinolone injections may still be beneficial.

Additional postoperative instructions are covered in Chapter 6.

Suggested Readings

Anderson, J. R.: The supratip in rhinoplasty, a dilemma. Laryngoscope 86:53–57, 1976.

Hoffman, D. F., et al: Steroids and rhinoplasty: A double-blind study. In Plastic and Reconstructive Surgery. Philadelphia: B. C. Decker, 1991.

McCollough, E. G.: Plastic Surgery. Birmingham, Ala.: Ebsco Publishing Co., 1991.

CHAPTER 20

Ethnic Rhinoplasty

In 1970, Fomon and Bell described three major categories of nasal features according to race:

1. Leptorrhine—usually found in members of the white race and characterized by a long, high narrow nose and nostrils (Fig. 20–1)
2. Mesorrhine—usually found among Orientals (Fig. 20–2)
3. Platyrrhines—usually found among members of the black race and characterized by a flat, broad nose and wide nostrils (Fig. 20–3)

Nasal architecture is not always related to the color of a person's skin. Some patients with white skin exhibit platyrrhine features, whereas others with brown or black skin have mesorrhine-like noses (Fig. 20–4). That is why critical evaluation of nasal architecture (and covering) override classification in the selection of surgical technique.

MESORRHINE AND PLATYRRHINE RHINOPLASTY

Because of the anatomic differences that exist in platyrrhine and mesorrhine noses, the surgeon must alter his approach from one of reduction to one of augmentation. Most non-Caucasians who seek nasal plastic surgery want refinement and wish to maintain most of their ethnic and racial characteristics. It is essential that the surgeon understand what the

Text continued on page 268

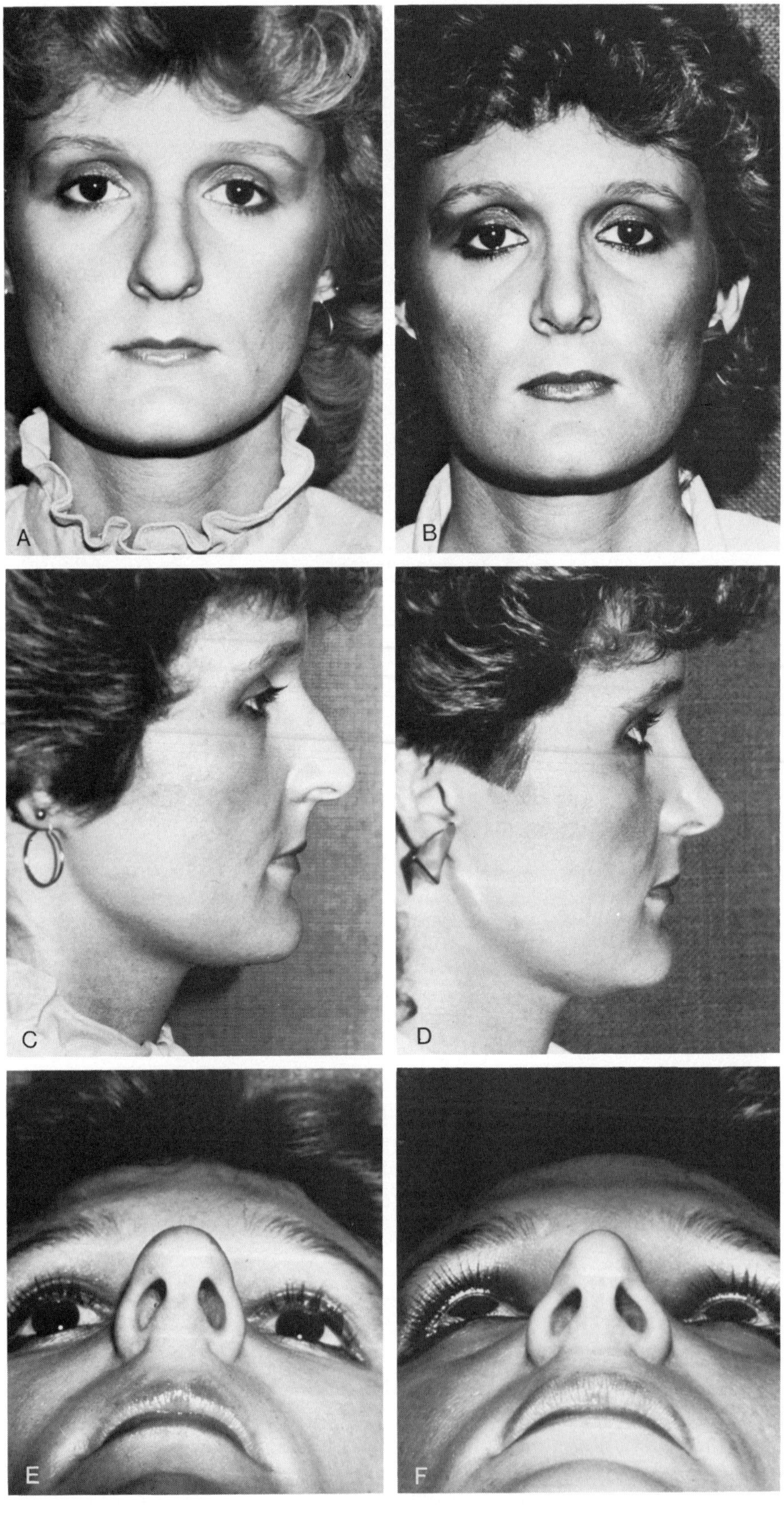

FIGURE 20–1. (*A* and *B*) Patient with a leptorrhine-type nose. (*C* and *D*) The characteristic high nasal dorsum and projecting tip was corrected. (*E* and *F*) Tip-plasty was accomplished with a double-dome procedure.

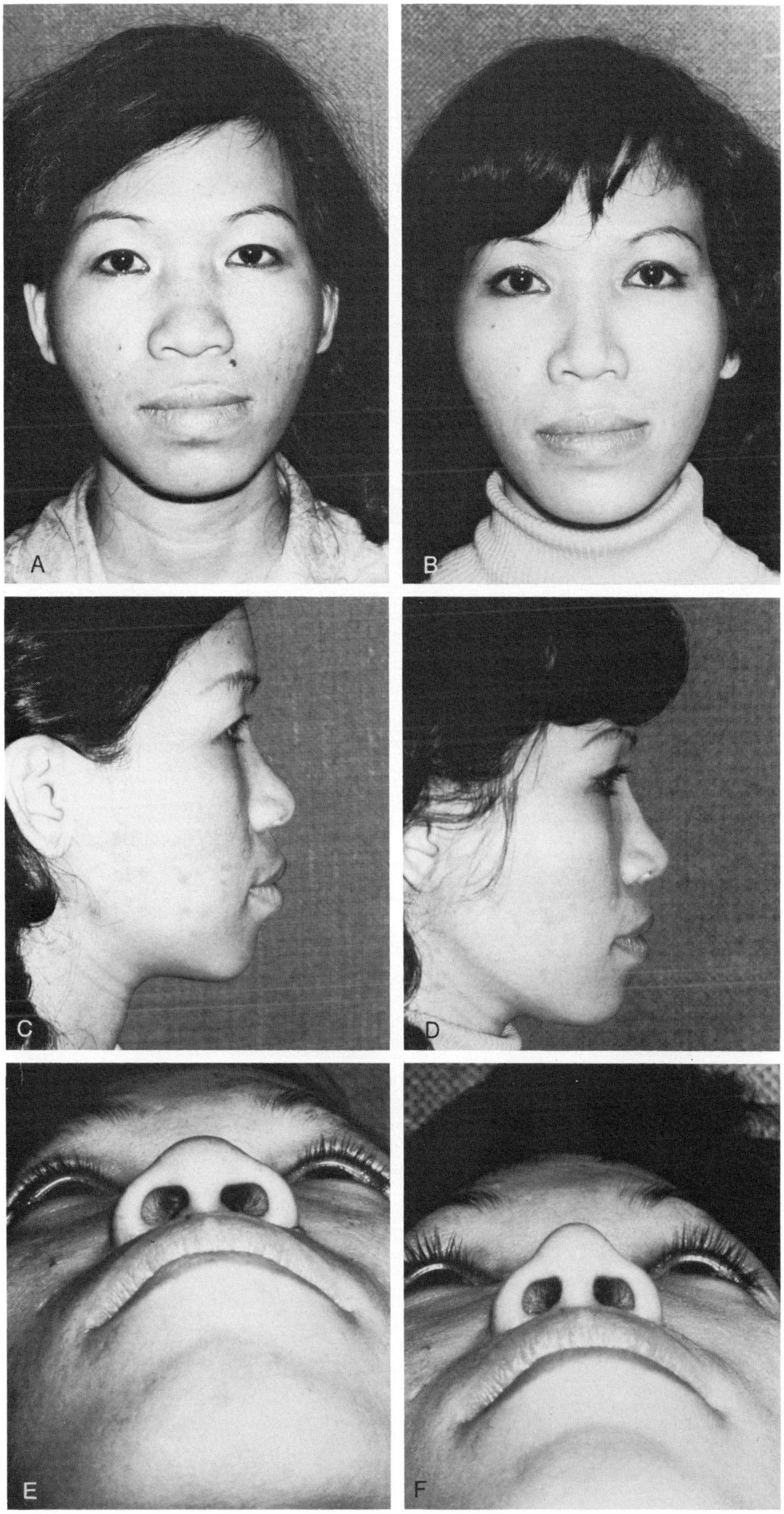

FIGURE 20–2. (*A* and *B*) An Oriental patient with the typical characteristics of a mesorrhine-type nose who desired aesthetic improvement. (*C* and *D*) The typical lack of dorsal height and columellar support require augmentation. Septal cartilage grafts were used in this case. (*E* and *F*) An I-beam tip-plasty and alar sil resections were performed.

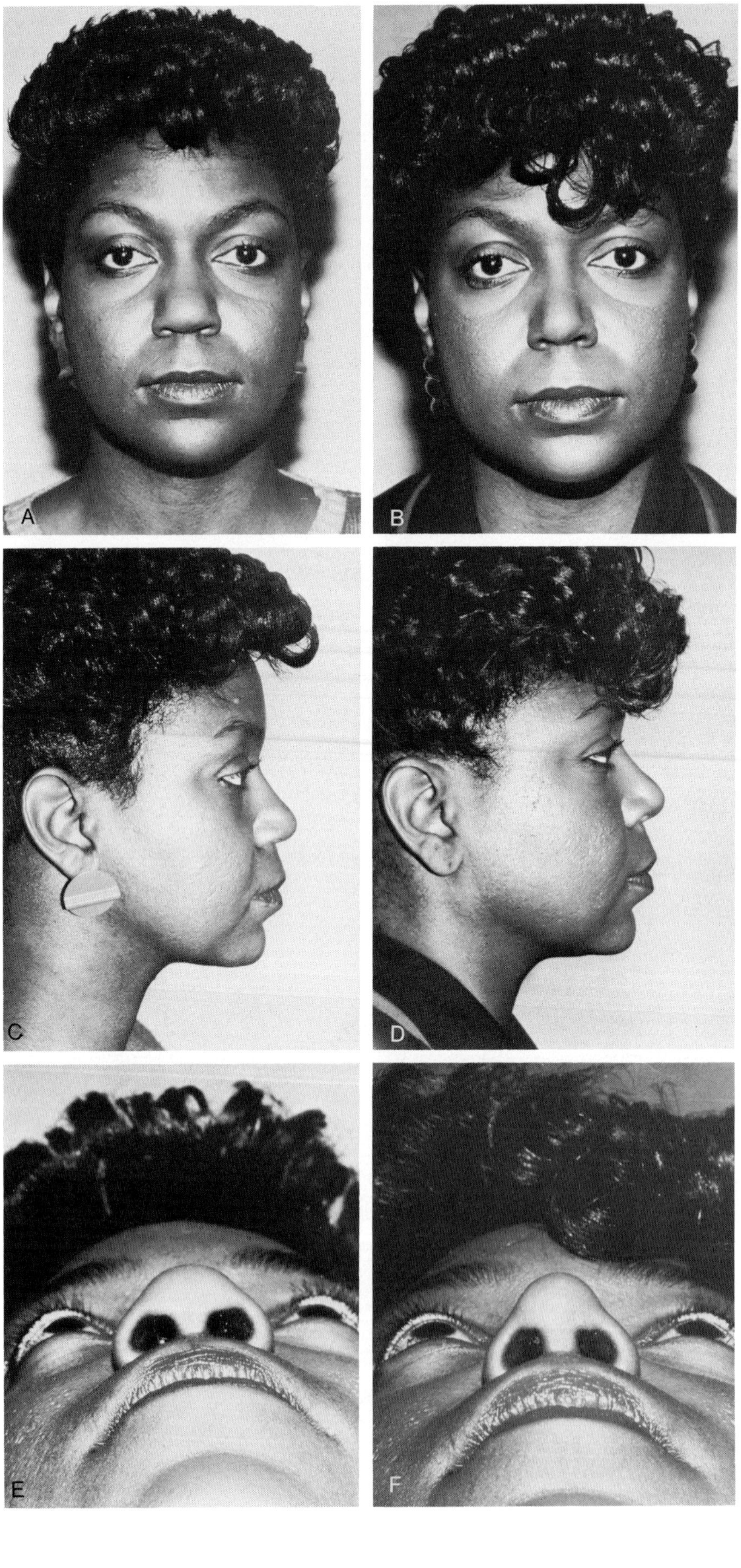

FIGURE 20–3. (*A* and *B*) The classic broad, flattened nose found in blacks requires osteotomy mobilization of the lateral walls and, oftentimes, dorsal augmentation, although in this case the dorsal height was satisfactory. (*C* and *D*) Nasolabial deficiency was augmented with septal cartilage. (*E* and *F*) Tipplasty was accomplished with vertical division and an I-beam cartilage sandwiched graft.

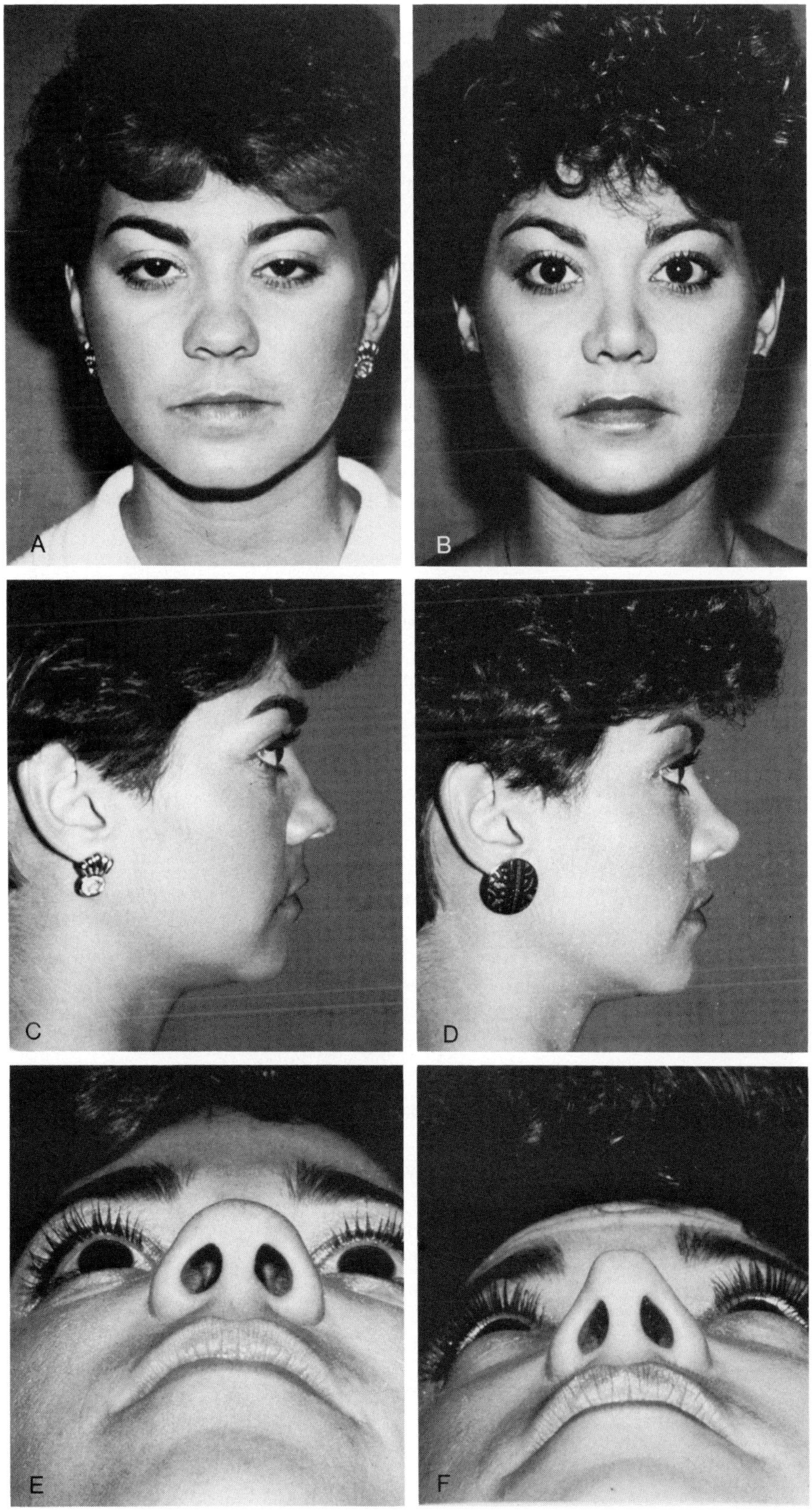

FIGURE 20–4. (*A* and *B*) Many Caucasian patients possess some of the characteristics of mesorrhine and platyrrhine noses. (*C* and *D*) In this case, dorsal augmentation was not necessary. (*E* and *F*) Because the tip cartilages were strong, correction was accomplished with vertical dome division and medial crural fixation without the use of supporting grafts.

patient hopes to achieve through plastic surgery and recognize his capabilities to achieve the mutual goals that have been established. The patient should understand the limitations of the surgery and consent with realistic expectations. The vagaries of augmentation rhinoplasty ought to be considered—and understood—by both patient and surgeon.

As previously stated, in three-dimensional artistic concepts, height and width are inseparable. Narrow noses are also well-projected noses. (Fig. 20–5).

The lack of bony and cartilaginous supporting elements accounts for the fact that most Asian and Negroid noses are broad and flat (see Figs. 20–2 and 20–3).

In the platyrrhine nose, alar cartilages usually are frail and seem to contribute little to tip support. The cartilaginous septum is also smaller and thinner, which accounts for a lower dorsum and greater columellar retraction accompanied by a more acute nasolabial angle. The nasal bones are smaller and wider and lack the height necessary to produce the necessary dorsal projection that helps most noses to appear narrow on frontal inspection. The nasal covering is thick and contains an abundance of subcutaneous tissue. The nostrils are wide, which is in part due to several factors, including insufficient tip projection, thick skin, and more lateral insertion at the nasofacial crease.

Aesthetic correction must include maneuvers that will correct or counter each of the above factors. Augmentation might require the use of grafts, implants, or a combination of both. And any of these could shift or become absorbed or infected.

The amount of projection that can be obtained with tip-plasty dictates what can and should be done to the nasal dorsum.

Platyrrhine Tip-Plasty

In most of these cases, a dome-division approach is preferred. It is possible to borrow 2 to 3 mm from the lateral crus and obtain additional height of the lobule as that portion of the lateral crus becomes part of the central I-beam complex. The most important aspect of tip-plasty in the Asian or Negroid nose is to provide a strong, central supporting strut coupled with augmentation of the premaxillary region (Fig. 20–6).

I-BEAM MEDIAL CRURAL FIXATION

The I-beam medial crural fixation with a central sandwiched tip graft is an excellent technique to use in mesorrhine and platyrrhine noses (see Ch. 14). The key element of tip projection is based on the augmented central limb of the tripod. When the medial crura are short or weak, additional support can be obtained by placing a cartilage strut graft between them. The medial crura are secured to the strut in a sandwich-like manner with two interrupted sutures of 5-0 polyglactin (Vicryl). The sandwiched graft creates a strong I-beam system. The graft ought to extend inferiorly past the columellar base and to within 3 mm of the premaxillary crest. Superiorly, the graft should extend at least to the transected ends of the medial crura, and higher when more projection is desirable (Fig. 20–7).

A straight piece of septal cartilage is preferred for the I-beam graft. The graft is fixed at at least two points with sutures until favorable fibrosis occurs.

Text continued on page 272

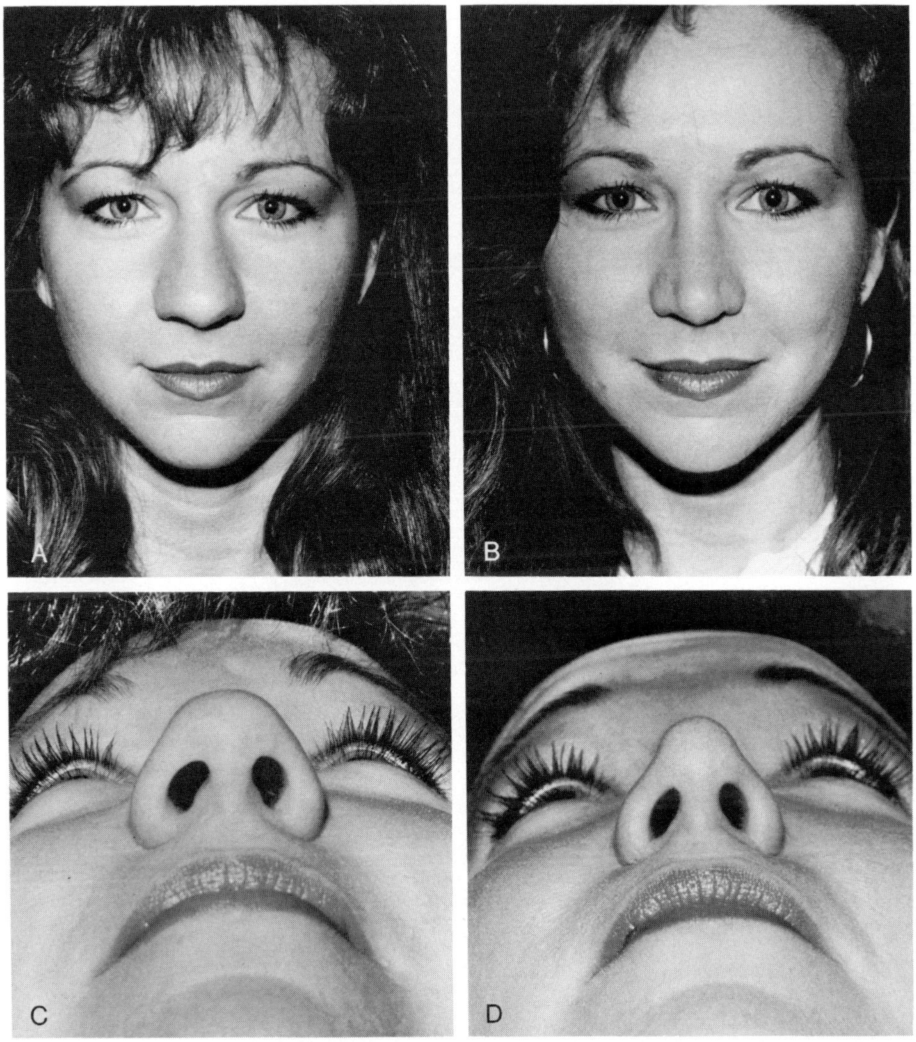

FIGURE 20–5. (*A* and *B*) In a wide nose, increasing the projection of and narrowing the lobule helps to eliminate some of the apparent width of the tip. (*C* and *D*) A large cartilaginous strut provides strength to increase tip projection. Alar sil resections narrowed the alar base.

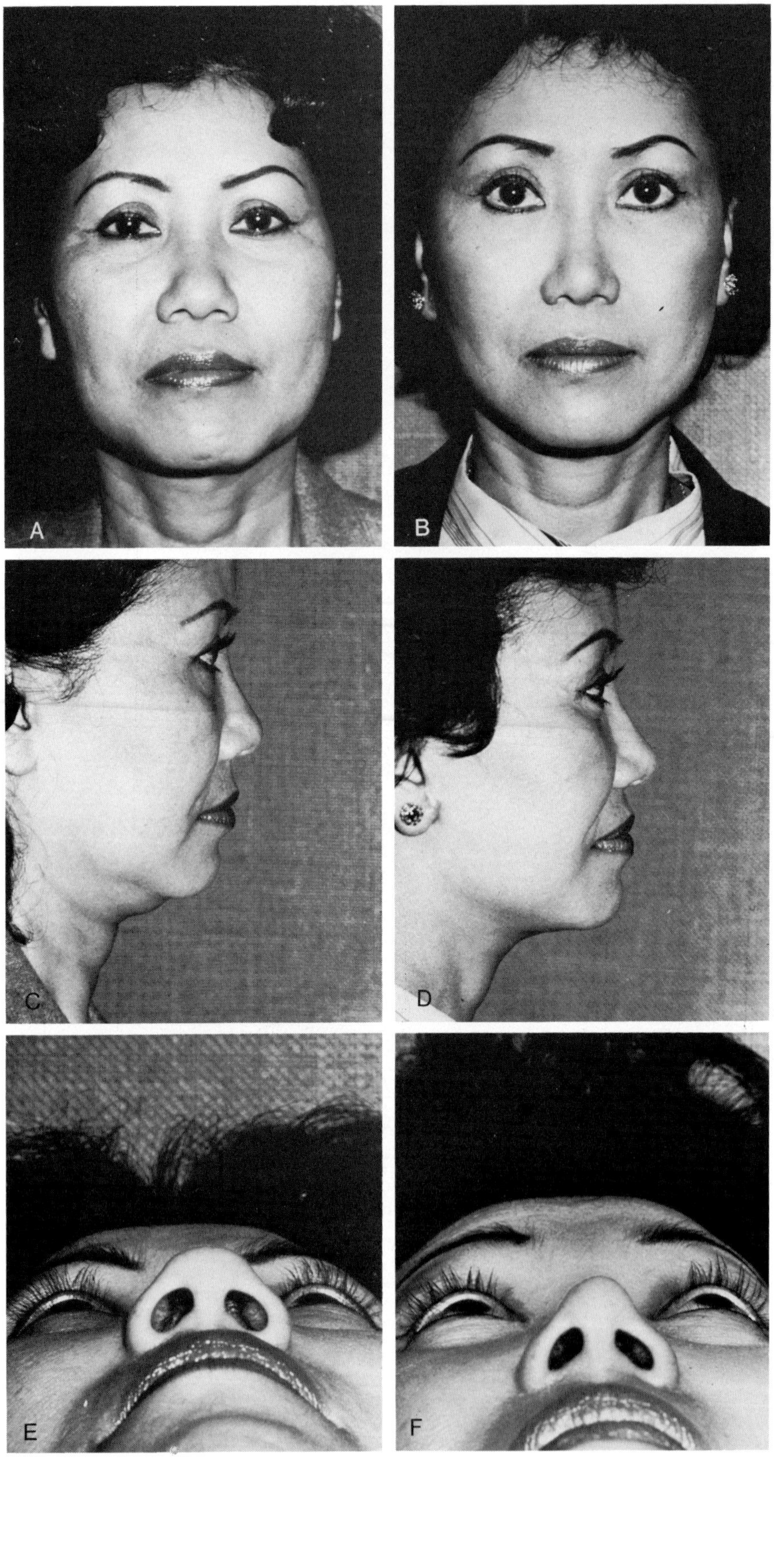

FIGURE 20–6. (*A* and *B*) Augmentation rhinoplasty commonly is indicated in the patient with mesorrhine features. (*C* and *D*) The premaxillary deficiency may be augmented with cartilage grafts. (*E* and *F*) Tipplasty required vertical dome division with I-beam sandwiched grafting.

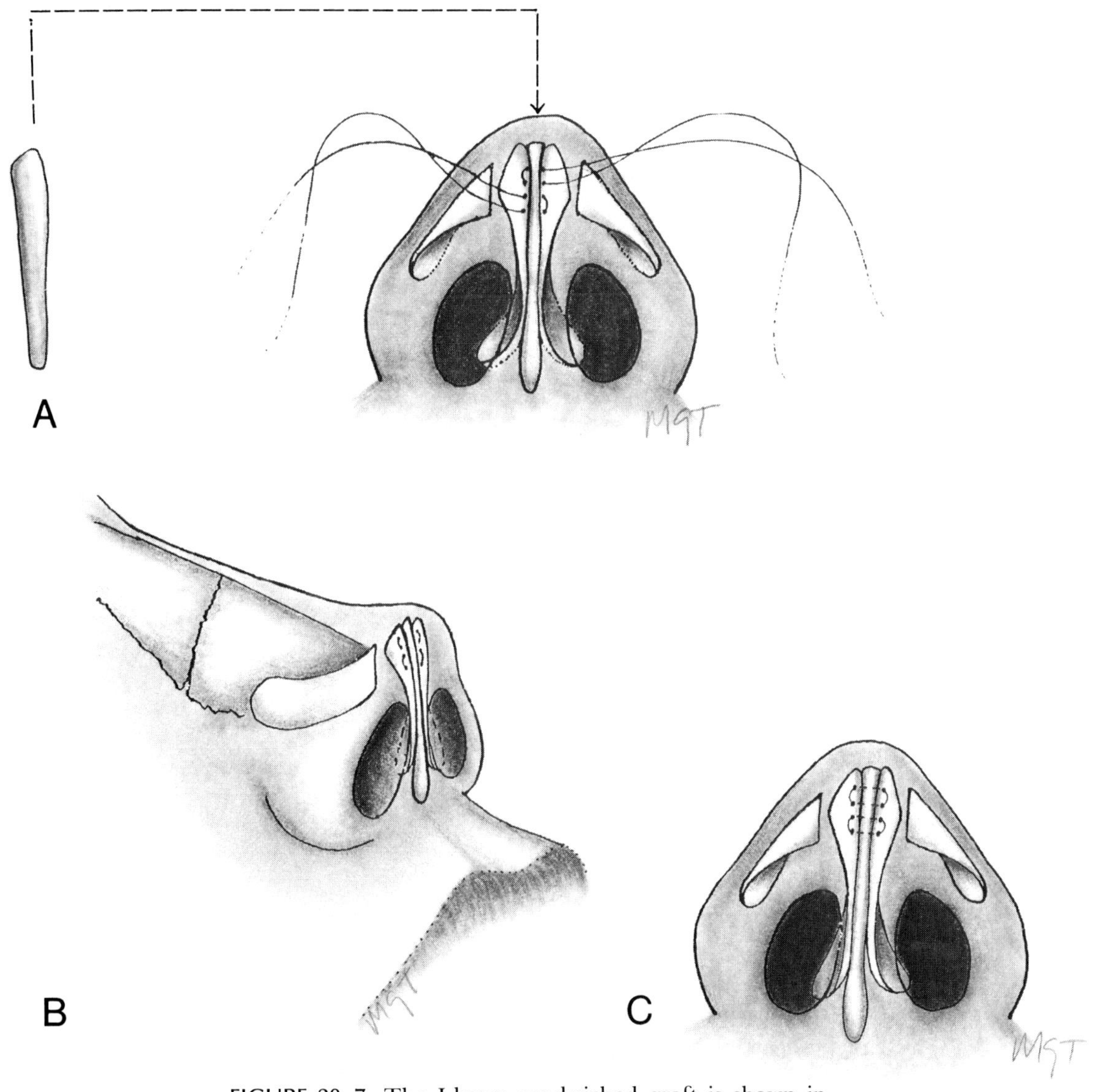

FIGURE 20–7. The I-beam sandwiched graft is shown in these drawings.

This technique is helpful not only in platyrrhine noses but also in patients with infantile-like tips, in revisional cases when large segments of alar cartilage have been previously removed, and in correcting cleft lip noses.

If additional projection is required in the patient with thick skin, the sandwiched tip graft can be extended 1 mm or more higher than the two transected ends of the medial crura.

By its nature, the I-beam sandwiched graft technique provides maximum structural support for tip projection and often straightens deformed medial crura (see Fig. 14–7*G–I*). The graft's secured position is more predictable than those of free shield grafts.

POSSIBLE SEQUELAE

Excess columellar show, alar notching, and pinched lobules are rare but potential sequelae. With experience, these problems occur less frequently.

Even if complete transection of the domes is not indicated, a sandwiched tip graft may be placed between and secured to the medial crura and/or domes to strengthen the medial tripod leg when single- or double-dome procedures are used (see Fig. 14–7).

When the alar cartilages are *strong,* a central support or sandwiched graft may not be necessary. Vertical transection of both the lower lateral cartilage and the vestibular skin at or near the dome was described by Goldman (see Figs. 14–37 and 14–38). The central support mechanism for the tip primarily depends on the two transected medial vestibulochondrial crural flaps, which are sutured to each other and to the caudal septum with two or three catgut sutures. When properly performed and when medial crural cartilages are strong, the procedure achieves projection, rotation, and lobular refinement (Fig. 20–8).

If additional narrowing and/or lobular height is desired, a 2- or 3-mm portion of the lateral crus can be "borrowed" by making the vertical division lateral to the dome (Figs. 20–9 and 20–10).

The length and strength of the medial crura often limit the amount of projection that can be obtained without adding additional support.

NARROWING THE BONY PYRAMID

Although the nasal bones are small in the mesorrhine and the platyrrhine nose, osteotomies and medial displacement provide an extra element of narrowing (Fig. 20–11).

Technique

A small incision is made perpendicular to the pyriform aperture at the anterior end of the right inferior turbinate with a No. 15 blade. The incision is carried through the mucosa and periosteum. Using a to-and-fro motion with the No. 15 blade, the periosteum on the undersurface of the frontal process of the maxilla is freed from the bones. A periosteal elevator (McCollough-Anderson) creates a subperiosteal tunnel on the medial surface of the frontal process of the maxilla and, more dorsally, the nasal bones.

Text continued on page 277

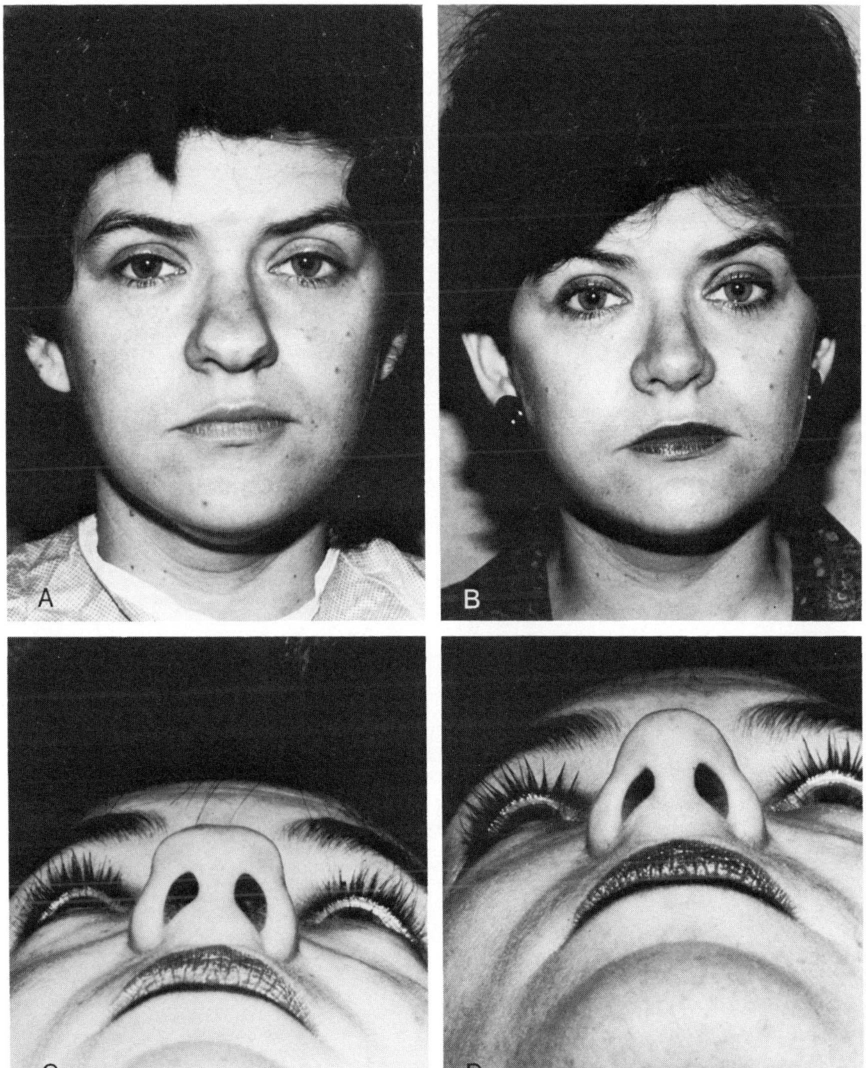

FIGURE 20–8. (*A* and *B*) A bulbous, bifid tip lends itself to a vertical dome-division (Goldman) procedure. (*C* and *D*) The bifidity is corrected when the two medial crural ends are sutured to each other.

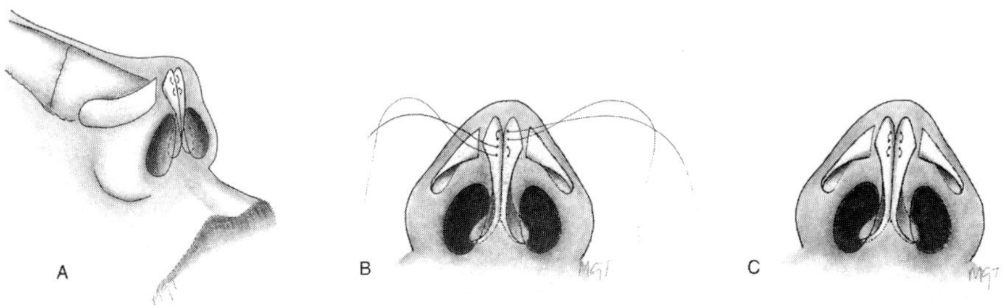

FIGURE 20–9. If the cartilages are strong, the two medial crura are sutured together with two mattress sutures of 5-0 Vicryl.

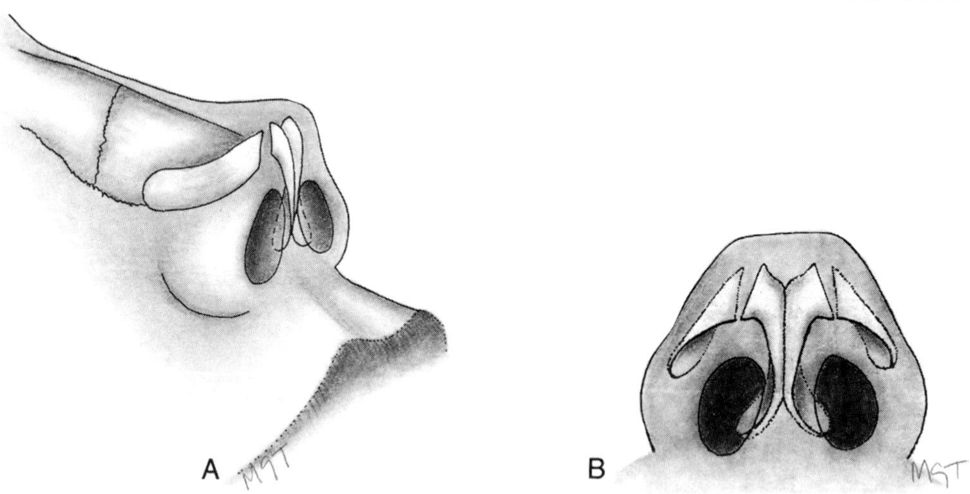

FIGURE 20–10. When it is desirable to increase the height of the lobule and obtain maximum narrowing, the lower lateral cartilage may be divided (including vestibular skin) 1 to 2 mm lateral to the dome.

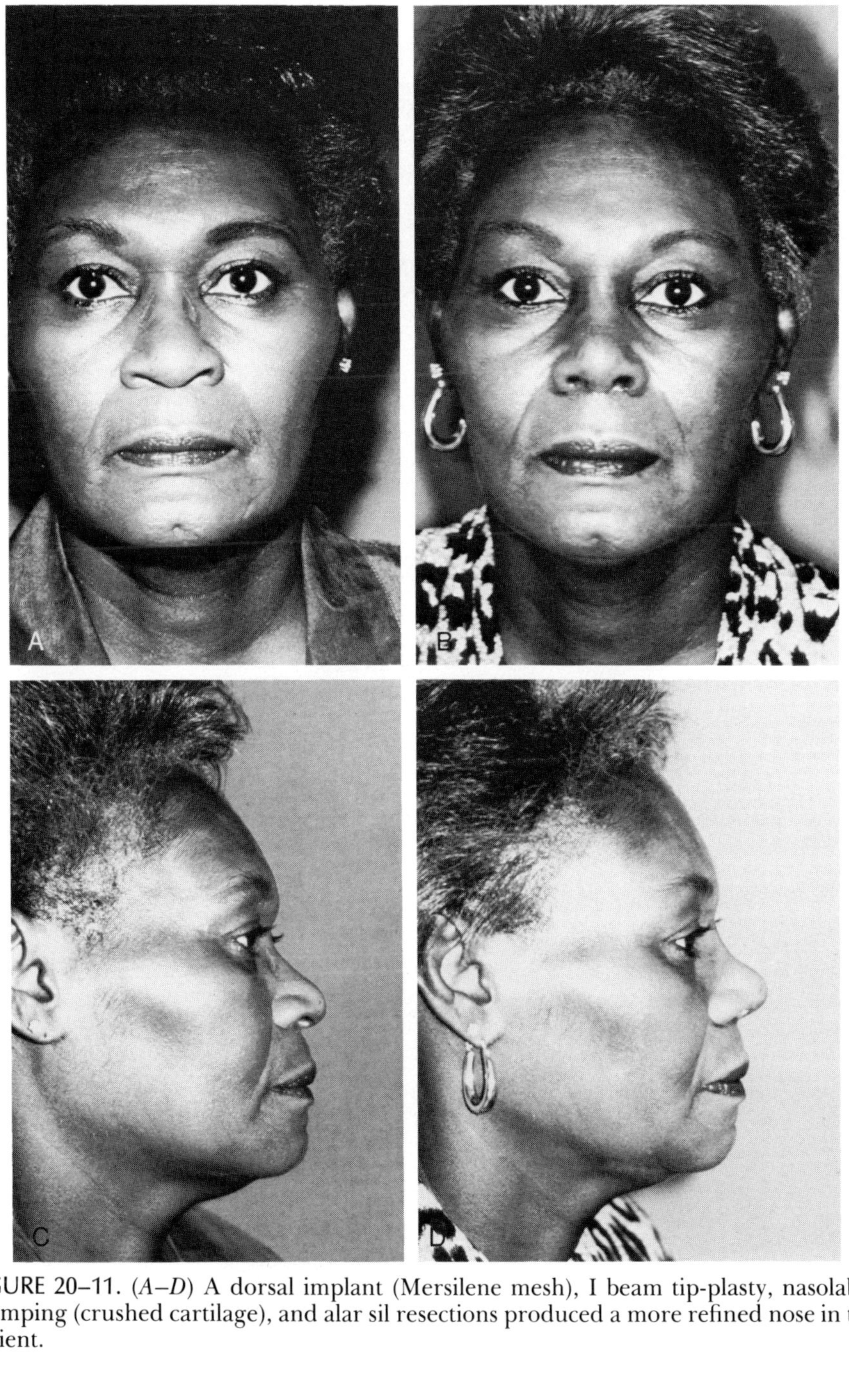

FIGURE 20–11. (*A–D*) A dorsal implant (Mersilene mesh), I beam tip-plasty, nasolabial plumping (crushed cartilage), and alar sil resections produced a more refined nose in this patient.

A guarded straight Neivert osteotome is inserted into the pocket. The assistant gently strikes the blunt end of the osteotome with a surgical mallet while the surgeon directs the cutting edge of the instrument along the desired path. The surgeon's opposite hand palpates the edge of the osteotome as the assistant's tapping drives it cephallically (Figs. 20–12 through 20–15).

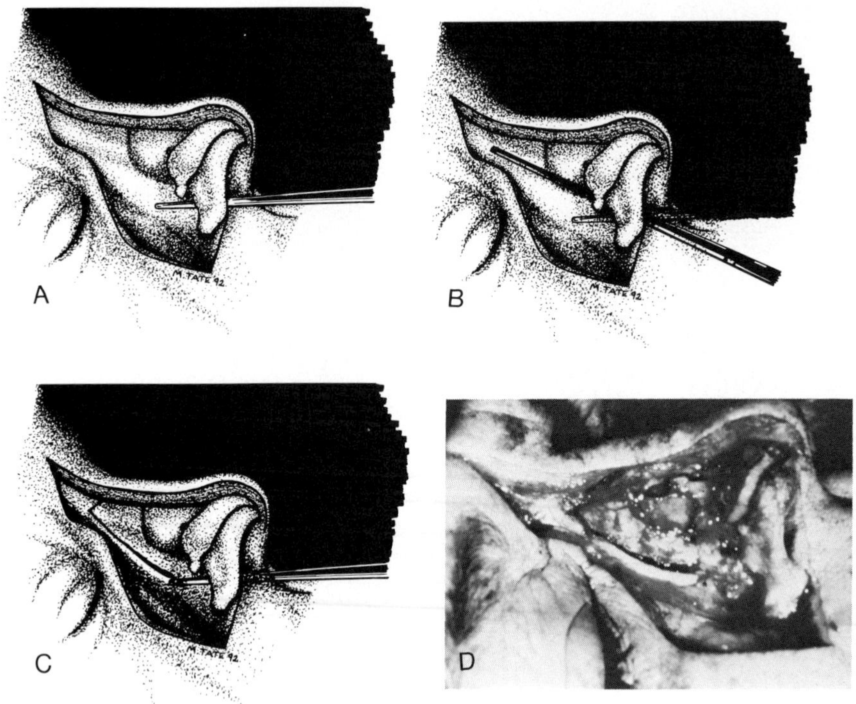

FIGURE 20–12. Complete mobilization of the lateral nasal walls is essential. (*A–C*) The desired technique of lateral osteotomy. (*D*) The desired result, i.e., complete mobilization.

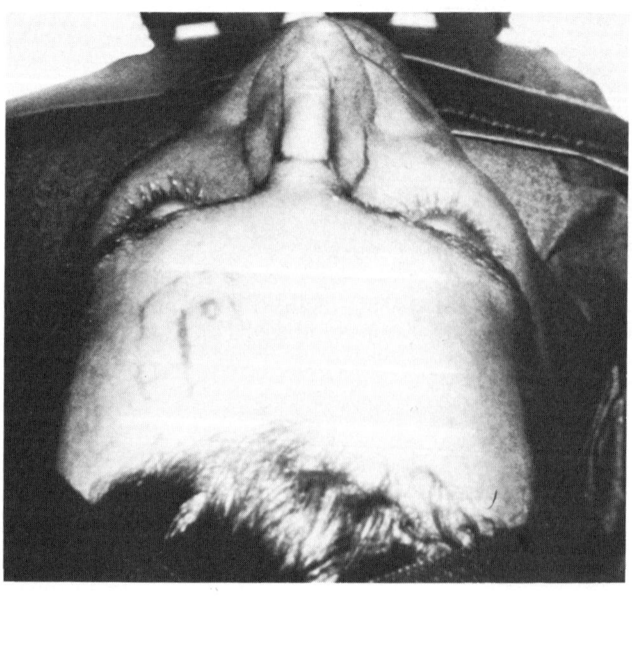

FIGURE 20–13. When both lateral walls have been mobilized, they are manipulated into their desired position.

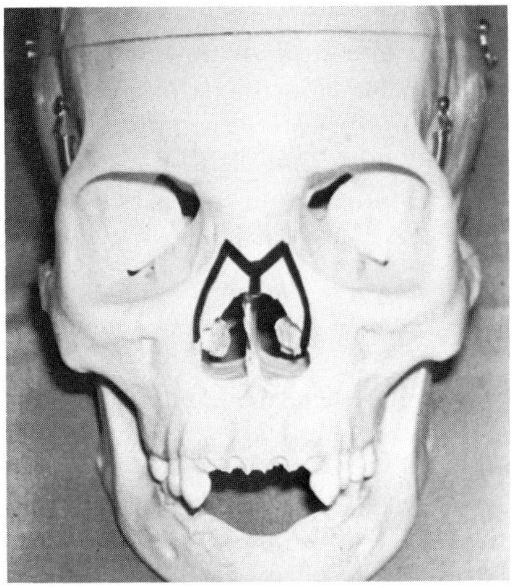

FIGURE 20–14. The desired path of osteotomy tracts in a patient who had no hump removal is shown on this human skull.

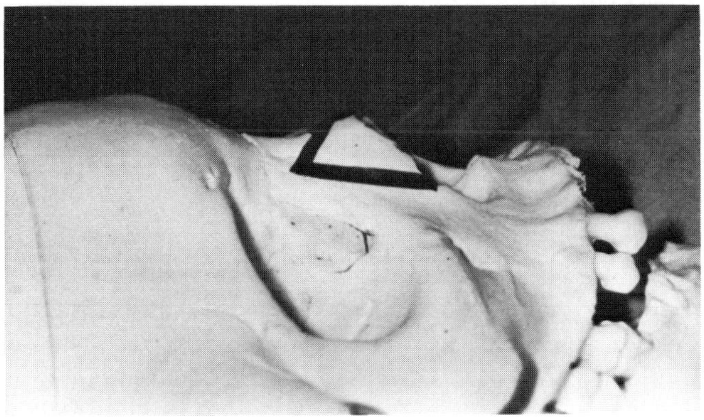

FIGURE 20–15. Lateral view of desired path of osteotomy tracts.

Provided the surgeon steers the osteotome along the path of least resistance and directs the blunt end laterally as the instrument moves along its path toward the medial canthal region, it is possible to create a desirable curved osteotomy with a straight osteotome (see Fig. 20–12).

When the guarded end of the osteotome has reached the desired position (usually designated by a change in the resonance of the tapping sound), the surgeon then manually rotates the osteotome medially to create the desired back fracture which should mobilize the lateral nasal walls (see Fig. 20–13). Manipulation with the thumb and index finger of the palpating hand should mold the mobilized bones into their desired position.

It is essential that the lateral walls be completely mobile. Incomplete mobilization may lead to postoperative widening, resulting in either an open-roof deformity or, in the case of unilateral widening, a crooked nose.

Medial osteotomies are not necessary when lateral osteotomies are performed as described.

If mobilization after lateral osteotomies is not complete, a long, flattened instrument (No. 3 Bard-Parker surgical knife handle) can be placed inside the nose against the lateral walls and a force directed laterally. In most cases, lateral displacement will complete the back fracture.

It is imperative that any initial greenstick fractures be completed; otherwise, the nasal bones tend to float laterally postoperatively, resulting in an open-roof deformity.

Excessive medially directed forces during mobilization of the lateral walls could inadvertently fracture the ethmoid bone and/or produce disarticulation at the ethmoid–quadrangular cartilage junction (rhinion). If this unfortunate event were to occur, a saddle deformity would immediately appear. Reconstruction should take place at this time. If the closed technique is being used for panoramic visibility and ease of reconstruction, the procedure should be converted to an external rhinoplasty.

DORSAL AUGMENTATION

The amount of augmentation required may dictate the material used.

Autografts

SEPTAL CARTILAGE

When sufficient septal cartilage is available, an autogenous graft is preferred. Several gently morselized stacked strips secured with an absorbable suture may suffice (Fig. 20–16).

AURICULAR CARTILAGE

Larger depressions may be augmented with auricular cartilage coupled with a strip of septal cartilage to provide a smoother dorsum (Fig. 20–17).

BONE GRAFTS

Cranial bone grafts are advocated by some surgeons, and although procurement of the grafting material is more complex, the results seem promising. Sometimes iliac bone grafts are used for dorsal augmentation, but postoperative pain and morbidity in the donor region make them less desirable.

For bone grafts to survive, it is essential that the cortical component of both the graft and the recipient site be removed so that medullary bone is in apposition to medullary bone. It is also imperative that the graft be absolutely fixed in position for 4 to 6 weeks.

Homografts

Irradiated bank cartilage is readily available and easy to sculpt. Large defects can quickly be augmented. The long-term survival of these grafts seems to be somewhat less predictable. Many surgeons advocate removing the outermost portions of the graft to help prevent twisting. Gentle morselization before insertion may help to facilitate survival.

IMPLANTATION MATERIALS

Silastic

Preformed Silastic implants are available from commercial suppliers or can be fashioned from blocks of material. Insertion and removal (if it should become necessary) are easy, but there are some drawbacks: The implant (1) is confined only by a fibrous capsule (free-floating); (2) is not attached to the skeletal framework; and (3) moves from side to side with manipulation (Fig. 20–18).

Text continued on page 282

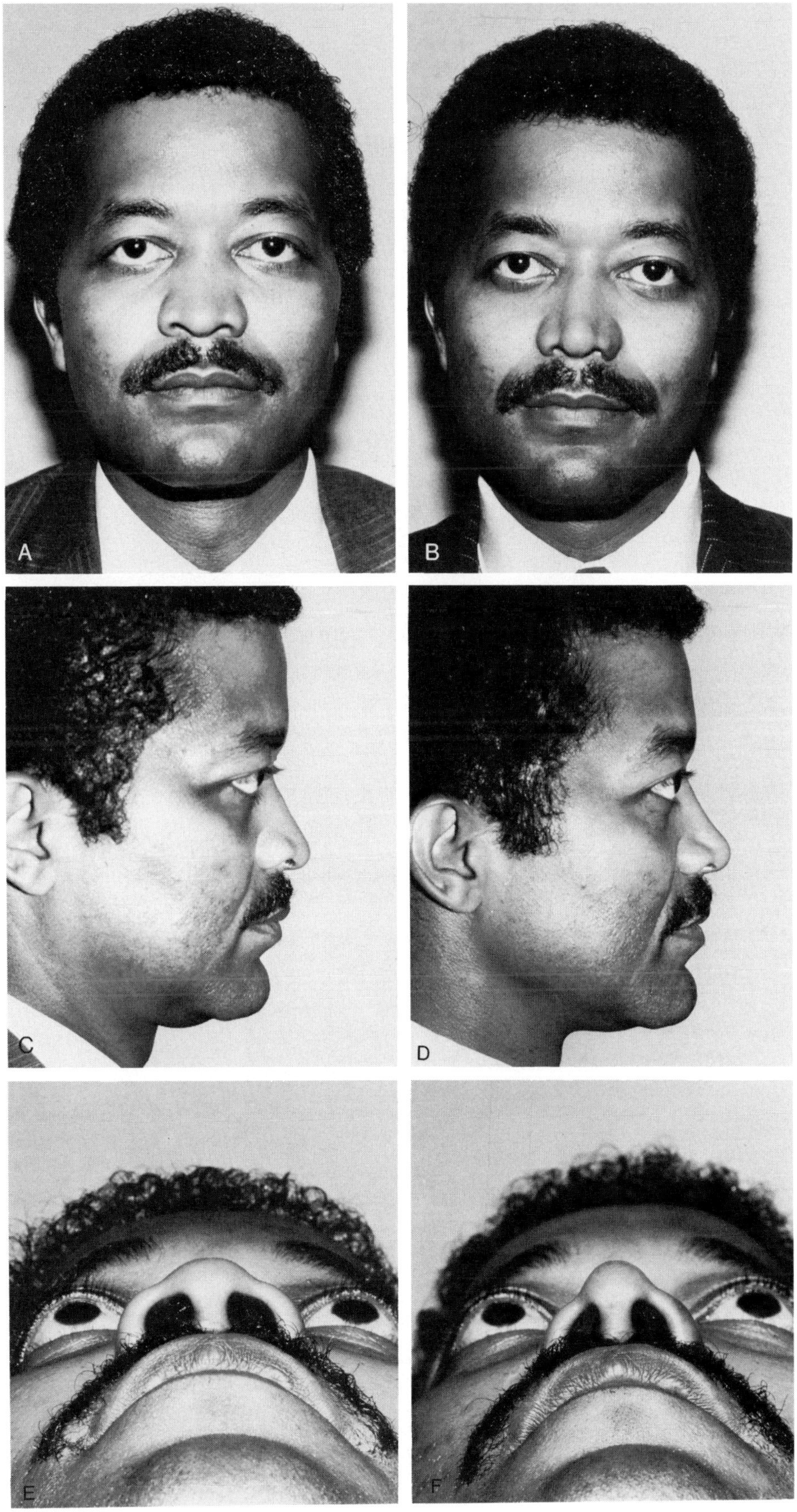

FIGURE 20–16. Platyrrhine nose augmented with stacked septal cartilage grafts to raise the height of the nasal dorsum. (*A*) Preoperative appearance of man with wide nose. (*B*) Narrowing was achieved with osteotomy and medial displacement of the lateral walls and by raising the bridge with stacked cartilage grafts. (*C*) Preoperative view of tip-lip relationship. (*D*) After tip elevation, the catrogenic saddle was corrected with grafting as described in *B*. (*E*) Note the flat lobule and wide alar. (*F*) Tip projection (I-beam technique) and alar base resections provide a more narrowed appearance.

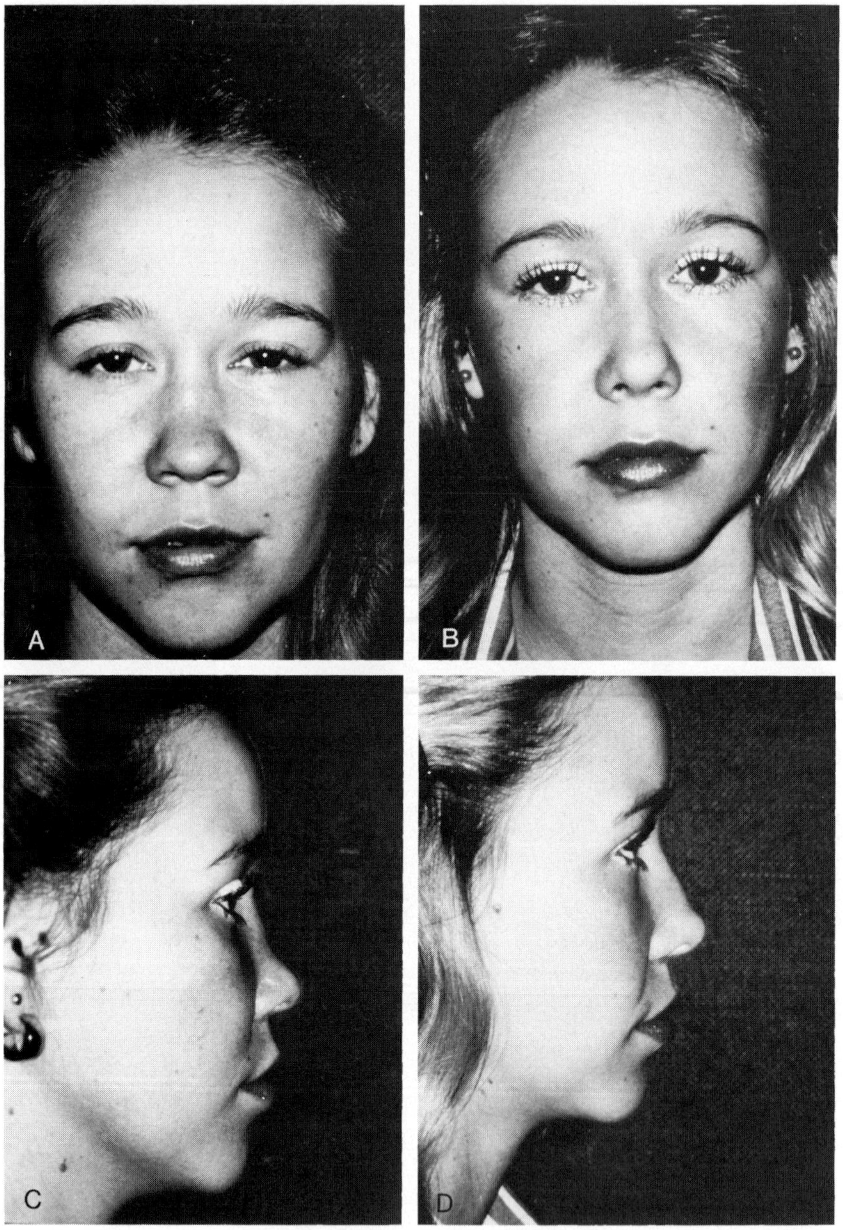

FIGURE 20–17. Patient whose saddle deformity was corrected with conchal cartilage taken from her ear. (*A*) The patient's wide nose is a result of loss of dorsal height and laterally displaced nasal walls. (*B*) Osteotomy medial positioning and dorsal augmentation improved her appearance. (*C*) Severe dorsal saddling and columella retraction are obvious. (*D*) Dorsal and premaxillary grafting were used to obtain this 12-month postoperative result.

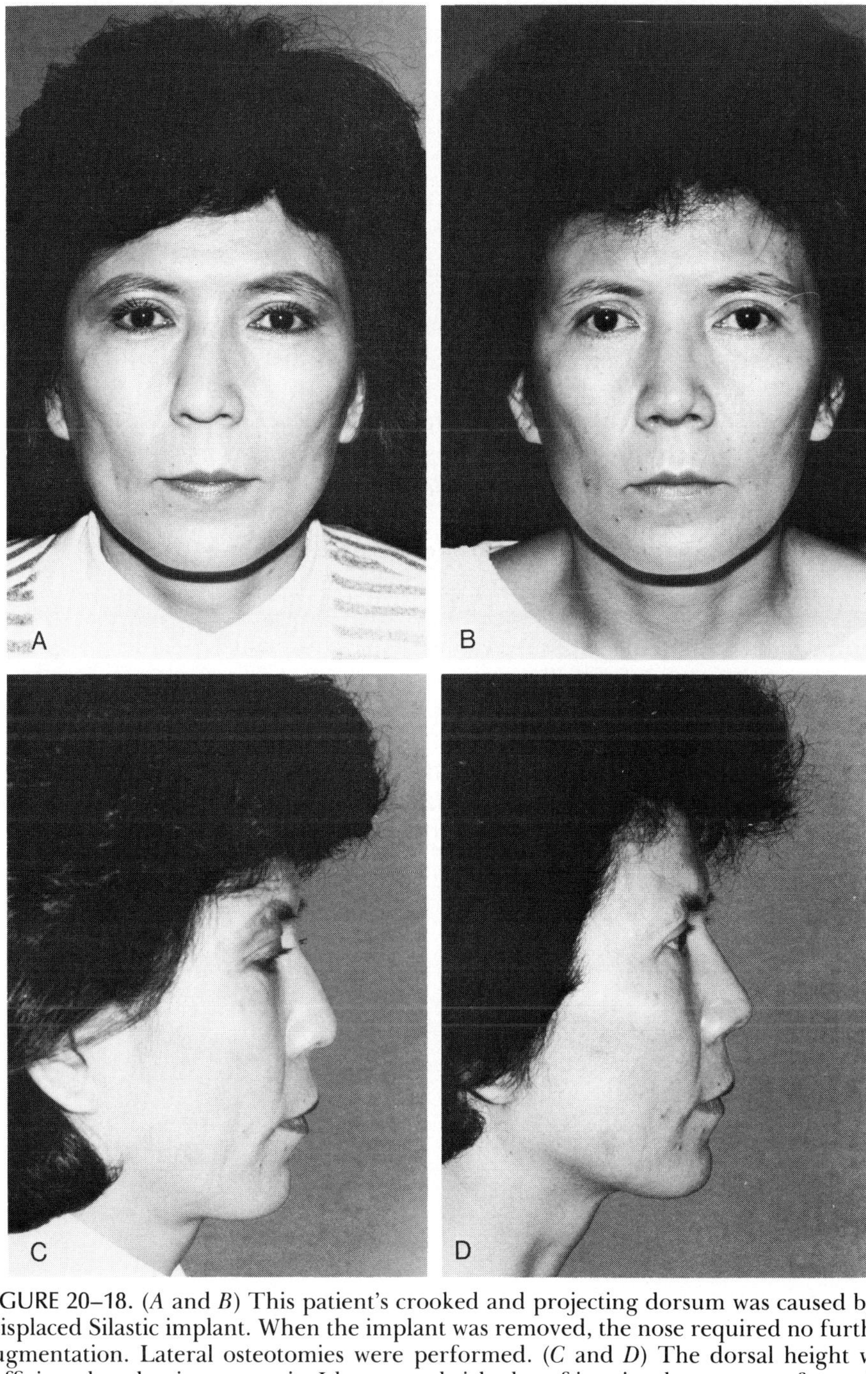

FIGURE 20–18. (*A* and *B*) This patient's crooked and projecting dorsum was caused by a misplaced Silastic implant. When the implant was removed, the nose required no further augmentation. Lateral osteotomies were performed. (*C* and *D*) The dorsal height was sufficient, but the tip was ptotic. I-beam sandwiched grafting tip-plasty was performed.

Mesh

For a number of years, rolled or folded mesh material has been used for facial augmentation. Both Beekhuis and Stucker popularized Supramid mesh implants for dorsal correction. In my experience, however, at least in the mandibular region, Supramid mesh may absorb. For that reason, I have used Mersilene mesh exclusively for chin augmentation. Mersilene has also been the material of choice when mesh is used for dorsal nasal augmentation (Figs. 20–19 and 20–20).

The sheet of mesh is cut in 3- to 4-cm-wide strips and folded to the desired thickness. To prevent unfolding, several absorbable mattress sutures are passed and tied.

INFECTION PREVENTION AND CONTROL

When a mesh implant fails, the cause usually is a postoperative infection. During preparation and insertion, the implant must not be handled with gloves that have previously come in contact with the skin or intranasal structures.

It is customary to soak the implant in an antibiotic solution (lincomycin [Lincocin] or gentamicin) before insertion. After insertion, all wounds are closed carefully and the patient is treated with prophylactic broad-spectrum antibiotics (cephalosporins).

If any portion of a mesh implant is exposed to the nasal vestibule, infection is assured, and at some point in time, removal will be necessary. Systemic antibiotic therapy and trimming any exposed portions may provide temporary improvement, but in my experience, once a mesh implant becomes infected or exposed, it ultimately will require removal.

Implant Removal. Unlike noninfected mesh implants (which are difficult to remove), an infected implant frees itself from its enveloping capsule and can be delivered with relative ease. When infection is present, antibiotic therapy is continued until seropurulent drainage subsides. When the infection has resolved, after 3 to 6 months, another implant or a graft can be inserted.

SUBTOTAL CORRECTION

If during the postoperative period smaller depressions become evident because of undercorrection or graft adsorption, additional measures can be considered.

Autografts

SEPTAL CARTILAGE

When sufficient septal cartilage is available, an autogenous graft is preferred. Several gently morselized stacked strips secured with an absorbable suture may suffice (see Figs. 20–2 and 20–6).

AURICULAR CARTILAGE

Larger depressions may be augmented with auricular cartilage coupled with a strip of septal cartilage to provide a smoother dorsum. (Fig. 20–21*A–F*).

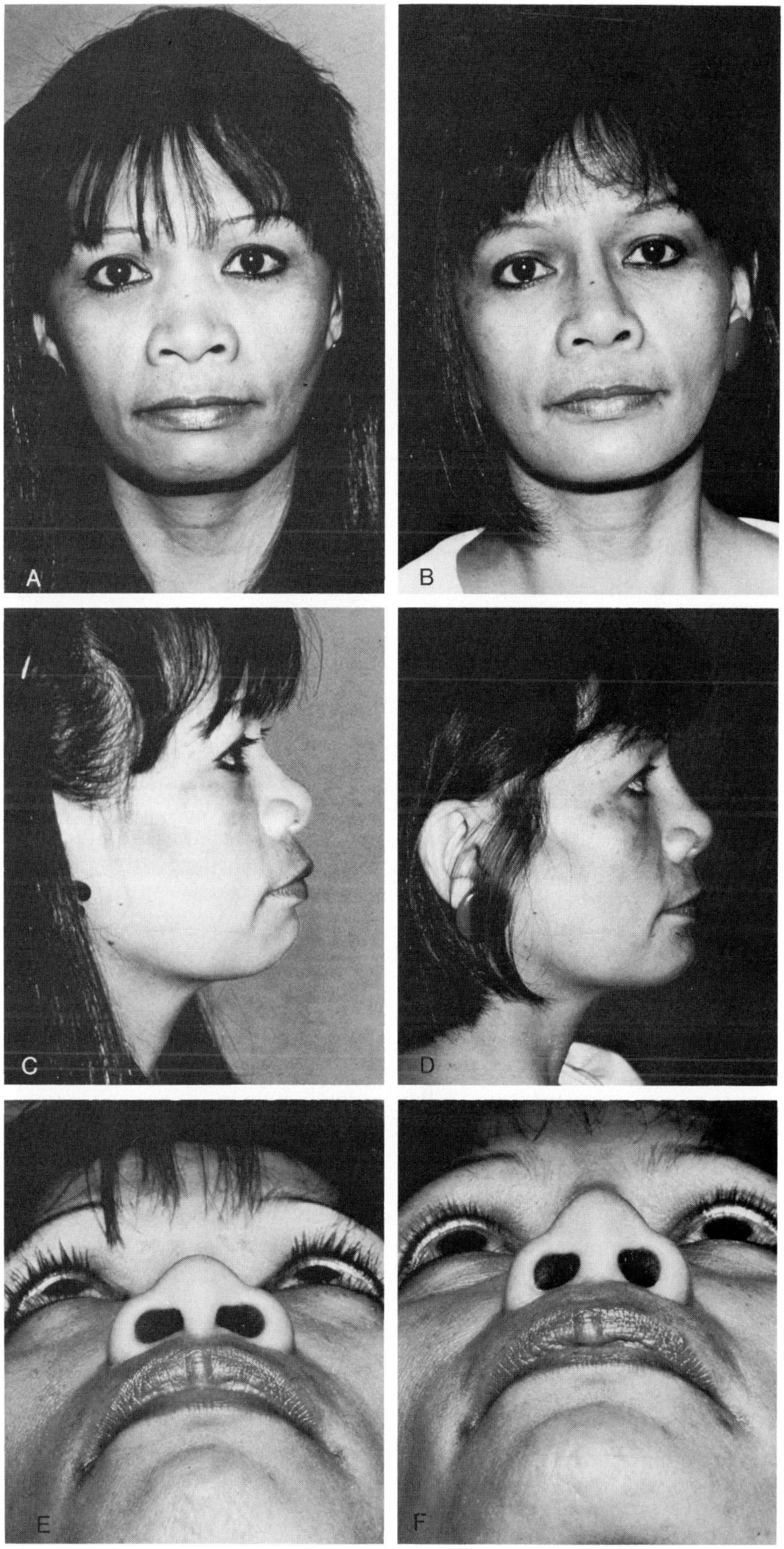

FIGURE 20–19. Dorsal augmentation may be achieved by Mersilene mesh implantation. (*A*, *C*, and *E*) Preoperative appearance of a patient with a broad, flat nose. (*B*, *D*, and *F*) The result shown was achieved with I-beam tip-plasty, a dorsal nasal Mersilene implant after lateral osteotomy with medial displacement, and alar sil resections.

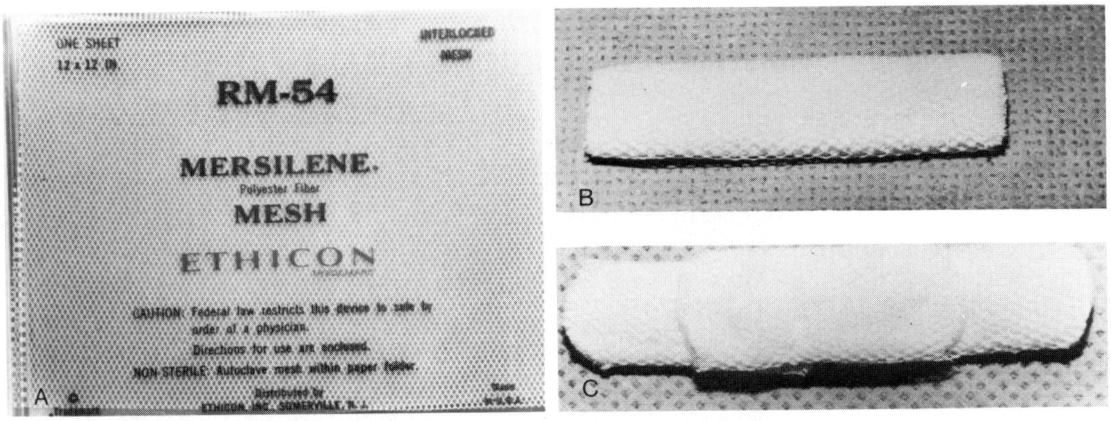

FIGURE 20–20. (*A*) A mesh implant can be fashioned from strips of Mersilene mesh. The lattice-like pattern of mesh allows for tissue ingrowth and secures the implant in the midline. (*B*) Typical implant used for chin and/or dorsal augmentation. (*C*) Compound implant fashioned from suturing two or more typical implants can be used when thicker and/or longer implants are required.

ALAR-PLASTY

If after obtaining maximum projection of the tip, additional narrowing is desired, an alar-plasty can be considered (see Fig. 19–5).

If possible, incisions and excisions should be restricted to the sil region. The incision should be planned to preserve a portion of the natural curvature of the alae.

An effective and efficient method of resecting the unwanted portion of tissue can be carried out with an Adson-Brown or Griffis-Brown forceps and a No. 11 blade (see Fig. 18–5).

Soft tissue resection should be carried into the floor of the vestibule. Only when a relatively large amount of tissue has been removed is an incision carried into the nasofacial crease. This extended maneuver can create an advancement-rotation flap and may help to prevent postoperative widening. Excision of a cresent-shaped portion of alae as described by Weir seldom is indicated. Complications can result when this type of excision is carried to the extreme.

Closure of the wound is a prerequisite to obtaining pleasing scars. Deep or buried sutures usually are not necessary. Accurate wound edge approximation and eversion can be accomplished with 5-0 plain catgut sutures. If the sutures are saturated with hydrogen peroxide six to eight times daily and kept moist with a mild ointment during the postoperative period, most of the suture material disintegrates during the first 5 to 6 days.

When tip projection is either maintained or increased, alar base resections are required less frequently. Conversely, as tip retrodisplacement occurs, the alae flare.

Keloids and/or hypertrophic scars seldom occur in the nasolabial fold. This dreaded complication, although it can be discussed with the patient, is highly unlikely, provided good plastic surgery principles are followed for wound closure.

Text continued on page 289

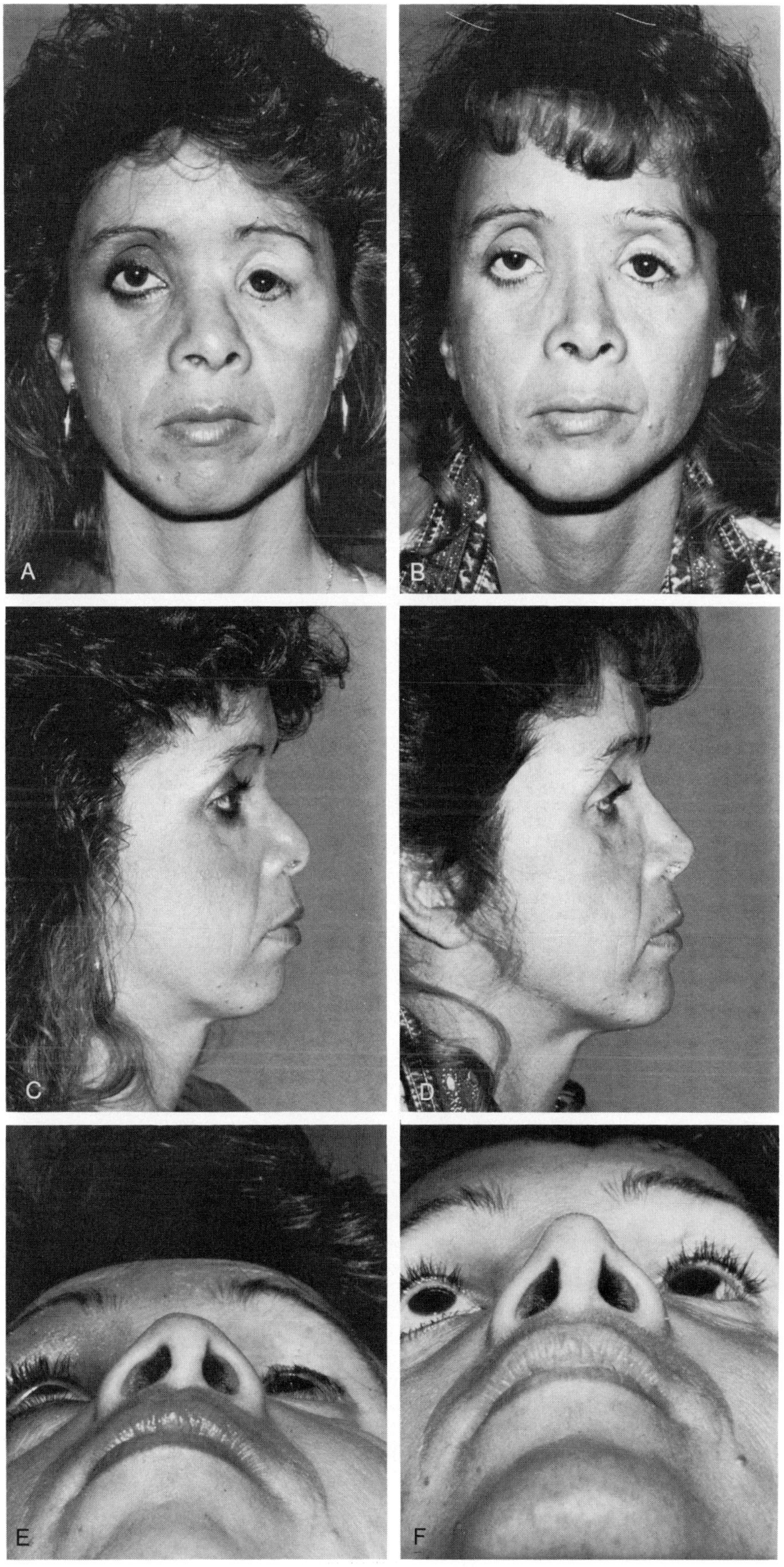

FIGURE 20–21. Autologous auricular cartilage taken from the patient's concha was used to correct deficient areas.

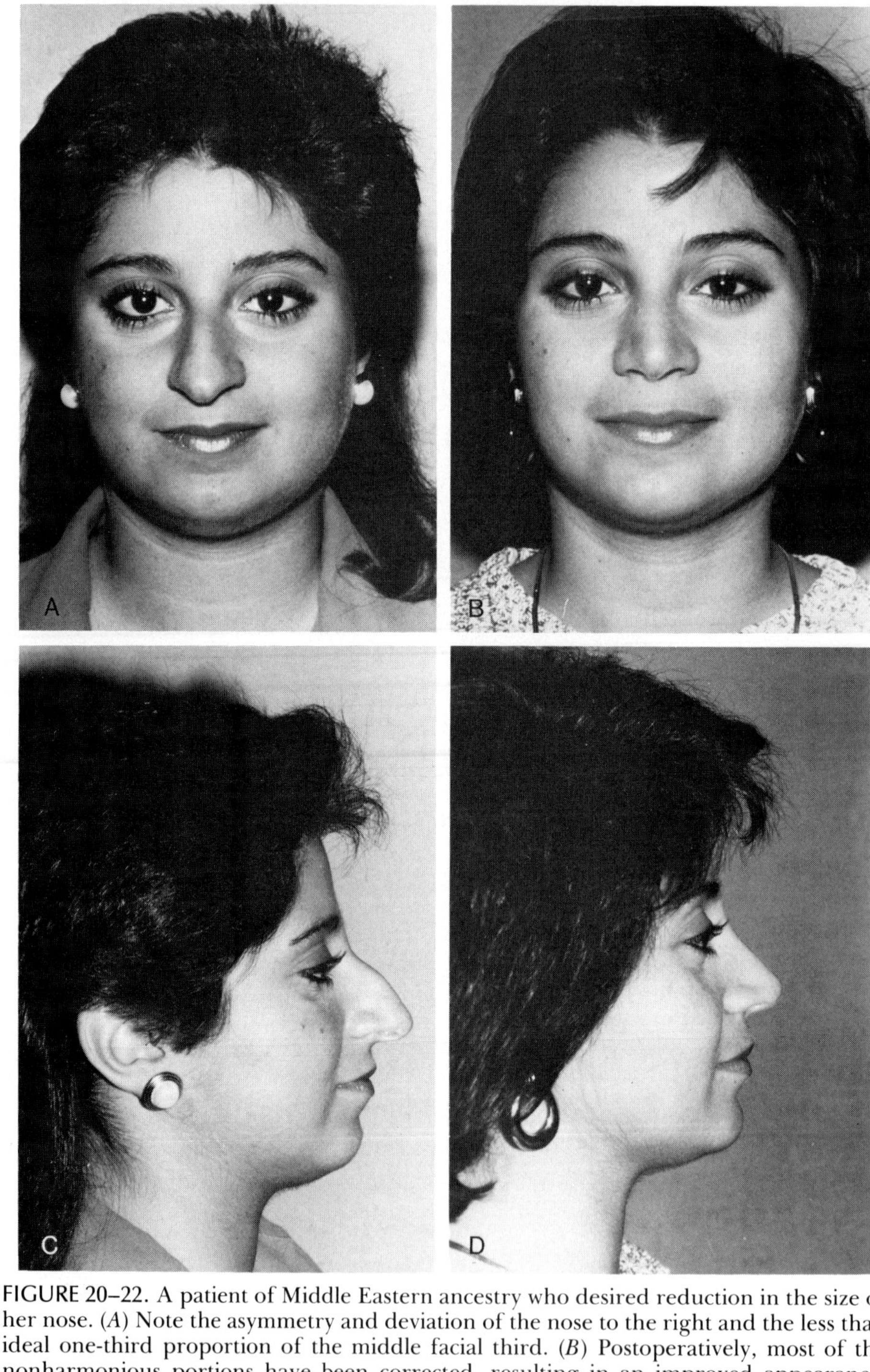

FIGURE 20–22. A patient of Middle Eastern ancestry who desired reduction in the size of her nose. (*A*) Note the asymmetry and deviation of the nose to the right and the less than ideal one-third proportion of the middle facial third. (*B*) Postoperatively, most of the nonharmonious portions have been corrected, resulting in an improved appearance. (*C*) The large dorsal hump and unaesthetic projecting tip are noted. (*D*) Tip-plasty coupled with caudal and dorsal septal reduction provide a natural, unoperated look. Only rhinoplasty was performed.

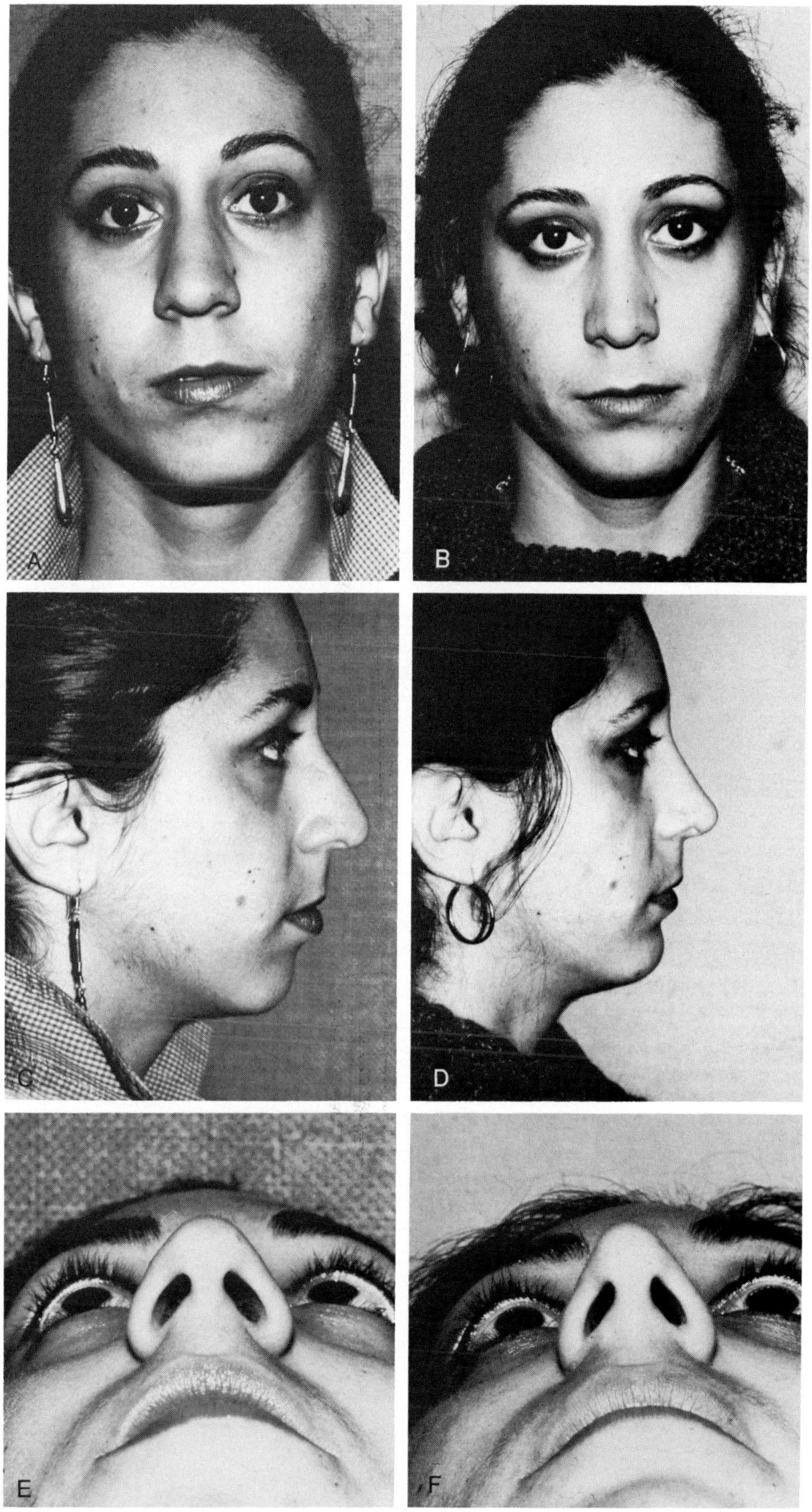

FIGURE 20–23. (*A* and *B*) Many patients desire enhancement in their facial features but want to maintain their ethnicity. (*C* and *D*) Minimal hump removal and chin augmentation were performed. (*E* and *F*) Tip-plasty was achieved with a double-dome procedure and a cartilaginous strut.

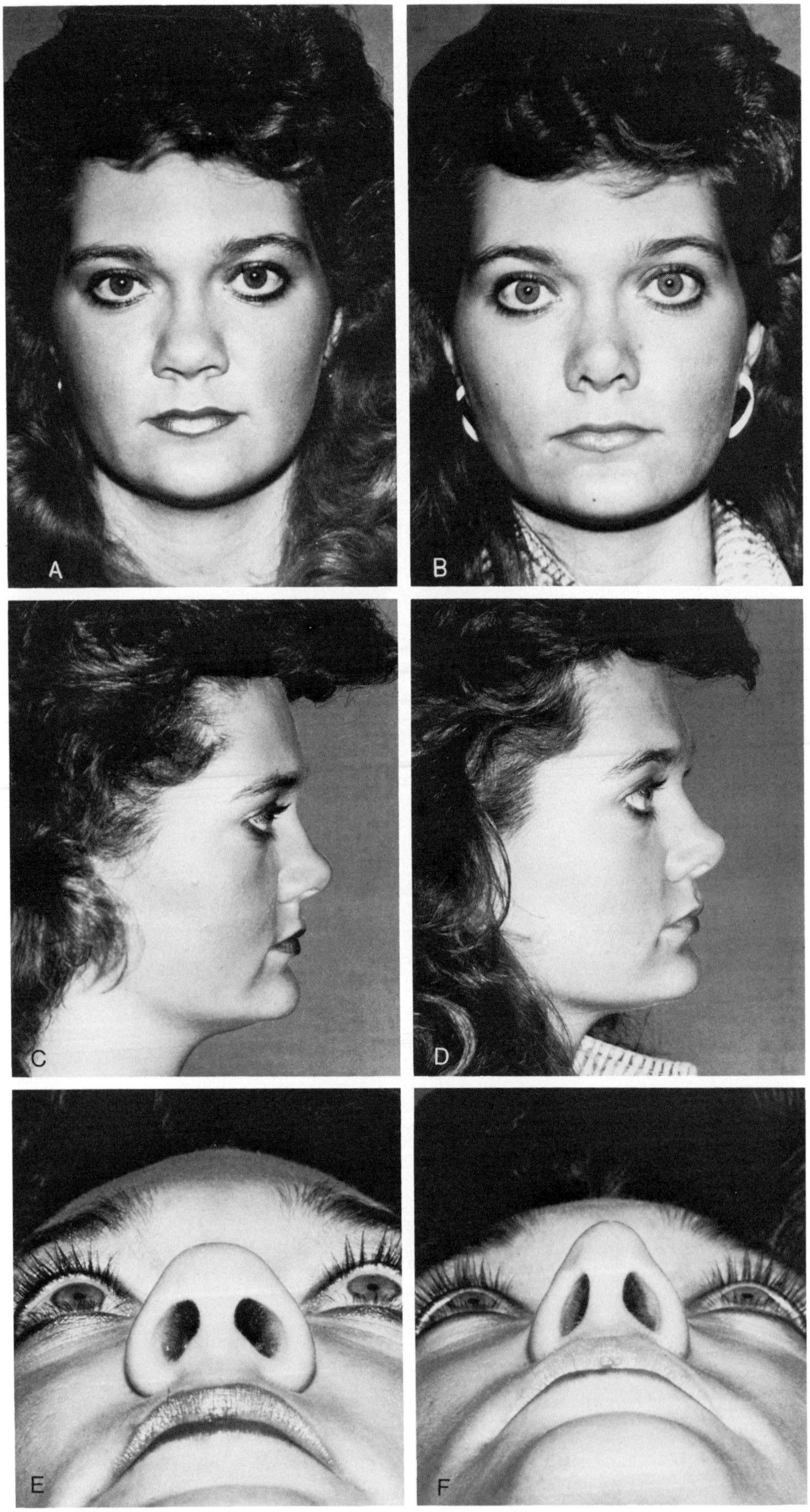

FIGURE 20–24. (*A* and *B*) A broad nose usually lacks projection in the dorsum and/or tip. The lateral walls must be narrowed and tip projection increased. (*C* and *D*) No hump removal was required. (*E* and *F*) Tip-plasty was performed with vertical dome division and medial crural fixation. No grafts were required. Alar sil resections also were performed.

ARABIC RHINOPLASTY

Many patients with characteristically large noses seek refinement without drastic change; others want to erase any stigma associated with their racial heritage. Once again, it is imperative that the surgeon and the patient have a meeting of the minds so that no misunderstanding exists as to what the patient is seeking.

In the typical patient of Arabic descent, the nasal skin is relatively thick, tip cartilages are soft and small, and the dorsal hump is large (Fig. 20–22).

Tip-plasty must incorporate techniques that provide maximum strength and support (i.e., dome division or double-dome unit with I-beam sandwiched grafts) and conservative hump removal. Figure 20–23 demonstrates what was accomplished in several patients with similar problems.

CAUCASIAN PLATYRRHINE NOSES

The anatomic variations commonly found in Asian and Negroid noses are not limited to people with black skin. These conditions often are seen in people with white skin. The principles of surgery described in this chapter apply to any person with a broad, flat nose, regardless of race or ethnicity (Fig. 20–24).

References

1. Denecke, HJ, Meyer R. Plastic Surgery of Head and Neck, Vol 1. Corrective and Reconstructive Rhinoplasty. New York, Springer-Verlag, 1967, pp 106–107.
2. Fomon, S., Bell, J. Rhinoplasty—New Concepts. Springfield, IL: Charles C Thomas, 1970, p. 16.

Suggested Readings

Baker, H. L., Kraruse, C. H. Update on the Negroid nose: An anatomic and anthropometric analysis. *In* Proceedings of the Fourth International Symposium, American Academy of Facial Plastic and Reconstructive Surgery. vol. 1. St. Louis, C. V. Mosby, 1984.

Pitanguy, I. The Negroid Nose: Plastic and Reconstructive Surgery of the Face and Neck. New York: Grune & Stratton, 1972.

Stucker, F. J. Non-Caucasian rhinoplasty. Trans Am Acad Ophthalmol Otolaryngol 82:417–422, 1976.

CHAPTER 21

Unsuccessful Rhinoplasty

Only in rare incidences is perfection achieved with nasal plastic surgery. Even so, some results are not acceptable to the patient or the surgeon or both. In 1974, between 5 and 12 per cent of rhinoplasties were reported to require revisional surgery.[1]

In some cases, the surgeon's trained eye sees imperfections that *are* acceptable to the patient. The decision to recommend additional surgery should be made with thoughtful consideration because after such surgery, the results can be worse rather than better.

On the other hand, some patients are unhappy with the outcome of their operation and seek additional surgery in an attempt to create something that the prudent surgeon knows is unobtainable or inadvisable. In such cases, additional surgery is contraindicated.

RECONSTRUCTION AND REVISIONAL SURGERY

Timing of Revision

A rule of thumb to follow is that a secondary procedure should not be attempted until at least 6 months after the primary operation (Fig. 21–1).

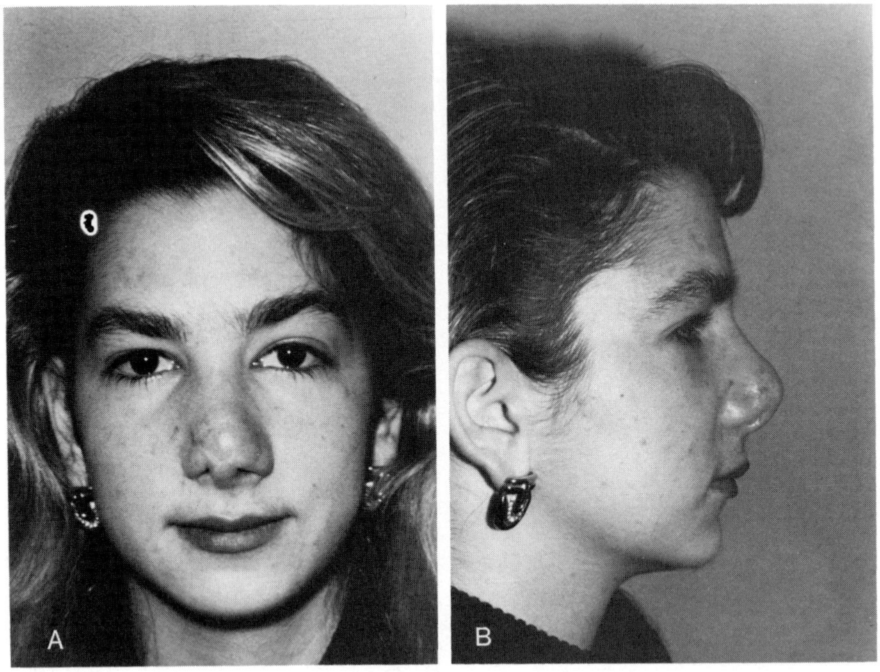

FIGURE 21–1. (*A* and *B*) This patient had undergone several nasal plastic operations within a few months of one another.

If the surgeon who will perform the revision also performed the first procedure, 6 to 9 months may be sufficient. If someone else performed the first operation, it is advisable to wait until virtually all post-operative edema has subsided so that even seemingly minor sequelae will become more evident.

To operate too early and too frequently might result in a downhill spiral of events that make the ultimate revision more difficult or impossible (Fig. 21–2).

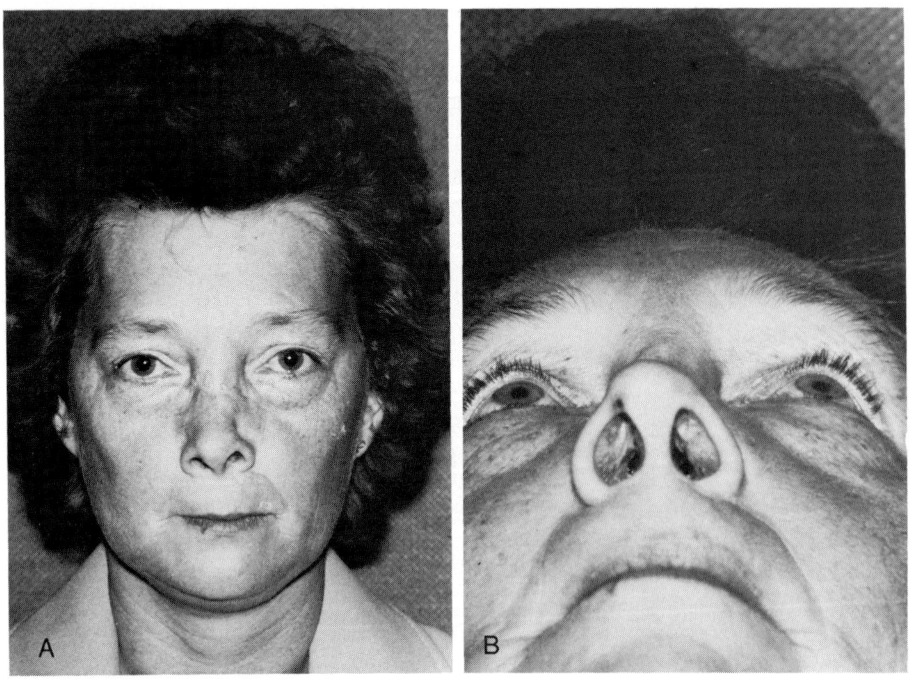

FIGURE 21–2. (*A* and *B*) This patient had undergone nine nasal procedures before she came to our clinic. External scarring, tissue deficiency, and nasal airway stenosis are evident.

What Went Wrong?

Iatrogenic nasal deformities not only cause the patient displeasure but also are damaging to the practice of nasal surgery as a whole. It has been proposed that every satisfied patient results in 5 other candidates having rhinoplasty, whereas each dissatisfied patient may keep 20 from consenting to surgery.

When the surgeon agrees that the result is unacceptable, he must first ask himself, "What went wrong?" and then, provided he knows the answer, determine if the deformity is one he is capable of correcting. If he believes that the patient's interests would best be served by referral to a colleague, he should take such action. If the surgeon decides to operate himself, the following fundamentals ought to be considered.

OMISSIONS AND COMMISSIONS

Unfavorable results usually are secondary to either errors of *omission* or errors of *commission.* The imponderables of healing, such as infection, scar formation, absorption, and/or rejection of grafts, are, for the most part, beyond the surgeon's control. Table 21–1 outlines some of the pitfalls and sequelae associated with misguided decisions at surgery.

Nasal deformities can further be categorized as those that result from undercorrection, those that result from overcorrection, and those that cannot be corrected with conventional rhinoplasty techniques.

1. The undercorrected nose simply requires completion of the operation (Fig. 21–3).

2. The overcorrected nose becomes a reconstructive operation (Figs. 21–4 and 21–5). Scar contracture must be freed by adequate undermining, and the nasal skeletal framework must be re-created (Figs. 21–6 and 21–7). *Text continued on page 297*

TABLE 21–1. PITFALLS AND SEQUELAE ASSOCIATED WITH REVISIONAL RHINOPLASTY

Pitfalls	Sequelae
a. Excessive removal of nasal lining	a. Scarring, stenosis, and retraction of the area
b. Nasal septum	b. Nasal septum
1. Improperly performed submucous resection	1. Persistent nasal obstruction or external deviation of the nose
2. Failure to lower cartilaginous dorsum	2. Cartilaginous hump
3. Improper shortening	3. Retraction or hanging columella, excessive nostril exposure
c. Upper lateral cartilages	c. Upper lateral cartilages
1. Detachment from nasal bone	1. Depression of lateral nasal wall
2. Excessive removal	2. Middle third saddle
3. Inadequate trimming	3. Middle third hump
d. Nasal bones	d. Nasal bones
1. Inadequate hump removal	1. Persistent bony hump
2. Excessive hump removal	2. Saddle deformity
3. Unequal hump removal	3. Asymmetry of the dorsum
4. Poorly placed lateral osteotomies	4. Asymmetry of bony framework or step deformity
5. Incomplete infracture laterally	5. Postoperative widening of bony dorsum
e. Nasal tip	e. Nasal tip
1. Improper trimming of the alar cartilages	1. Asymmetry of the tip—boxed tip
2. Unequal excision of alar cartilage	2. Asymmetry of the tip
3. Excessive resection of alar domes	3. Pinched tip
f. Nares	f. Nares
1. Failure to perform alar resection	1. Flaring nostrils
2. Unequal alar resections	2. Asymmetry of nares
g. Failure to use columella strut	g. Poor projection of tip or ptosis of tip
h. Failure to recognize temporary distortion from injection of local anesthetic	h. Poor projection of tip with pseudohump
i. Failure to remove debris	i. Osteogenic proliferation or foreign body granuloma

From Kerth, J. D., Bytell, D. E. Revision in unsuccessful rhinoplasty. Otolaryngol Clin North Am (1)7:67, 1974.

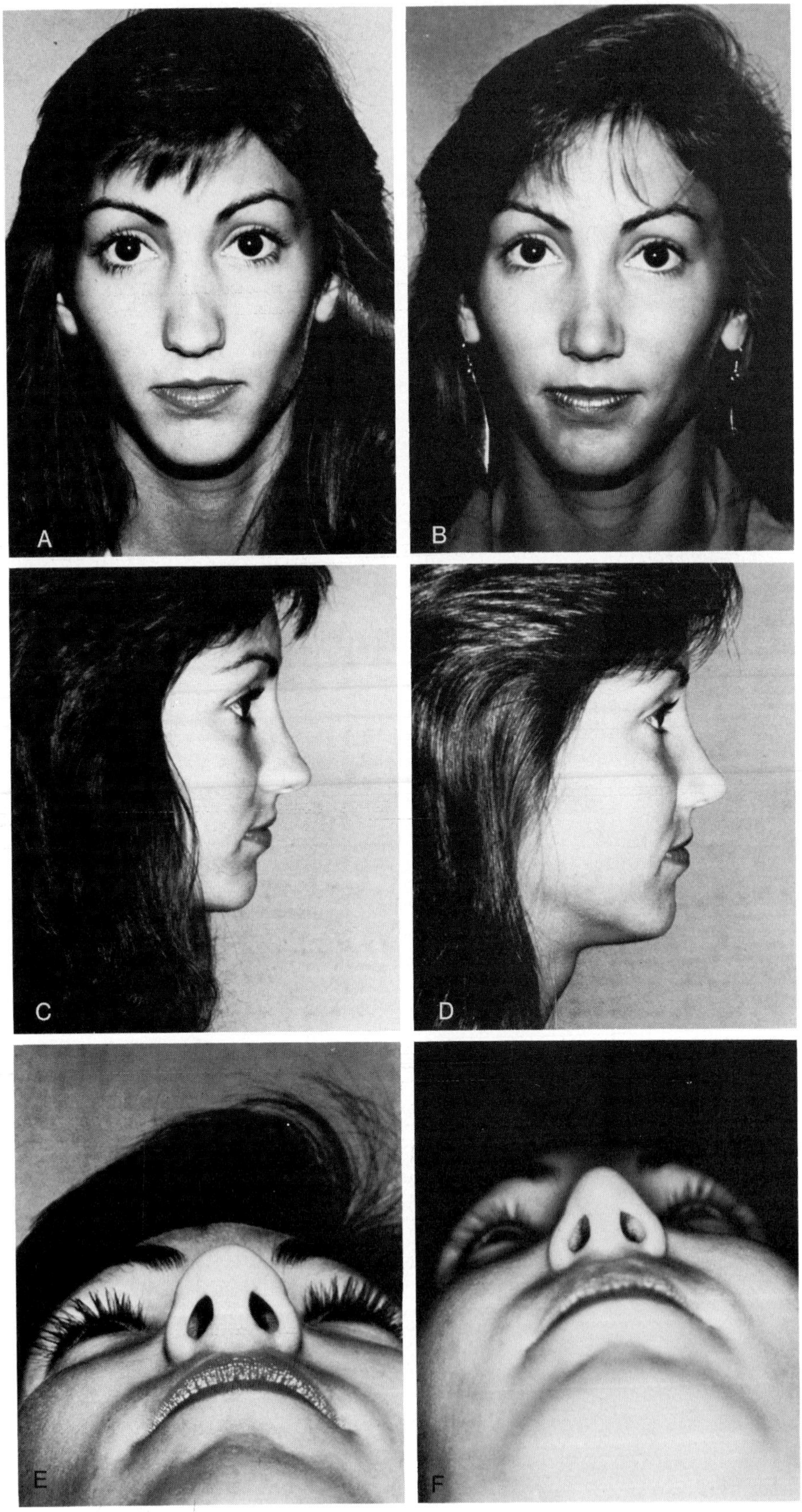

FIGURE 21–3. (*A*) An underlying septal deviation resulted in asymmetry and an open-roof deformity in this patient. (*B*) Septoplasty, osteotomies, and dorsal augmentation with cartilaginous grafts from the septum and a double-dome unit were required. (*C*) Prerevision irregularity of the cartilaginous dorsum is noted. (*D*) A No. 15 blade was used to remove the offending cartilage. (*E*) Preoperative asymmetry of the lobule can be seen. (*F*) Symmetry and refinement occurred after a double-dome unit tip-plasty.

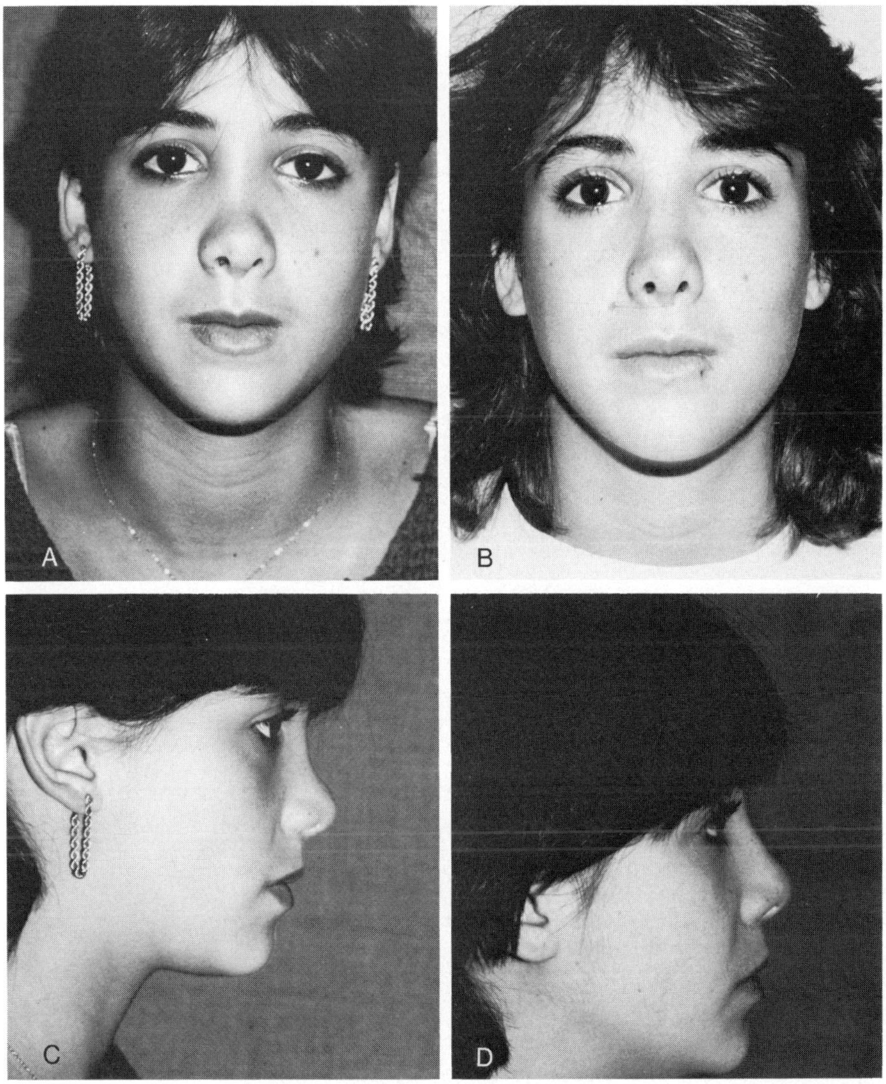

FIGURE 21–4. (*A* and *C*) This patient had undergone a rhinoplasty that resulted in saddling of the dorsum. Note the loss of nasal definition because of the lack of dorsal bridge. Correction was carried out with a Mersilene mesh implant. (*B* and *D*) Augmentation of the dorsum helped to reestablish the upper and middle third architecture.

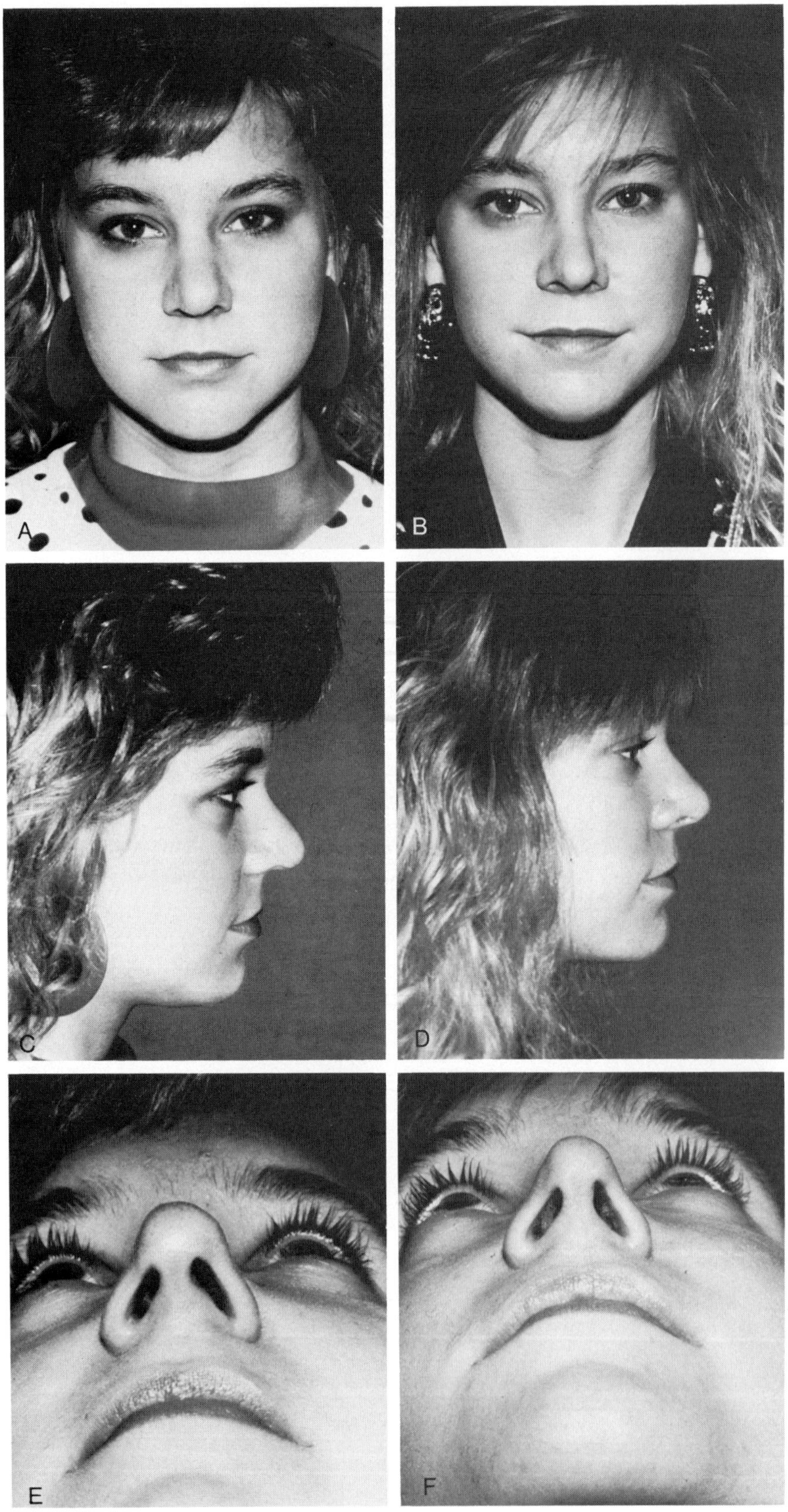

FIGURE 21–5. When it is necessary to reconstruct the tip with cartilaginous grafts, external rhinoplasty conversion provides a panoramic exposure so that grafts can be accurately secured into position. (*A, C,* and *E*) Prerevisional deformities are detectable. (*B, D,* and *F*) The right lateral crus was missing. Septal cartilage was used for reconstruction. The dorsum and tip projection was adjusted accordingly. Portions of the remaining left alar cartilage were refashioned to provide symmetry.

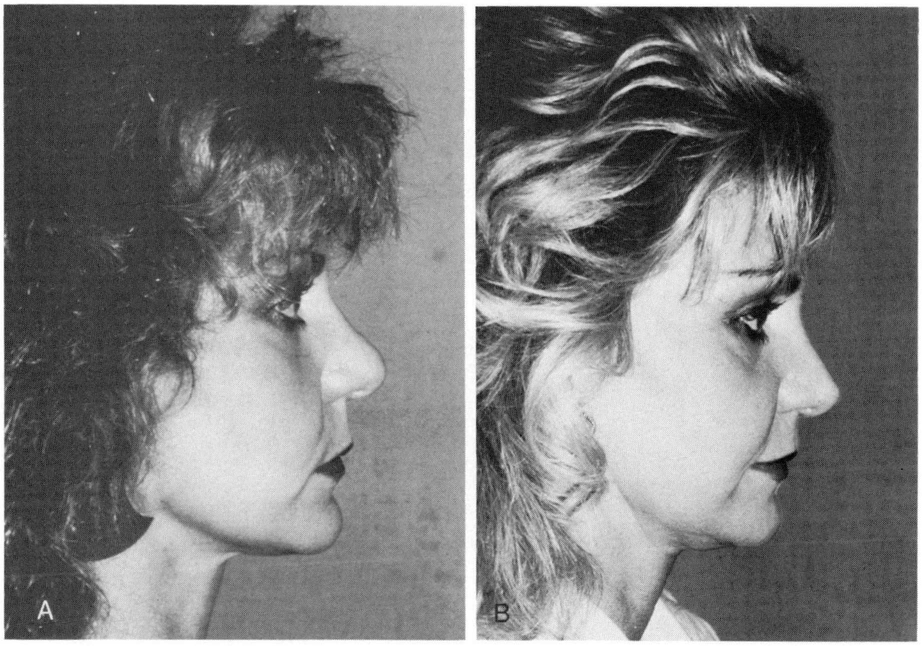

FIGURE 21–6. (*A*) Previous nasal plastic surgery left this patient with a large mass of scar tissue in the tip and supratip regions. (*B*) Through an external rhinoplasty, the mass of scar was excised (see Fig. 21–7). Other than a dermabrasion performed 18 months later, no additional surgical maneuvers were required.

3. Many severely maimed and/or scarred noses require total or subtotal reconstruction with regional flaps and/or composite grafts (see Fig. 22–14).

Dissection and Undermining

When correction calls for a minor procedure, such as rasping of a small irregularity of the bony dorsum or excision of a piece of alar cartilage that is projecting into the nasal airway, dissection is limited to allowing the introduction of the rasp or to removing the offending portions of tissue.

The role of proper draping of the nasal skin over the architectural framework of the nose often is underestimated. The removal of a cartilaginous polly beak or undercorrected nasal dorsum often calls for wide undermining of the dorsal and lateral nasal skin to allow for redraping. Likewise, even minor corrections of the alar cartilages are best performed by delivery, so that the soft tissues can be molded to the alar cartilaginous framework.

Meticulous placement of the nasal dressing helps to create a form for all components to heal in the desired positions. Conversely, an improperly applied dressing can tent the skin and create a permanent postoperative deformity (Fig. 21–8).

External Rhinoplasty

The role of raising a dorsal nasal flap in revisional rhinoplasty must not be underestimated. The primary advantage of this approach is that maximum exposure is available for diagnosis and reconstruction. Excessive scar tissue can be excised directly and accurately.

In many cases, normal anatomic relations must be reestablished. Grafts to reconstruct the skeletal framework can be accurately placed and secured with suturing techniques (see Fig. 21–11).

The advantages and timing of external rhinoplasty conversion are covered in more detail in the section on tip modification.

Text continued on page 300

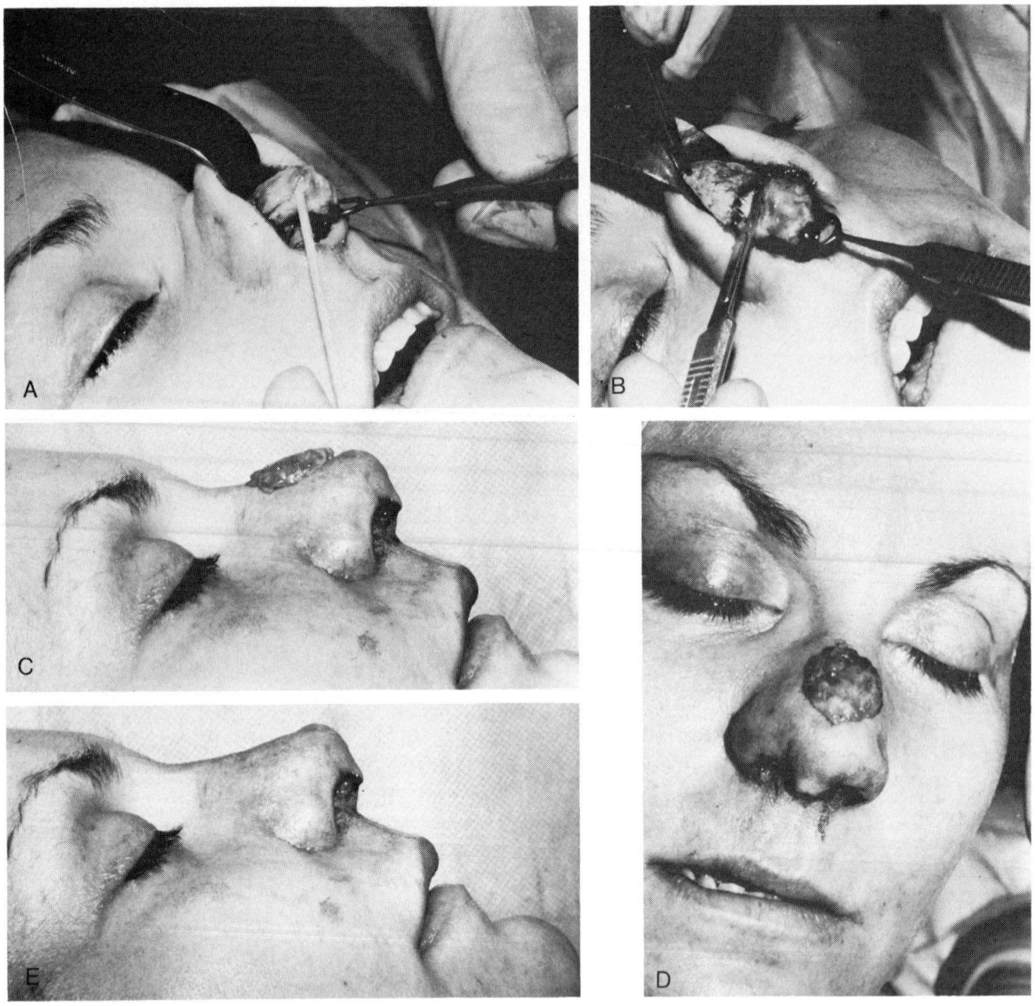

FIGURE 21–7. (*A*) When the dorsal skin flap is retracted, the mass of scar tissue is readily identified. (*B*) The cartilaginous structures of the tip are identified and the scar dissected free. (*C* and *D*) The mass of scar is placed on the nasal skin. (*E*) Appearance of the nose at operation's end. The final appearance after rhinoplasty and dermabrasion is shown in Figure 22–6*B*.

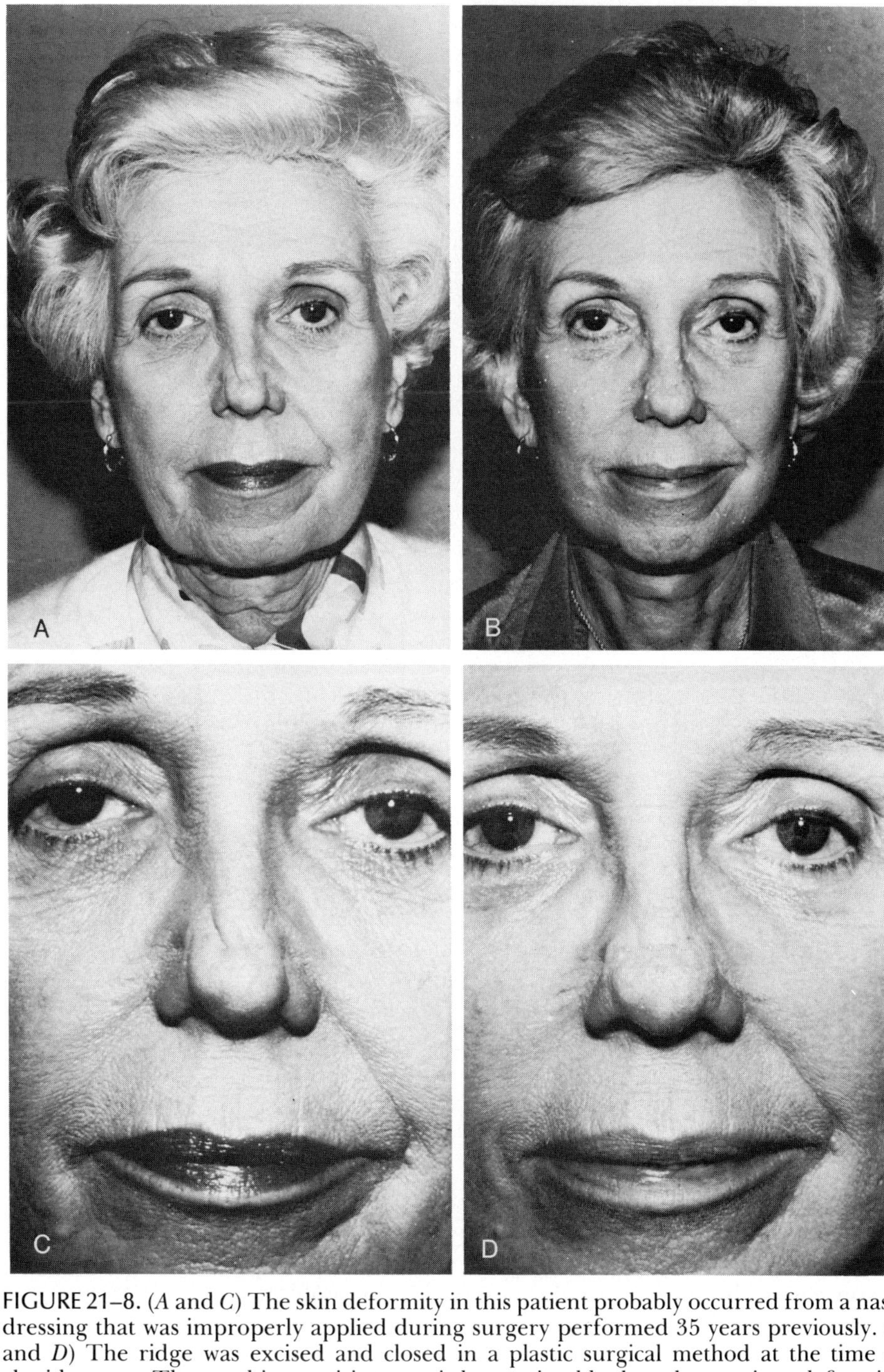

FIGURE 21–8. (*A* and *C*) The skin deformity in this patient probably occurred from a nasal dressing that was improperly applied during surgery performed 35 years previously. (*B* and *D*) The ridge was excised and closed in a plastic surgical method at the time of rhytidectomy. The resulting excision scar is less noticeable than the previous deformity. This patient refused dermabrasion, which could have provided additional camouflaging (see Ch. 25).

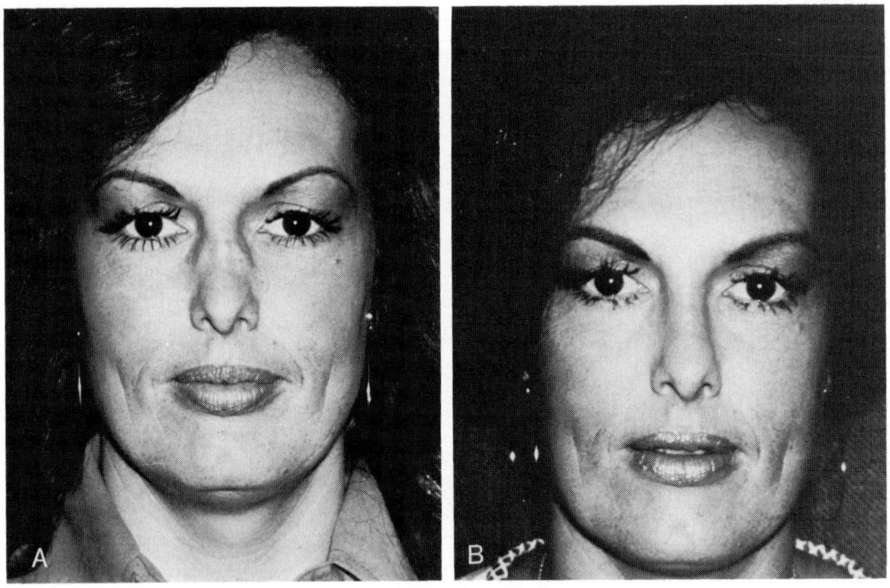

FIGURE 21–9. (*A*) Failure to completely mobilize and secure the position of the lateral walls can result in an open-roof deformity. (*B*) This problem can be corrected by performing bilateral lateral osteotomies.

CORRECTING THE UPPER THIRD OF THE NOSE

The upper one third of the nose comprises the bony vault, consisting of nasal bones, frontal processes of the maxillary bones, and perpendicular plate of the ethmoid.

Errors of Omission

DORSAL PROJECTION

Undercorrection of the bony dorsum may require further deepening of the nasofrontal angle with a sharp osteotome. It is difficult to deepen the nasofrontal angle with a rasp. On the other hand, a rasp is recommended for lowering the bony dorsum in the patient whose lateral bony walls were previously mobilized with osteotomies.

WIDTH

Excessive width of the upper one third may be secondary to inadequate mobilization of the lateral walls at the time of rhinoplasty or widening in the postoperative period (Fig. 21–9).

Correction is accomplished by complete mobilization with osteotomies. The new osteotomy tract should be placed as close as possible to the nasofacial crease and, it is hoped, below the primary track. Complete mobilization at the time of surgery coupled with proper application of splints and dressings is advisable.

Most greenstick fractures return to their original preoperative position. Excessive internal nasal packing may cause the lateral walls to widen, even if complete mobilization was accomplished at surgery. In some cases, molding techniques can be practiced by the patient if the lateral wall should begin to “float” outward in the postoperative period (Fig. 21–10).

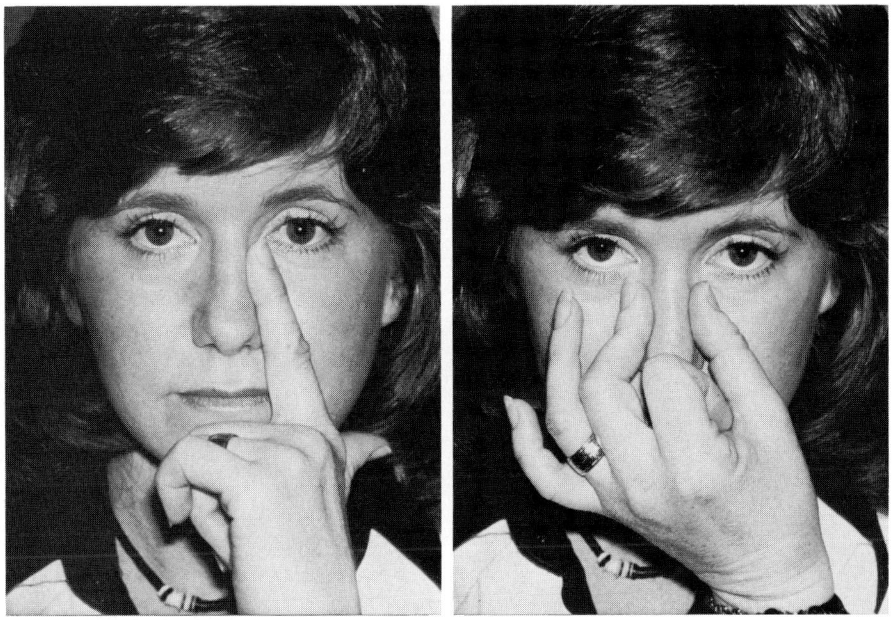

FIGURE 21–10. Finger pressure applied for 1 to 2 minutes and repeated 20 times daily for 4 to 6 weeks may help to prevent widening of the lateral nasal walls.

ASYMMETRY

Unevenly performed hump removal, paramedian healing of the lateral walls, or failure to straighten a deviated perpendicular plate of the ethmoid during septoplasty can cause asymmetry of the upper one third of the nose.

Errors of Commission

Overly aggressive removal of the bony dorsum at the time of rhinoplasty reduces the height of the nasal dorsum from the lateral view, produces upper third saddling from the lateral view, and results in a nose that appears wide from the front (Fig. 21–11). Removal of the central support of the upper one third with hump removal (or septoplasty) and/or fracture of the dorsal cantilever (ethmoid–quadrangular cartilage complex) at the time of surgery results in an iatrogenic saddle deformity. Trauma can also cause the collapse of the upper one third of the pyramid (Fig. 21–12).

Regardless of the cause, the dorsal height must be reestablished by augmentation. A number of materials are available for reconstruction. Those most commonly used at our clinic are discussed below.

CARTILAGINOUS GRAFTS

Autogenous septum is the material of choice if an adequate amount of cartilage is available. For large defects, the cartilage can be stacked and secured with absorbable sutures. Gentle morselization of cartilaginous grafts is recommended (Fig. 21–13). When septal cartilage is inadequate or not present, auricular conchal cartilage may be used. Pronounced saddling of the upper one third of the nose may require conchal cartilage from both ears (Fig. 21–14). Minor depressions or irregularities can be corrected with excised portions of alar cartilage removed during tip-plasty.

Homologous cartilage grafts are less predictable, but I prefer them over bone grafts.

Text continued on page 305

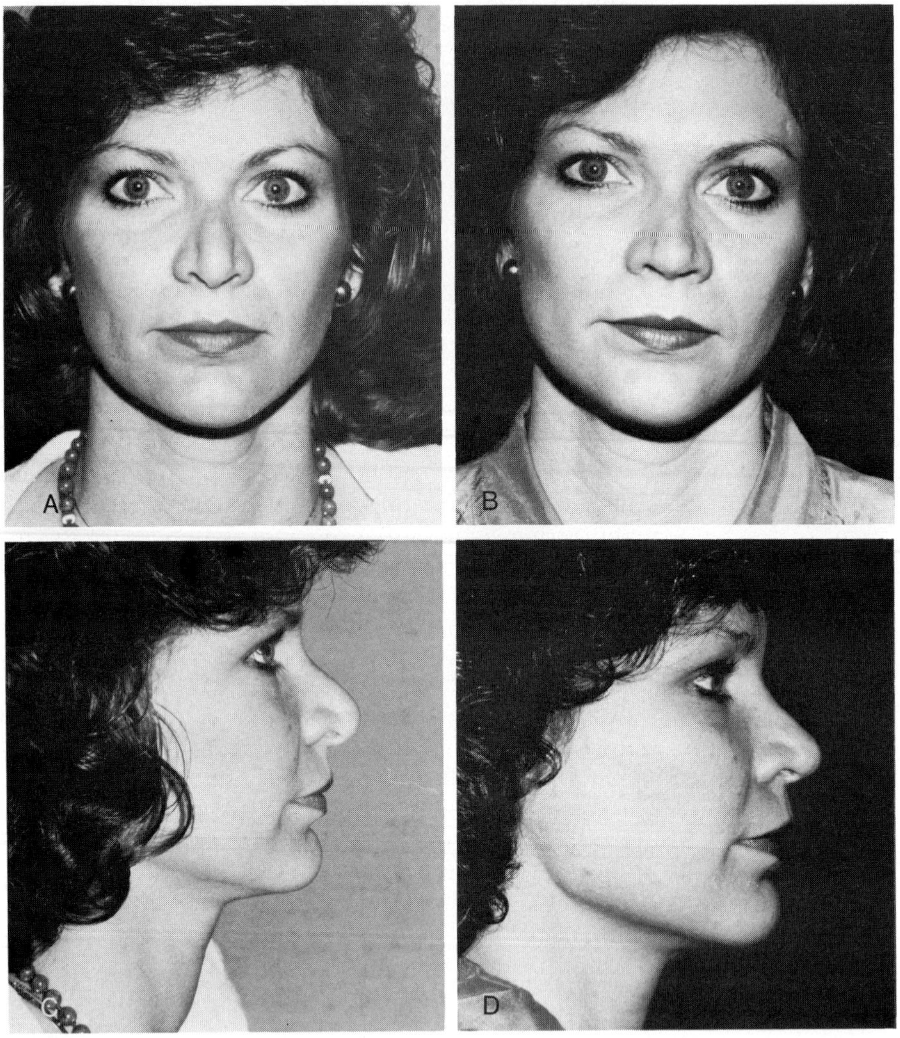

FIGURE 21–11. (*A* and *C*) Excessive removal of bone and tip cartilages coupled with a loss of support and scar tissue buildup in the supratip region are telltale signs of unsuccessful nasal plastic surgery. (*B* and *D*) Augmentation, scar tissue excision, and tip-plasty provide a more natural appearance.

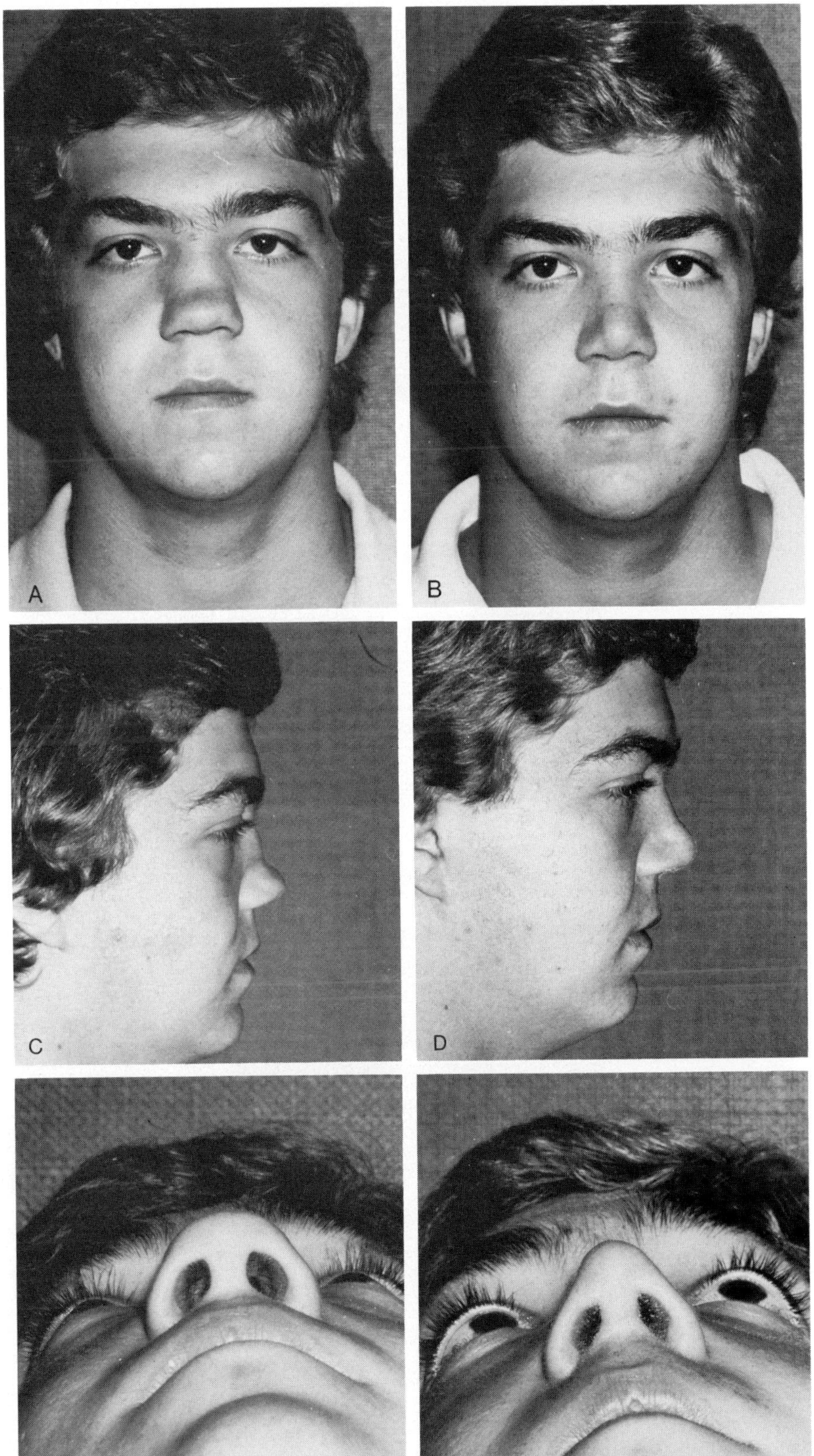

FIGURE 21–12. (*A* and *C*) Early trauma damaged most of the skeletal support in this young man's nose. (*B* and *D*) Augmentation was achieved with conchal cartilaginous grafts. Nasal osteotomies were also required. (*E* and *F*) Dome-division (Goldman-type) tip-plasty and alar sil resections were performed.

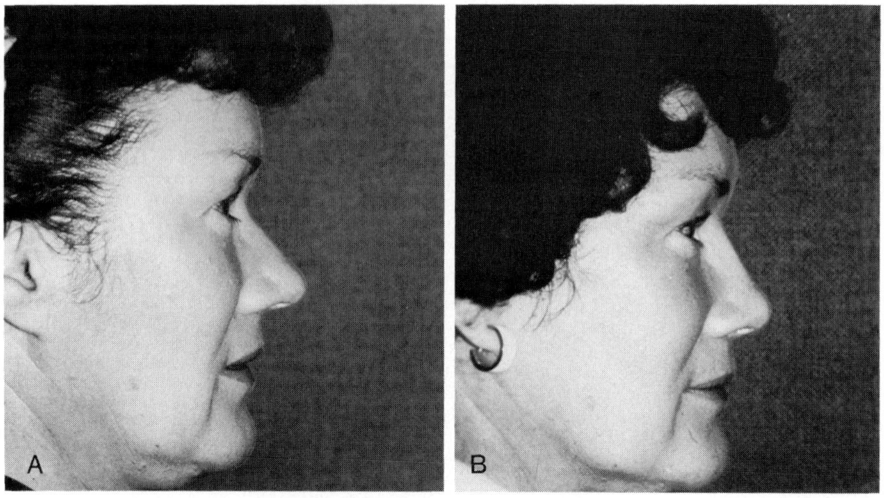

FIGURE 21–13. (*A* and *B*) Septal cartilage grafts may be used over the bony dorsum for augmentation.

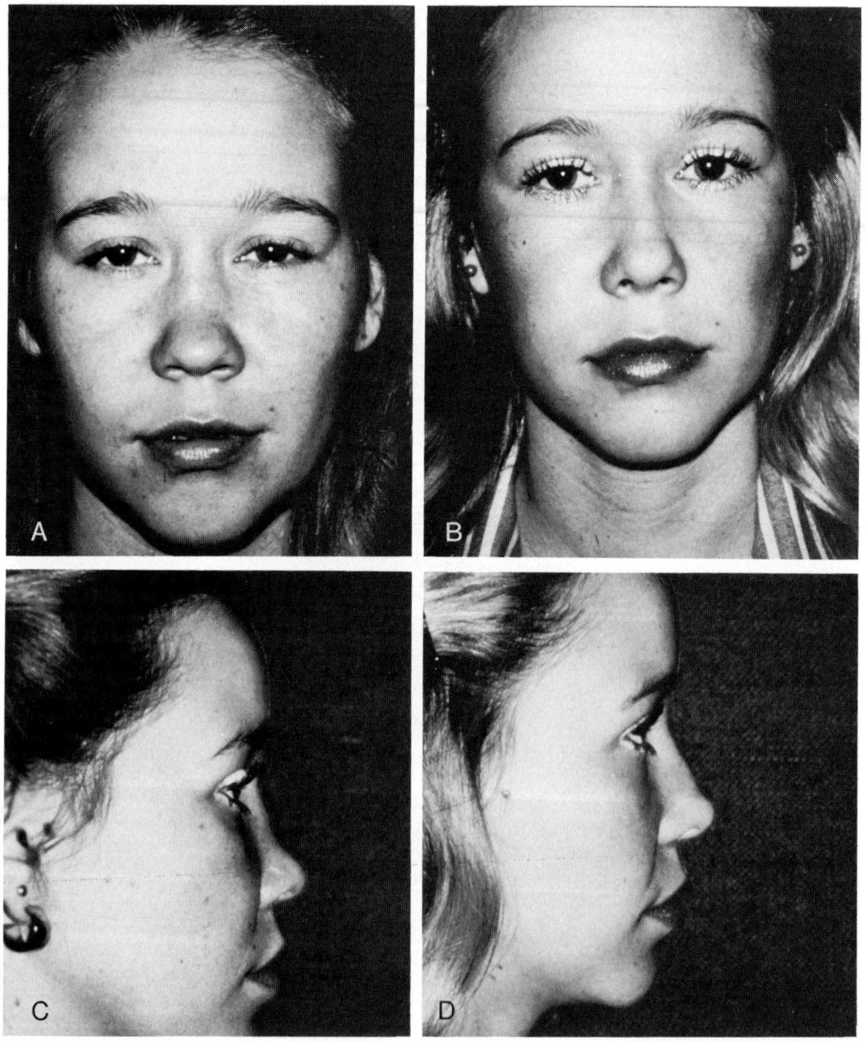

FIGURE 21–14. Auricular cartilage grafts from both ears were required to correct the saddle deformity in this young woman. (*A* and *C*) Postinjury deformities are obvious. (*B* and *D*) Postsurgical correction.

IMPLANTS

An abundance of alloplastic materials are available for dorsal augmentation. Implants that closely simulate the tissues they are designed to replace are best. Mersilene mesh, when placed subperiosteally, becomes intimately attached to the nasal bony dorsum and firmly attached in its new bed. Fibrous ingrowth into the lattice pattern of a mesh implant produces a consistency not unlike bone (Fig. 21–15).

Meticulous antiseptic handling of the implant before insertion reduces the possibility of infection. The implant must not be handled with gloves that have come in contact with the patient's skin or with instruments used earlier in the operation. Soaking the implant in a broad-spectrum antibiotic (lincomycin or gentamicin) may also reduce the incidence of infection. Prophylactic antibiotic therapy is indicated when alloplastic materials are used for reconstruction. All intranasal incisions must be closed completely to minimize the opportunity for intranasal organisms to come in contact with the implant. An exposed implant eventually will become an infected implant.

INJECTABLE GRAFTS

Collagen and fibrin complex materials are helpful for the short term, but they eventually are destroyed by the body's immune system. Fat cells transferred from one part of the body to another, especially when injected, seldom survive the tranfer. Although Fibril (a bovine extract used as a temporary injectable tissue filler) contains some of the patient's own tissues, the initial improvement seen after injection seems to be short-lived.

CORRECTING THE MIDDLE THIRD OF THE NOSE

The middle one third is composed of the cartilaginous dorsum and the upper lateral cartilages.

Errors of Omission

Insufficient or irregular removal of cartilage at the time of surgery may be the easiest "deformity" to revise. Correction is accomplished by elevating the dorsal soft tissue and shaving the projecting portions with a No. 15 blade or angulated scissors (Figs. 21–16 and 21–17).

Errors of Commission

DORSAL PROJECTION

As is the case with the bony dorsum, saddle deformities or insufficient height of the cartilaginous dorsum must be augmented (see Fig. 21–18). The principles and techniques described for augmenting the upper one third of the nose are applicable to the middle one third.

Text continued on page 310

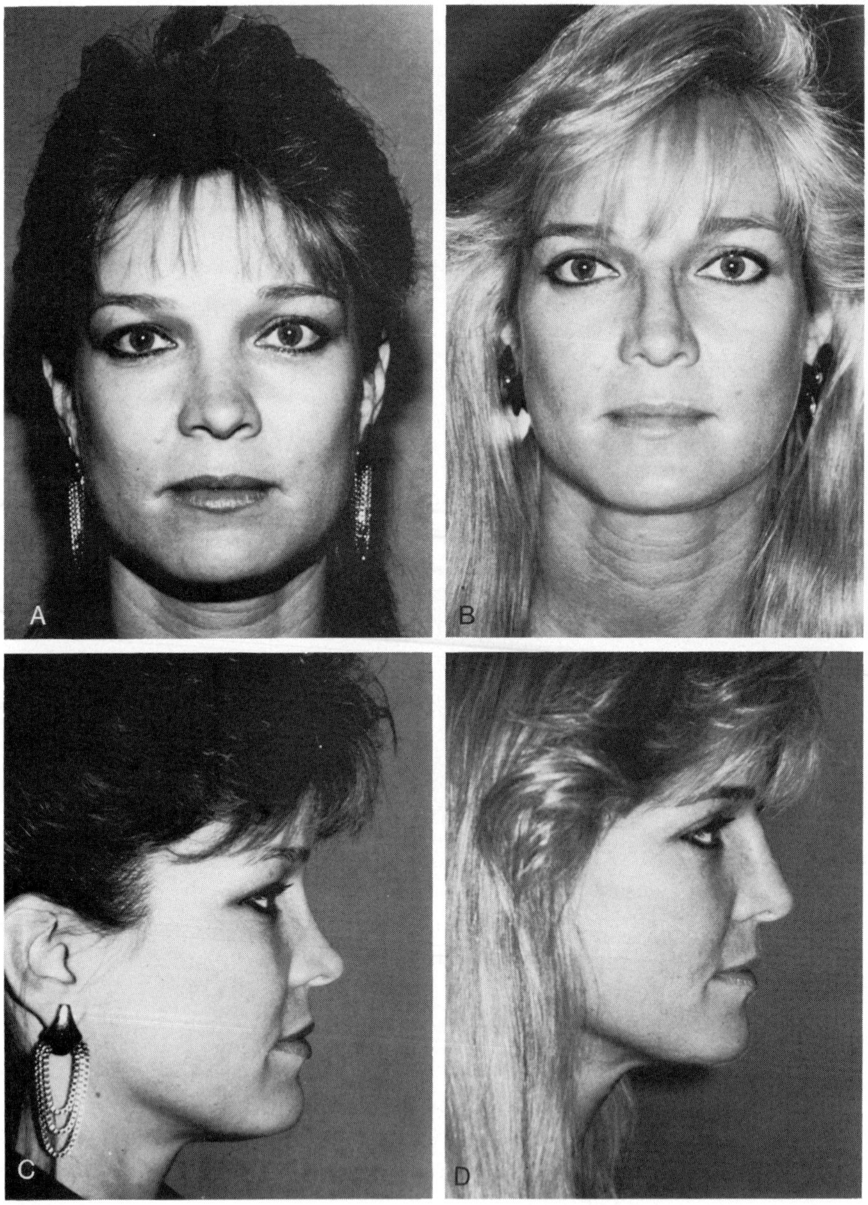

FIGURE 21–15. (*A* and *C*) A Mersilene mesh dorsal implant was used in this tall woman to restore the height of her nasal dorsum. (*B* and *D*) Septal cartilage was used to correct the retracted columella.

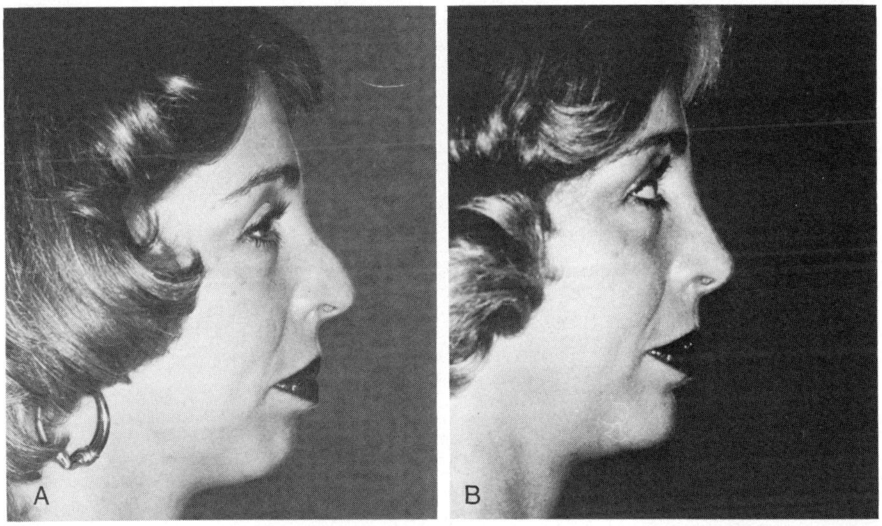

FIGURE 21–16. (*A*) Failure to lower the dorsum in the area of the cartilaginous superior septal angle can result in a polly-beak deformity. (*B*) Removal of the excessive cartilage coupled with a cartilaginous columellar strut for support corrected the polly beak.

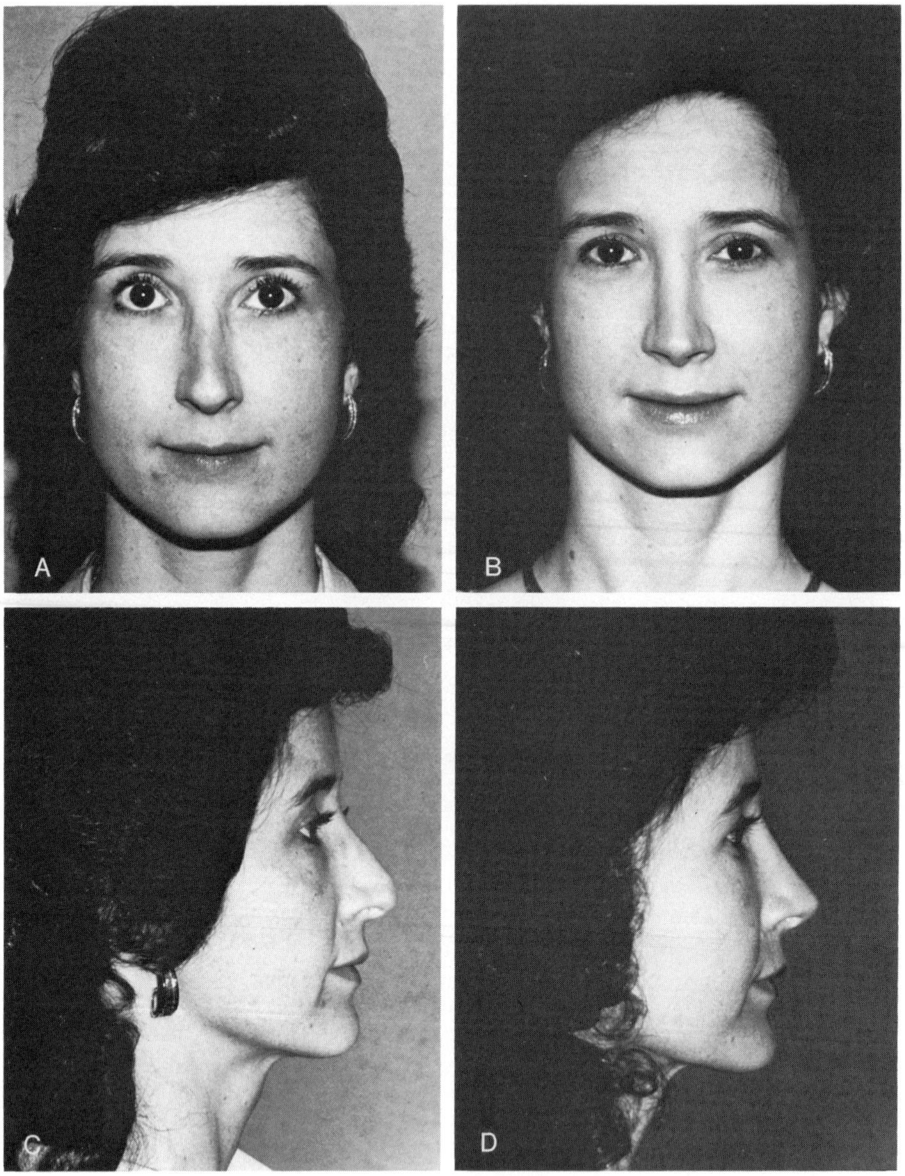

FIGURE 21–17. (*A* and *C*) Prerevision photographs show loss of tip support. (*B* and *D*) Correction of a polly-beak deformity may involve excision of excessive supratip scar, additional lowering of the cartilaginous septum, and tip reconstruction with an I-beam–type tip-plasty.

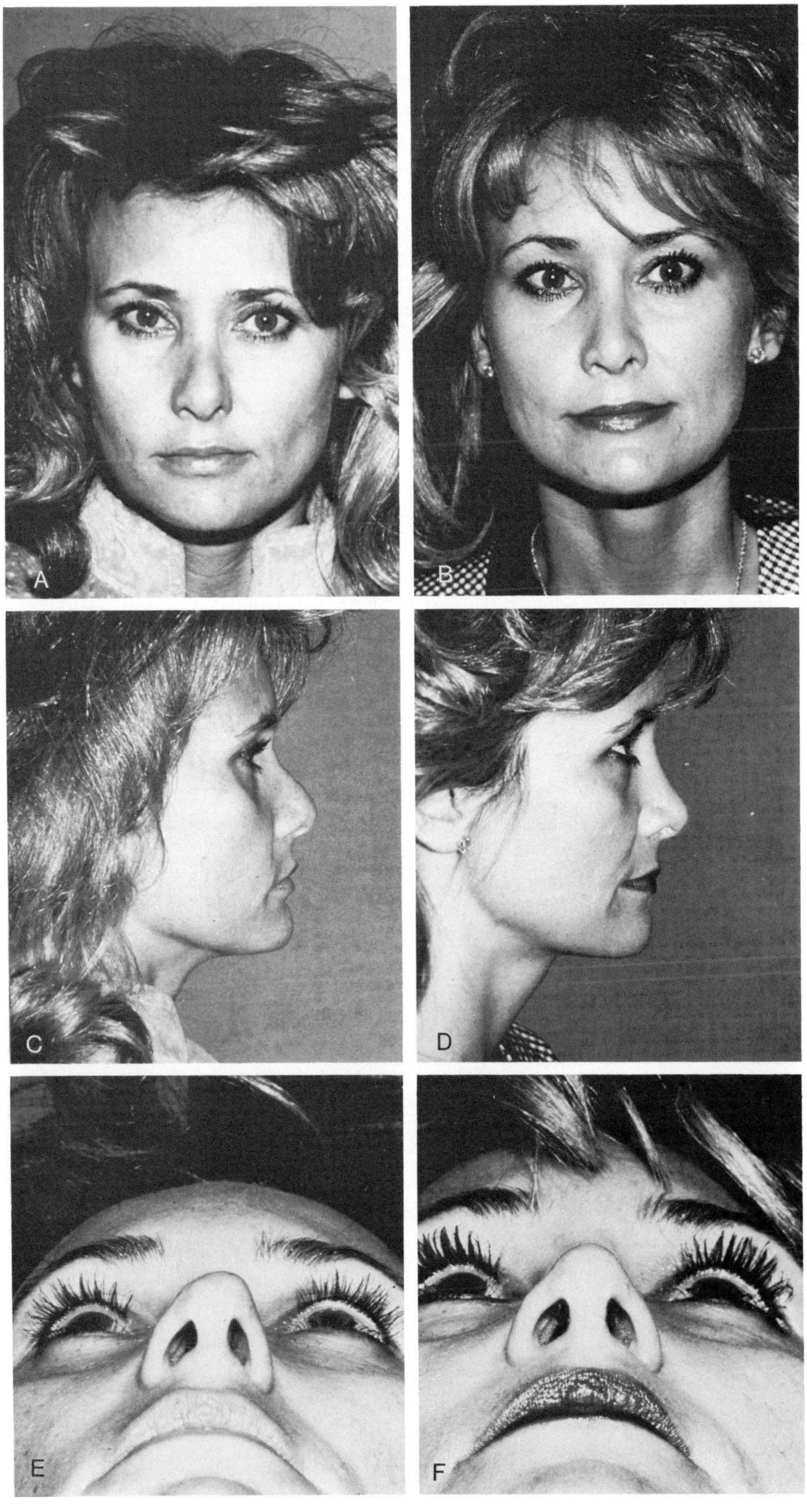

FIGURE 21–18. (*A*, *C*, and *E*) Overresection of the dorsal bone and cartilage and failure to close the open-roof deformity and correct a septal deviation led to the problems seen in this patient. (*B*, *D*, and *F*) Osteotomies, dorsal augmentation, and septoplasty provide improvement in both appearance and function. Dome-division (I-beam–type) tip-plasty helped to provide symmetry and support to the lobule.

WIDTH

A wide middle one third often is caused by a loss in dorsal height. Correction is accomplished, in part, by dorsal augmentation (Fig. 21–19).

Lateralization of the nasal bones during healing also causes widening of the upper lateral cartilages. After adequate freeing of the cicatrix and the surrounding soft tissues, mobilization with osteotomies followed by medial displacement will narrow the middle one third.

Inadvertent disarticulation of the upper lateral cartilages from their attachment to the undersurface of the nasal bones creates the unmistakable inverted V deformity of the middle one third.

Loss of tip projection causes the middle one third to have a widened appearance. Correction and prevention include maintaining and/or reestablishing tip projection coupled with sufficient undermining over the middle one third to allow for proper draping (Fig. 21–20).

ASYMMETRY

Although uneven excision of the dorsum of the upper lateral cartilages may lead to postoperative asymmetry of the middle one third of the nose, failure to recognize or correct a deviation of the nasal septum is the most common cause of this deformity (Fig. 21–21).

Correction involves separating the upper lateral cartilages from the dorsal septum coupled with the appropriate septoplasty (see Ch. 10).

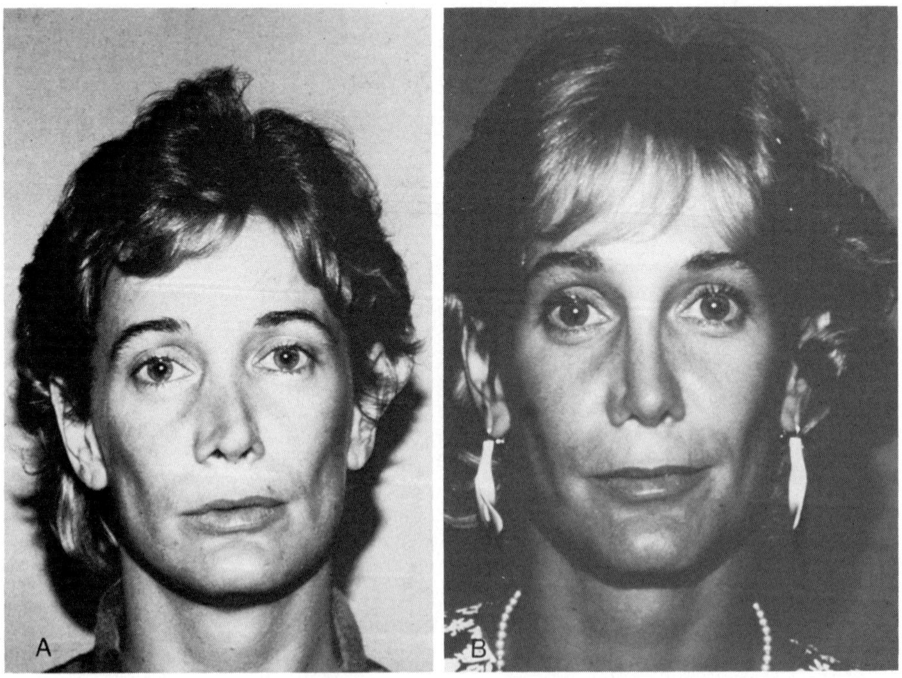

FIGURE 21–19. (*A*) After several unsuccessful attempts, this patient had been left with a deviated septum, collapse of the lateral lower one third, and a severe saddle. (*B*) Augmentation with a Mersilene mesh dorsal implant helped to correct the saddling of both bony and cartilaginous components of the nasal dorsum. Cartilage grafting was required in the tip.

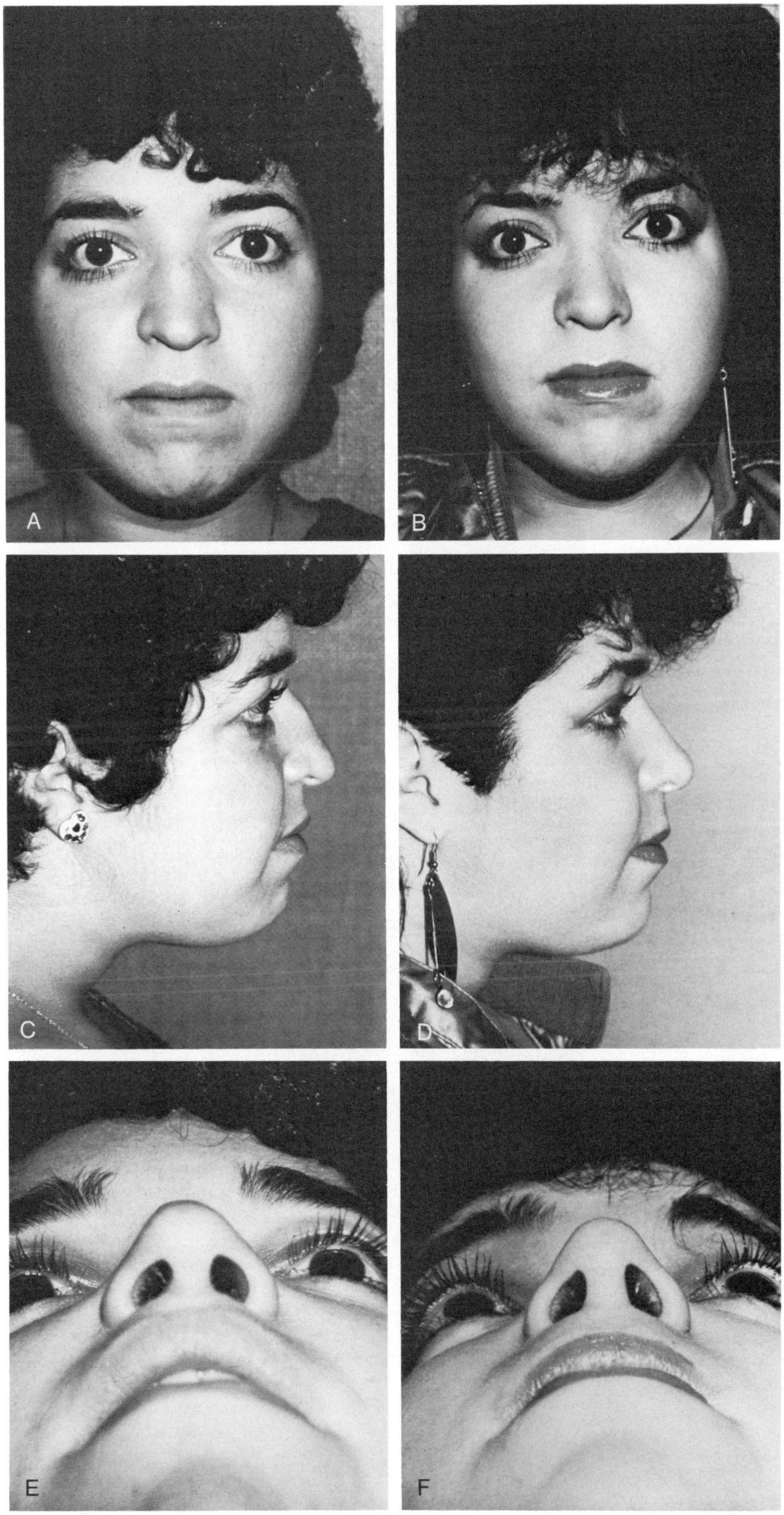

FIGURE 21–20. (*A*, *C*, and *E*) Loss of tip support produces a widened lower third of the face. (*B*, *D*, and *F*) These conditions were corrected in this patient with an I-beam–type tip-plasty. Cartilage grafting to the premaxilla was also performed, as was Mersilene mesh chin augmentation.

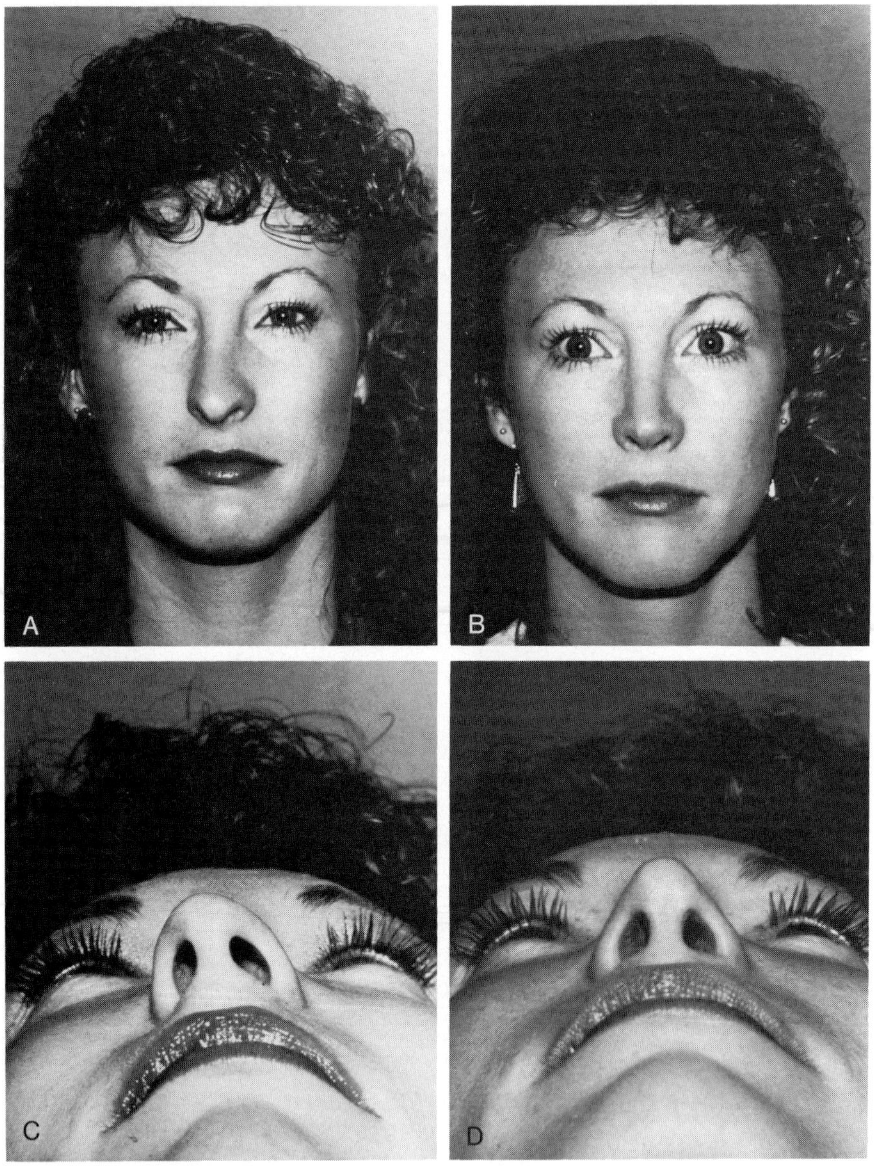

FIGURE 21–21. (*A* and *C*) Failure to correct a deviated septum at the time of rhinoplasty resulted in a persistent twist in the nose. (*B* and *D*) A Metzenbaum swinging-door septoplasty and I-beam–type tip-plasty corrected her problem.

CORRECTING THE LOWER ONE THIRD OF THE NOSE

The lower one third, the nasal tip, comprises the lower lateral cartilages, columella, and alae. Correcting deformities or asymmetries of the nasal tip may involve minor excision of excessive cartilage, insertion of camouflaging grafts, or total reconstruction of the cartilaginous skeletal framework. Any of the techniques for tip-plasty may need to be considered. For more complicated deformities, the following techniques may prove helpful (Fig. 21–22). Alterations to the nasal skeleton when coupled with an understanding of the anatomy, physiology, and vagaries of healing allow the surgeon-artist to achieve predictably good results.

After marginal and intracartilaginous incisions have been made, bipedical vestibulochondrial flaps can be developed with scissors dissection. Cartilage delivery and inspection can then be achieved (see Fig. 14–4). Incisions should not limit or dictate which technique the surgeon might select. Most of the surgical maneuvers presented in this chapter can be performed through closed rhinoplasty.

With primary rhinoplasty, revisional nasal tip surgery is a surgical progression. A number of individual factors may cause the surgeon to modify his plan. At any point in the progressive system when the desired result has been achieved, the tip-plasty should be terminated.

When more complex reconstructive techniques are indicated, an external approach might provide the additional exposure needed to facilitate correction. The classic delivery procedure can be converted to an external rhinoplasty at any time during the operation.

Tip Projection, Support, and Rotation

The length and strength of the medial crura play a more crucial role in tip support than often is appreciated. This central limb of the tripod often is deficient or retrodisplaced in noses that require revisional surgery (Figs. 21–23 and 21–24).

A complete and bilateral septal transfixion incision may have destroyed much of this critical central support mechanism. When the medial crura extend only a fraction of the length of the columella, disruption of their attachment to the caudal septum may allow them to settle during healing until they come to rest at a level that will become the new columellar base. As this phenomenon occurs, the tip assumes a more retrodisplaced position.

Support can be reestablished by plumping grafts inserted beneath the feet of the medial crura (Fig. 21–25) or by cartilaginous struts placed between the medial crura to effectively lengthen and strengthen them (Fig. 21–26). Anatomically, the medial lateral crura are longer than the medial crura. As previously described, the central (medial crural) leg is supported by a number of elements, including the fibrous attachment to the inferior (caudal) margin of the nasal septum and the superior suspension of Pitanguy's ligament. Destruction of Pitanguy's ligament usually occurs during a previous operation.

Retrodisplacement coupled with tip ptosis and the emergence of a more acute nasolabial angle is an expected and predictable sequela of rhinoplasty if forward support is not reestablished at the end of operation (Fig. 21–27).

If a bilateral transfixion incision were extended inferiorly past the attachment of the medial crural footplates and both lateral crura were shortened

Text continued on page 319

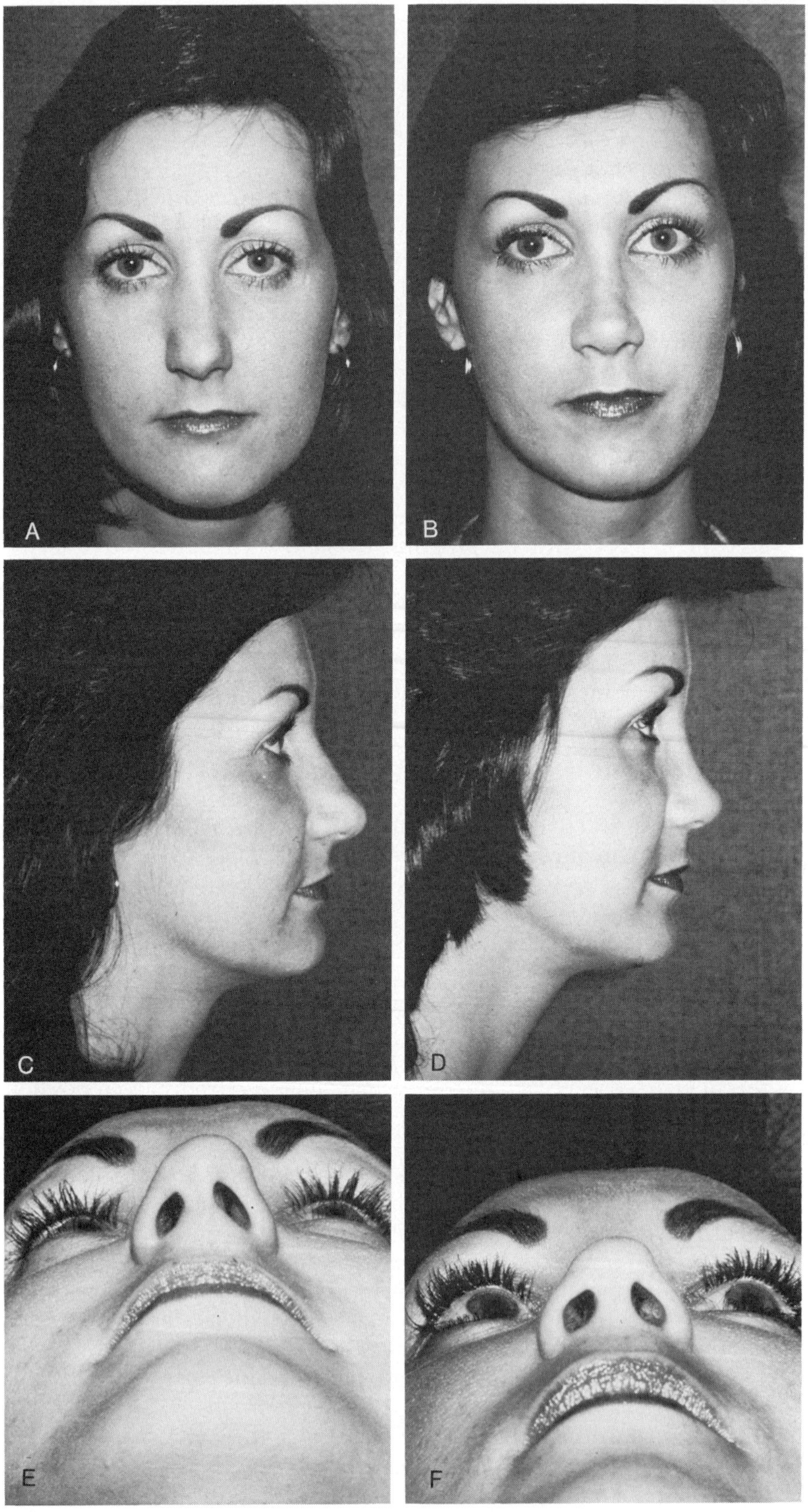

FIGURE 21–22. (*A, C,* and *E*) Asymmetric excision of tip cartilages, failure to correct a septal deviation, and a decision not to perform osteotomies produced the defects seen in this patient. (*B, D,* and *F*) Correction was carried out by performing septoplasty, osteotomies, and tipplasty with onlay cartilage grafts over the right dome area.

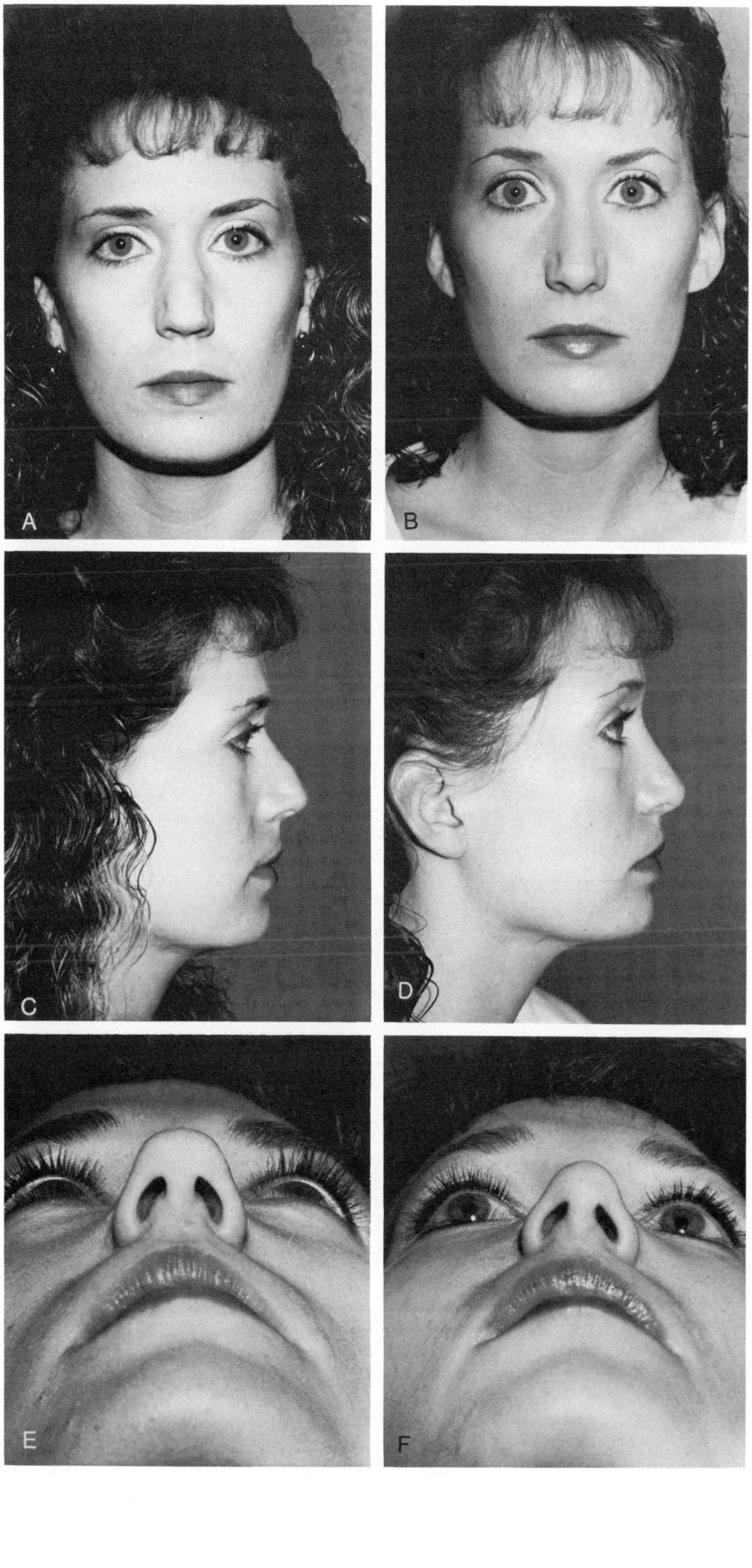

FIGURE 21–23. (*A, C,* and *E*) This twin previously underwent a rhinoplasty during which much of the tip cartilages were removed, resulting in a loss of tip support and a polly beak. (*B, D,* and *F*) After resection of the supratip scar, an I-beam–type tip-plasty was performed.

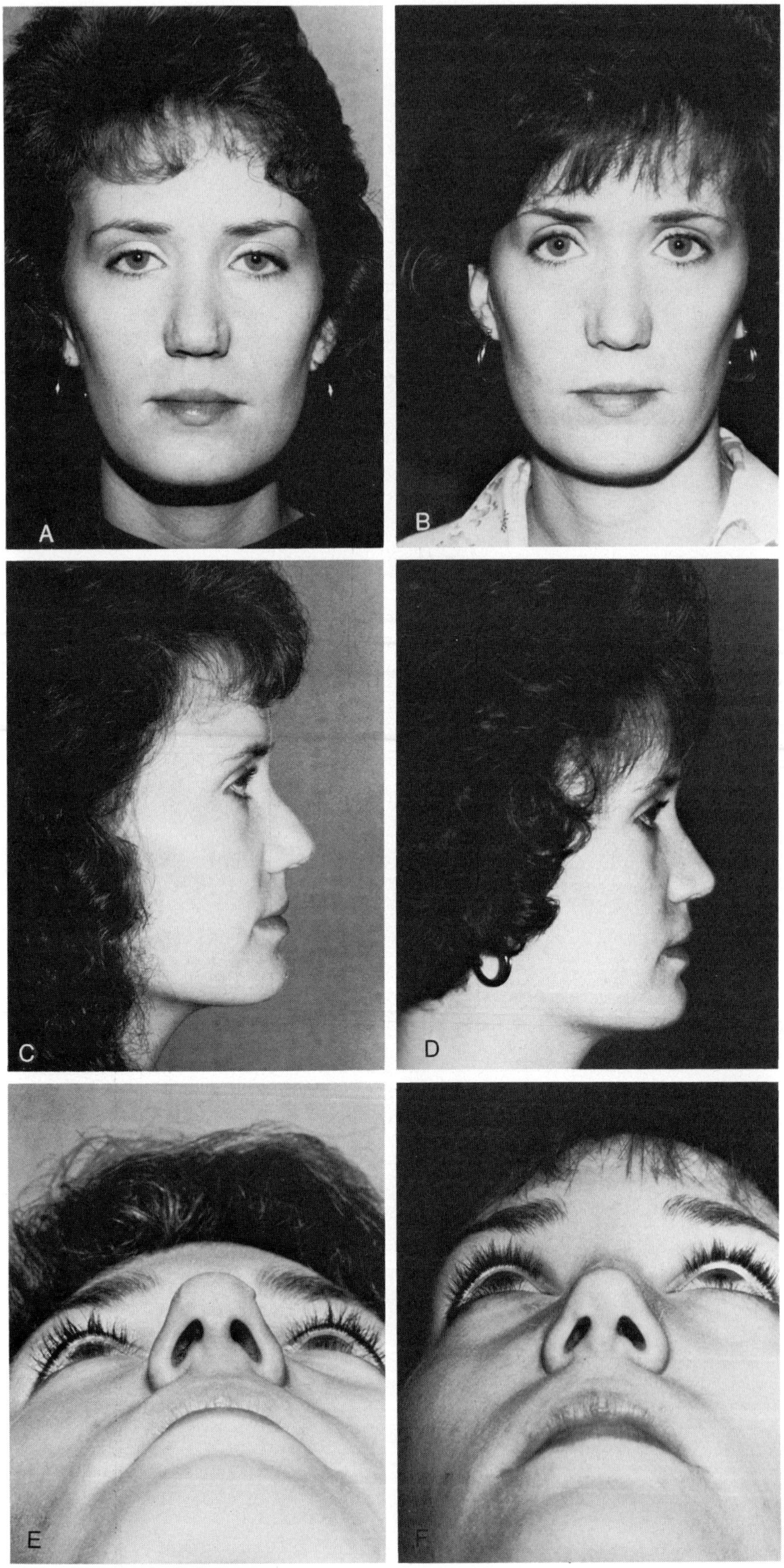

FIGURE 21–24. (*A, C,* and *E*) The patient shown in Figure 21–23 had an identical twin sister who underwent surgery by the same surgeon, resulting in a similar deformity plus an external scar in each supra-alar region. (*B, D,* and *F*) This patient required reconstruction of all three legs of the tip tripod with cartilaginous grafting and staged scar revision with dermabrasion.

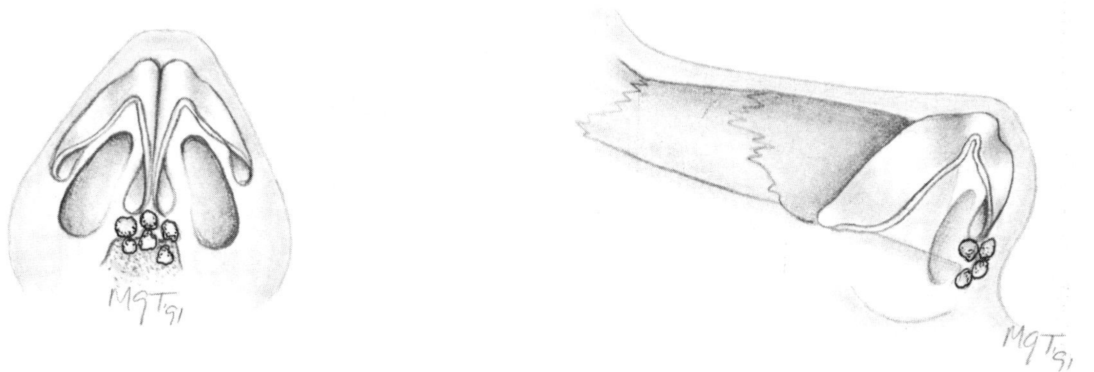

FIGURE 21–25. Fragments of morselized cartilage may be inserted beneath the feet of the medial crura to provide support to the tip.

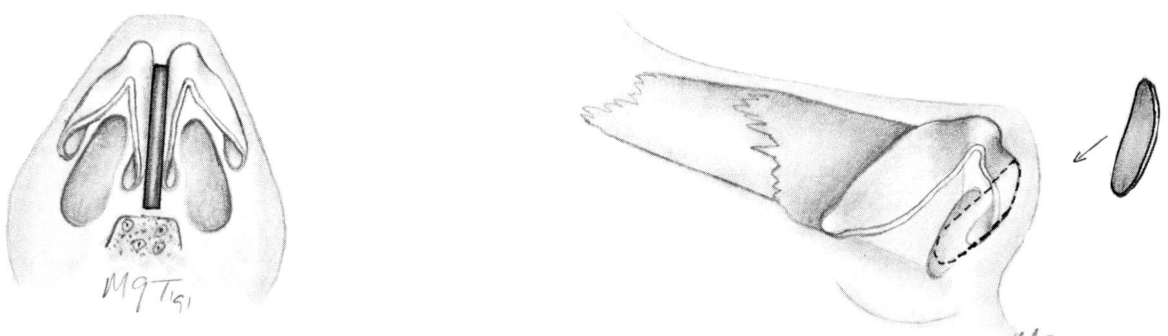

FIGURE 21–26. A strong, straight piece of septal cartilage may be inserted between the medial crura and extended to within 2 to 3 mm of the premaxillary crest to provide support to the tip.

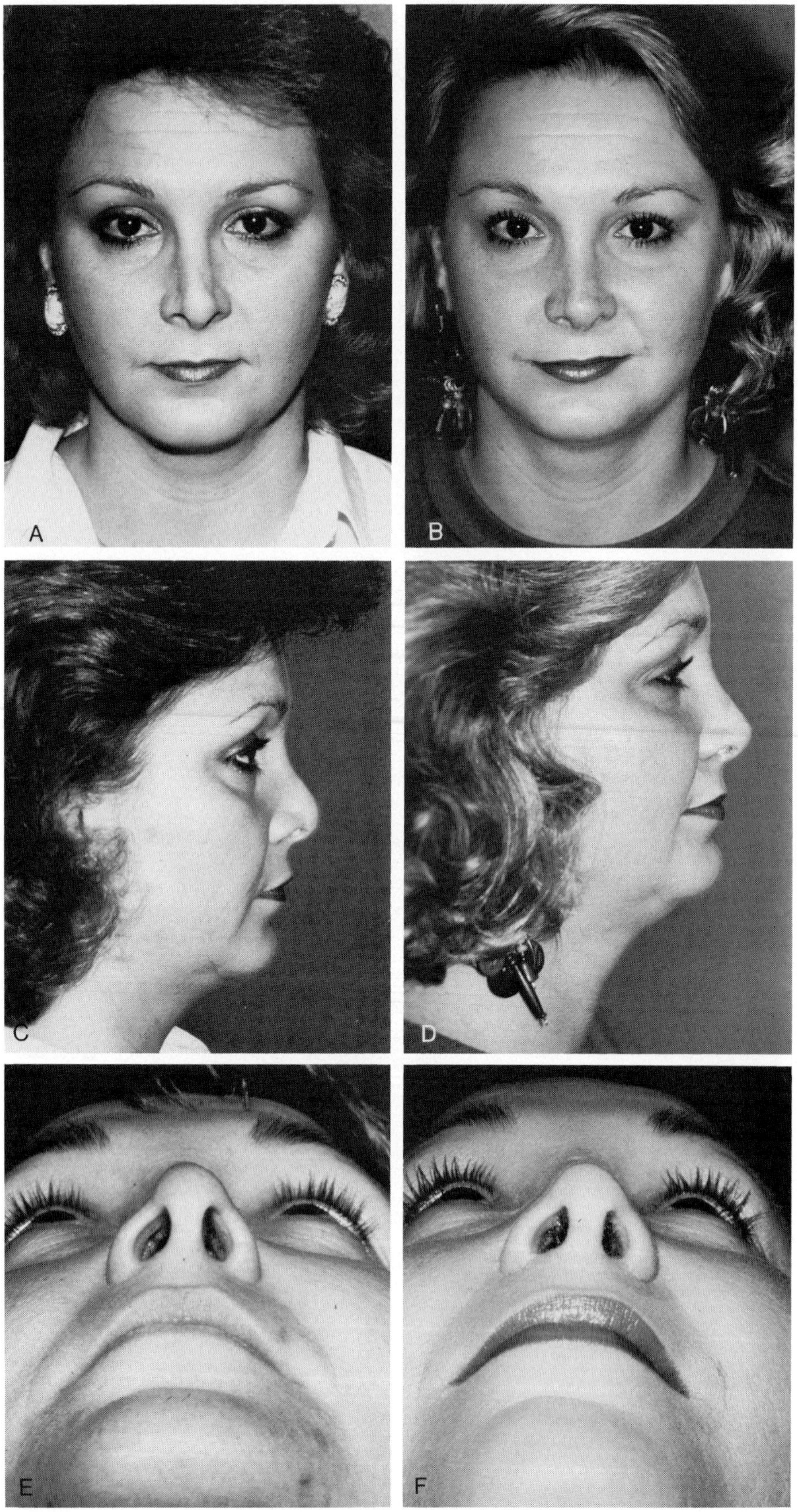

FIGURE 21–27. (*A, C,* and *E*) The ability to produce tip projection is the key to performing revisional rhinoplasty. The prerevision state of the patient shows over-resection of tip cartilages with loss of support. (*B, D,* and *F*) Revisional result obtained with an I beam technique with a sandwich tip graft. This maneuver is the workhorse of revisional tipplasty. A shield-type graft may also be sutured to the caudal and superior extent of the I beam.

or weakened, loss of tip projection would follow. Tip ptosis and acute angulation of the nasolabial complex are minimized, however, because a taller tripod has been effectively and dynamically converted on all three sides to one with shorter legs. The net effect is tip retrodisplacement without significant rotation or ptosis; such was the case in the patient in Figure 21–27.

When the skin and soft tissue covering the tip of the nose are deprived of their support, the base of the nose widens and nostril flaring is noted. Alar sil resections should be considered if this phenomenon occurs.

When upward rotation of the tip is desirable, cartilaginous columellar struts, plumping grafts, or permanent buried septocolumellar sutures can be used to support the central leg of the tripod. As its central component becomes the dominant leg, the tip rotates superiorly toward the forehead (Fig. 21–28).

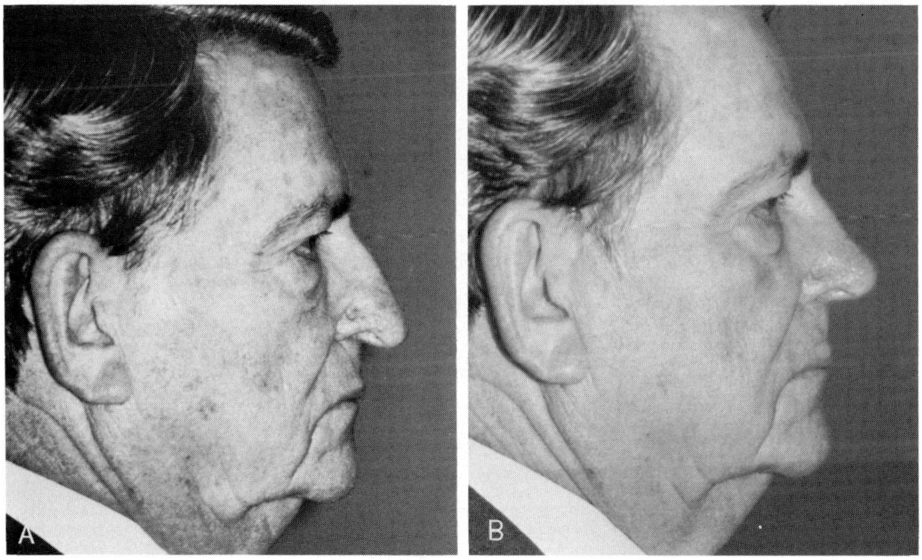

FIGURE 21–28. (*A*) As some people age, the tip becomes severely ptotic, resulting in a less than desirable appearance and altered nasal air flow. (*B*) Reconstruction of the central dominant leg of the tripod with plumping grafts and I-beam tip-plasty provides the desired projection and rotation in most cases. Many patients also obtain better airways.

Techniques Used for Tip Modification

The cascading approach to the nasal tip described in Chapter 14 affords the surgeon the opportunity to recognize the point in the operation when the best result that can be provided to the patient has been achieved. With experience, the surgeon learns to select the simplest technique that will accomplish the desired outcome while minimizing the risk of revision.

Most cases that require revisional surgery involve reconstruction of more than one third of the nose. Severely maimed noses require total or subtotal reconstruction.

At best, the goal in revisional rhinoplasty should be to improve the appearance and function of the nose. Perfection seldom is achievable when the result depends on reconstruction with grafts and implants. Patients should be forewarned that postoperative imperfections may exist and that more than one operation might be required to achieve a satisfactory result. The degree of improvement seems to be directly proportional to the experience and skills of the surgeon; therefore, early in one's career, it may be advisable to refer complicated reconstructions to a more experienced colleague.

References

1. Kerth, J.D., Bytell, D.E. Revision in unsuccessful rhinoplasty. Otolaryngol Clin North Am 7(1):67, 1974.

Suggested Readings

McCollough, E.G. Rhinoplasty: A humbling experience. J Oral Maxillofac Surg 47:1132–1141, 1989.

Rogers, B.O. Rhinoplasty, The Unfavorable Result in Plastic Surgery. Boston: Little, Brown, 1972, pp. 283–319.

Tobin, H.A. Revision of the failed rhinoplasty. Current Therapy in Otolaryngology—Head and Neck Surgery 3:137–141, 1987.

Toruimi, D.M., Johnson, C.M. Revision rhinoplasty using open structure rhinoplasty technique. In Goldwyn, R.M., ed. Plastic and Reconstructive Surgery of the Head and Neck. Proceedings of the Fifth International Symposium. Philadelphia: B.C. Decker, 1991, pp. 27–31.

Wright, M.R. Management of patient dissatisfaction with results of cosmetic procedures. Arch Otolaryngol 106:486–471, 1980.

CHAPTER 22

Nasal Reconstruction

Daniel E. Rousso and Fred G. Fedok

The reconstruction of the nose was among the earliest plastic surgical procedures performed.[1–3] The Indian origins of this are well known and have been described. This early and enduring interest in the reconstruction of this facial region is directly related to the importance of the nose in the normal human visage. The nose occupies the central portion of the face; any imperfection is immediately recognized and impacts the overall facial appearance. The configuration and appearance of the nose convey both the personality and the state of being of the person. Accordingly, one's nose may influence how one is regarded and how successful one is in social and business interactions. The nose, with its delicate, detailed anatomy, provides a formidable challenge to the reconstructive surgeon.

As one examines the various regions of the nose, significant differences in the properties of the skin and the underlying skeleton as well as in the basic topographical contours are noted. A technique to reconstruct the upper dorsum of the nose may not be appropriate to reconstruct the lower third, or the tip, of the nose. Techniques as varied as skin grafting, skin flaps, composite grafts, myocutaneous flaps, and microvascular tissue transfers have been described in nasal reconstruction.[4–10] These are appropriately used only after consideration of the multitude of factors that constitute an effective reconstructive strategy.

NASAL ANATOMY

A thorough understanding of the complex and varied anatomy of the nose is fundamental in planning a reconstructive procedure. A more complete description is offered elsewhere in this text. The interrelation of skin, skeletal support, and lining often must be addressed, depending on the size and location of the defect. The skin of the tip typically is thick and sebaceous, although it can be thin and almost transparent. The skin over the dorsum usually is thinner than that of the tip, which is an important consideration when using local flaps.

Replacement of the skeletal support and mucosal lining should be thin and delicate to allow for the preservation of an adequate airway. The function of the nose should be restored, not hampered, by the reconstruction.

TIMING OF RECONSTRUCTION

The timing of reconstruction is based on several factors. In the case of small traumatic defects or the removal of low-grade cancers, the reconstruction can be attempted almost immediately. Alternatively, if the defect is secondary to the removal of an aggressive squamous cell carcinoma or recurrent basal cell carcinoma, then the reconstruction may need to be delayed from 6 months to 1 year. The patient's underlying physical health and psychological status in accepting the reconstructive results must also be considered. The delay in reconstruction frequently allows the patient to accept the reality of the nasal defect and, subsequently, better accept the limitations of nasal reconstruction. Finally, the timing of reconstruction may depend on the condition of the tissues in the area to be reconstructed as well as the condition of the prospective tissue donor area. For instance, in the case of trauma, local tissue contusions and lacerations may delay reconstruction. When a large part of the nose is missing, the patient may elect to use a prosthesis until the formal reconstruction is attempted (Fig. 22–1).

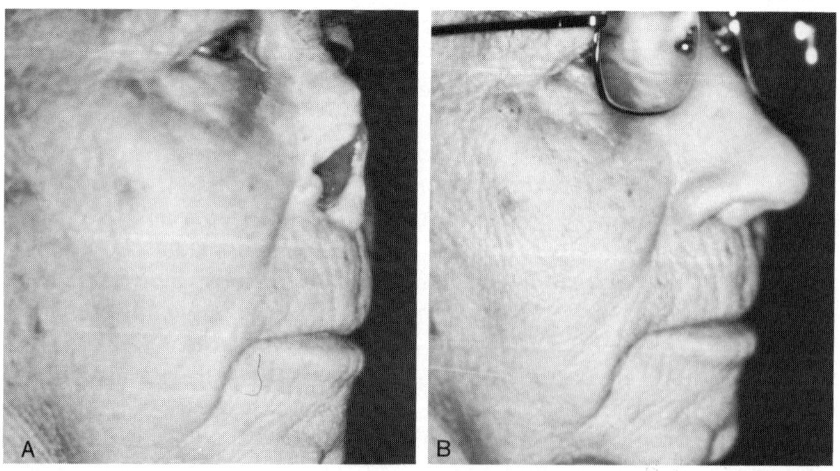

FIGURE 22–1. A nasal prosthesis may be useful, especially if formal reconstruction procedures need to be delayed for a prolonged period. (*A*) Defect after resection of recurrent basal cell carcinoma. (*B*) Prosthesis in place. (Prosthesis created by Dr. M. Mazaher, Lancaster Cleft Palate Clinic, Lancaster, PA.)

REPLACEMENT OF TISSUE WITH LIKE TISSUE

The concept of dividing the nose into aesthetic units has helped surgeons to achieve results that are more natural, allowing incision to fall along junctures of contour and shadowing.[11] The units are the nasal tip, alae, dorsum, and lateral side walls of the nose (Fig. 22–2).

Any reconstruction of the nose must strive to mimic the normal anatomy. One must, therefore, attend to the basic aesthetic components of the area involved and the associated aesthetic units. The method of reconstruction should preserve the color, thickness, and texture of the regional skin. The texture and thickness of the adjacent skin must be matched or the reconstruction will be obvious and inferior. Replacement of actinically damaged skin of the nasal dorsum with undamaged skin from the postauricular area may prove to be a glaring mismatch. The reconstruction should not distort the normal anatomy and in fact should merge with the remaining native tissue in the aesthetic unit. If this is not possible, then reconstruction of the entire aesthetic unit should be considered. At times, an optimal reconstruction may require the removal of normal tissue and reconstruction of the aesthetic unit as a whole.

When the underlying skeleton is missing, an effort must be made to reconstruct that skeleton. Over time, as edema subsides and wounds contract, the soft tissue of the reconstructed nose will reveal an absence of skeletal support. Finally, previous therapy may limit the availability of donor tissue. For instance, the use of a nasolabial flap may be prevented by the previous excision of a skin cancer or by radiation therapy. Such situations compel the reconstructive surgeon to be well versed in various reconstructive techniques.

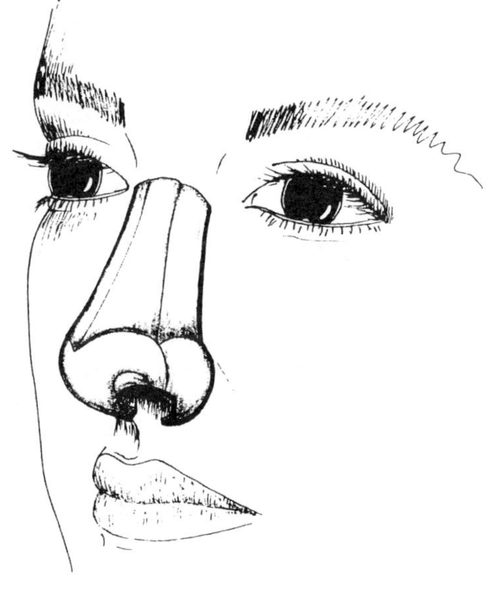

FIGURE 22–2. Aesthetic units of the nose.

PATIENT'S ROLE IN RECONSTRUCTION

The decision to use a particular flap or graft may be influenced by donor site availability as well as by patient choice or medical condition. Each decision in reconstruction must involve the patient. The patient's physical or psychological status may dictate that a lesser procedure be performed for a small defect and may not allow the conversion to a defect that incorporates the entire aesthetic unit or requires multiple stages.

TECHNIQUES

The following examples illustrate various techniques that can be used in nasal reconstruction. The format is an orderly progression of techniques from the simplest to the more technically challenging. In practice, as the nasal defects become more extensive or complicated, the reconstructive surgeon has to resort to more technically challenging reconstructive techniques.

Secondary Intention

In some circumstances, acceptable results may be achieved by simply allowing the wound to heal secondarily. Small medial canthal defects that spare the eyelids and are symmetrically located above and below the medial canthus can be left to heal secondarily. This increases the healing time, but the ultimate result can be satisfactory.

If the defect is more inferior or superior to the medial canthus, then the resulting cicatricial contracture results in pulling or distortion of the eyelid. Similarly, a defect near the tip or alar margin also results in contracture and distortion of the inferior aspect of the nose if healing occurs through secondary intention. For this reason, a graft or flap is necessary for the repair of most nasal defects.

Use of Dermabrasion in Partial-Thickness Defects

The removal of a superficial lesion (or trauma) may result in a partial-thickness defect of the nasal skin, leaving much of the dermis intact. In these limited cases, dermabrasion is a viable technique. It may be used to locally contour the tissue around the defect, or it can be used to blend the defect with the entire aesthetic unit. The case shown in Figure 22–3 illustrates the use of dermabrasion in this situation. Dermabrasion can play a crucial role in the final result of any technique of nasal reconstruction, especially in the refinement of scars involving thick, sebaceous skin.

Direct Primary Closure

Because of the paucity of available redundant skin on the nose, most defects do not lend themselves to simple fusiform closure. The simplest method of repair often is the best. Small (1-cm) full-thickness skin defects over the superior dorsum, lateral nasal wall, supratip, and infratip areas may be closed primarily (Figs. 22–4 and 22–5). Care must be taken to preserve symmetry and avoid distortion. If the defect is much larger than 1 cm, a graft or flap usually is necessary to avoid undue tip rotation or alar retraction.

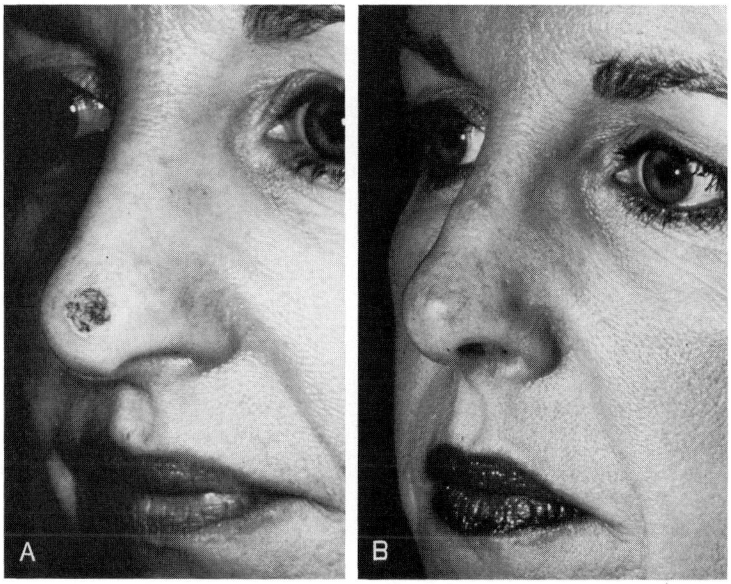

FIGURE 22–3. Dermabrasion alone may be enough to correct a partial-thickness skin defect. (*A*) Preoperative view of defect. (*B*) Postoperative view after dermabrasion of nasal skin to the level of the Mohs defect.

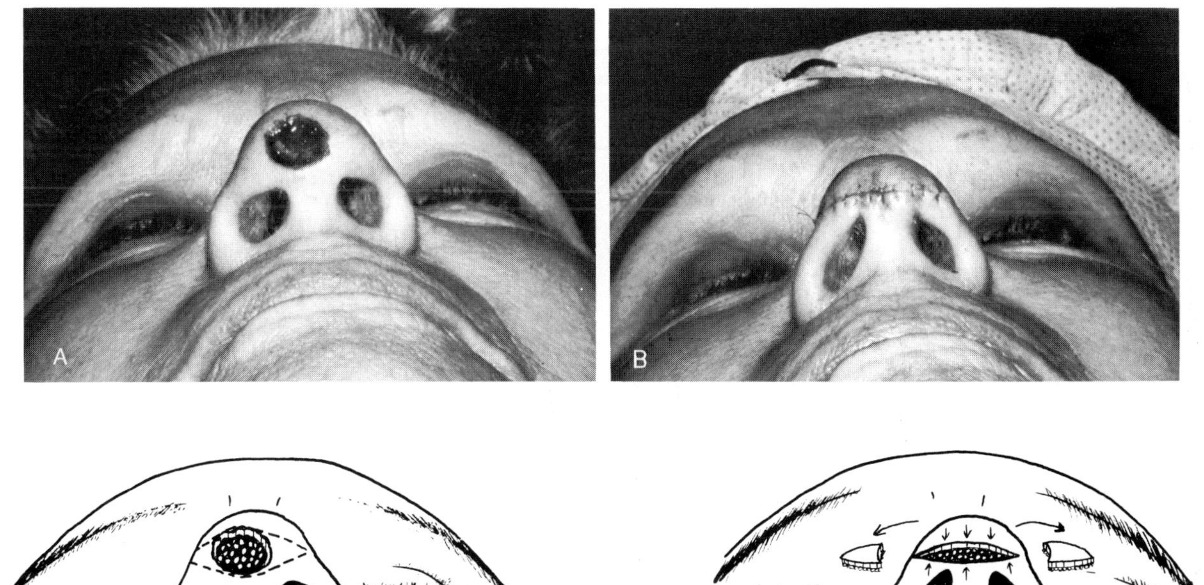

FIGURE 22–4. Infratip defects occasionally can be closed primarily. Note the improvement in this patient's nostril shape postoperatively. (*A*) Preoperative view of defect. (*B*) Intraoperative repair. (*C* and *D*) Schematics of *A* and *B*.

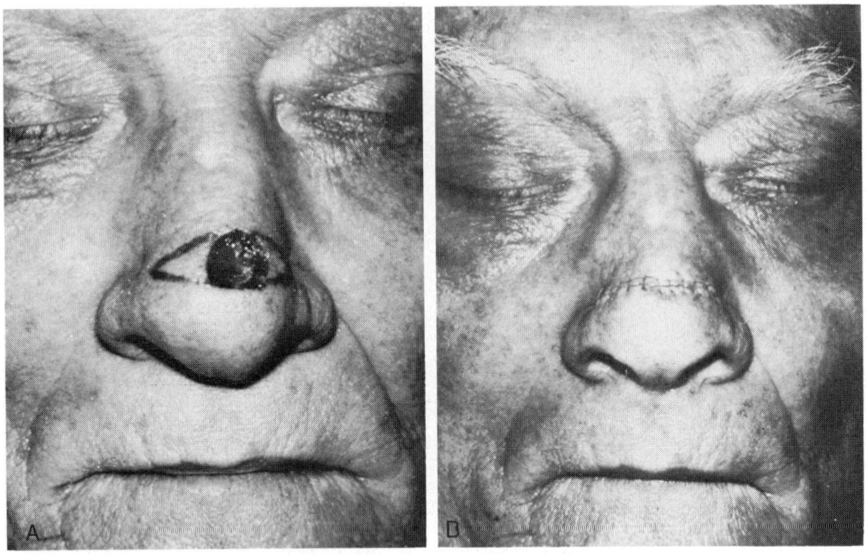

FIGURE 22–5. Supratip defects, when closed primarily, often can improve tip ptosis. This may not be a viable alternative in a young patient with a short nose. Also, the resulting horizontal scar usually requires follow-up dermabrasion in the patient with thick, sebaceous skin. (*A*) Resulting Mohs defect before reconstruction. Areas to be discarded are outlined. (*B*) Closed defect with improvement in senile tip ptosis.

Grafts and Flaps

If the defect is large enough or involves crucial tissues, then flaps, grafts, or a combination of these must be used. The decision as to which technique to use depends on a number of factors, including size and location of the defect, skin color and texture, and the patient's age and associated medical problems (Table 22–1). Each technique has advantages and disadvantages. One must analyze the particular problem and choose the technique that will achieve the best aesthetic and functional result.

TABLE 22–1. COMPARISON OF ADVANTAGES OF GRAFTS AND FLAPS

Grafts	Flaps
Availability of distal donor site tissue	Similar color and texture
Better in young patients	Good survival rate
Technically easy	Less contracture
Failure does not result in additional local deformity	Direct closure of secondary defects
	Good in older patients

FULL-THICKNESS SKIN GRAFTS

Full-thickness skin grafts are most effectively used in two circumstances. The first is in the case of a traumatic skin avulsion in which the tissue is available and in satisfactory condition for replantation. The second is in the case of a full-thickness skin defect with an intact cartilaginous and bony skeleton. A younger patient with a relatively small defect and thin skin often is a good candidate for a full-thickness skin graft. Full-thickness grafts are preferable to split-thickness grafts on the nose. Unless severe trauma or burns prevent their availability, full-thickness grafts should be used to avoid the contraction and deformity associated with split-thickness grafts. Donor site selection depends on the need to achieve optimal skin color and texture match. Typical donor sites are the postauricular, nasolabial, preauricular, and supraclavicular areas and the lobule of the ear (Fig. 22–6).[6, 12]

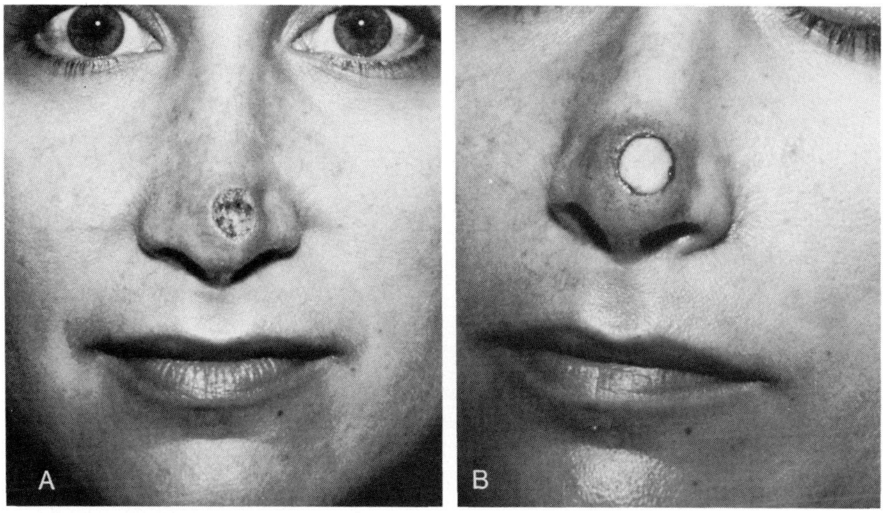

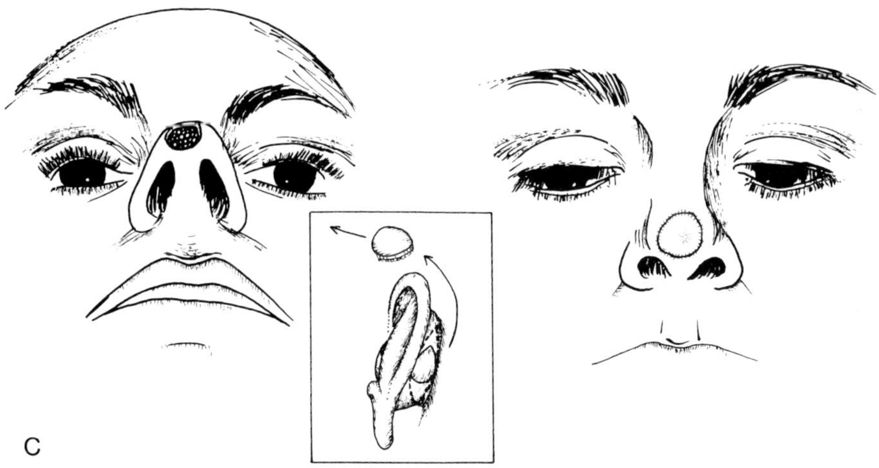

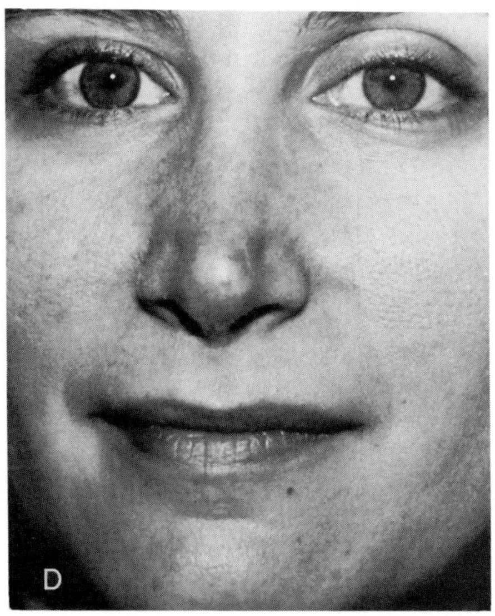

FIGURE 22–6. A full-thickness skin graft was used for the isolated skin defect in this young patient with thin skin. Her fair complexion and minimal actinic changes made this a viable reconstructive technique. (*A*) Preoperative view of defect. (*B*) Skin graft in place intraoperatively. (*C*) Postauricular donor site (inset). (*D*) Two-year follow-up shows acceptable texture and color match.

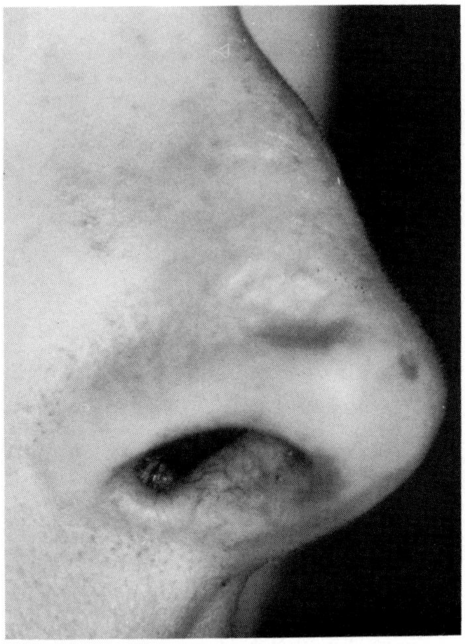

FIGURE 22–7. A thin skin graft may result in a depressed area if the recipient skin is thick and sebaceous.

Certain advantages are associated with the use of full-thickness skin grafts. The technique is easy to perform, and there usually is little donor site morbidity. Because younger patients do not have an excessive amount of loose adjacent skin, a local flap may not be available. A full-thickness skin graft may be a preferable choice. The disadvantages of full-thickness skin grafts include the possibility of poor color and texture match and the risk of pincushioning (convexity of a flap or graft occurring secondary to wound contracture). Skin grafts may remain erythematous or violaceous for prolonged periods, making the use of makeup or dermapigmentation necessary. If the patient has extremely thick nasal skin, the resulting graft may appear too thin or concave (Fig. 22–7). An ancillary technique, such as dermabrasion, may be necessary if the entire aesthetic unit is not replaced.

COMPOSITE, CHONDROCUTANEOUS, AND PERICHONDRIAL-CUTANEOUS FREE GRAFTS

These grafts are a further extension of the use of free full-thickness skin grafts. Composite and chondrocutaneous grafts include full-thickness skin and accompanying perichondrium and cartilage. They can be used when both the soft tissue and the underlying cartilaginous skeleton has been lost. The auricle is the usual donor site, using the conchal bowl, root of the helix, or helical rim. In general, the smaller the size of the composite graft, the greater the chance for successful revascularization and graft survival. Composite grafts designed with a maximal diameter of 1 cm are successful. It is recommended that a graft larger than 2 cm in diameter not be attempted. Others report success of larger grafts when the graft is designed with a larger skin component to promote earlier revascularization. Cooling with iced saline-soaked gauze pads may increase graft survival.[5, 8, 13]

The advantages of using composite grafts are that they maintain the shape and the support of the soft tissue. They frequently are used to reconstruct defects that involve the alar rim or columella. A disadvantage of using these grafts is the size limitation, although several techniques are described that may extend this limitation. Also, depending on the patient's age and actinic damage, the skin of the auricle may be a poor match for the nasal skin. Finally, larger grafts result in difficulty in obtaining a satisfactory closure of the ear donor site (Fig. 22–8; see also Fig. 22–15).

Some authors advocate the use of perichondrial-cutaneous grafts,[14] which contain full-thickness skin and accompanying perichondrium. The donor site, as in chondrocutaneous grafts, usually is the external ear. The reported advantage of these grafts is that they provide more bulk than full-thickness skin grafts. The perichondrium may enhance revascularization of the grafted skin and, hence, lessen the risk of graft loss. There may also be less graft shrinkage and contracture.

LOCAL SKIN FLAPS

The use of local flaps may represent the most favorable method for reconstructing small to moderate-sized defects.[15–18] The transposed tissue usually provides the best texture, color, and thickness match for the missing tissue. If the flaps are properly designed, there is minimal donor site morbidity, and additional scars are placed within the local region to be reconstructed.

Bilobed and rhomboid flaps are ideal for such reconstructions. The advantage of these local flap techniques is that the tissue donor site is in the same general anatomic area of the nose in which the defect is located. Similar tissue, therefore, is brought into the area. The vectors of tension commonly are directed horizontally, thereby avoiding retraction of the nasal tip and alae. Skin defects that are between 2 and 3 cm in diameter and involve the nasal tip respond well to the use of a bilobed flap. Rhomboid flaps are useful for smaller defects. The disadvantages of using these local flaps include pincushioning and the creation of larger and more complex scars on the nose. The size of the defect to be reconstructed is also limited by the amount of laxity of available tissue on the nose and adjacent structures (Figs. 22–9 through 22–11).

The proper design of these flaps is the most critical step in their use. The design of the flap must address the following issues: the ability to transfer the necessary amount of tissue to the area to be reconstructed without producing distortion and undue tension, appropriate tissue match, and proper placement of incisions to produce the least noticeable scars in the recipient and donor sites.

When the defect is too large or in a poor location for reconstruction with local nasal tissue, then nasolabial flaps frequently are used.[8, 19] They have many uses in moderate to large reconstructions but have only limited use in tip reconstructions.

Nasolabial flaps offer several advantages when compared with more distant flaps. The donor site is in an area that is adjacent to the patient's nasal defect. Skin texture usually is similar to that of the nose. Furthermore, age-related skin laxity provides an abundance of available tissue. The resultant incisions are easy to camouflage in an elderly patient (Fig. 22–12; see also Fig. 22–15). Because the vascularity of the flap is extremely reliable, flap failure seldom is a problem. Skeletal support frequently can be supplied with the use of septal and conchal cartilage grafts. Lining can be provided by folding the flap or using other local turn-in flaps as well as by composite grafts.

Although the nasolabial area can supply tissue that is similar to that of distal nasal skin, a major disadvantage is that these flaps usually are bulky and prone to developing prolonged edema. If the flap cannot be designed with a pedicle that is incorporated into the nasal reconstruction, a second stage is required to sever the pedicle. Improper flap design also distorts the normal anatomic features, such as the nasal-facial junction. Finally, the flap is difficult to design without significant donor site morbidity in the younger patient.

Text continued on page 335

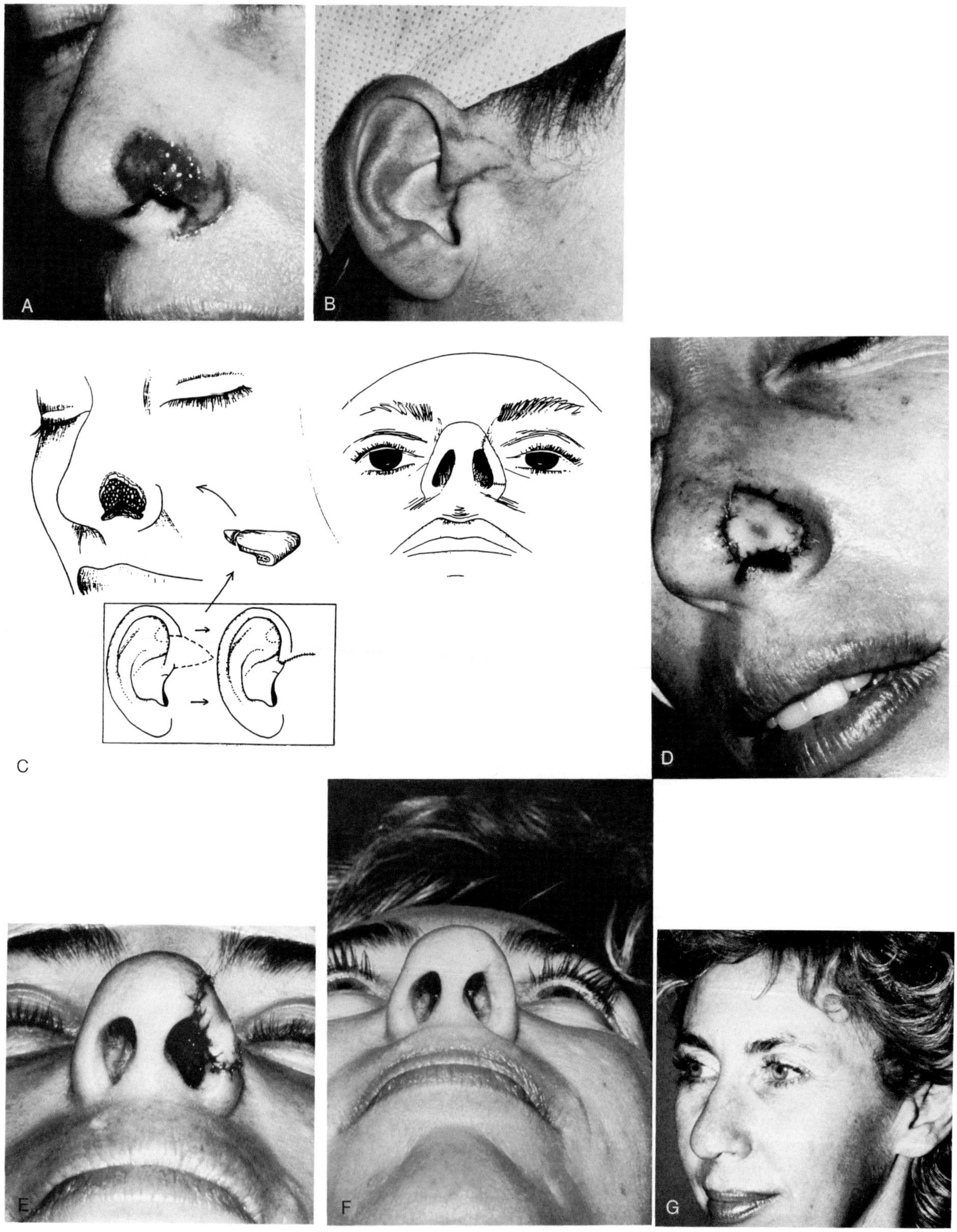

FIGURE 22–8. A composite graft from the contralateral auricular helical root was used to reconstruct this alar defect. (*A*) Preoperative view of defect. (*B*) Preoperative view of donor site. (*C*) Donor site may be closed primarily. (*D* and *E*) Intraoperative view with graft in place. Larger skin paddle may increase the chance for graft survival. (*F* and *G*) One-year postoperative outcome.

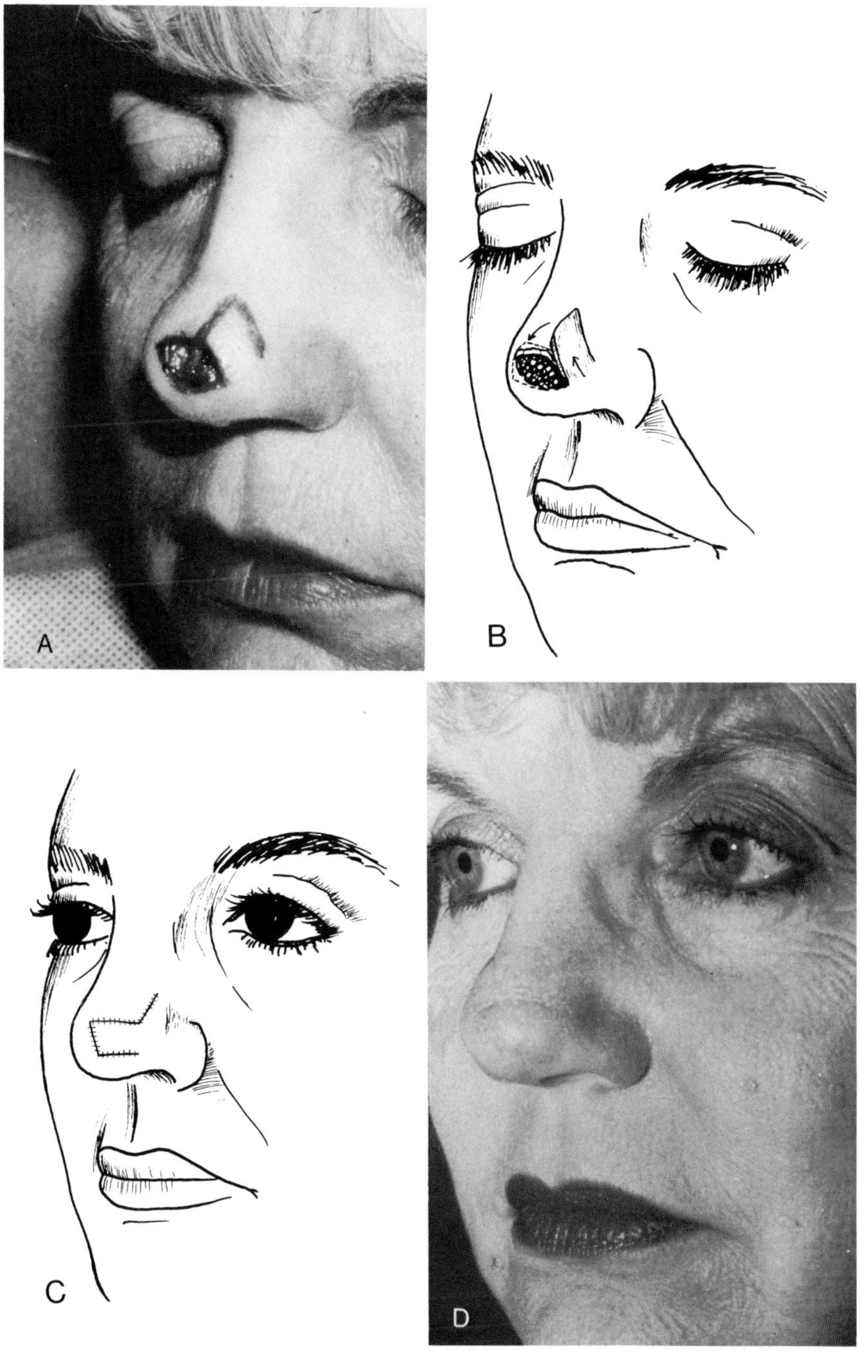

FIGURE 22–9. A rhomboid flap was used for this tip defect, thereby reducing the potential for alar and tip retraction. (*A* and *B*) Preoperative view of defect. (*C*) Postoperative view. (*D*) One-year follow-up without dermabrasion.

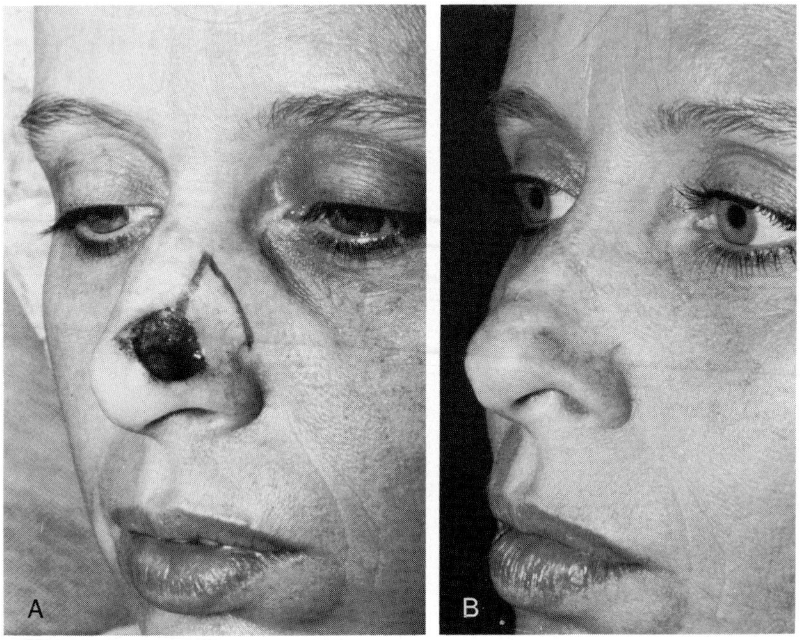

FIGURE 22–10. A supratip defect corrected with a rhomboid flap. Larger defects than this may require an alternative method. (*A*) Preoperative view. (*B*) One-year postoperative outcome without dermabrasion.

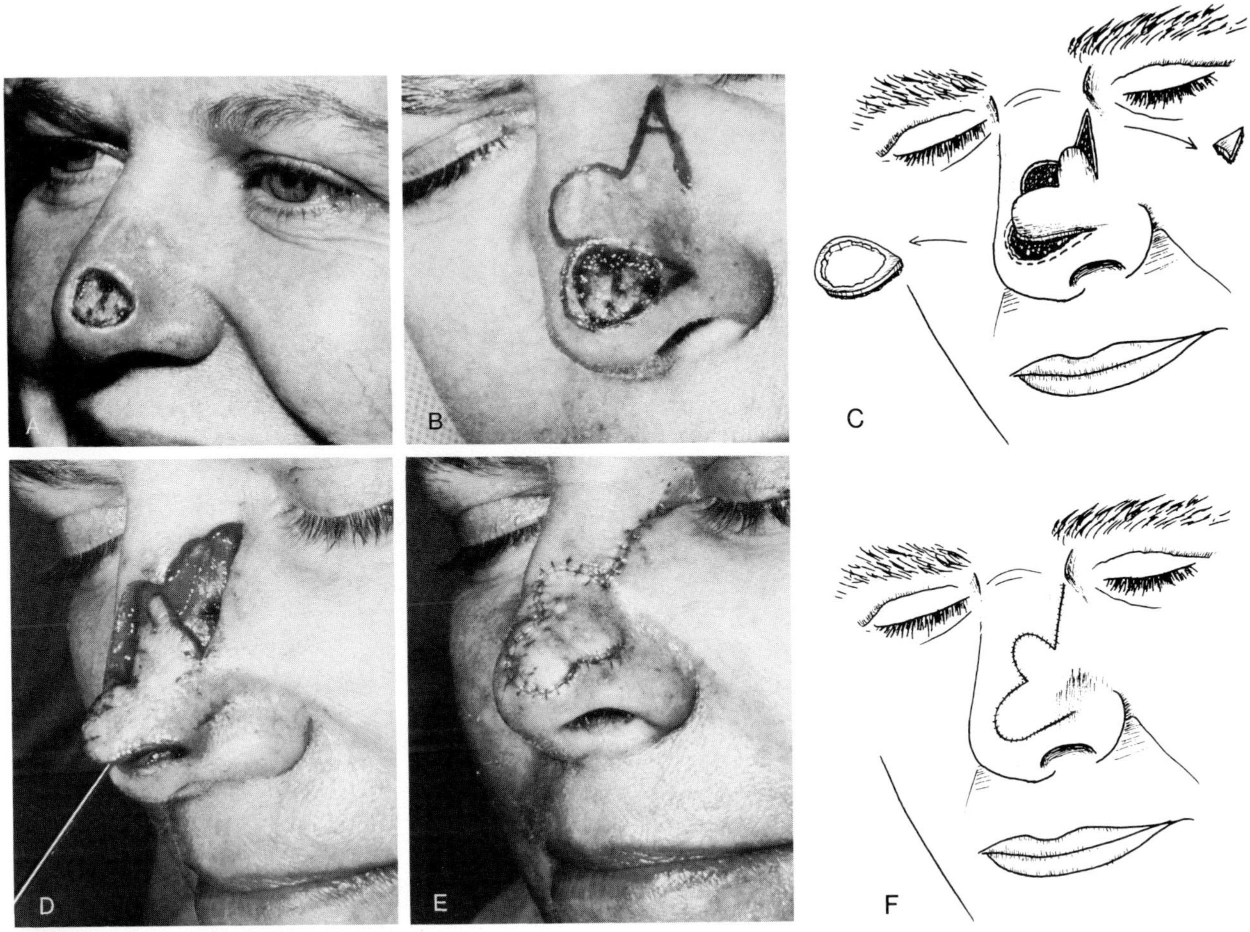

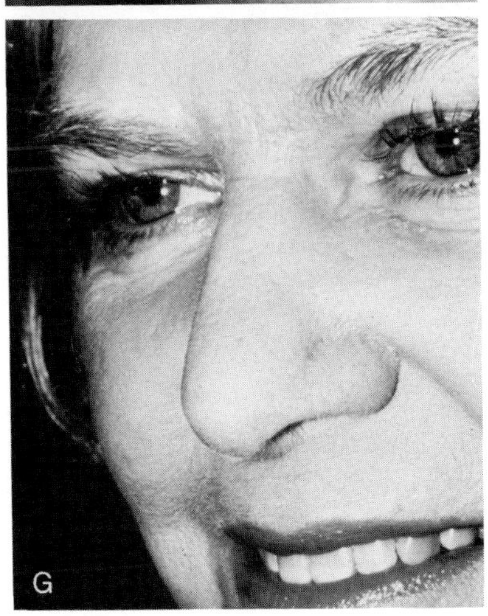

FIGURE 22–11. A bilobed flap was used for this 2.5-cm tip defect. (*A*) Preoperative view. (*B, C, D, E,* and *F*) Intraoperative views. (*G*) Two-year post-operative outcome. Dermabrasion was performed 3 months after the flap was transferred.

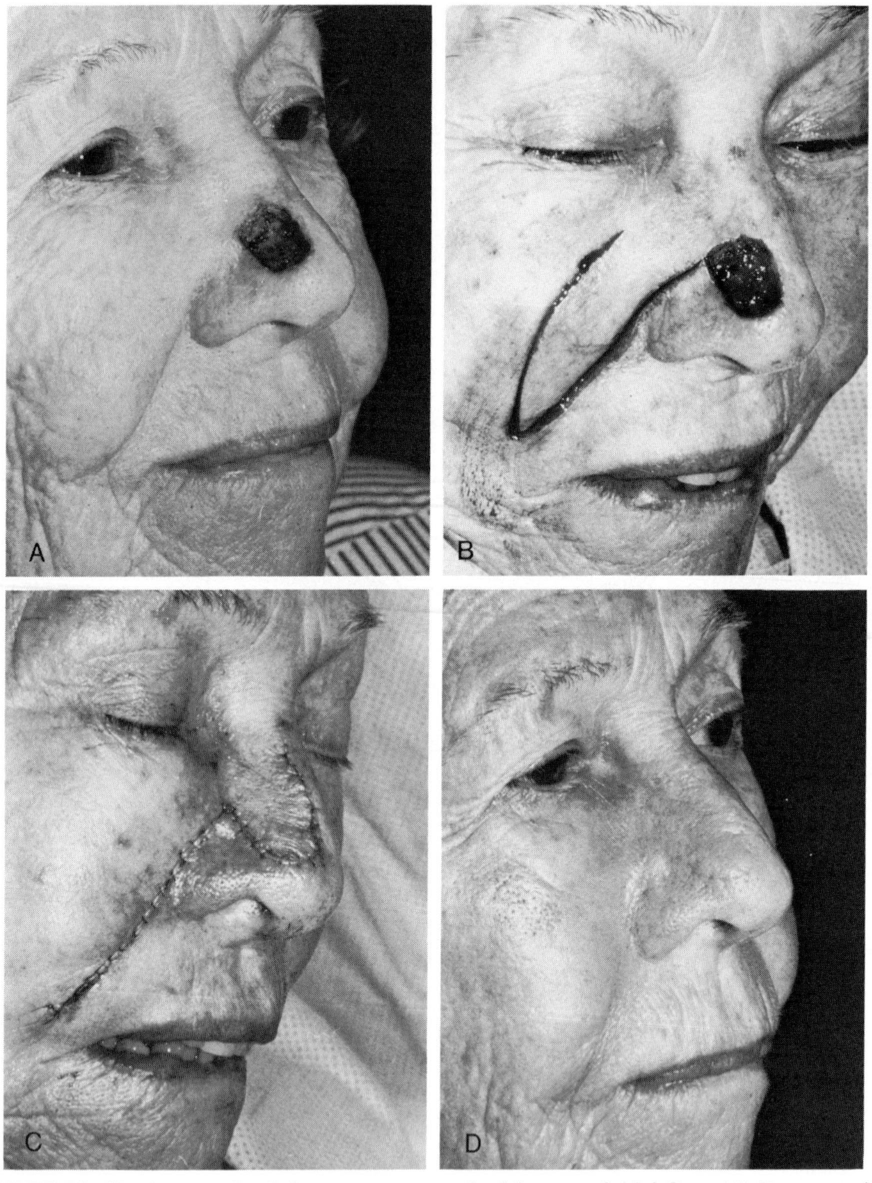

FIGURE 22–12. A supratip defect reconstructed with a nasolabial flap. (*A*) Preoperative view. (*B* and *C*) Intraoperative views. (*D*) One-year postoperative outcome.

A modification of the nasolabial flap is the island pedicle flap.[20] The main advantages of this technique are that it eliminates the need to divide a flap pedicle at a later step and that it preserves the crucial alar-facial groove that often is obliterated when using the standard nasolabial flap. By tunneling under the remaining bridge of alar skin, the groove between the alae and the cheek is retained. The island pedicle flap is useful for skin defects over the alae but usually does not extend to the nasal tip (Fig. 22–13).

FOREHEAD FLAPS

The forehead flap is among the earlier methods of nasal reconstruction that have endured over time. When a defect is too large to allow the use of local flaps or the reasonable use of a free graft, then a more distant flap has to be used. If a defect occupies more than 50 per cent of the aesthetic unit, the removal of the remaining skin from the aesthetic unit and reconstruction of the entire aesthetic unit should be considered.[12, 21]

The forehead flap is probably the most frequently used distant flap for nasal reconstruction.[22–25] Several alternative designs allow for lengthening of the pedicle and for various positions of the donor site on the forehead. An advantage of these flaps is their ability to supply large amounts of tissue with a reliable axial blood supply usually based on the supratrochlear artery and vein. Some designs also incorporate the supraorbital vessels. The converse scalping forehead flap has an alternative design and incorporates the supratrochlear, supraorbital, and superficial temporal vessels.[26] The disadvantages of using forehead flaps are that they usually require at least two stages and subsequent procedures need to be performed to refine the result. The donor site area is outside the area to be reconstructed and produces a vertical or an oblique forehead scar that may heal poorly in the younger patient. Although the forehead provides an abundance of tissue for reconstruction, its color and texture can be different from those of the native nasal tissue. Despite these drawbacks, it usually is the flap of choice for larger nasal defects (Fig. 22–14).

The Washio flap is mentioned as an alternative flap that may be used in the younger patient or in other situations in which a forehead donor site cannot be used.[27] This flap allows the transfer of retroauricular skin to the nose and avoids a forehead scar. The major disadvantage of the flap is that it has a more tenuous blood supply based on the superficial temporal vessels and sometimes requires a delay, or staged revascularization of the flap.

LINING AND SKELETAL SUPPORT

Full-thickness nasal defects require replacement of not only external skin but also lining and skeletal support. This repair is more complex and necessitates the use of multiple flaps and/or grafts.

The lining should be replaced with tissues that closely resemble those that were removed—ideally, mucosa. Multiple techniques can be used, including mucosal advancement flaps, septal chondromucosal flaps, infolded tips of forehead or nasolabial flaps, or skin grafts.

Local turned-in flaps are easiest to perform but may be too bulky, depending on the thickness of the adjacent skin. These flaps must be designed to avoid airway obstruction. Mucosal advancement or septal chondromucosal flaps may achieve a more functional airway but can be more technically difficult to perform.

Defects extending from the alar margin to the inferior edge of the upper lateral cartilages are of great consequence, and without proper lining,

Text continued on page 338

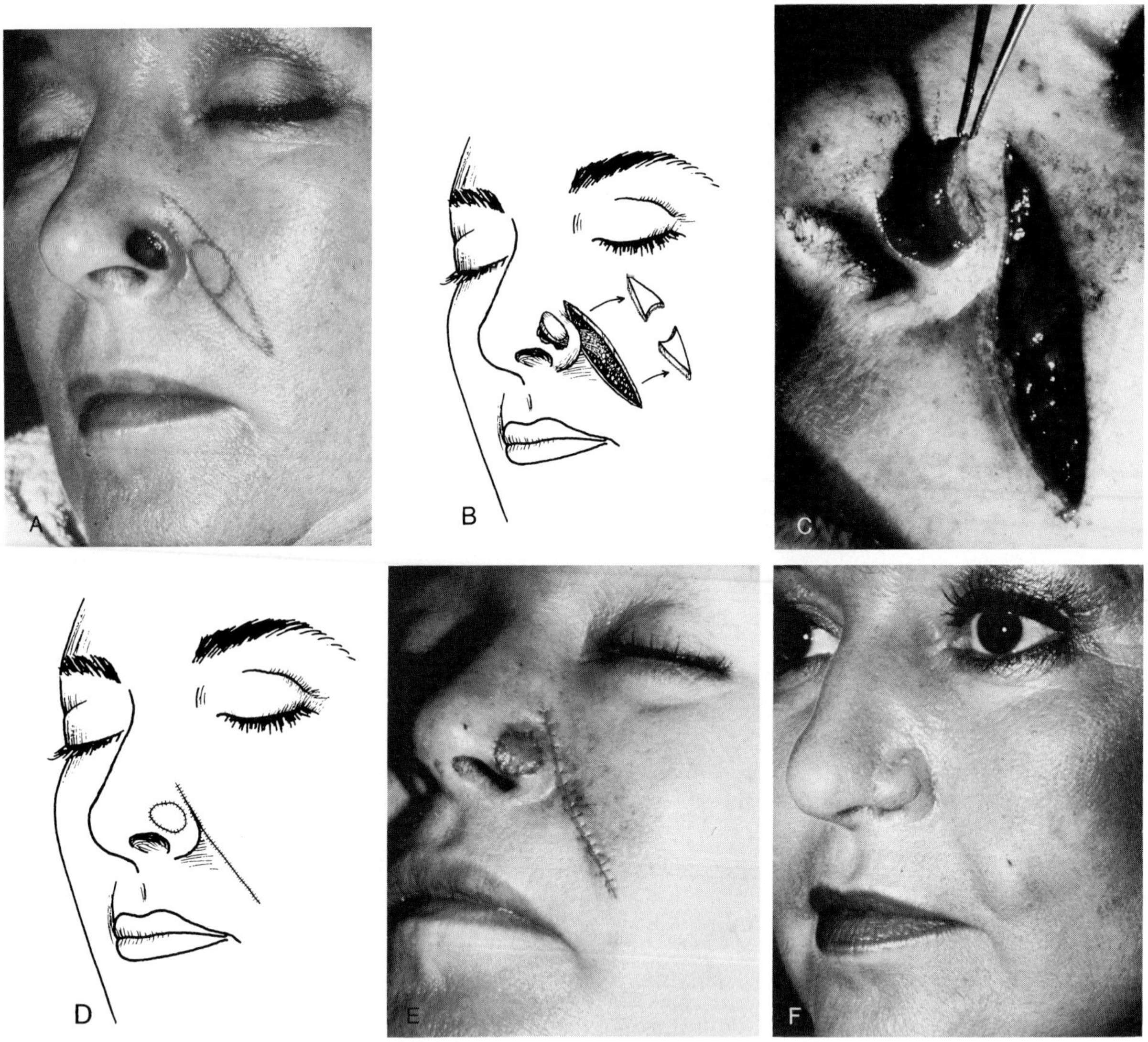

FIGURE 22–13. An island pedicle flap was used for this alar skin defect. The alar facial groove is preserved without the need for secondary procedures. (*A*) Preoperative view. (*B, C, D,* and *E*) Intraoperative views. (*F*) One-year postoperative outcome. Further improvement could be obtained with dermabrasion, but the patient declined further refinement.

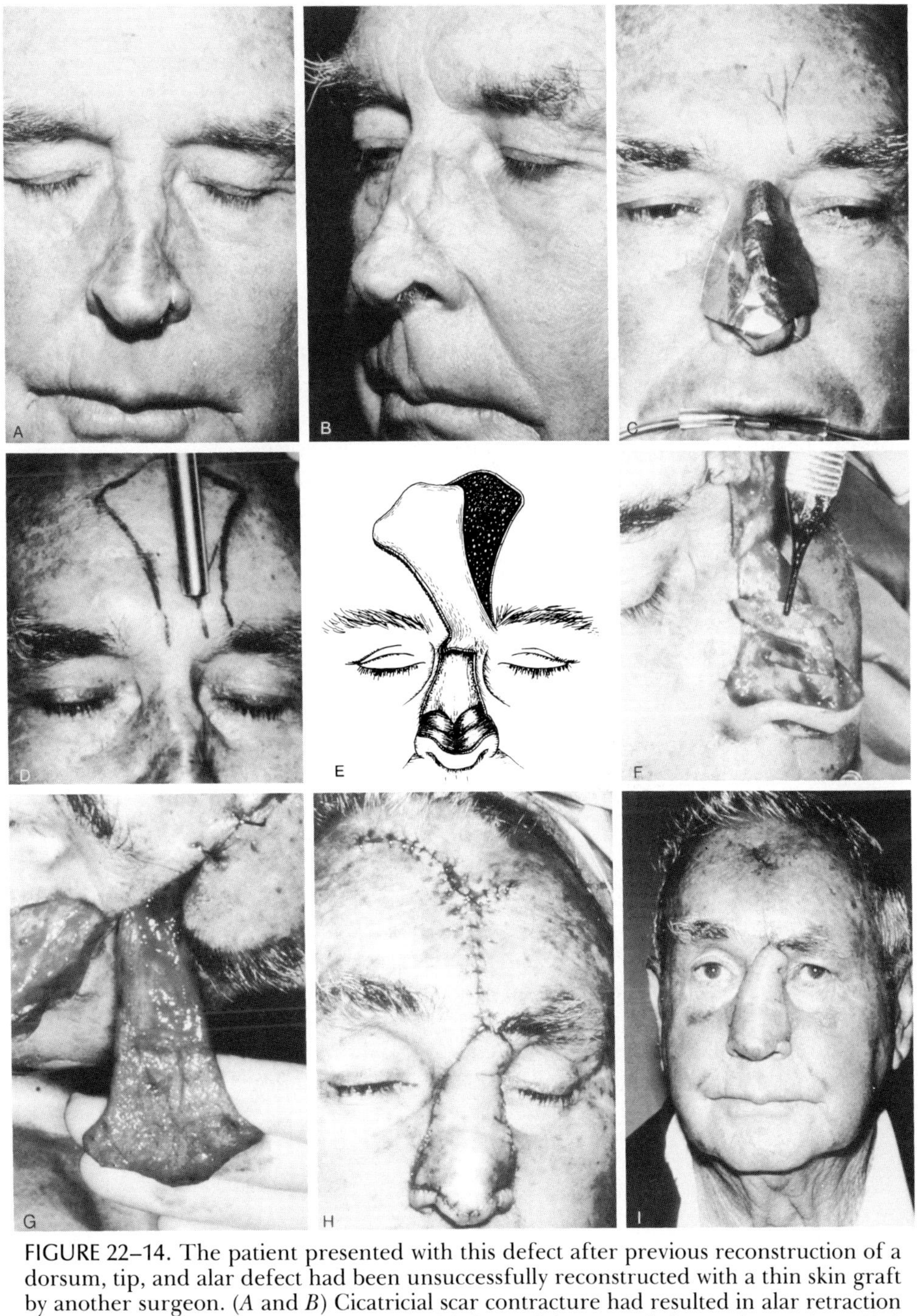

FIGURE 22–14. The patient presented with this defect after previous reconstruction of a dorsum, tip, and alar defect had been unsuccessfully reconstructed with a thin skin graft by another surgeon. (*A* and *B*) Cicatricial scar contracture had resulted in alar retraction and vestibular stenosis, which caused his chief complaint—nasal airway obstruction. (*C*) A template is used to outline the aesthetic units for resurfacing with a forehead flap. (*D*) The Doppler is used to identify and preserve the supratrochlear vessels. (*E* and *F*) Convex auricular conchal cartilage grafts are used to support the weakness in the nasal valve area. The mucosa remains intact. (*G*) The flap is thinned distally. (*H*) The donor site is closed primarily. (*I*) One week follow-up. The flap pedicle is divided at 3 weeks. *Illustration continued on following page.*

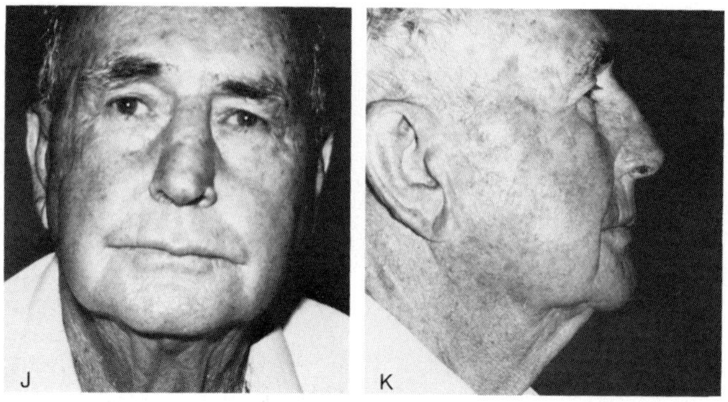

FIGURE 22–14 *Continued* (*J* and *K*) One-year postoperative outcome.

there will, ultimately, be wound contracture, distortion, and, possibly, airway compromise. More proximal defects are less critical and can be treated with skin grafts on the undersurface of the overlying flap.

Skeletal support can be achieved by cartilage or bone grafts. The choice largely depends on the defect's location. For defects that involve the distal nose, cartilage grafts are preferable. Donor sites include conchal cartilage, septal cartilage, and costal cartilage. Irradiated costal cartilage homograft may be used, but it frequently is resorbed to some degree after many years; autologous cartilage is preferred.

Conchal cartilage graft is ideal for replacing the convexity of the lower lateral cartilages. It can be used as a free cartilage graft or with its associated skin used for lining (Figs. 22–15 and 22–16; see also Fig. 22–14).

Defects that involve the total nose require more complicated bony and/or cartilage replacement. These commonly include cantilevered bone grafts, nasal septal hinge flaps, and various struts.

The cantilever bone graft is preferably harvested as a split calvarial graft and fixed into position with small metal plates. Split calvarial bone is less readily resorbed than iliac or costal bone and is thought to be a superior donor site, if available.

Inferior and superior septal hinge flaps incorporate full-thickness septal bone or cartilage with accompanying bilateral septal mucosal flaps. The septum is swung anteriorly to create a foundation on which the new nose is reconstructed.[2, 3, 21, 28–30] The use of the septal hinge flap has virtually revolutionized the concept of total nasal reconstruction and should be considered when one is faced with such an extensive defect. A thorough discussion of this technique is beyond the scope of this text.

SUMMARY

The nose occupies such a critical aspect of the human face that reconstruction of defects commands an astute appreciation of both reconstructive principles and the delicate aesthetics of the area. The surgeon who attempts nasal reconstruction must, therefore, have various techniques at his disposal.

Although nasal reconstruction is as much a surgical art as it is a science, the following generalizations can be delineated.

1. The technique that causes the least morbidity (i.e., the least additional incisions and scarring) frequently is the method that is best chosen. Simple is best.

Text continued on page 342

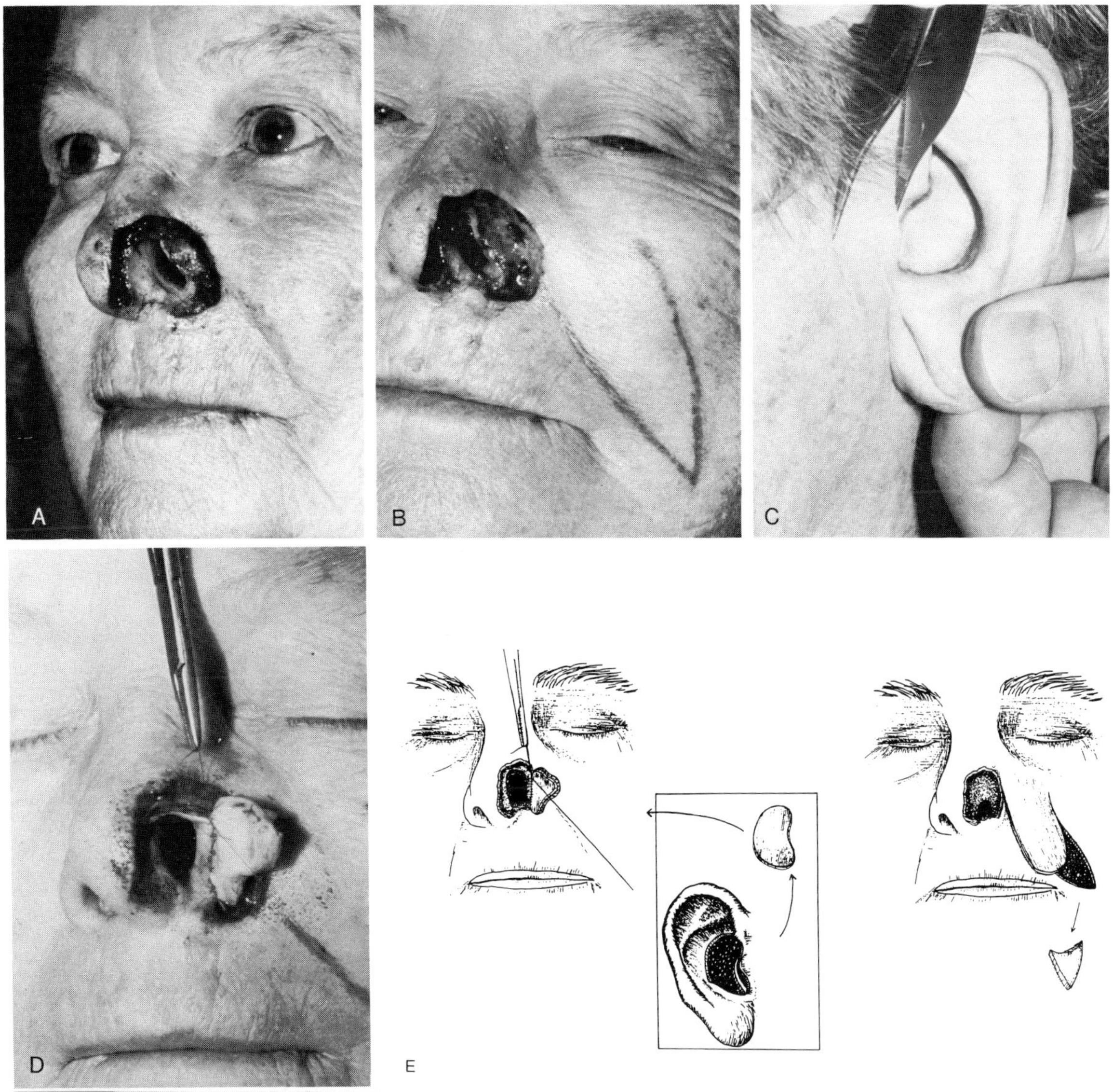

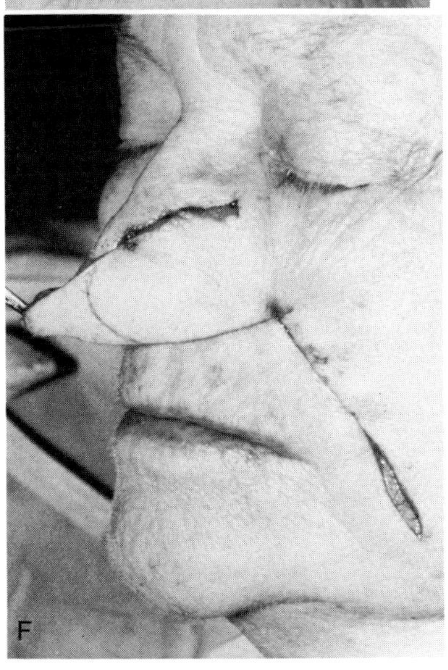

FIGURE 22–15. This alar, tip, and lateral wall defect required lining, skeletal support, and skin coverage. (*A*) Preoperative view. (*B*, *C*, *D*, *E*, and *F*) Intraoperative views. A chondrocutaneous auricular conchal graft is used for lining and support. A nasolabial flap is used for skin coverage. *Illustration continued on following page.*

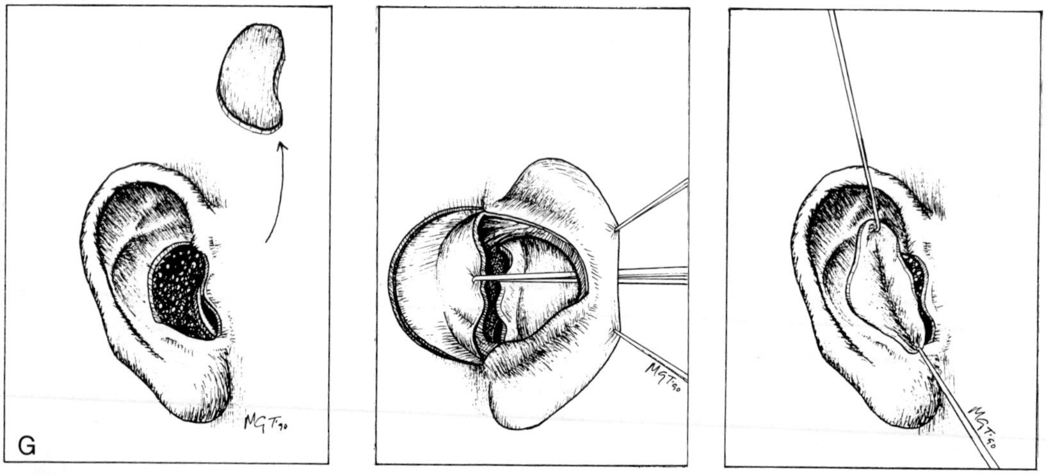

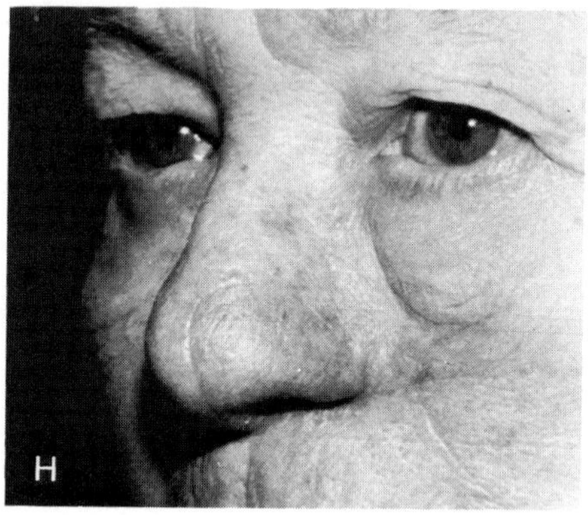

FIGURE 22–15 *Continued* (*G*) The auricular donor defect is closed with a postauricular-island pedicle flap. (*H*) Two-year follow-up after staged revision of the alar facial groove.

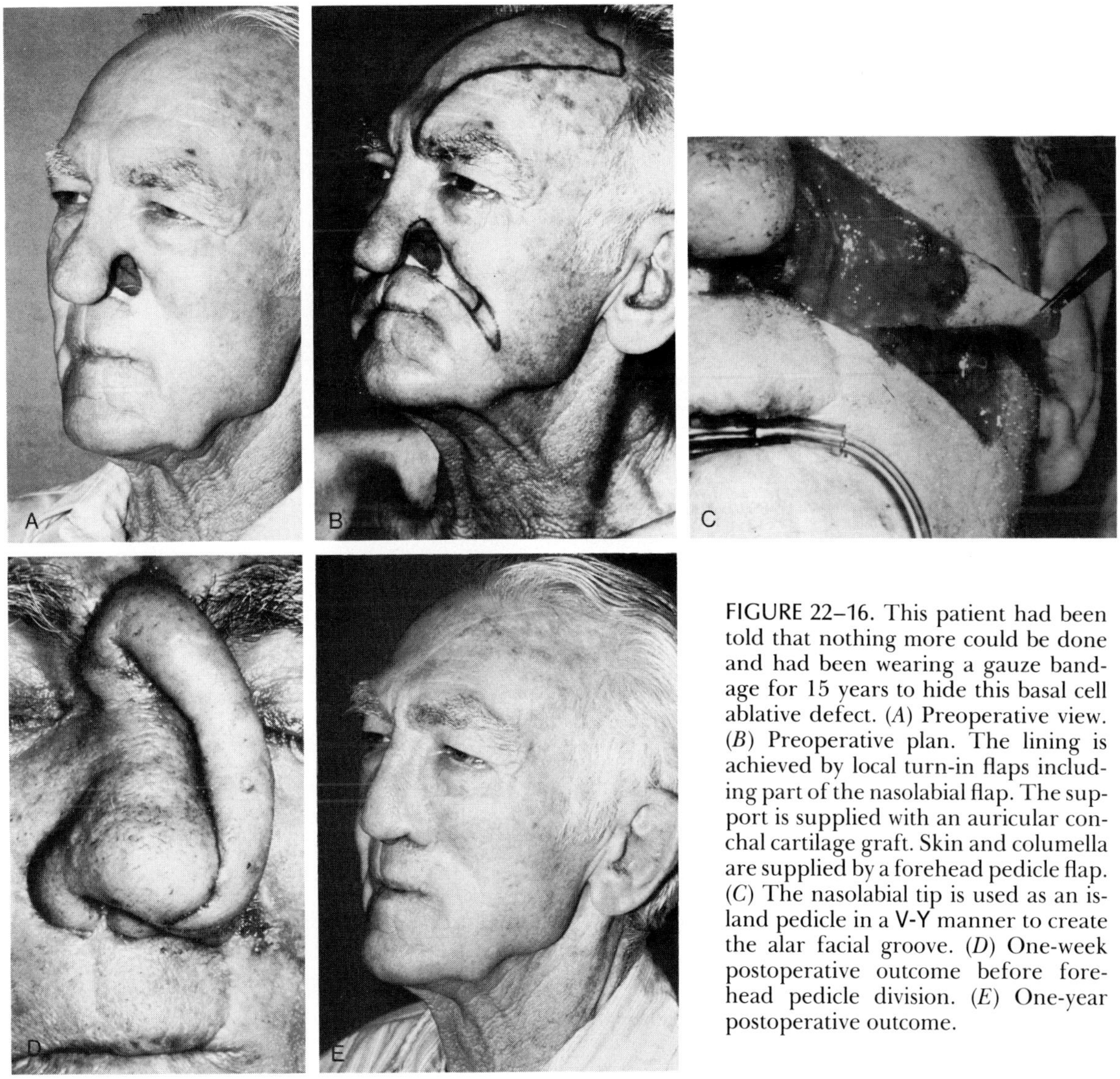

FIGURE 22–16. This patient had been told that nothing more could be done and had been wearing a gauze bandage for 15 years to hide this basal cell ablative defect. (*A*) Preoperative view. (*B*) Preoperative plan. The lining is achieved by local turn-in flaps including part of the nasolabial flap. The support is supplied with an auricular conchal cartilage graft. Skin and columella are supplied by a forehead pedicle flap. (*C*) The nasolabial tip is used as an island pedicle in a V-Y manner to create the alar facial groove. (*D*) One-week postoperative outcome before forehead pedicle division. (*E*) One-year postoperative outcome.

2. Reconstruction of nasal defects often is optimized by staged procedures such as scar revision and dermabrasion. Because the goals are not only to restore nasal function but also to create a natural appearance, methods that enhance results should be used.

3. In choosing a reconstructive technique, especially in the design of flaps and grafts, one should plan a backup procedure if the primary technique fails to satisfy the goal of reconstruction.

4. Whenever possible, patients should have an active part in choosing a particular reconstructive technique. They should understand the risks, limits, and alternatives to the procedures proposed.

References

1. Mazzola, R.F., Marcus, S. History of nasal reconstruction with particular emphasis on the folded forehead flap technique. Plast Reconstr Surg 72:408–414, 1983.
2. Gullane, P.J. Nasal reconstruction. J Otolaryngol 9:455–461, 1980.
3. Millard, D.R. Total reconstructive rhinoplasty and a missing link. Plast Reconstr Surg 37:167–183, 1966.
4. Miller, T.A. Nasal reconstruction. Surg Clin North Am 66:189–200, 1986.
5. Maves, M.D., Yessenow, R.S. The use of composite auricular grafts in nasal reconstruction. J Dermatol Surg Oncol 14:994–999, 1988.
6. Manson, P.N., Hoopes, J.E., Chambers, R.G., Jaques, D.A. Algorithm for nasal reconstruction. Am J Surg 138:528–532, 1979.
7. Miller, T.A. The Tagliacozzi flap as a method of nasal and palatal reconstruction. Plast Reconstr Surg 76:870–874, 1985.
8. Bennett, J.E. Reconstruction of lateral nasal defects. Clin Plast Surg 8:597–598, 1981.
9. Ohmori, K., Sekiquchi, J., Ohmori, S. Total rhinoplasty with free osteocutaneous flap. Plast Reconstr Surg 63:387–394, 1979.
10. Panje, W.R. A new method for total nasal reconstruction: The trapezius myocutaneous island paddle flap. Arch Otolaryngol 108:156–161, 1982.
11. Burget, G.C., Menick, F.J., The subunit principle in nasal reconstruction. Plast Reconstr Surg 76:239–247, 1985.
12. Millard, D.R. Reconstructive rhinoplasty of the tip. Clin Plast Surg 8:507–520, 1981.
13. Barton, F.E. Aesthetic aspects of partial nasal reconstruction. Clin Plast Surg 8:177–191, 1981.
14. Brent, B., Ott, R. Perichondro-cutaneous graft. Plast Reconstr Surg 62:1–4, 1978.
15. McGregor, J.C., Soutar, D.S. A critical assessment of the bilobed flap. Br J Plast Surg 34:197–205, 1981.
16. Borges, A.F. Choosing the correct Limberg flap. Plast Reconstr Surg 62:542–545, 1978.
17. Elliot, R.A. Rotation flaps of the nose. Plast Reconstr Surg 44:146–149, 1969.
18. Rigg, B.M. The dorsal nasal flap. Plast Reconstr Surg 52:361–364, 1973.
19. Guerrerosantos, J., Dicksheet, S. Nasolabial flap with simultaneous cartilage graft in nasal alar reconstruction. Clin Plast Surg 8:599–602, 1981.
20. Herbert, D.C. A subcutaneous pedicled cheek flap for reconstruction of alar defects. Br J Plast Surg 31:79–92, 1978.
21. Millard, D.R. Aesthetic reconstructive rhinoplasty. Clin Plast Surg 8:169–175, 1981.
22. Thomas, J.R., Griner, N., Cook, T.A. The precise midline forehead flap as a musculocutaneous flap. Arch Otolaryngol Head Neck Surg 114:79–84, 1988.
23. Adamson, J.E. Nasal reconstruction with the expanded forehead flap. Plast Reconstr Surg 81:12–20, 1988.
24. Millard, D.R. Reconstructive rhinoplasty for the lower two-thirds of the nose. Plast Reconstr Surg 57:722–728, 1976.
25. Mendleson, B.C., Masson, J.K., Arnold, P.G., Erich, J.B. Flaps used for nasal reconstruction: A perspective based on 180 cases. Mayo Clin Proc 54:91–96, 1979.
26. Converse, J.M. New forehead flap for nasal reconstruction. Proc R Soc Med 35:811–812, 1942.
27. Washio, H. Retroauricular-temporal flap. Plast Reconstr Surg 43:162–166, 1969.
27a. Millard, D.R. Various uses of the septum in rhinoplasty. Plast Reconstr Surg 81: 112–129, 1988.
28. Burget, G.C., Menick, F.J. Nasal reconstruction: Seeking a fourth dimension. Plast Reconstr Surg 78:145–157, 1986.
29. Burget, G.C., Menick, F.J. Nasal support and lining: The marriage of beauty and blood supply. Plast Reconstr Surg 84:189–203, 1989.

CHAPTER 23

Surgical Scar Revision

Unsightly, disfiguring scars or defects on the face can be disconcerting as well as devastating to one's self-image. The appearance of most scars or blemishes may be improved by well-planned and carefully executed surgery, but there are some important facts patients contemplating such procedures should know.

Scars are unsightly because they may be wide or longer than 1 inch; they may be elevated above or depressed below adjacent skin; or they may cross natural creases or facial contours or be a different color from adjacent tissues. An improvement in any one of these characteristics should make the scar less conspicuous. The correction of two or three of these factors often results in dramatic improvement of the appearance of the scar and relieves unwanted traction on surrounding tissues. Surgical treatment for deep scars and skin defects implies that incisions usually are made to remove the existing scar or blemish. Superficial scars may be improved with dermabrasion alone (Fig. 23–1).

Patients should be reminded that when an incision is made into the skin, regardless of where it is placed, who makes it, for what purpose it is made, or whether it is deliberate or accidental, it heals in the same manner as any other cut; that is, it produces scar tissue, nature's method of healing. This simple fact frequently is forgotten or ignored by some people who think that a plastic surgeon can make an incision and leave no visible scars and that he can in fact eliminate existing scars.

The surgeon's goal is to replace an unsightly or disfiguring scar with a better scar, one that is more narrow and more level, that blends with the

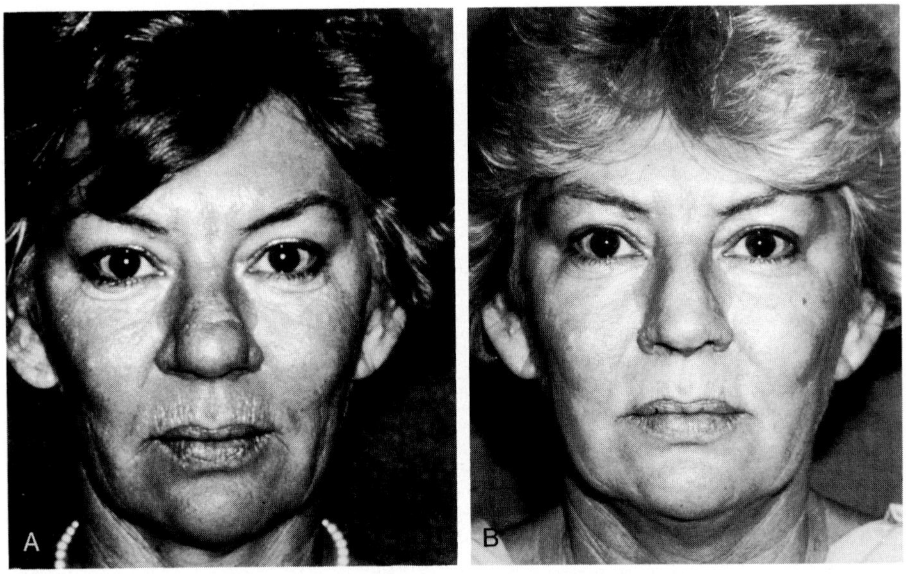

FIGURE 23–1. (*A*) A depressed scar is present in a patient with early rhinophyma. (*B*) Dermabrasion may virtually eliminate the depression and improve the texture of the surrounding skin.

surrounding skin surface, and that causes no contracture or pull on the surrounding structures: in short, a scar that is as inconspicuous as possible. The final appearance of any scar depends on many factors, particularly the patient's own healing capability (Fig. 23–2).

The maturation of scars may take from 6 to 18 months and sometimes longer, especially in young children. Initially, a freshly repaired scar usually looks acceptable. Then it reddens, may be somewhat raised above the surrounding skin, and frequently is hard or lumpy. The firmness and redness gradually lessen and should disappear, leaving a softer scar that is more level and lighter in color than the adjacent skin.

Patients seeking scar revision should be emotionally prepared to accept the fact that the removal of a scar will result in another (one hopes) improved scar and that the final appearance will not be evident for 6 to 18 months. Also, in most cases, more than one procedure may be required.

Most people with recent scarring want repair immediately; however, scar revision, except in selected cases, should not be undertaken too soon. The passage of time is the best, kindest, and, in the long run, simplest treatment to give a scar of recent origin because most undergo spontaneous improvement if given enough time to do so (often 6 to 18 months).

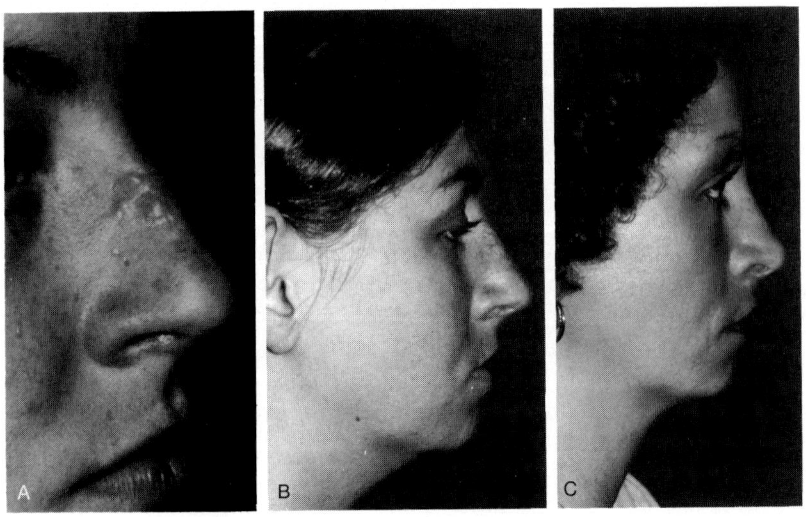

FIGURE 23–2. This patient sustained an injury to her nose that resulted in a deviation in the septum and pyramid. (*A* and *B*) Staged reconstruction, including scar revision, was planned, but after septorhinoplasty, the scar softened and flattened and the redness faded. (*C*) No additional surgery was desired.

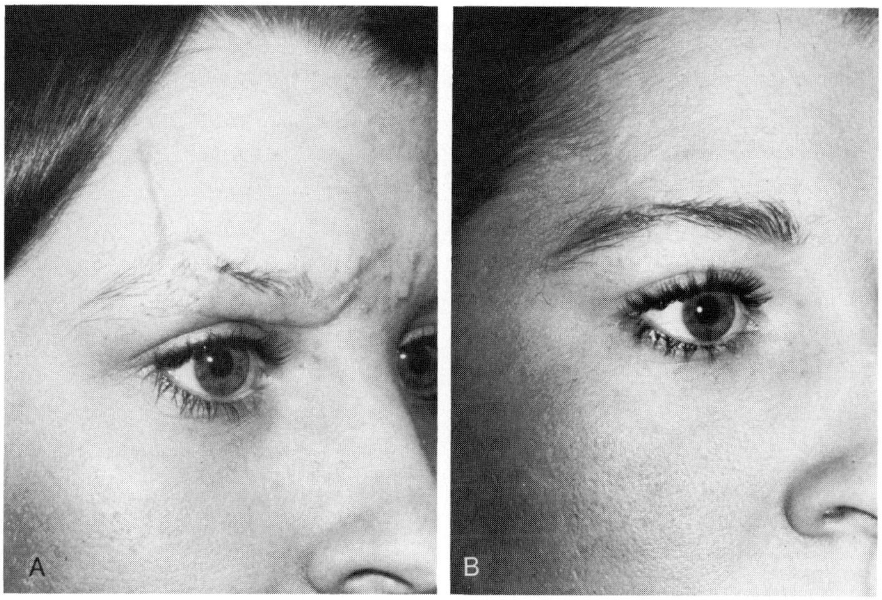

FIGURE 23–3. (*A*) Traumatic injuries often produce irregular scarring, as seen in this patient. (*B*) Surgical scar camouflaging may require excision of the existing scar with geometric broken-line closure, dermabrasion, and intralesional steroid injections. Several procedures performed at 3- to 6-month intervals usually are necessary. Only dermabrasion was performed on the scars of the glabella.

Only after the scar has become soft and white is it mature. A decision regarding a second-stage revision may be delayed until this time. Scars that distort normal structures (e.g., lips, nostrils), those that spread widely or produce deformity by contraction, and U- or J-shaped scars may be repaired earlier because little or no improvement in the basic problem can be anticipated with the passage of time (Fig. 23–3).

When removing an existing scar or blemish by excision, the surgeon should make every effort to place the line of incision in or parallel to a normal crease line of the face or body (Fig. 23–4). Sometimes it may be necessary to change the direction of a scar so that it will follow these lines.

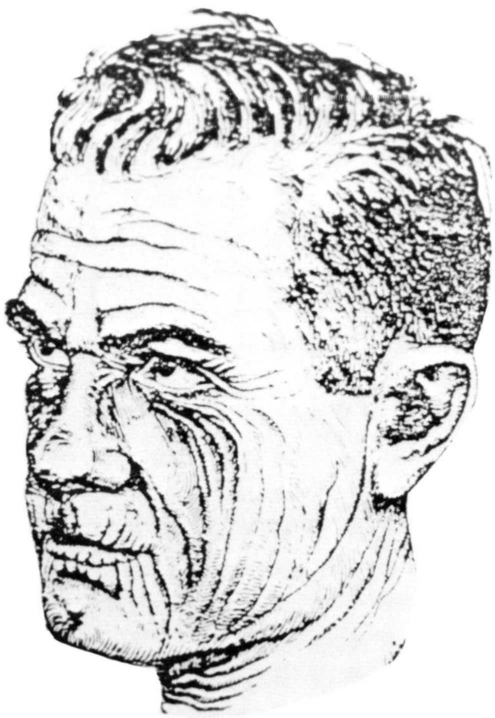

FIGURE 23–4. The relaxed skin tension lines of the face are demonstrated.

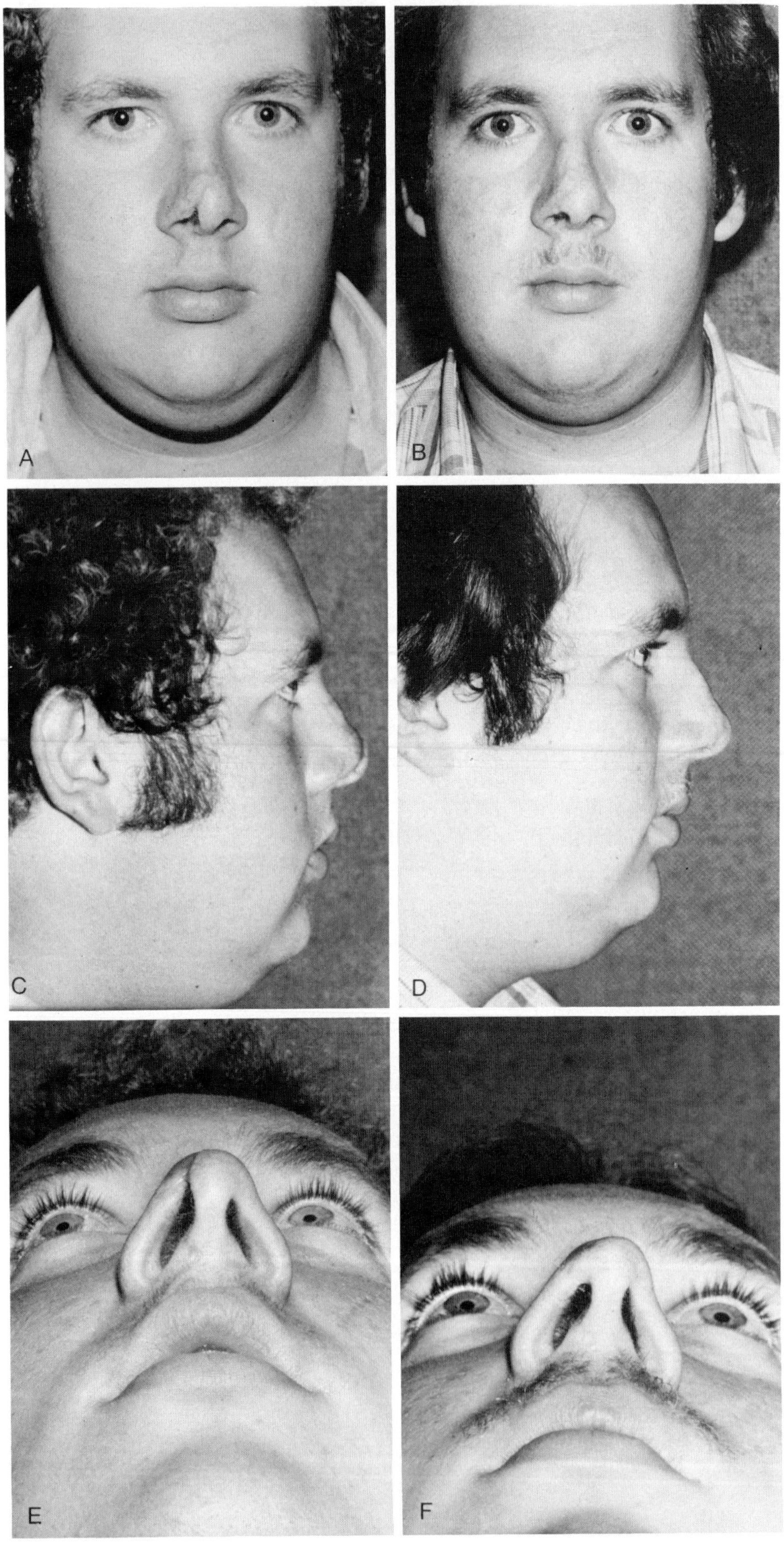

FIGURE 23–5. (*A, C,* and *E*) A traumatic deficiency of the right alar margin is noted. (*B, D,* and *F*) The defect was corrected with an auricular composite graft. The patient refused dermabrasion, which might have provided additional improvement.

Excision of large, unsightly scars may require multiple operations over a period of time (i.e., serial excisions). It may be necessary to shift surrounding tissue to fill a defect or, rarely, resort to skin grafting or tissue expansion (Fig. 23–5).

STAGES OF RECONSTRUCTION

Scar revision often requires at least two and frequently three surgical procedures to obtain the best achievable result. Each stage usually is separated by 6 to 12 months. Because some scars mature more quickly than others, subsequent stages may be performed sooner. One of the paradoxes of healing is that scars on younger children may take 18 to 24 months and sometimes longer to mature, whereas the same scar on an elderly patient may be flatter, thinner, and softer within 3 months. This unpredictable factor often accounts for the variability in the final result that occurs with scar revision and wound healing.

POSTOPERATIVE CONSIDERATIONS FOR SCAR REVISION

When incisions have been made into the skin to remove existing scars, the new skin edges are carefully approximated with fine, delicate sutures. Because it takes several days for the wound edges to mend, the immediate postoperative period is crucial in getting the best possible result. Patients must be willing to accept the temporary swelling and discoloration that occur after such operations. Although these effects usually are visually disconcerting, most people consider them a negligible inconvenience for the physical and psychological improvement.

When lacerations are sutured, scar revisional techniques after maturation might provide additional improvement in the appearance of scars (see Ch. 24). In many situations, a tape dressing is placed over the suture to help protect it. The tape is removed during the 1-week postoperative visit. The incision sites may be retaped for an additional week.

A dissolvable suture (6-0 fast-absorbing catgut) is used to close surgical incisions. If a tape dressing is placed over the suture line, the surface suture material ordinarily comes off when the tape is removed. If it does not, it can be gently removed with delicate instruments.

If no tape has been placed over the suture line, six times daily the patient should perform the following routine:

- Saturate a cotton-tipped applicator with full-strength hydrogen peroxide.
- Gently bathe the suture line with the peroxide-moistened applicator for 3 minutes.
- Always stroke along (parallel to) the suture line—never across (perpendicular to) it.
- After each peroxide treatment, apply a thin layer of a topical antibiotic ointment to the suture line.

The ritual should be repeated until the sutures have been removed and there is no longer crusting along the suture line.

If a tape dressing was applied to the surgical area, residual suture material should be removed from the wound when the tape is removed.

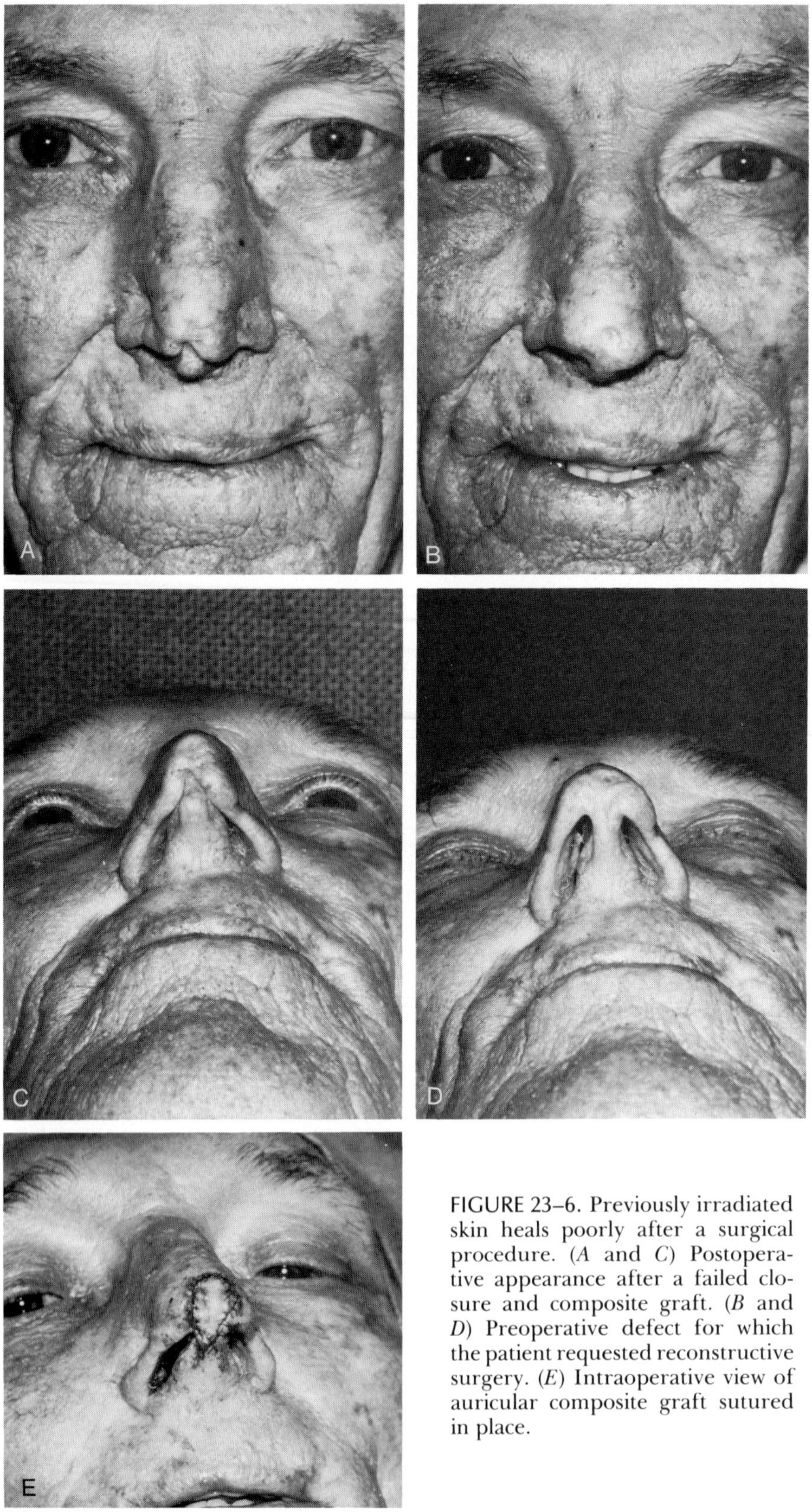

FIGURE 23–6. Previously irradiated skin heals poorly after a surgical procedure. (*A* and *C*) Postoperative appearance after a failed closure and composite graft. (*B* and *D*) Preoperative defect for which the patient requested reconstructive surgery. (*E*) Intraoperative view of auricular composite graft sutured in place.

Retaping the area for another 5 to 7 days provides support to the new healing scar and may help to prevent widening.

Make-up may be applied to the surgical area for camouflaging within 2 to 3 days after the tapes and/or sutures are removed.

It may be beneficial for the patient to tape the incision site at night or whenever possible for at least 6 months. Pulling or exerting tension on a scar promotes the formation of unwanted scar tissue. Properly applied crosstaping relieves some of the tendency for additional scar formation. Whenever tapes are removed, they should be gently pulled along (parallel to) the lines of the incisions, not across them.

Patients should be reminded that it takes 6 to 12 months for the scar to mature. Most scars become red and lumpy before they begin to flatten and lighten in color. In Caucasians, not until a scar is white and flat is it mature. In blacks, a mature, nonhypertrophied scar is flat and tan. If excess lumpiness or firmness should occur in a scar, intralesional steroids can help. Triamcinolone (10 to 20 mg/mL) can be injected into a raised, thickened scar every 3 to 4 weeks until it flattens. The steroid should not be placed into the subcutaneous tissues because dimpling caused by fat necrosis may occur. If dimpling should appear, the condition usually is self-limiting, but it might take 12 to 24 months for the depression to subside.

More than one scar revision operation usually is necessary to obtain the best possible result. The first two procedures require excisional surgery with suture repair; later stages usually require dermabrasion.

Some patients withhold valuable information from their surgeons that can be crucial to their care. In patients who have received irradiation therapy for acne, the tissues may not heal after surgery. Such was the case in the gentleman whose photographs are shown in Figure 23–6.

Suggested Readings

Kazanjian, V.H., Converse, J.M. Surgical Treatment of Facial Injuries. 3rd ed. Baltimore: Williams & Wilkins, 1974, 600.

McCollough, E.G., Chatham, D.R. The art and science of wound healing. Ala Med 54:26–38, 1985.

McCollough, E.G., Langsdon, P.R. Dermabrasion and Chemical Peeling. New York: Thieme Medical Publishers, 1988.

Webster, R.C., McCollough, E.G. Skin wound approximation with new absorbable suture material. Arch Otolaryngol 111:577, 1985.

Wolfe, D., Davidson, T.M. Scar revision. In Roenigk, R.K. and Roenigk, H.H., eds., Dermatologic Surgery. New York: Marcel Dekker, 935–957.

CHAPTER 24

Dermabrasion

In some noses, a planned dermabrasion after rhinoplasty can provide the finishing touches. Such was the case in the patient shown in Figure 24–1.

The technique of dermabrasion is similar to that of sanding a scratch from a wooden table, in that the work is done on the elevated areas around the scar. The objective is to take down the edges surrounding a depression so that they are closer to the level of the defect. When successful, this process diminishes the high-low junctions that are responsible for casting shadows made by light striking the skin from an angle.

The skin of the nose is relatively thick, especially at the tip. It thins out over the rhinion and thickens again in the nasion. This must be remembered when performing dermabrasion (Fig. 24–2). When the texture of the nasal skin is irregular from excessive or deep scarring, a second dermabrasion may be required 6 to 12 months after the initial treatment.

Some superficial scars might be removed by dermabrasion, and those that are moderately deep may be improved but not removed. Some of the deep or ice pick–type scars may not be improved and may require punch grafting, in which skin craters (e.g., chickenpox scars) are surgically removed and replaced by small circular full-thickness skin grafts from the back of the ear. Dermabrasion is required 3 to 6 months later.

In some cases, a second dermabrasion within 6 to 12 months can provide additional improvement to moderately deep scars. On rare occasions, dermabrasion can be done a third time, but there is a limit. Before surgery, it is difficult to predict the degree of improvement one might receive.

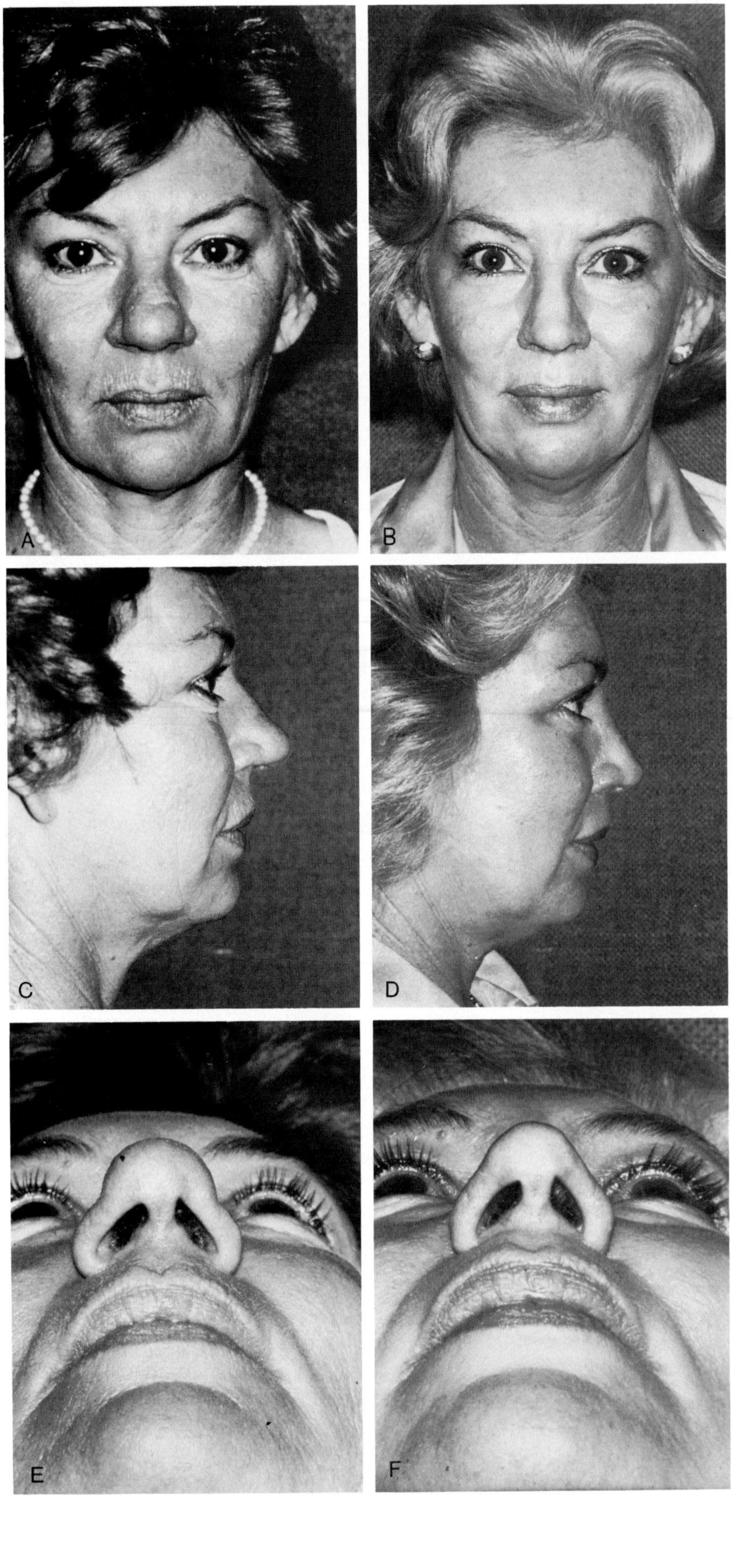

FIGURE 24–1. A two-staged nasal plastic operation was planned and performed in this patient with early rhinophyma. (*A, C,* and *E*) A rhinoplasty was carried out first. Six weeks after surgery, the nose was improved. (*B, D,* and *F*) A dermabrasion of the nose provided additional refinement. A full-face chemical peel was performed at the same time.

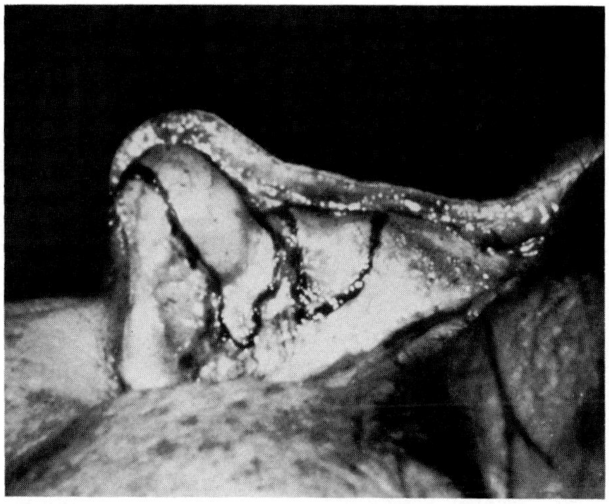

FIGURE 24–2. This cadaver slide demonstrates how skin and soft tissue thickness affect the dorsal profile.

Every case is different, and each patient's skin responds to the same treatment by the same surgeon in a different manner.

Orentreich emphasizes that skin pores are the surface openings of the oil glands. Neither dermabrasion nor a peel is designed to alter them (see Fig. 24–10*A*, *D*, and *E*).

APPLICATIONS

Finishing Touches

When dermabrasion is done as part of a revision of surgical or accidental scars, it can provide the finishing touch to help smooth the tissues out after the initial procedures have been completed (Fig. 24–1). In some cases, only dermabrasion may be required for scars resulting from accidents.

Rhinophyma

When acne rosacea has been long-standing, progressive surgical planing followed by dermabrasion can provide dramatic improvement. The excessive sebaceous-containing tissues are removed down to the normal dermis (Figs. 24–3 through 24–5). Early rhinophyma often can be improved to prevent an unsightly appearance.

Hyperpigmentation

Because dermabrasion can eradicate melanocytes, the procedure can be used to intentionally produce hypopigmentation in some patients (Fig. 24–6).

Telangiectasia

A number of methods are effective against superficial telangiectasia, including lasers and hyfrecation. (Hyfrecation is destruction of tissue with an electrical hyfrecator.) Dermabrasion can also remove superficial blood vessels and improve both the texture and the quality of the skin of the nose.

Text continued on page 359

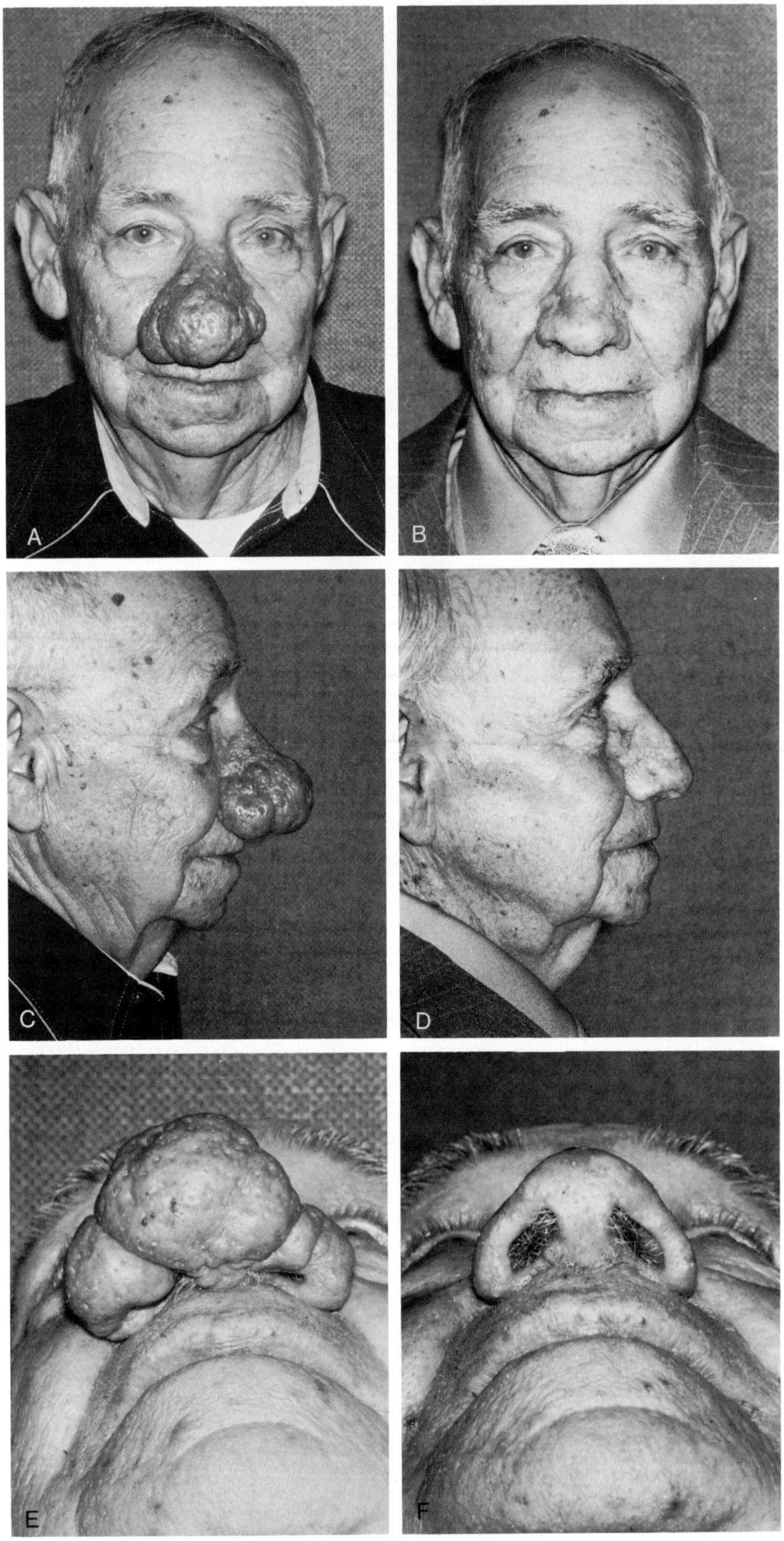

FIGURE 24–3. (*A*, *C*, and *E*) The rhinophymatous condition of this man's nose was far advanced. (*B*, *D*, and *F*) Cold-knife shave excision (shown in Fig. 24–4) removed the bulk of the offensive tissues. Final contouring was performed with wire-brush dermabrasion.

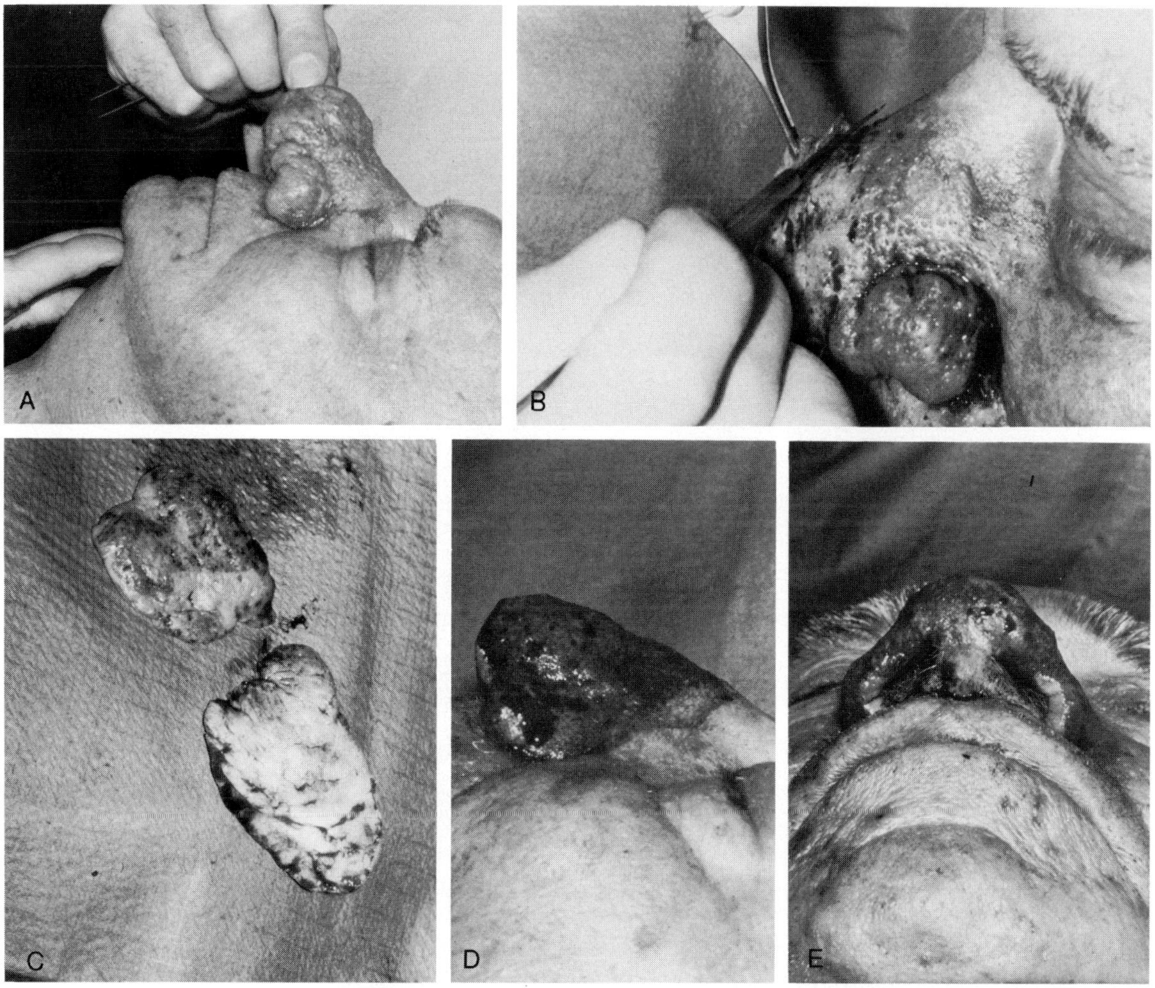

FIGURE 24–4. (*A*) The thickness of the sebaceous-filled skin is estimated, and shave excision is begun with sharp dissection. (*B*) Excisional contouring begins until the surgeon believes that he is approaching normal dermis. (*C*) Examples of portions of the specimen removed. (*D*) Final honing is achieved with wire-brush dermabrasion. (*E*) The result at end of operation is shown.

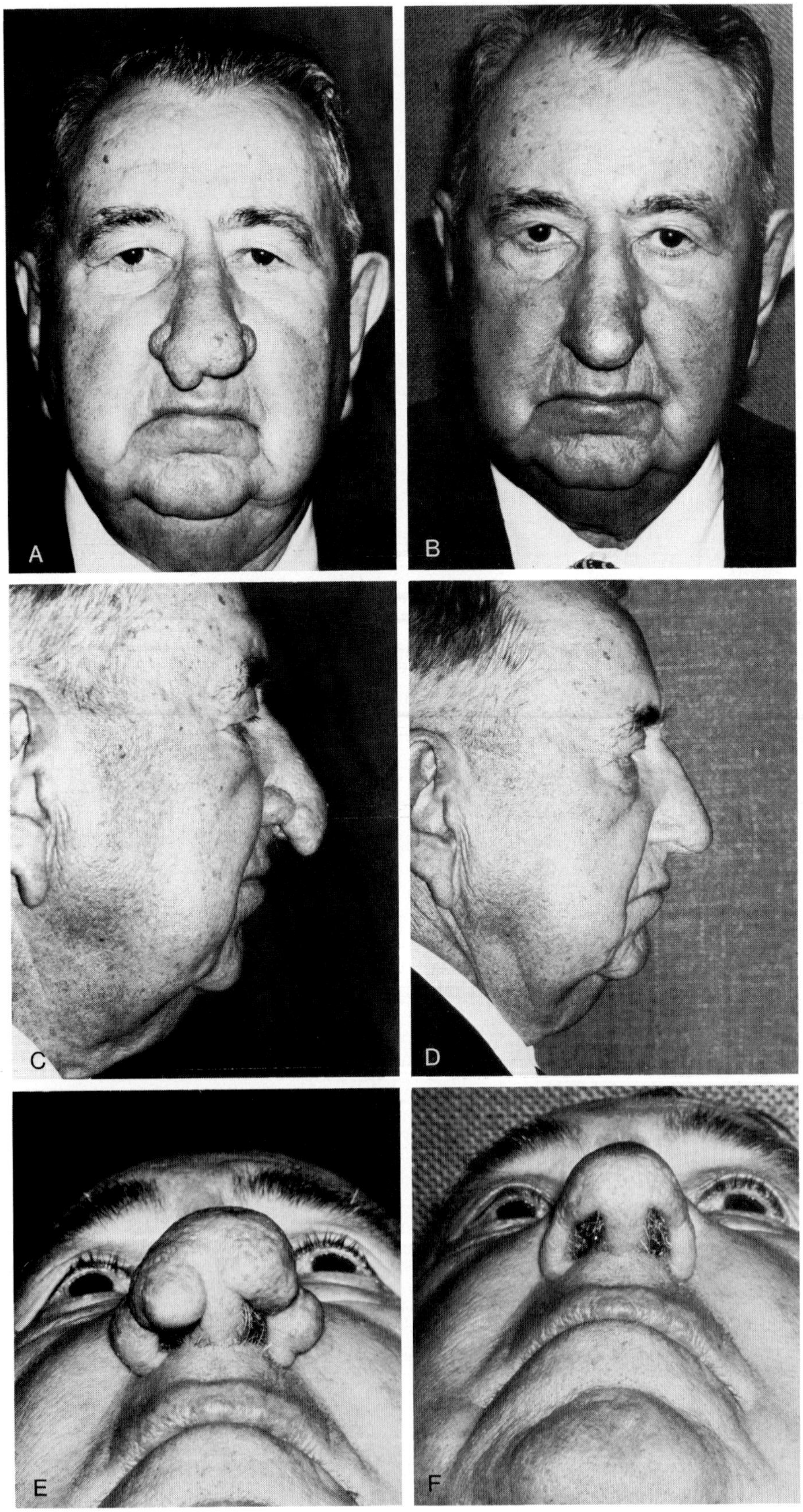

FIGURE 24–5. (*A, C,* and *E*) This gentleman suffered with progressive rhinophyma. (*B, D,* and *F*) After cold-knife excision and intraoperative wire-brush dermabrasion to remove the excessive sebaceous-laced and thickened skin of his nose, marked improvement was shown.

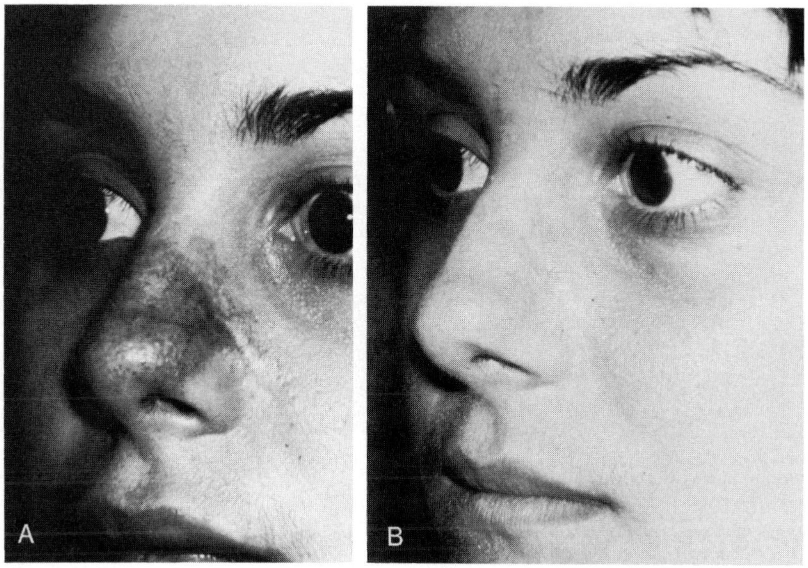

FIGURE 24–6. (*A*) Pigmented lesions on the nose lend themselves to treatment with dermabrasion. (*B*) Only one procedure was required in this patient.

TECHNIQUE

Dermabrasion is carried out with a round wire brush inserted into the handpiece of a motorized instrument (Fig. 24–7). In the nasofacial crease, a pear-shaped diamond fraise sometimes is used (Fig. 24–8).

Because the risk of blood-borne infections is at an all-time high, it is advisable to wear protective shields and garments. Skin debris, blood, and tissue fluids are scattered around the field throughout the procedure (Fig. 24–9).

The superficial layers of skin are progressively removed down to the upper dermis. A distinctive bleeding pattern apprises the surgeon that he has reached the appropriate level, the junction of the papillary dermis (Fig. 24–10). At the conclusion of the procedure, sponges moistened with saline solution are applied over the abraided regions until bleeding stops.

For additional description of the surgical procedure, the reader is directed to a textbook (*Dermabrasion and Chemical Peeling*) written by the author on the subject.

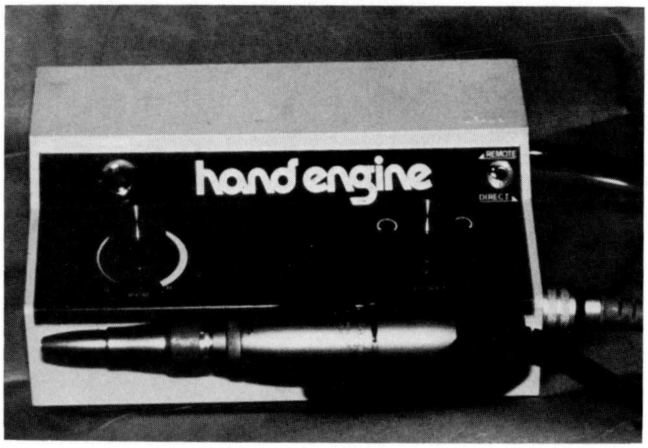

FIGURE 24–7. Dermabrasion is performed with a motorized hand instrument.

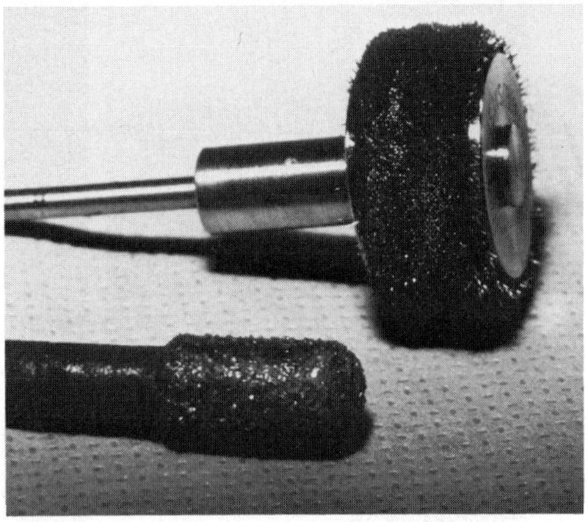

FIGURE 24–8. A wire brush is preferred for most areas. The rounded diamond fraise works well in the nasofacial and nasolabial creases.

POSTOPERATIVE INSTRUCTIONS

It has been shown by Maibach and Rovee that abraded wounds which are kept moist and free of crusting heal more rapidly. This is most easily accomplished by having the patient stand in a shower and use the fingertips to gently agitate the wound. This washing must be repeated six times per day. After each wash, an ointment (or cream) must be applied to the dermabraded areas. The ointment acts as a moisturizer and prevents dryness and crusting.

At this stage in the healing process, new, delicate skin is being formed, and premature removal of the crusts may damage it and delay healing.

By about the 8th to the 10th day, most of the crusting should have disappeared. The new skin appears intensely pink. At this stage, the moistening agent should be applied more sparingly but gently rubbed in, much in the manner one would use a moisturizing cream.

Within about 14 days, the patient should be able to use makeup over the dermabraided areas. Although they usually do not cover as well, water-based makeups are more easily removed and are, therefore, recommended for the 1st week or so that makeup is used. Makeup should never be applied to unhealed areas or crusts.

The intense pink color usually fades after the 2nd week, but some pink remains for about 6 to 8 weeks. After the pink color disappears, the skin usually remains tenser and somewhat smoother.

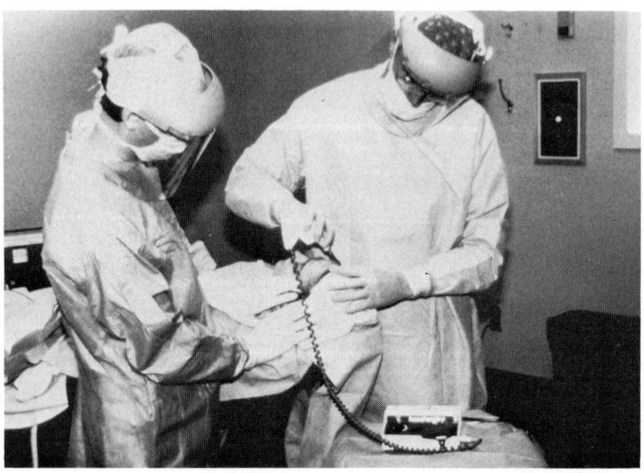

FIGURE 24–9. Universal precautions are exercised by the entire staff during dermabrasion to reduce the risk of transmitting blood-borne infections.

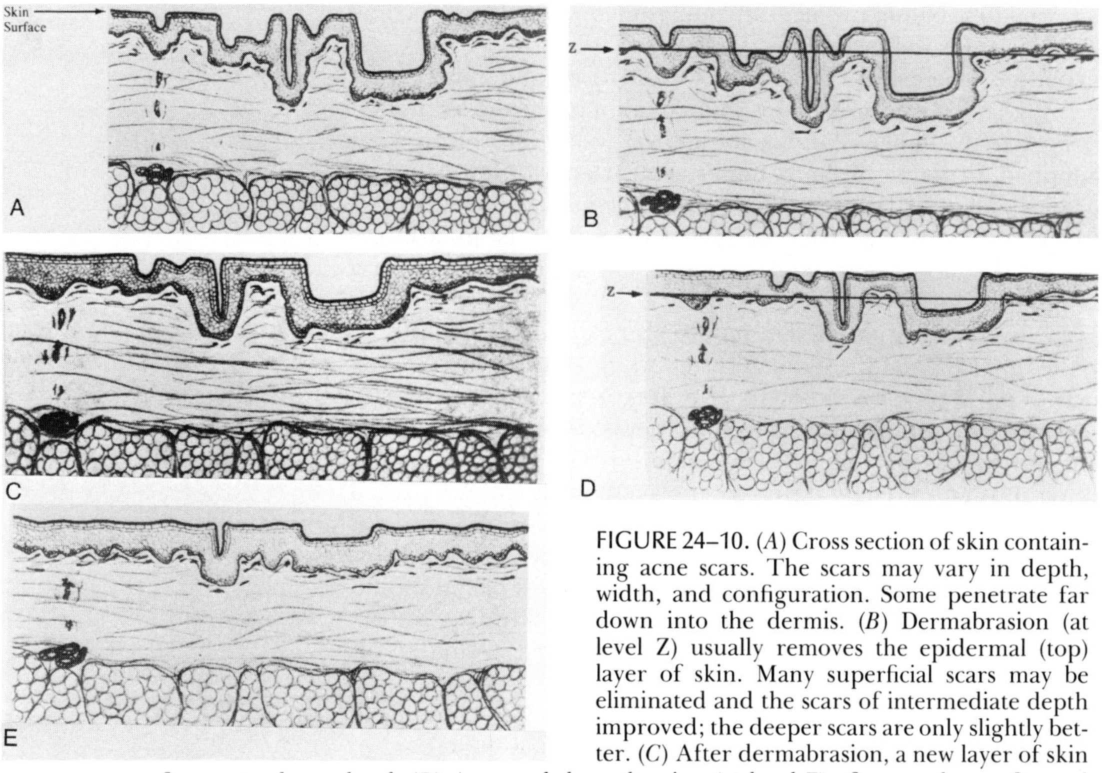

FIGURE 24–10. (*A*) Cross section of skin containing acne scars. The scars may vary in depth, width, and configuration. Some penetrate far down into the dermis. (*B*) Dermabrasion (at level Z) usually removes the epidermal (top) layer of skin. Many superficial scars may be eliminated and the scars of intermediate depth improved; the deeper scars are only slightly better. (*C*) After dermabrasion, a new layer of skin forms at a lower level. (*D*) A second dermabrasion (at level Z) often can be performed within 6 to 12 months. (*E*) After two procedures, some scars still exist, but improvement can be seen in the overall texture and consistency of the skin.

Small white cysts (i.e., milia) may appear in the treated areas. These usually disappear in 2 to 3 weeks without specific treatment. If they do not, they can be marsupialized with a No. 18 needle.

Early in the healing process, exposure to heat, cold, wind, or emotional upset (i.e., fear, anger, crying) causes the skin to temporarily become intensely pink. This results from increased blood flow or blushing. After 3 to 4 months, this phenomenon should disappear.

The delicate new skin toughens with time. Makeup, nail polish products, astringents, detergents, hair sprays, and so on could produce contact dermatitis during the first few weeks after the procedure. The skin gradually toughens and can tolerate most of a patient's presurgical activities.

Resuming Activities of Daily Living

Wearing Eyeglasses. If the nose area has been dermabraded, patients should wait 2 weeks before wearing eyeglasses. The pressure of glasses resting on the dermabraded nose skin (except for brief periods) should be avoided. Contact lenses may be inserted the day after surgery.

The patient should be reminded that swelling, crusting, and redness are expected with dermabrasion. His or her facial appearance may be alarming for a week or so, but time and diligent skin care will help to ensure the most favorable surgical result. Close adherence to the postoperative instructions is vital to avoiding problems that might jeopardize the outcome of a well-executed surgical procedure.

Sun Exposure. The patient should try to avoid direct and indirect rays of the sun for at least 8 weeks. Blotchy pigmentation of the dermabraded areas may appear if the new skin is exposed too soon. This means that being outdoors (i.e., golfing, fishing, tennis, similar activities) during the sunny part of the day should be avoided during the initial 8-week period. The dermabraded areas should be protected for 6 months by a large-brimmed hat and a sunscreen product if the patient will be exposed for a prolonged period.

Skin Care. Continued use of skin moisturizers is the best adjunct in nurturing the new skin and preserving its smooth, soft texture.

Returning to Work or School and Resuming Social Activities. When the patient may return to work depends on the amount of public contact as well as the amount of sun exposure the job involves plus how much redness and swelling develop. The average patient can return to work or go out socially about 2 weeks after dermabrasion.

Athletics. Exposure to extremes of heat, cold, or wind (as in snow skiing or other such outdoor sports) may damage the new skin and should be avoided for 6 months. No swimming, gym, or strenuous athletic activity should be undertaken for 2 weeks, and no diving or skiing is permitted for 2 months.

Medications. After surgery, the patient is advised to begin taking all the medications that were being taken before surgery (see Chapter 6).

Weakness. It is not unusual for a person who has had an anesthetic or an operation to feel weak and dizzy, have a rapid pulse rate, or break out in a cold sweat. These effects gradually clear up in a few days without further treatment.

Suggested Readings

Maibach, H.I., Rovee, D.T. (eds.). Epidermal Wound Healing. Chicago: Year Book Medical Publishers, 1972.

McCollough, E.G., Langsdon, P.R. Dermabrasion and Chemical Peeling. New York: Thieme Medical Publishers, 1988.

Roenigk, H.H., Jr., Roenigk, R.K. Dermatologic Surgery. New York: Marcel Dekker, 959–991, 1989.

CHAPTER 25

Rhinoplasty and Facial Rejuvenation

Rhinoplasty can be an integral part of restoring the appearance of youth to an aging face.

AGING OF THE NOSE

Throughout life, the nose changes. In early childhood, the nose is short and soft and lacks a significant bridge (Fig. 25–1). During puberty, the nose begins to assume the characteristics of the person's ancestors. Development continues until a person becomes a physical adult. The age at which this occurs varies from person to person but usually it happens at an earlier age in women than in men. Some young women are physically mature at age 13 and some men at 15. Growth charts and a careful documentation of menstrual and shaving histories have proved to be more practical parameters than arbitrary chronologic criteria.

Once adulthood has been reached, the nose usually maintains its predetermined size and shape until conspicuous signs of aging begin to appear. Redundant skin eventually appears over and below the eyelids along with herniated periorbital fat. The brows become ptotic, jowls develop along the mandibular margin as the face loses its full appearance, and loose skin hangs below the chin (Fig. 25–2).

While these unwanted sequelae of aging are occurring, physical changes are occurring in the nose as well. The architectural integrity of the nasal

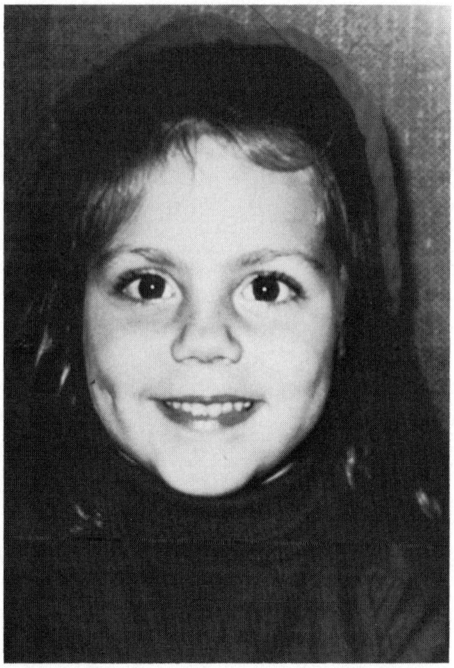

FIGURE 25–1. Characteristics of a youthful face: large eyes and lips, rounded cheeks, and a short nose.

skeleton begins to deteriorate. Some of the structural alterations include the physical separation of the interlocking scrolls of the upper lateral and alar cartilages, loss of soft tissue padding below the feet of the medial crura, loss of tone and elasticity of the dorsal nasal skin to which Pitanguy's suspensory ligament is attached, and thickening of the skin of the lobule. The cumulative effect is that a heavier tip has lost much of its support and, naturally, ptosis occurs.

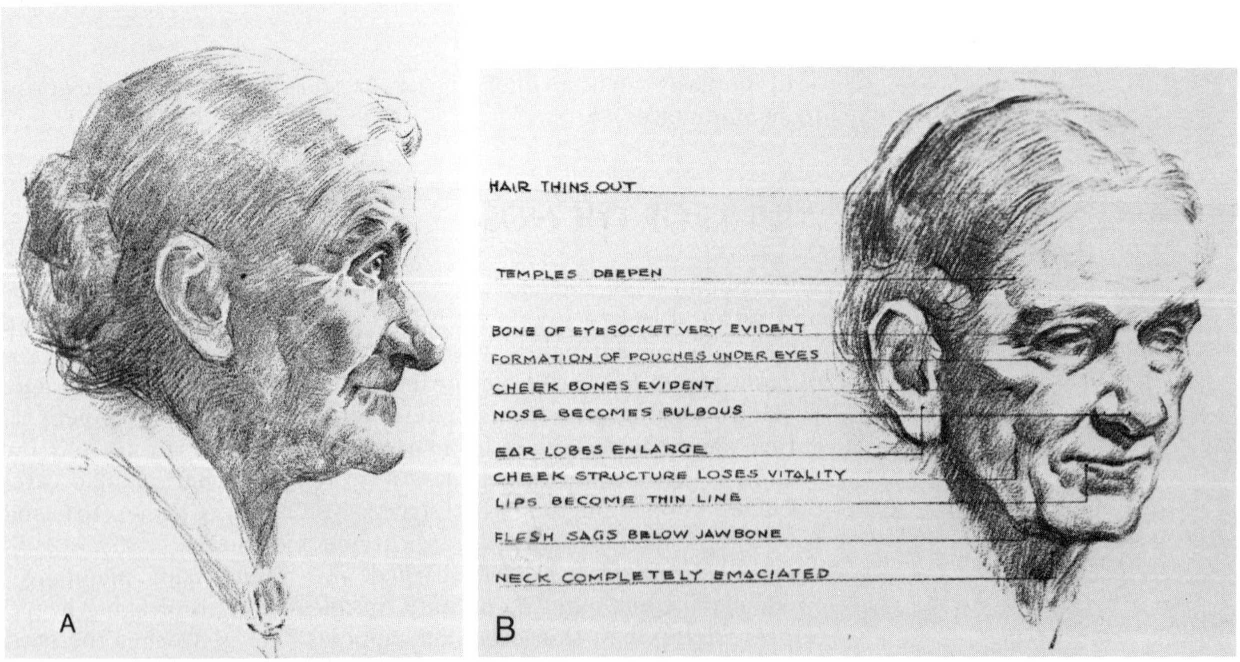

FIGURE 25–2. (*A*) Profile appearance of advanced aging changes as support is lost at the base of the columella and upper lip. (*B*) Corresponding changes in the aging face are demonstrated. (From Drawing the Head and Hands by Andrew Loomis and Ethel Loomis. Copyright © 1956 by Andrew Loomis. Used by permission of Viking Penguin, a division of Penguin Books USA, Inc.)

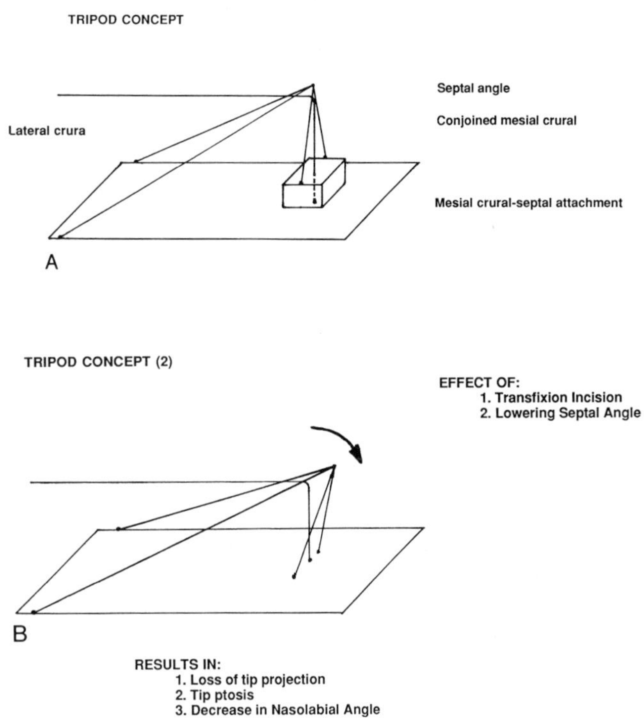

FIGURE 25–3. Tripod concept of tip support. (*A*) Ideal tip-supporting anatomic mechanisms. (*B*) The changes associated with aging are demonstrated (i.e., loss of medial crural support at nasolabial angle results in ptosis).

Schematically, the central leg (conjoined medial crura) loses much of its foundation and the tripod falls to the shorter leg (Fig. 25–3). As this phenomenon occurs, the nasolabial angle becomes more acute and changes occur in the nasal introitus. The nasal internal junctional angles are altered in the region of the nasal valve (Fig. 25–4).

The development of a larger dorsal hump is an illusion created by the altered tip projection that has occurred as a result of the changes noted.

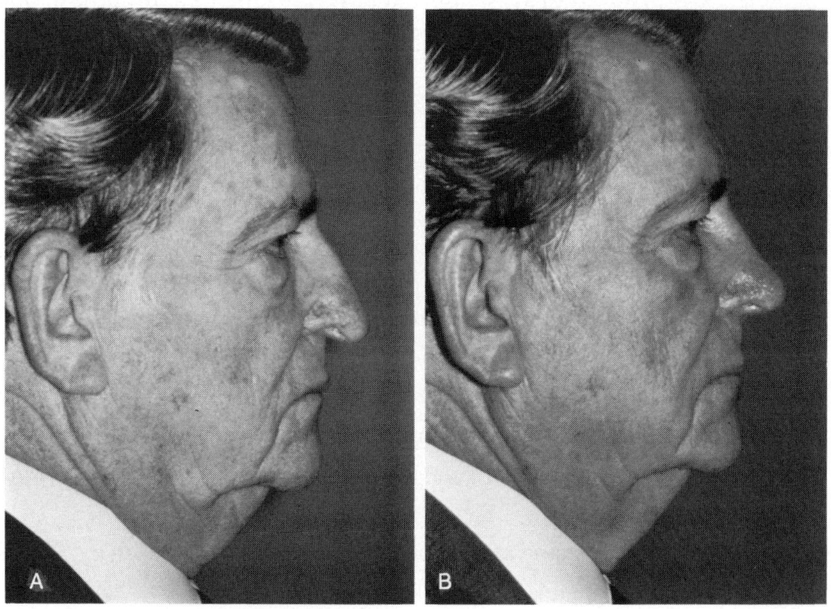

FIGURE 25–4. A severely ptotic tip can be supported with columellar plumping grafts and struts. (*A*) Preoperative state of tip in an aged patient. (*B*) Postoperative correction.

PLANNING THE APPROPRIATE OPERATION

In many cases, it is not necessary to perform a complete rhinoplasty. A thoughtful and well-executed tip-plasty technique that provides maximum support and/or rotation may be all that is required.

If the skin has become heavier and thicker because of acne rosacea, with or without frank rhinophyma, planing and dermabrasion may provide additional improvement. These procedures usually are deferred to a second operation performed 3 to 6 months after rhinoplasty. The exception is in the case of severe rhinophyma. When the condition is far advanced, the skin should be treated before alteration of the nasal skeleton is attempted (see Fig. 24–3).

When it has been determined that the dorsal bony and/or cartilaginous hump is to be reduced in size, caution must be exercised. Removal of too much of the hump is ill-advised. The older or more mature patient typically seeks refinement. A strong dorsum is associated with an elegant appearance. A "cute" nose on an older patient seems inappropriate. A good philosophy when operating on an older patient with a large nose is not to make it a small nose but to make it a more aesthetically pleasing large nose (Fig. 25–5).

ANATOMIC CONSIDERATIONS

When a large amount of hump is removed, the older, inelastic skin cannot accommodate to the new framework. In the event that the skin does not contract sufficiently, external incisions to remove tissue redundancy might become necessary.

Wider undermining toward the nasofacial junction may help redundant skin to drape laterally into this anatomic groove. As one ages, the bones in and about the nose become more brittle. Because of this phenomenon, care must be taken during the portions of the operation in which the nasal bones are manipulated (i.e., hump removal, osteotomies, and septal surgery).

Because many older patients have some degree of pulmonary compromise, it is prudent to keep internal nasal packing to a minimum. Some techniques can virtually eliminate internal packing and ought to be considered in this group of patients.

REJUVENATION PLAN

Many older patients seek only a rhinoplasty, whereas others present for total facial rejuvenation. The point in the master plan at which nasal plastic surgery is performed depends on a number of factors, including the following:

- Patient's health
- Degree of rejuvenation sought
- Time required for the surgeon to perform the individual rejuvenation procedures
- Patient's comfort and safety for a lengthy operating room experience
- Total cost of surgery and facilities fees

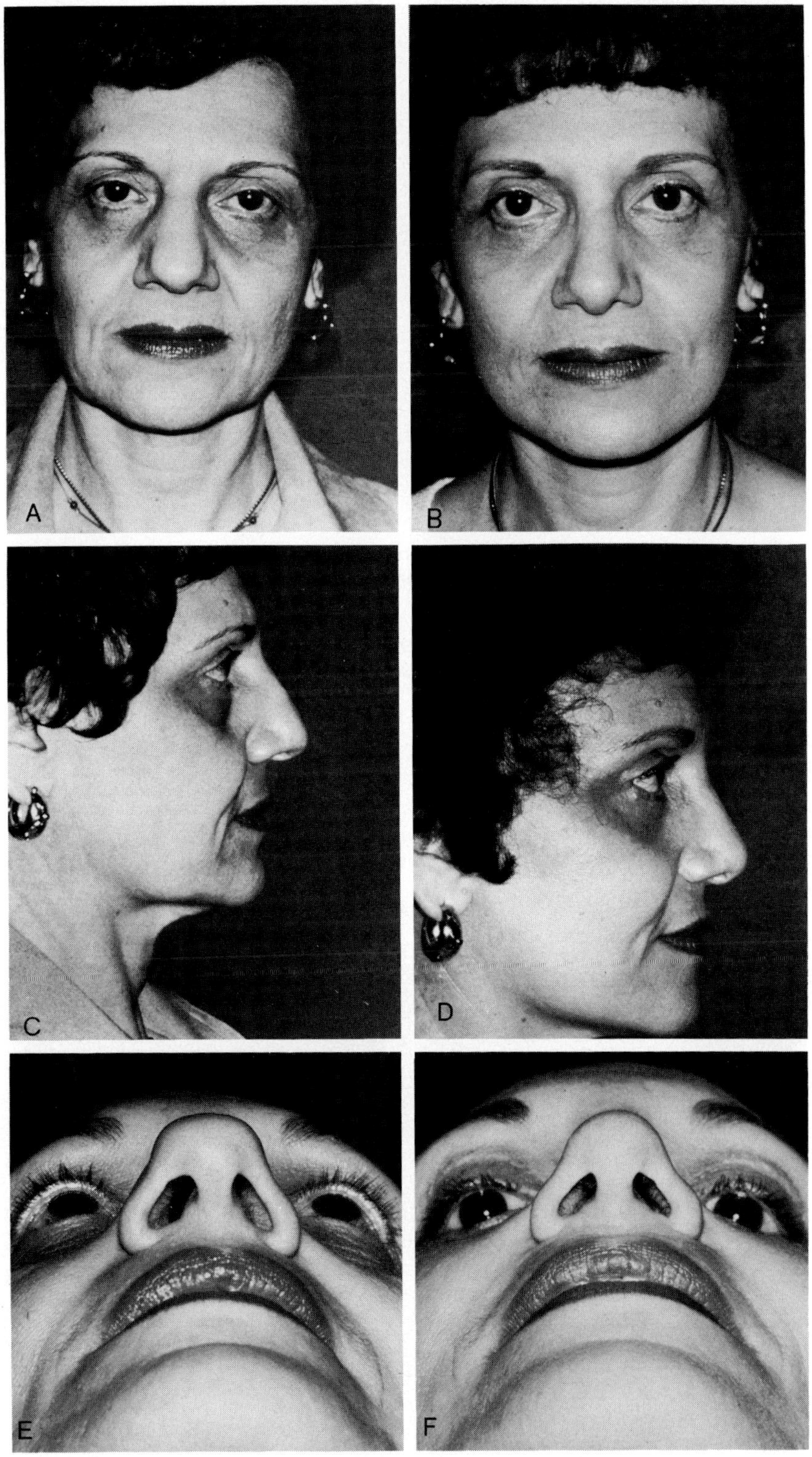

FIGURE 25–5. In older patients with a strong ethnic background and a large nose, it is best to attempt to produce a better-looking large nose than to make a smaller nose. (*A, C,* and *E*) Preoperative appearance of patient with large nose and typical signs of aging. (*B, D,* and *F*) After reduction rhinoplasty, blepharoplasty, and face lifting, the result is a more youthful appearance.

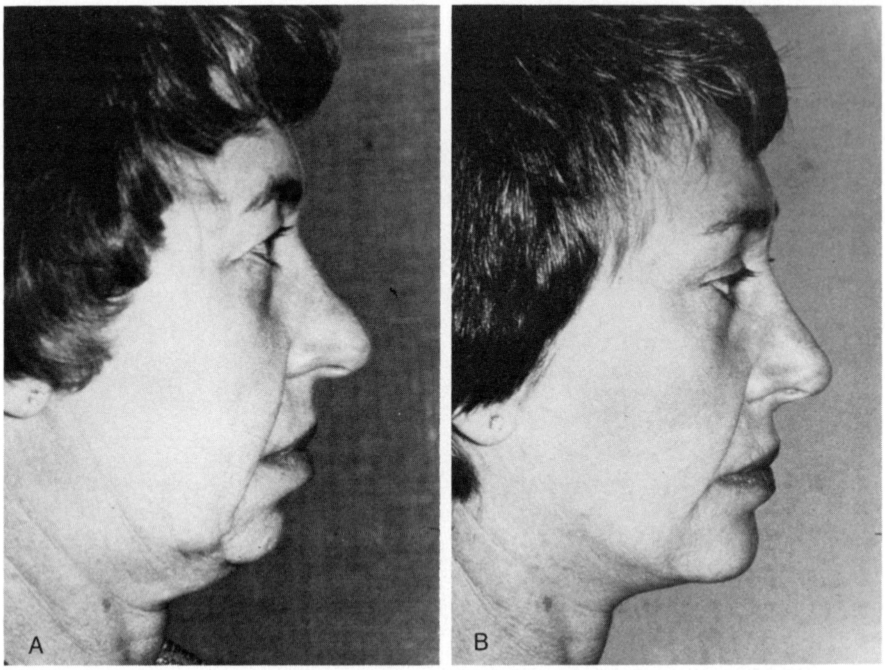

FIGURE 25–6. (*A*) Some patients who present for facial rejuvenation surgery may be unaware of the subtle changes occurring in their noses. (*B*) This patient required only a tip-plasty. No hump was removed. Chin augmentation blepharoplasty, and face lifting were also performed.

Because of the anesthetic program, physical plant, and supporting staff, I perform several surgical procedures at the same setting on a patient who is in good health.

The order of events, if all these procedures should be desired and/or required, might be as follows:

1. Upper and lower lid blepharoplasties
2. Forehead, cheek, and neck facelift
3. Septorhinoplasty
4. Chin augmentation
5. Perioral—chemical peel (Figs. 25–6 and 25–7).

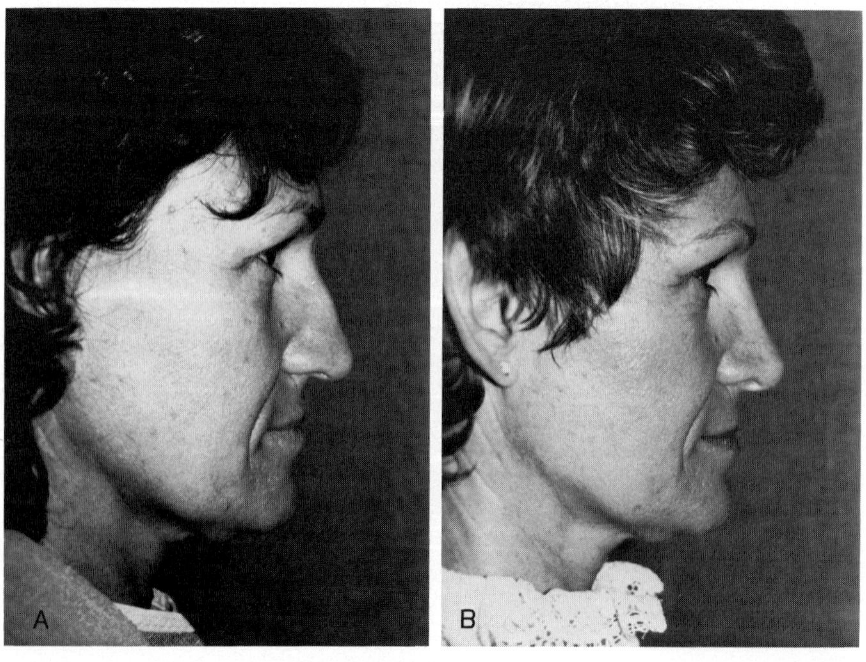

FIGURE 25–7. (*A*) Loss of premaxillary soft tissue support and upper lateral–lower lateral cartilage attachments produced a prematurely acute nasolabial angle. (*B*) Tip rotation was accomplished with a large cartilaginous strut and premaxillary crushed cartilage plumping grafts.

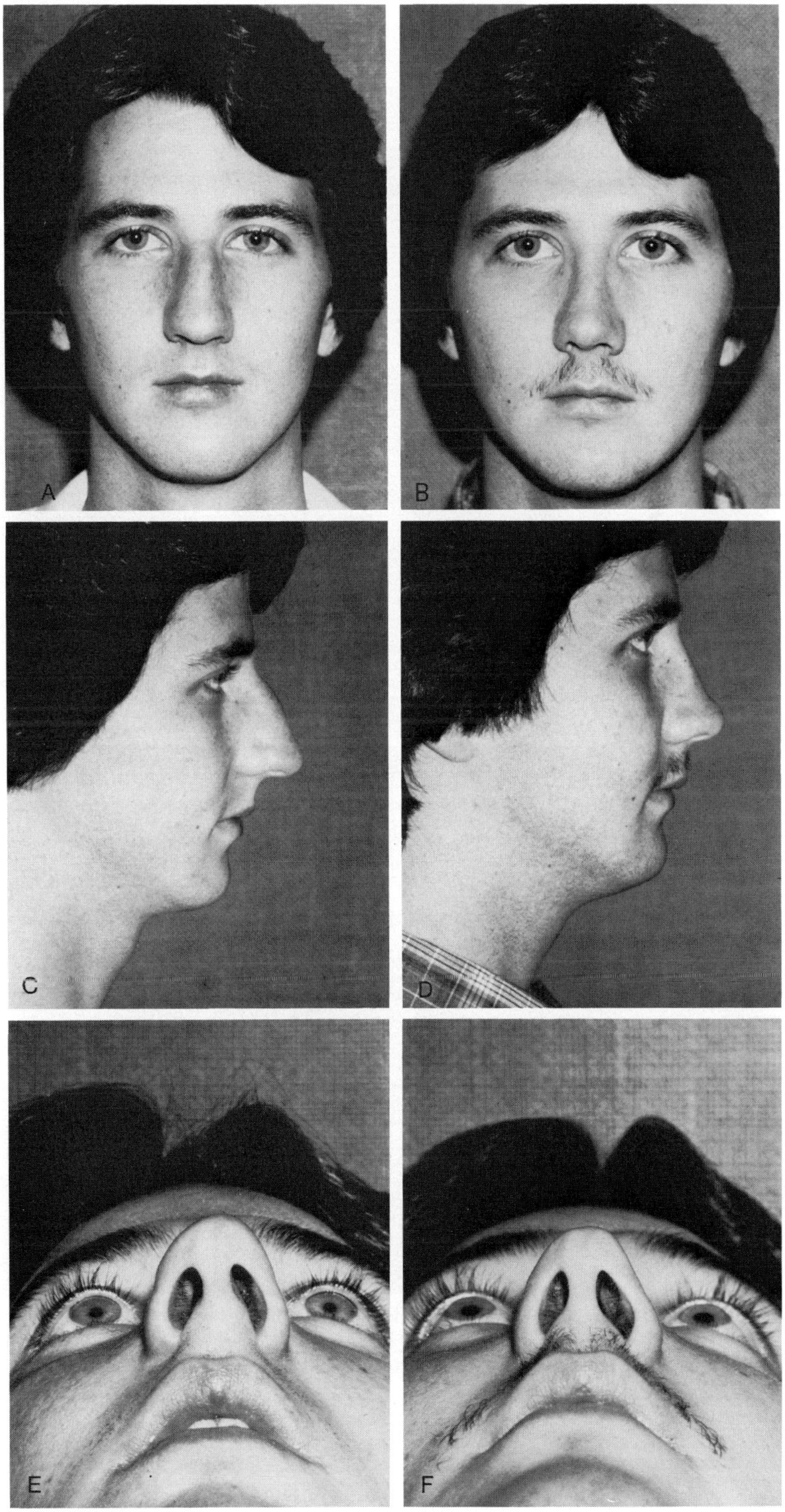

FIGURE 25–8. (*A, C,* and *E*) A ptotic tip makes this patient appear older than his chronologic age. (*B, D,* and *F*) Reduction rhinoplasty with tip-supporting and rotational maneuvers were performed along with septoplasty.

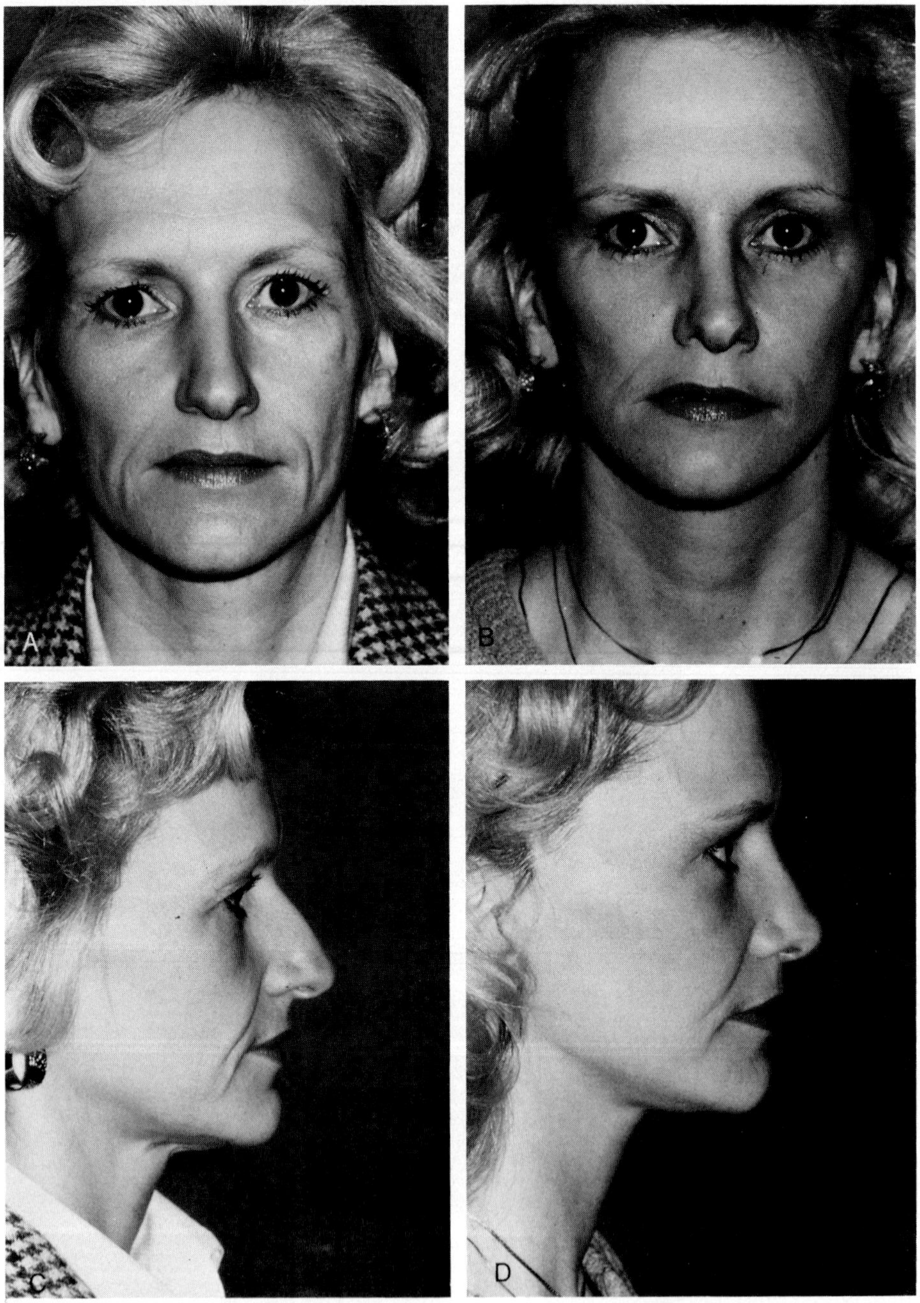

FIGURE 25–9. This patient had multiple facial rejuvenation procedures at the time of rhinoplasty. (*A* and *C*) Preoperative views. (*B* and *D*) Postoperative outcome of rhinoplasty, blepharoplasty, and rhytidectomy.

AGE PARAMETERS

Many patients develop ptotic tips at a young age, before other characteristic signs of aging appear. Early correction can prevent severe tip ptosis as aging progresses (Fig. 25–8).

At midlife, rhinoplasty often can be combined with a maintenance program for the person who does not want to be overtaken by the ravages of aging (Fig. 25–9).

Because of a lack of finances, a fear of plastic surgery resulting from misinformation, job constraints, or an unsuccessful search for the "right" surgeon, many patients do not seek their first plastic operation until late in life. As long as a patient is in good health, is cleared for elective surgery by her or his personal physician, has realistic expectations, and, statistically, might have another 10 to 15 years of quality life to enjoy, it is not too late to have surgery.

When a mother who had previously brought three daughters and a son to me for septorhinoplasty surgery was asked, "Why do you want to have surgery?" she answered, "It's my turn." Some people have disliked the appearance of their noses since adolescence or have lived with breathing difficulties for many years but have not found the right combination of circumstances to cause them to make the commitment to proceed with surgery. Helping people to correct a disfigurement that may have bothered them for most of their lives can be a gratifying experience. When rhinoplasty is combined with other rejuvenation surgery, it often can be the "crème de la crème."

Suggested Readings

McCollough, E. G., Mangate, D. Systematic approach to correction of the nasal tip in rhinoplasty. Arch Laryngol 107:12, 1981.

Pitanguy, I. Aging face surgery. In Plastic and Reconstructive Surgery of the Head and Neck. Proceedings of the Fifth International Symposium. Philadelphia: B.C. Decker, 1991, pp. 145–148.

Simmons, R. L., Beeson, W. H. Aesthetic Surgery of the Aging Face. St. Louis: C.V. Mosby, 1986, pp. 296–305.

CHAPTER 26

Chin Augmentation

In the Western hemisphere, a facial profile is considered aesthetically balanced when the chin approximates a vertical line dropped from the lower lip while the head is in the Frankfort position (Fig. 26–1). Alteration of the chin can greatly enhance this facial balance, especially in patients seeking rhinoplasty. About 20 per cent of patients who request rhinoplasty can also benefit from augmentation mentoplasty. Most who require chin augmentation have an underdeveloped mandibular symphysis (microgenia) with normal occlusion (angle, class 1; Figs. 26–2 through 26–4). As long as no major malocclusion exists, chin augmentation can be performed by implant insertion or sliding osteotomy.

AUGMENTATION MATERIALS

Many materials have been used for augmentation, for example, ivory, gold, silver, and paraffin. Because these materials often caused tissue reactions that led to unfavorable results, many surgeons opted to use autografts. Since the early 1980s, allograft materials have become more popular than autograft materials because of their ready availability, ease of tailoring, lack of donor site morbidity, lower rate of resorption, and relative postoperative tissue tolerance. Implant materials such as acrylics, silicones, Silastic, polyamide mesh, and Teflon are also commercially available (Fig. 26–5).

Text continued on page 378

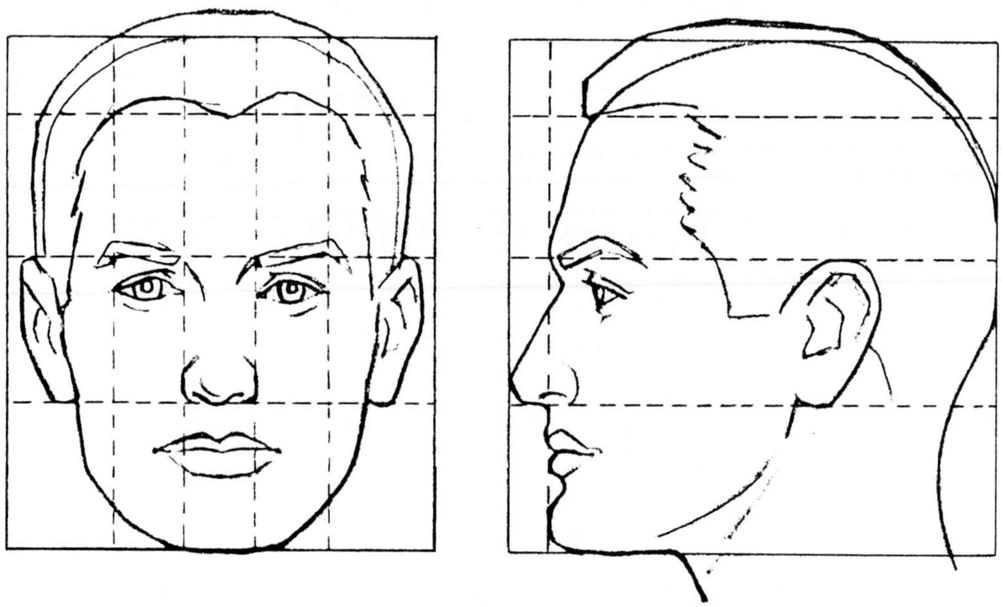

FIGURE 26–1. The ideal projection and relation of the chin were described by Leonardo da Vinci.

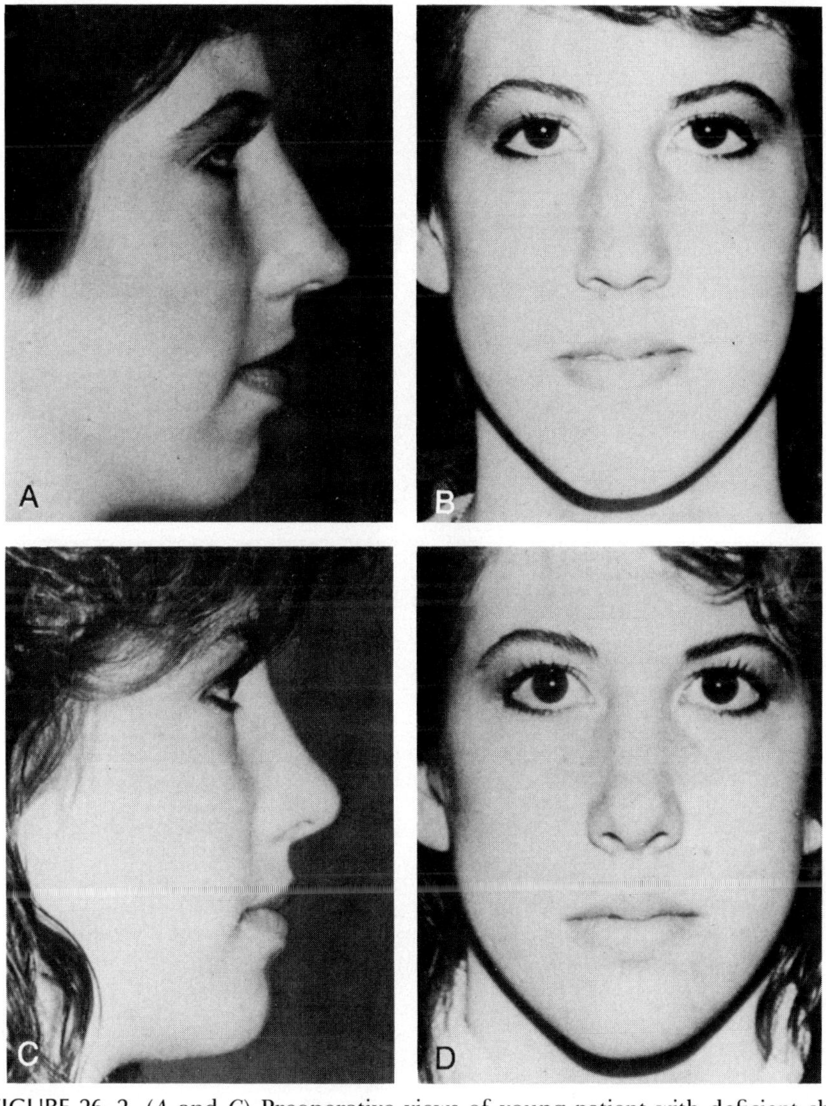

FIGURE 26–2. (*A* and *C*) Preoperative views of young patient with deficient chin projection. (*B* and *D*) Correction with Mersilene mesh implant. (From McCollough, E.G., et al: Augmentation mentoplasty using Mersilene mesh. Arch Otolaryngol Head Neck Surg 116:1154–1158, 1990. Copyright 1990, American Medical Association.)

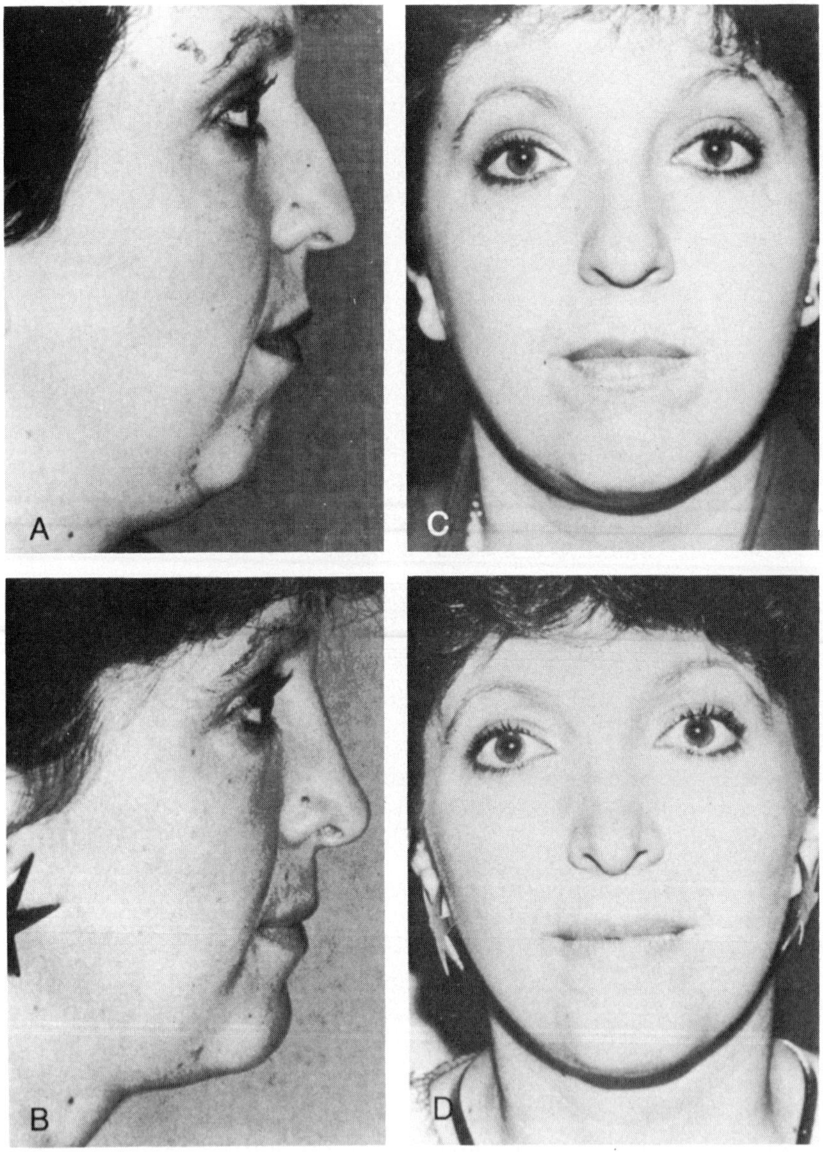

FIGURE 26–3. (*A* and *C*) Preoperative views of middle-aged patient with deficient chin and obtuse cervicomental angle. (*B* and *D*) Rhinoplasty and chin augmentation (mesh) only were performed in the 1970s. Today, suction-assisted lipectomy could have improved the appearance of the submental region. (From McCollough, E.G., et al: Augmentation mentoplasty using Mersilene mesh. Arch Otolaryngol Head Neck Surg 116:1154–1158, 1990. Copyright 1990, American Medical Association.)

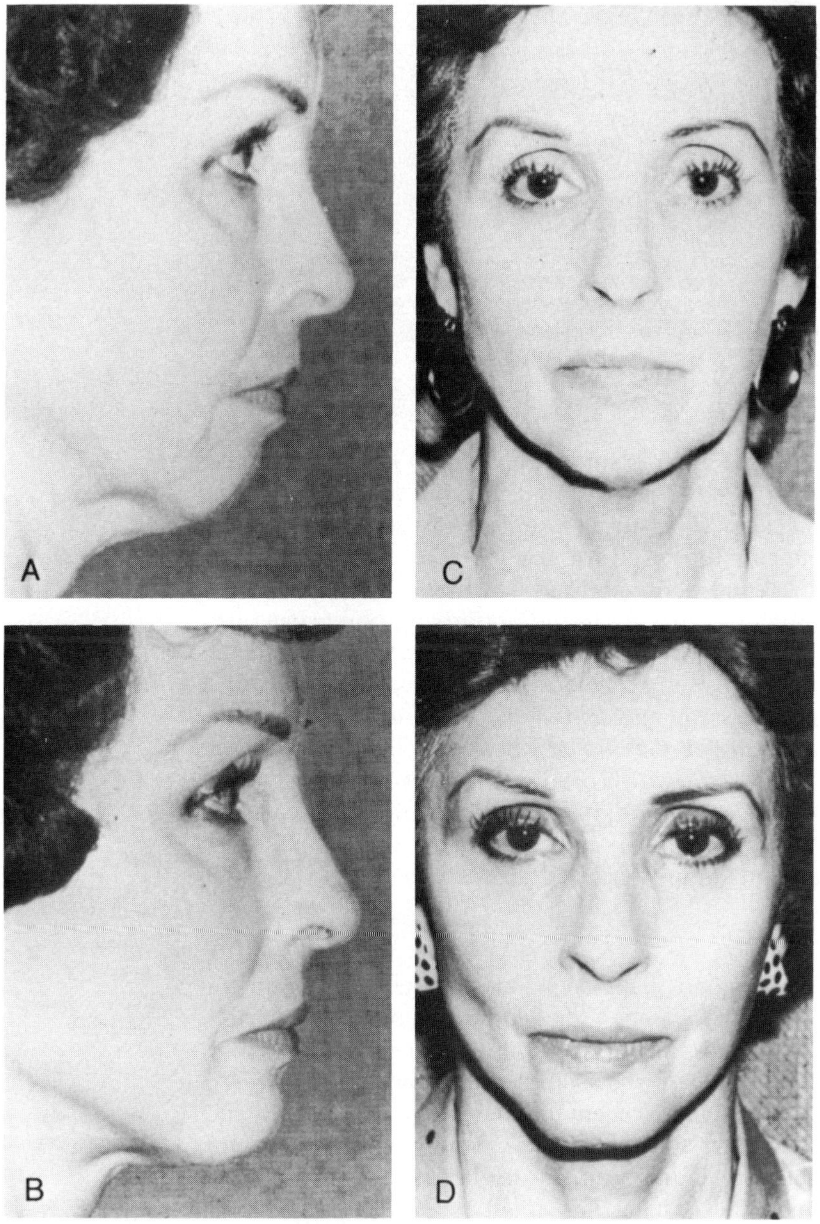

FIGURE 26–4. (*A* and *C*) Hypogenia can produce unbalance to ideal facial proportions. (*B* and *D*) Longer (wider) implants often are required to augment paramedian deficiency. Complex mesh implants may be required. (From McCollough, E.G., et al: Augmentation mentoplasty using Mersilene mesh. Arch Otolaryngol Head Neck Surg 116:1154–1158, 1990. Copyright 1990, American Medical Association.)

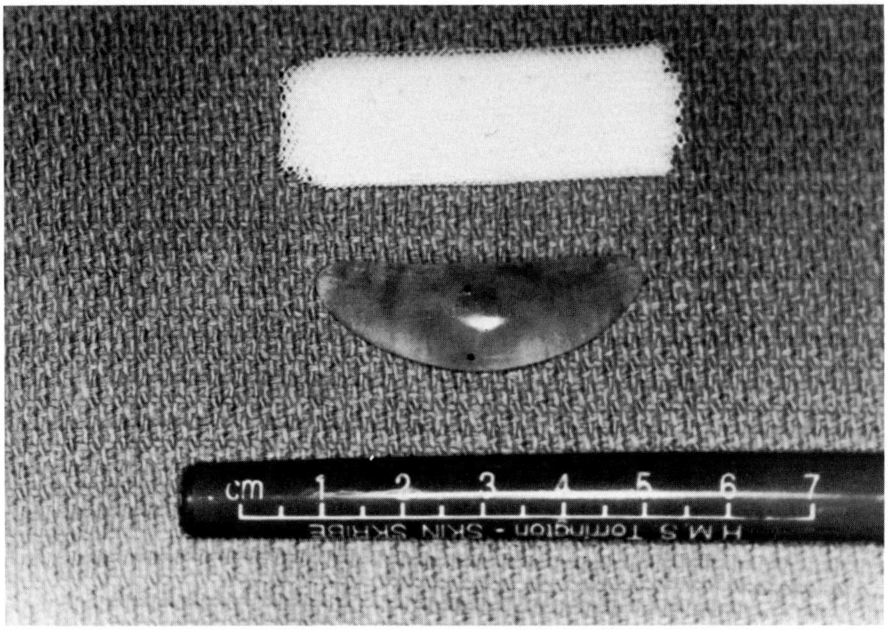

FIGURE 26–5. Comparison of preformed silicone implant with typical Mersilene mesh implant.

The optimal implant material for chin augmentation has not yet been found. Whenever foreign bodies are inserted into human tissues, some problems can be anticipated. The surgeon must try to select an implant with high host acceptability that produces a good aesthetic result. Hard implants, such as acrylics, are dense and can be difficult to shape, which prevents them from fully conforming to the underlying bony structure. Silicone rubber implants are easier to sculpt and shape than the acrylic implants, but they can easily slip out of position. Also, silicone rubber implants have a higher infection and extrusion rate than the acrylic implants. A major shortcoming of Teflon and silicone sponge implants has been their continued shrinkage, which produces asymmetry and changes in chin profile. Polyamide mesh undergoes hydrolytic degradation and gradually loses its bulk. These factors have fueled the search for better allograft materials for chin augmentation.

MERSILENE MESH

A number of plastic surgeons have begun using Mersilene mesh for augmentation procedures. Mersilene mesh is composed of nonabsorbable Dacron polyester fibers that are woven into multifilament strands of polyethylene terephthalate. It can easily be layered and tailored to the desired size and shape. This material has excellent tensile strength, durability, and surgical adaptability. A major advantage is its porosity, which allows for tissue ingrowth, thereby preventing implant displacement. Within 3 to 6 months, upon palpation the implant has much of the consistency and texture of a bone graft. The 30 × 30-cm sheets can be cut to the desired width and folded to the necessary thickness to produce various sized implants. Mersilene implants are probably best sterilized in a gas autoclave. Other advantages of using Mersilene are its inertness (it does not elicit a profound inflammatory response), pliability (it easily conforms to the contour of the mandible and does not erode neighboring structures), and resiliency (it maintains its structural integrity). No significant clinical adverse effects of Mersilene's component fibers have been reported in its common use for fascia repair.[1] Because of its construction, the mesh can be cut to achieve the appropriate configuration without unraveling or fraying.

IMPLANT CONSTRUCTION

My observations on the use of Mersilene for augmentation are based on 10 years' experience. I have used this material exclusively in augmentation mentoplasty.

From 1978 to 1988, 277 patients underwent chin augmentation at the McCollough Plastic Surgery Clinic, Birmingham, Alabama, by the technique described below. Ninety-five per cent of these procedures were performed on an outpatient basis in the clinic's operating room.

For implant construction, a sheet of Mersilene mesh is patterned and cut from a 4 × 15-cm template strip. The mesh is folded onto itself to achieve a rectangular configuration measuring about 4.0 × 1.5 cm (see Fig. 20–20).

Three different thicknesses (thin, No. 1; medium, No. 2; and thick, No. 3) can be fashioned by using one strip (28 layers), one and one-half strips (30 layers), and two strips (50 layers), respectively. Using a 4-0 polyglycolic acid suture, the implant material is sewn in a running horizontal mattress manner to prevent unfolding during preparation, sterilization, and implantation.

At surgery, the appropriate implant size is chosen, and the edges are trimmed to create a tapered lateral border. Before insertion, the implant material is soaked in a gentamicin solution (4 mg/mL). Throughout the procedure, the mesh is not touched by the surgeon's hand. Instead, sterile curved hemostats are used to hold the implant and maneuver it into the recipient site (no-touch technique).

SURGICAL TECHNIQUES

Implants may be inserted either through an intraoral approach or through an incision made in the submental skin crease. The intraoral incision is favored when no submental surgery is performed. No significant difference in infection rates exists between the intraoral and the external approach. The no-touch technique for inserting the implant significantly reduces the risk of contamination that may have resulted from touching the mouth or face earlier during the procedure.

INTRAORAL APPROACH

A 2.5-cm horizontal incision is made through the inner aspect of the lower lip at least 1 cm above and parallel to the gingivolabial sulcus. Sharp and blunt supraperiosteal dissection is performed in the midline of the symphyseal area to avoid the nerves of the chin (second premolar area).

To prepare the implant for placement, a 3-0 chromic suture on a Keith needle is passed through each end of the implant and tied. The needle is then passed into the lateral end of the pocket through the skin.

Immediately before final placement, the implant is again saturated with the gentamicin solution. Using the no-touch technique, the implant is carefully placed in the subperiosteal pocket with curved hemostats on each end, allowing the 3-0 chromic guide sutures to further position the implant. Size, contour, and positioning of the implant depend upon the conditions present. The objective is simple—fill the deficiency.

The correct implant positioning is confirmed by close inspection and palpation, and the guide sutures are trimmed under tension so that they retract below the skin's surface. Three buried interrupted 5-0 polyglycolic acid sutures are placed deep in the soft tissue over the implant to close the pocket. The mucosa is then closed with 5-0 plain catgut in a running lock-stitch suture.

EXTERNAL APPROACH

Candidates for an external approach include patients who have significant intraoral pathologic damage and patients who wear dentures. The principal disadvantage of the external approach is the external scar, which is minimal in most cases.

A horizontal 2-cm submental incision is made through the skin to the periosteal layer of the lower symphysis. The midline dissection is carried subperiosteally, creating a pocket just medial to the mental nerves. The remaining procedure and positioning are then performed in a manner similar to that described for the intraoral approach.

The implant should be positioned between the pogonion and menton level to achieve the most natural chin profile.

After closing the incision with a 5-0 fast-absorbing catgut suture, Micropore paper tape is applied to the skin overlying the anterior aspect of the chin. Finally, an elastic bandage (Elastoplast) is applied. The dressing remains in place for 1 week. The patient is instructed not to brush the lower teeth and to eat a soft, debris-free diet for 5 days postoperatively.

COMPLEX IMPLANTS

For marked microgenia, three implants sutured in a staggered lengthwise manner with a 4-0 polyglycolic acid suture provide adequate projection. This longer and thicker implant produces a smooth, lateral contour over the anterior mandibular body, preventing a "button chin" (see Fig. 20–20).

POSTOPERATIVE COMPLICATIONS

As is the case with other foreign materials inserted into the human body, there are some disadvantages to the use of Mersilene mesh. Of concern is that on two occasions, patients who had undergone their postoperative courses uneventfully later presented with sterile abscesses after facial trauma. These patients presented 2 years and 4 years after the mesh was implanted.

In these instances, cultures did not yield microorganisms. Thus, it must be concluded that inflammation of the Mersilene implant can occur several years after its insertion, especially after facial trauma.

If an infection or serious inflammatory response develops in the operative site, the implant can easily be removed intact. A smooth, fibrous capsule usually surrounds the implant. Evidence of bone resorption beneath alloplastic implants in the chin has been reported in a number of cases. Resorption occurred principally in implants placed subperiosteally, with some cases reported in those placed supraperiosteally. No clinically significant bone resorption has occurred in the cases I have been fortunate to follow up.[2]

References

1. Package insert for Mersilene polyester fiber mesh. Ethicon, Inc., Somerville, NJ.
2. McCollough, E.G., Hom, D.B., Weigel, M.T., Anderson, J.R.: Augmentation mentoplasty using Mersilene mesh. Arch Otolaryngol Head Neck Surg 116:1154–1158, 1990.

Suggested Readings

McCollough, E.G.: Rhinoplasty: A humbling experience. J Oral Maxillofac Surg 47:1132–1141, 1989.

McCollough, E.G., Magat, D.S.: Augmentation mentoplasty. Laryngoscope 89:2008–2010, 1989.

INDEX

Note: Page numbers in *italics* refer to illustrations